An Atlas of Imaging of the Paranasal Sinuses

Second Edition

An Atlas of Imaging of the Paranasal Sinuses

Second Edition

Lalitha Shankar
University of Toronto
Toronto, Canada

Kate Evans
Ear, Nose and Throat Department
Gloucestershire Royal Hospital
Gloucester, UK

With contributions from

Thomas R Marotta
St. Michael's Hospital
University of Toronto
Toronto, Canada

Eugene Yu
University of Toronto
University Health Network
Toronto, Canada

Michael Hawke
University of Toronto
Toronto, Canada

Heinz Stammberger
University ENT Clinic
Graz, Austria

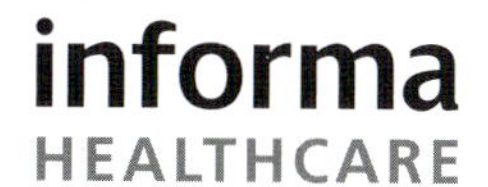

First published in 1994 by Martin Dunitz Limited, London
2nd edition © 2006 Informa Healthcare, an imprint of Informa UK Ltd
4 Park Square, Milton Park, Abingdon,
Oxon OX14 4RN
Color photographs © Lalitha Shankar, Kathryn Evans, Michael Hawke, Heinz Stammberger 2006

Tel.: +44 (0)20 7017 6000
Fax.: +44 (0)20 7017 6699
E-mail: info.medicine@tandf.co.uk
Website: www.tandf.co.uk/medicine

Bristish Library Cataloguing in Publication Data

A CIP record for this book is available from the British Library.

Library of Congress Cataloging-in-Publication Data

Data available on application

ISBN 10: 1-84184-448-9
ISBN 13: 978-1-84184-448-0

Distributed in North and South America by

Taylor & Francis
6000 Broken Sound Parkway, NW, (Suite 300)
Boca Raton, FL 33487, USA

Within Continental USA
Tel.: 1(800)272-7737; Fax: 1(800)374-3401
Outside Continental USA
Tel.: (561)994-0555; Fax: (561)361-6018
E-mail: orders@crcpress.com

Distributed in the rest of the world by
Thomson Publishing Services
Cheriton House
North Way
Andover, Hampshire SP10 5BE, UK
Tel.: +44 (0)1264 332424
E-mail: tps.tandfsalesorder@thomson.com

Composition by Parthenon Publishing

Printed and bound by T. G. Hostench S.A., Spain

Contents

Contributors

Kate Evans MB FRCS
Ear, Nose and Throat Department
Gloucestershire Royal Hospital
Gloucester, UK

Michael Hawke MD FRCS(C)
University of Toronto
Toronto, Canada

William Hodge
North Bay General Hospital
North Bay, Ontario
Canada

Cameron Hunter
North Bay General Hospital
North Bay, Ontario
Canada

Edward Kassel MD
Mount Sinai Hospital
University of Toronto
Toronto, Canada

Walter Kucharczyk MD
Division of Applied and Interventional Research
Toronto Western Research Unit
Toronto, Canada

Thomas R Marotta MD FRCP(C)
St. Michael's Hospital
University of Toronto
Toronto, Canada

Hemant Parwar MBBS
Hospital for Sick Children
University of Toronto
Toronto, Canada

Lalitha Shankar MD FRCP(C)
University of Toronto
Toronto, Canada

Samantha Shankar BSc
Albany Medical College
Albany, NY, USA

Manohar Schroff
Hospital for Sick Children
University of Toronto
Toronto, Canada

Herman M Schuttevaer MD
Department of Radiology
Rijnland Hospital
Leiderdorp
The Netherlands

Heinz Stammberger MD
University ENT Clinic
Graz, Austria

Robert Wilinsky MD FRCP(C)
University of Toronto
Toronto, Canada

Eugene Yu MD FRCP(C)
University of Toronto
University Health Network
Toronto, Canada

Preface

This Second Edition of *An Atlas of Imaging of the Paranasal Sinuses* attempts to provide a comprehensive overview of the imaging modalities that are currently regarded as the gold standard in the management of diseases of the paranasal sinuses. Both computerized tomography (CT) and magnetic resonance imaging (MRI) have revolutionized the diagnosis of diseases of the paranasal sinuses. The ability to reformat images in any plane and in three-dimensions has added an enormous value both in diagnosis, staging and the planning of surgical resection or reconstruction. This Atlas aims to increase the understanding of both radiologists and otorhinolaryngologists of the complex anatomy of the paranasal sinuses when normal and when affected by anatomical variation, surgery or disease.

Lalitha Shankar
Kate Evans
Michael Hawke
Heinz Stammberger
Thomas R Marotta
Eugene Yu

Acknowledgments

This book is dedicated to all of our spouses and children, who have in their own way assisted us with this project – some by helping to get this book on the way, while others stayed out of the way! Radiology is all about observation.

'This observation is more than seeing; it is knowing what you see and comprehending its significance.' (Anonymous)

We also dedicate this book to all of our teachers.

Contributors to the second edition

Chapter 1: K Evans, L Shankar, H Stammberger
Chapter 2: K Evans, L Shankar, M Hawke, S Shankar, H Stammberger
Chapter 3: K Evans, L Shankar, M Hawke, S Shankar, H Stammberger
Chapter 4: E Yu, L Shankar, T Marotta
Chapter 5: K Evans, L Shankar, M Hawke
Chapter 6: L Shankar, K Evans, M Hawke
Chapter 7: K Evans, L Shankar, M Hawke, E Yu
Chapter 8: L Shankar, K Evans, M Hawke, T Marotta
Chapter 9: E Yu, T Marotta, L Shankar, K Evans
Chapter 10: K Evans, L Shankar, M Hawke, E Yu, T Marotta
Chapter 11: H Parwar, M Schroff
Chapter 12: EE Kassel

Images: W Kucharczyk, HM Schuttevaer, R Wilinsky, C Hunter, W Hodge
Diagrams: S Shankar – frontal recess, cribriform plate, ostiomeatal complex, arteries of the sinus

1

Introduction

The concept of functional endoscopic sinus surgery was developed by Walter Messerklinger in Graz, Austria in the early 1970s following extensive research into the pathophysiology and anatomy of the paranasal sinuses. Messerklinger's concepts have revolutionized, improved, and radically altered the techniques used for the diagnosis and treatment of patients with sinus disease. The concepts of functional endoscopic sinus surgery were popularized and exported from the German-speaking countries by Heinz Stammberger in 1984 and David Kennedy in 1985.

Endoscopic sinus surgery evolved from a combination of the techniques of intranasal surgery, which originated in the 19th century, and endoscopy of the lateral nasal wall, which was initially used only as a diagnostic tool.

Intranasal surgery to facilitate the drainage of purulent secretions was initially reported in the late 19th century. Inferior meatal antrostomy (fenestration) was described in the late 1890s, and middle meatal antrostomy was described in 1886 by Mikulicz and again in 1899 by Siebenmann. At that time, it was noted that middle meatal antrostomies did not stenose with the same rapidity as those performed in the inferior meatus; however, the surgeons of those pre-antibiotic times were deterred by the close anatomical relationship of the orbit to the site of the middle meatal antrostomy.

Hirschmann first described endoscopy of the nasal cavities in 1903. He used an instrument that had originally been designed as a cystoscope. There were many subsequent attempts by a variety of rhinologists to develop a more sophisticated instrument. The development of the operating microscope in the late 1950s improved the peroperative view of the nasal cavity, especially that of the posterior ethmoid and sphenoid sinuses. The main disadvantage of the microscope was its straight visual field, which did not permit an adequate view into the ethmoid clefts. The development of the fiberoptic rod telescope by Hopkins in the early 1950s was a dramatic advance. This optical system includes a light source distant from the instrument and a quartz rod air lens system that provides excellent resolution with high contrast, and (despite the small diameter of the endoscope) a wide field of vision. With the addition of angled lenses, these endoscopes have made it possible to examine in detail the clefts and recesses of the nasal cavity (Figures 1.1 and 1.2). Initially, they were used only for diagnostic purposes. Messerklinger showed that it was possible to introduce appropriately designed instruments alongside the endoscopes to perform precise surgical resection under direct vision.

Until the development of endoscopic sinus surgery, inflammatory disease of the paranasal sinuses requiring surgery was treated using radical procedures such as the Caldwell–Luc radical antrostomy, intranasal ethmoidectomy, and external frontoethmoidectomy. All of these radical surgical procedures involve the extensive removal of diseased mucosa. While a working knowledge of these procedures is still required as surgical options for the treatment of benign sinus disease, the majority of patients with chronic sinusitis are more appropriately treated with the minimally invasive and more conservative technique of functional endoscopic sinus surgery.

In 1944, Hilding demonstrated elegantly in animals that there were definite pathways along which the cilia transported and cleared the mucus produced within a sinus, and that the mucus would inevitably pass to and through the natural ostium, despite the presence of an inferior meatal intranasal antrostomy, which would be circumnavigated. The importance of this work was not realized at the time, and intranasal antrostomies and the Caldwell–Luc procedure remained the mainstays of surgical treatment.

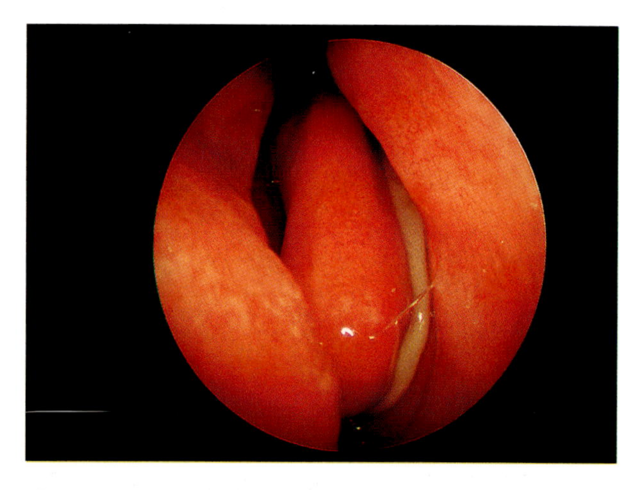

Figure 1.1 *Endoscopic image of chronic sinusitis.* This patient presented with left-sided chronic maxillary sinusitis. Note the creamy white purulent material draining from the left semilunar hiatus.

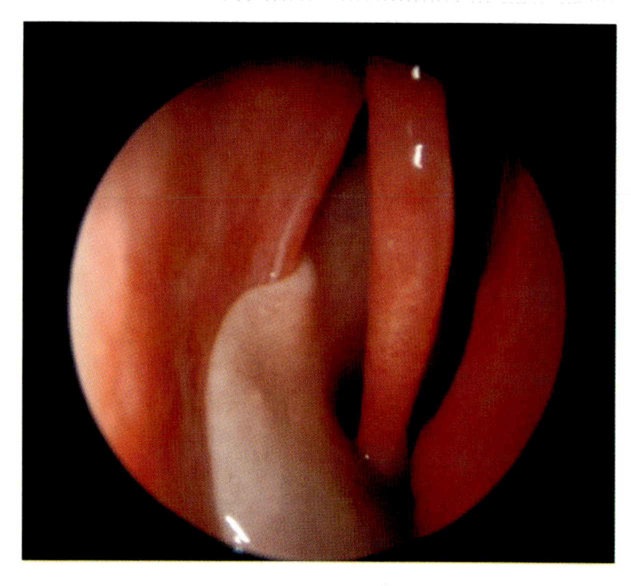

Figure 1.2 *Endoscopic image of nasal polyps.* Several yellowish nasal polyps can be seen arising from the right middle meatus.

Messerklinger established that the health of the frontal and maxillary sinuses is subordinate to that of the anterior ethmoid sinus, as these are ventilated from and drain into the nasal cavity via their prechambers (the frontal recess at the entrance to the frontal sinus and the infundibulum at the entrance to the maxillary sinus), which connect their ostia to the anterior ethmoid sinus. He also demonstrated that occlusion of the narrow and stenotic clefts (prechambers) of the ethmoid labyrinth, which connect the ostia of the frontal and maxillary sinuses to the anterior ethmoid, led to disordered ventilation and decreased mucociliary clearance from the larger (frontal and maxillary) paranasal sinuses and therefore predisposed the patient to recurrent infections.

Messerklinger noted that infection of these larger sinuses was usually rhinogenic in origin, spreading from the nose through the anterior ethmoid to involve the frontal and maxillary sinuses secondarily. He also demonstrated that, despite the fact that the symptoms of infection in these larger sinuses were usually clinically dominant, the underlying cause was generally not to be found in the larger sinuses themselves, but instead in the clefts of the anterior ethmoid sinuses in the lateral nasal wall (Figure 1.3). Messerklinger observed that when infections in the frontal and maxillary sinuses did not heal or when they recurred promptly, a focus of infection usually persisted in one of the narrow clefts of the anterior ethmoid sinus; this infection interfered with the normal ventilation and drainage of the sinuses, and spread locally to involve the prechambers and secondarily the larger sinuses.

Messerklinger also noted that, after a limited endoscopic resection of the disease within the anterior ethmoid that was responsible for obstruction of the ventilation and drainage pathways of the larger paranasal sinuses, and with re-establishment of drainage and ventilation through the natural pathways, even massive mucosal pathology within the frontal and maxillary sinuses usually healed without direct surgical intervention involving the

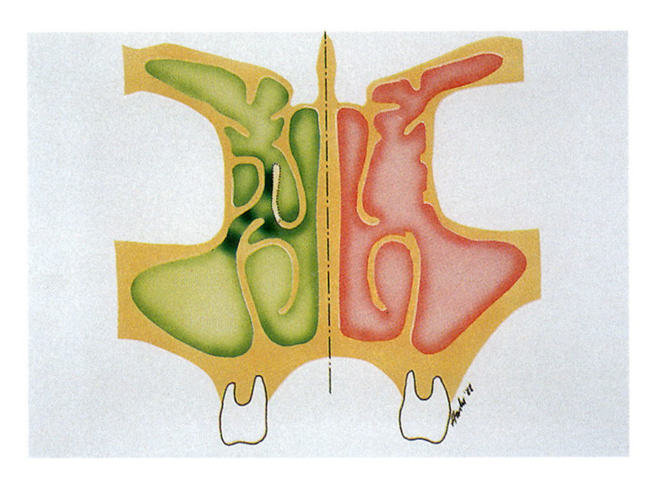

Figure 1.3 *Schematic drawing demonstrating the key diseased area of the anterior ethmoid on the left*. The anatomy after functional endoscopic sinus surgery is shown on the right. From: Functional Endoscopic Sinus Surgery: The Messerklinger Technique, by Professor Heinz Stammberger, with kind permission of the publisher Mosby-Year Book.

larger sinuses (Figure 1.3). Mucosal changes within the frontal and maxillary sinuses that had previously been regarded as irreversible returned to normal several weeks following what was essentially a minimal, endoscopically controlled resection of disease.

In summary, the key theory of endoscopic sinus surgery is that, by removing localized disease obstructing the narrow ethmoid clefts, and thereby restoring normal mucociliary clearance and ventilation, spontaneous resolution of the mucosal disease in the maxillary and frontal sinuses will follow without the need for radical mucosal excision.

Developments both in the design of diagnostic endoscopes and in the re-evaluation of radiographic imaging have been instrumental in the evolution of these endoscopic surgical techniques.

Precise surgical techniques aimed at restoring normal physiological conditions and the preservation of as much mucosa as possible have only developed with the additional anatomical and pathophysiological information that has been provided by radiographic imaging. Indeed, functional endoscopic sinus surgery has only been able to develop to its current level because of the advances that have occurred in the field of radiology.

Messerklinger's initial work in Graz was conducted with information derived from conventional tomography. This technique has now been superseded by computed tomography (CT), which is now considered an essential component of the diagnostic investigation of patients presenting with symptoms suggestive of disease of the paranasal sinuses. CT is an ideal method for the demonstration of the delicate bony leaflets of the ethmoid labyrinth. It also identifies those anatomical variants that may compromise the ventilation of the sinuses and it can demonstrate those discrete areas of diseased mucosa that are responsible for recurrent disease in the larger paranasal sinuses (the frontal and the maxillary sinuses). The majority of these latter abnormalities will not be evident, even on careful diagnostic endoscopic assessment. Because the rhinologist is interested in the detail of the fine structures within the lateral wall of the nose, radiologists will have to direct their attention towards the drainage pathways and prechambers of the larger paranasal sinuses and away from the more obvious abnormalities that may be secondarily present in the larger paranasal sinuses. CT is now regarded as essential when the patient has undergone previous sinus surgery. In this situation, CT scans will provide valuable information about the presence of potentially hazardous situations, such as a dehiscence of the lamina papyracea, the proximity of the orbit to areas of disease, septation of the frontal or sphenoid sinuses, and the location of the internal carotid artery and optic nerve.

Systematic endoscopic assessment of the lateral nasal wall in conjunction with CT of the nose and paranasal sinuses allows precise localization of the underlying disease processes and thus aids the clinician in planning appropriate therapy. The ability to identify radiologically those abnormalities that may increase surgical morbidity prior to commencing surgical dissection is important for both the surgeon and the patient.

The development of image guidance for endoscopic sinus surgery, also known as computer-assisted sinus surgery (CASS), is a fairly new technology that can help to reduce intraoperative complications as well as playing a valuable role in the planning of complex surgical resections. The system depends on accurate placement of a reference frame on the patient's head, linked to preoperative multiplanar CT images by either an optical or an electromagnetic system. Special instruments allow the surgeon to have a real-time endoscopic view of the operative site correlated with axial, coronal, and sagittal images (Figure 1.4). There are particular benefits in training ENT surgeons, in reducing intraoperative injury to the orbit and brain, in revision surgery, and during complex procedures involving dehiscence of the optic nerve or internal carotid artery and other anomalies pre-existent in the sinus walls. These benefits need to be considered against an initial increase in operative time and cost.

Understandably, there is considerable interest among both radiologists and rhinologists in the radiological anatomy of the paranasal region. More recently, knowledge of the required radiographic techniques, anatomy, and significant pathology of the structures identified by CT has been included in the training curriculum for radiologists.

This book is intended as a simple concise atlas to introduce both rhinologists and radiologists to the essential concepts of endoscopic sinus surgery, and to identify the relevant anatomy and variations that may influence disease and surgery. This information is important to both surgeons and radiologists so that CT scans can be interpreted accurately prior to and at the time of surgery.

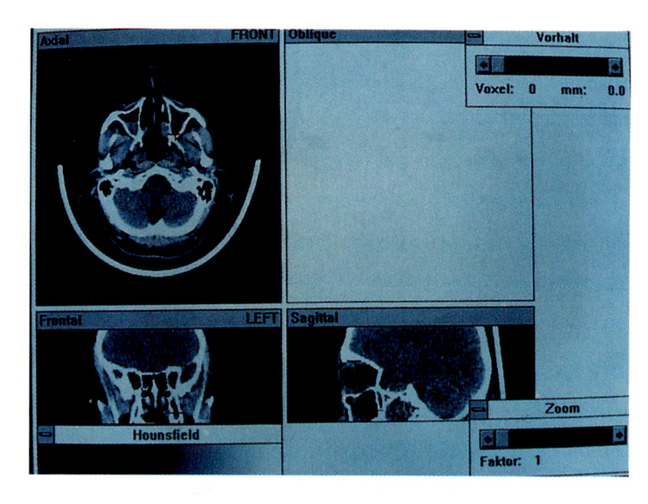

Figure 1.4 Screen of image-guided system indicating the multiplanar CT images.

2

Nasal physiology

The nose and paranasal sinuses have multiple functions including the provision of an upper respiratory air channel, filtering and humidification of inspired air, olfaction, vocal resonance, speech, and nasal reflex functions. For the purpose of this text, attention will be drawn only towards those functions that are of significance in the pathogenesis of sinusitis, or in the interpretation of sinus radiographs and computed tomography (CT) images of the paranasal sinuses.

The nose and paranasal sinuses are lined with a ciliated, pseudostratified columnar epithelium, beneath which lies the tunica propria containing serous and mucous glands. The main function of the nose is to transmit, filter, warm, and humidify inspired air. The most important factors contributing to the maintenance of the normal physiology of the paranasal sinuses and their lining mucous membranes are mucous secretion, clearance and ventilation. Normal drainage of the paranasal sinuses requires a complex balance between the production of mucus and its transportation through and out of the sinus. This balance is to a large extent dependent upon the amount of mucus produced within the sinus, its composition and viscosity, the effectiveness of the ciliary beat, mucosal reabsorption, and the condition of the ostia and the ethmoid clefts through which the mucus must pass on its way into the nasal cavity. Ventilation and drainage of the frontal and maxillary sinuses depend primarily upon the patency of both the actual sinus ostia and their ethmoid prechambers that connect the ostia with the nasal cavity via the anterior ethmoid.

MUCOUS SECRETION

Under normal conditions, the mucous blanket that covers and protects the nasal mucosa is produced continuously by the mucoserous nasal glands and the intraepithelial goblet cells. The mucous blanket has two layers: an inner serous layer, the sol phase, in which the cilia beat, and an outer more viscous layer, the gel phase, which is transported on top of the sol phase by the ciliary beat. The balance between the underlying sol phase and the outer gel phase is critically important for the maintenance of normal mucociliary clearance. Under normal conditions, dust and other fine particles become incorporated into the gel phase and are transported with the mucus out of the sinuses. The mucous layer is produced continuously and transported steadily away from the sinus. A healthy maxillary sinus renews its mucous layer on average every 20–30 minutes.

VENTILATION AND DRAINAGE

The ostia of the two largest and clinically most important sinuses, the frontal and maxillary sinuses, communicate with the middle meatus by very narrow and delicate prechambers. The frontal sinus opens into an hourglass-shaped cleft, the frontal recess (Figure 2.1). The maxillary sinus ostium opens into a cleft in the lateral nasal wall, the ethmoid infundibulum (Figure 2.2). Both the frontal recess and the infundibulum are parts of the anterior ethmoid complex. If these prechambers become obstructed, then the drainage and ventilation of the frontal and maxillary sinuses will be impaired and a secondary infection within these sinuses is more likely to develop.

The nasal mucosa is innervated by the autonomic nervous system, with parasympathetic stimulation causing an increased serous type of secretion and sympathetic stimulation causing an increased mucinous secretion.

NASAL BLOOD FLOW

The nasal mucosa has an abundant blood flow, which is derived from both the internal and the external carotid arterial systems. The main arterial supply is derived from the sphenopalatine branch of the maxillary artery, as well as having contributions from the anterior and posterior ethmoidal branches of the ophthalmic artery.

Venous sinusoids form special areas of erectile cavernous tissue overlying the inferior turbinate and the inferior margin and posterior end of the middle turbinate. Similar tissue may also be present in the submucosa of the nasal septum anteriorly, where it is known variously as the septal swell body, the tuberculum septi, and the tumescence of Zuckerkandl (Figure 2.3).

The autonomic nerve supply of the blood vessels is derived from the superior cervical sympathetic ganglion and from the sphenopalatine ganglion, which relays the parasympathetic nerve fibers.

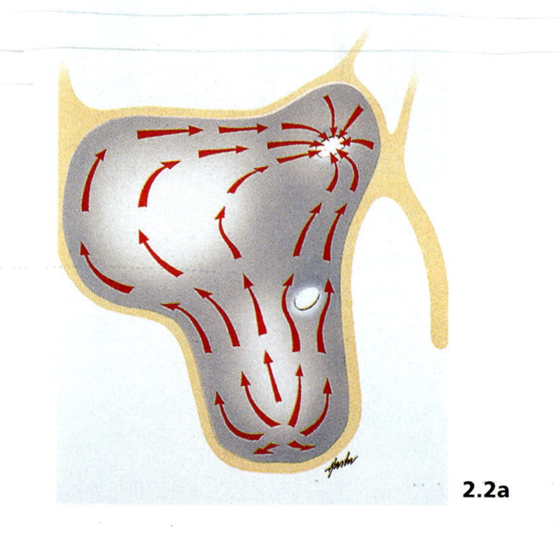

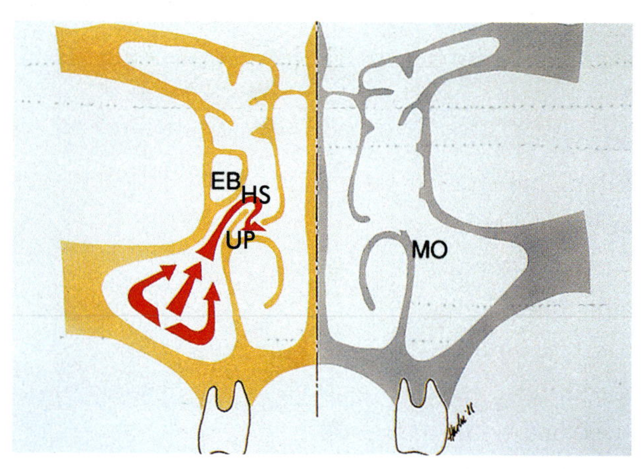

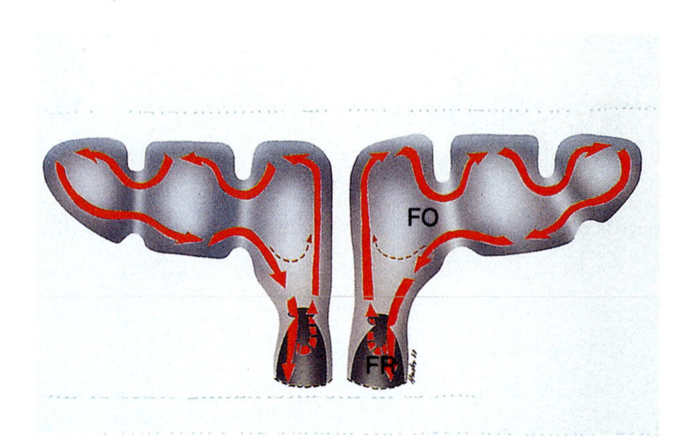

Figure 2.1 Schematic drawing showing the normal mucociliary transportation route within and exiting the frontal sinuses. FO, frontal sinus ostium; FR, frontal recess, which is the ethmoid prechamber connecting the frontal sinus ostium to the anterior ethmoid. From: Functional Endoscopic Sinus Surgery: The Messerklinger Technique, by Professor Heinz Stammberger, with kind permission of the publisher Mosby-Year Book.

Figure 2.2 Schematic drawings showing the normal transportation pathways of mucus inside (a) and exiting (b) the right maxillary sinus. EB, ethmoid bulla; HS, hiatus semilunaris; MO, maxillary sinus ostium. Note the infundibulum, the prechamber connecting the maxillary sinus ostium with the nasal cavity via the hiatus semilunaris. The infundibulum is the space lying between the uncinate process (UP) and the ethmoid bulla (EB). Modified after W Messerklinger. From: Endoscopic Sinus Surgery: The Messerklinger Technique, by Professor Heinz Stammberger with kind permission of the publisher Mosby-Year Book.

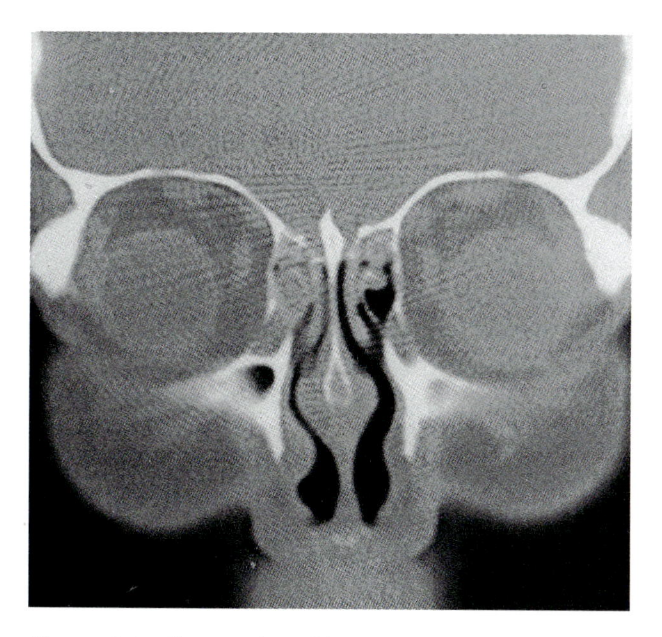

Figure 2.3 *The septal swell body*. The bulbous swelling on the anterior nasal septum in this coronal CT scan is produced by an area of submucosal erectile tissue known variously as the nasal septal swell body, the tuberculum septi, and the tumescence of Zuckerkandl.

Sympathetic stimulation causes vasoconstriction and parasympathetic stimulation causes vasodilatation. Blood flow can be affected by a variety of local factors, including temperature, humidity, trauma, and infection, as well as by the administration of vasodilator or vasoconstrictor drugs. Blood flow is also altered by hormonal changes (i.e. hyper- and hypothyroidism), as well as by increased levels of estrogens during menstruation and pregnancy. Emotional stress may cause either vasoconstriction or vasodilatation.

The administration of topical nasal decongestants such as 0.1% xylometazoline hydrochloride nasal solution USP prior to CT examination leads to shrinking of the inferior turbinates and of the nasal swell body. The middle turbinates and the ethmoid prechambers remain unaffected.

The degree of vasodilatation (swelling) of the nasal mucosa has a great effect upon the resistance of the nasal airway. Vasodilatation is dependent both on autonomic control of the blood flow and on the nasal cycle. The nasal cycle is the term used to describe the normal paradoxical opening and partial obstruction of alternate sides of the nasal airway. This normally alternates from side to side approximately every 2–3 hours. The factors controlling the nasal cycle are at present unknown (Figure 2.4).

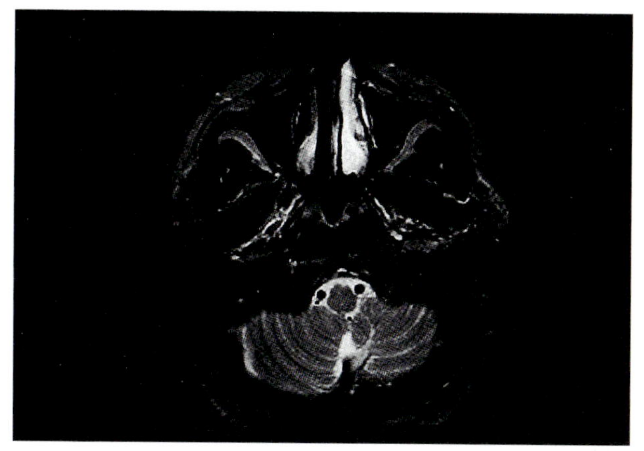

Figure 2.4 *The nasal cycle*. The engorgement and vasodilatation of the left inferior turbinate from the normal nasal cycle can be seen on this T2-weighted MRI scan as a hyperintense (white) area.

Zinreich and Kennedy have demonstrated the cyclical changes of the nasal cycle in normal volunteers using magnetic resonance imaging (MRI). On T2-weighted scans, the increase in signal intensity and mucosal volume was seen to be limited to the inferior and middle turbinates, the ethmoid prechambers, and the nasal septum. These changes alternated from side to side over the course of the day. This increased signal intensity is indistinguishable from inflamed mucosa. To define the extent of inflammation separate from the normal nasal cycle, topical decongestants can be administered. This results in a prompt vasoconstriction. Malignancy, such as squamous cell carcinoma, has a low signal intensity on T2-weighted images, and thus can easily be differentiated from the normal nasal cycle and from inflamed mucosa.

The nasal cycle is associated with a number of physiological changes in the alternating sides of the nose. Studies of nasal physiology are currently being undertaken using acoustic rhinometry and rhinoresistometry. Cyclic changes in the width of the nasal cavity and airflow resistance have been observed. Turbulent airflow is necessary for sufficient contact between inspired air and nasal mucosa. The initially laminar airflow entering the decongested or 'working phase' side quickly becomes turbulent, and this effect is enhanced by the greater width of the nasal airway. On the congested or 'resting phase' side, the airflow is found to remain mainly laminar. This rhythmic cycling between patency and obstruction diminishes with age.

The cycle of decongestion and congestion has been shown to have an impact on mucociliary clearance. Research by Soane and co-workers, demonstrated that the clearance of a radiopharmaceutical agent was more rapid in the patent side of the nose as compared with the congested side. It is thought that the nasal cycle allows the nose to reload the nasal mucus with water lost when the mucosa is in the decongested state. When the cycle reverses leading to nasal obstruction, the viscosity of the mucus is increased, causing a decreased ciliary beat frequency and the resulting slowed clearance.

The erectile tissue of the nasal cavity is also affected by postural changes, for example by lying on one's side in bed. Here, the mucosa of the dependent nasal cavity slowly undergoes engorgement as gravity causes blood to pool in the venous sinusoids.

MRI OF NORMAL PARANASAL SINUSES

Both CT and MRI both demonstrate sinonasal mucosa. The high incidence of asymptomatic abnormalities of the paranasal sinuses observed during routine CT imaging of the head is well known. MRI is more sensitive than CT because it detects mucosal thickening in addition to changes in the nasal cavity resulting from the normal nasal cycle (Figure 2.4). The mucosa of the nasal cavity, the turbinates, and the ethmoid complex are seen as low signal intensity on T1-weighted scans, intermediate signal intensity on proton density (PD)-weighted scans, and hyperintense (i.e. brighter) on T2-weighted scans. The alternating nasal cycle is seen as increased brightness of the turbinates, the ethmoid sinuses, and the mucosa overlying the nasal septum on T2-weighted scans. As a result of the normal nasal cycle the inferior turbinates appear larger and brighter when the mucosal volume is greater. Up to 3 mm thickness in the sinonasal mucosa is considered to be clinically insignificant. These cyclical changes are only seen in the ethmoid sinuses and do not occur in the larger paranasal sinuses. The normal sinuses are seen as signal-void cavities.

Anything greater than 4 mm thickness is more likely to be pathological, although it is not uncommon to see patients with hyperintense mucosa less than 3 mm thick who have symptoms of rhinosinusitis. The MRI changes that are observed in the sinonasal mucosa must be correlated with the patient's clinical history and physical findings. Neither bone nor the air within the sinuses produces a signal, and demarcation between air and bone is not possible on MRI scans. The major disadvantage of MRI is that air, bone, calcification, and metallic densities are all seen as signal-void areas, and consequently the subtle calcifications that characterize certain tumors remain undetected on MRI. Thin healthy mucosa may on occasion be seen as a thin layer of low signal intensity on T1-weighted sequences. The turbinates and the nasal septum are isointense with brain, or of intermediate signal intensity on normal MRI sequences.

3

Gross and sectional anatomy of the nasal cavity and paranasal sinuses

This chapter is subdivided as follows in order to simplify the description of the complex nasal and paranasal sinus anatomy and the surrounding structures:

- Nasal bone, cavity, and septum
  - Nasal bone
  - Nasal cavity
  - Nasal septum
  - Superior turbinate
  - Middle turbinate and ground lamella
  - Inferior turbinate
- Structures of lateral nasal wall
  - Ostiomeatal complex (uncinate process, ethmoid infundibulum, hiatus semilunaris, lateral sinus)
  - Superior meatus and sphenoethmoid recess
  - Middle meatus
  - Inferior meatus
  - Lacrimal apparatus and nasolacrimal duct
- Paranasal sinuses
  - Frontal bone and sinus
  - Frontal recess and drainage
  - Maxilla and maxillary sinus
  - Ethmoid bone
  - Ethmoid sinuses (anterior ethmoid sinus, agger nasi, ethmoid bulla, Haller's cells, posterior ethmoid sinus)
  - Sphenoid bone, sinus, and drainage
- Structures surrounding paranasal sinuses
  - Pterygopalatine fossa
  - Orbital apex
- Vascular supply of nasal cavity and paranasal sinuses
  - Anterior and posterior ethmoidal arteries
  - Splenopalatine artery
- Nerve supply of paranasal sinuses

NASAL BONE, NASAL CAVITY, AND NASAL SEPTUM

Nasal bone

The paired nasal bones articulate at their medial borders. Laterally, the nasal bone articulates with the frontal process of the maxilla; superiorly, it articulates with the frontal bone. Inferiorly, the nasal bones are attached to the upper lateral nasal cartilage. The internal surface has a groove that transmits the anterior ethmoid nerve. The external surface offers attachment to the nasalis muscle.

Nasal cavity (Figures 3.1–3.7; Table 3.1)

The nasal cavity is a midline structure extending from the base of the skull to the roof of the mouth. Air passes through both the oral cavity and the nasal cavity during respiration. The structures within the nasal cavity warm, humidify, and filter inspired air before it reaches the lower respiratory tract. The nasal cavity is divided by the nasal septum into two symmetrical nasal fossae.

The roof of the nasal cavity is formed by the nasal and frontal bones anteriorly, by the cribriform plate of the ethmoid bone in the middle portion, and by the sphenoid, the alae of the vomer, and the sphenoidal process of the palatine bone posteriorly.

The cribriform plate, which is only 2–3 mm wide, is perforated by approximately 20 foramina, which transmit fibers of the olfactory nerve. The thin lateral lamina of the cribriform plate is the most vulnerable area surgically.

The floor of the nasal cavity is formed by the bones of the hard palate, namely the palatine process of the maxilla anteriorly and the horizontal plate of the palatine bone posteriorly.

The lateral wall of the nasal cavity can be divided into three parts. The anterior part is formed by the frontal process of the maxilla and the lacrimal bone. The middle part is formed by the ethmoid labyrinth, the maxilla, and the inferior turbinate. The posterior part is formed by the perpendicular plate of the palatine bone and the medial pterygoid plate of the sphenoid. The inferior turbinate protrudes from the lateral wall with the posterior part of the middle turbinate. The anterior part of the middle turbinate and the superior turbinate arise from the skull base. Below and lateral to each turbinate there is the corresponding meatus. The lateral wall of the nasal cavity will be discussed in detail later.

Anteriorly, the nasal cavity communicates with the exterior through the nasal vestibule which lies between the alar cartilage and the anterior nasal septum. Posteriorly, the nasal cavity communicates with the nasopharynx through the choanae. These are bounded superiorly by the body of the sphenoid and the alae of the vomer, inferiorly by the posterior border of the horizontal process of the palatine bone and soft palate, laterally by the medial pterygoid

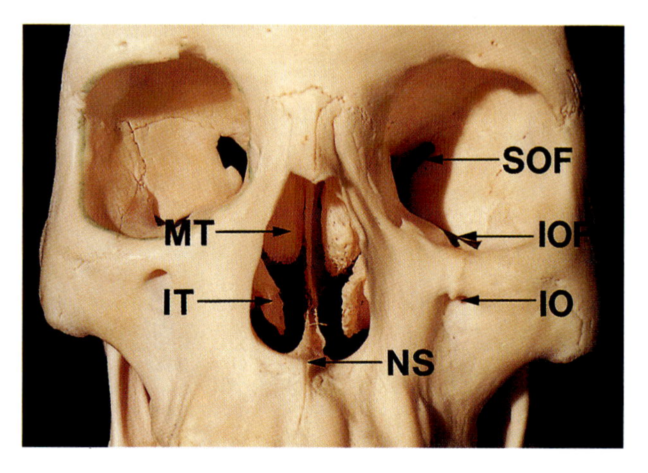

Figure 3.1 *Osteology*. Anterior view of the skull demonstrating some of the bony features of the nasal cavity and orbit. The nasal spine (NS) can be seen at the base of the bony nasal septum. The prominent middle turbinate (MT) and the inferior turbinate (IT) are shown. The superior orbital fissure (SOF) and inferior orbital fissure (IOF) are demonstrated. The inferior orbital foramen (IO) transmits the infraorbital nerve.

Table 3.1 Bony walls of the nasal cavity

Roof
- Anterior roof: nasal and frontal bone
- Middle roof: cribriform plate of ethmoid bone
- Posterior roof: sphenoid, alae of vomer, and sphenoidal process of palatine bone

Floor
- Anterior floor: palatine process of maxilla
- Posterior floor: horizontal process of palatine bone

Lateral wall
- Anterior: frontal process of maxilla and lacrimal bone
- Middle: ethmoid labyrinth, three turbinates and meati, and medial wall of maxilla
- Posterior: perpendicular plate of palatine bone and medial pterygoid plate of sphenoid

Medial wall or the nasal septum
- Quadrilateral cartilage
- Palatine bones
- Vomer
- Perpendicular plate of ethmoid bone
- Maxillary crest

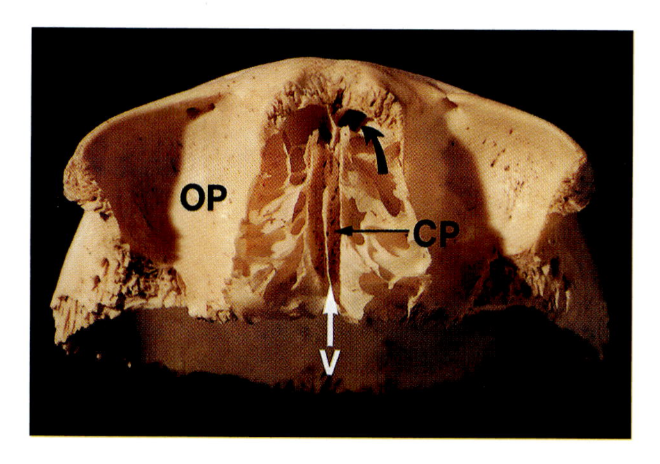

Figure 3.2 *Inferior aspect of frontal bone*. Inferior view of the frontal bone showing the ethmoid notch with the depressions of the ethmoid foveolae (foveolae ethmoidales ossis frontalis) *in situ*. The relationship of the vomer (V) and the cribriform plate (CP) to the foveolae ethmoidales, seen in Figure 3.21, is demonstrated. The curved arrow indicates the frontal recess entering the frontal sinus. The orbital plate (OP) is also shown.

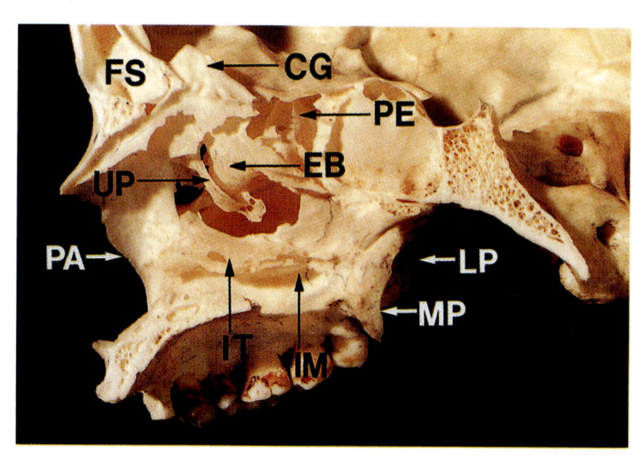

Figure 3.4 *Lateral wall of nose.* Half-skull showing the bony features of the lateral wall of the nose. The middle turbinate and superior turbinate have been removed, opening the posterior ethmoid air cells (PE). Features demonstrated include the frontal sinus (FS), crista galli (CG), pyriform aperture (PA), medial (MP) and lateral (LP) pterygoid plates, inferior turbinate (IT), and inferior meatus (IM). The uncinate process (UP) lies anterior to the ethmoid bulla (EB). The hiatus semilunaris is the two-dimensional cleft lying between these two structures.

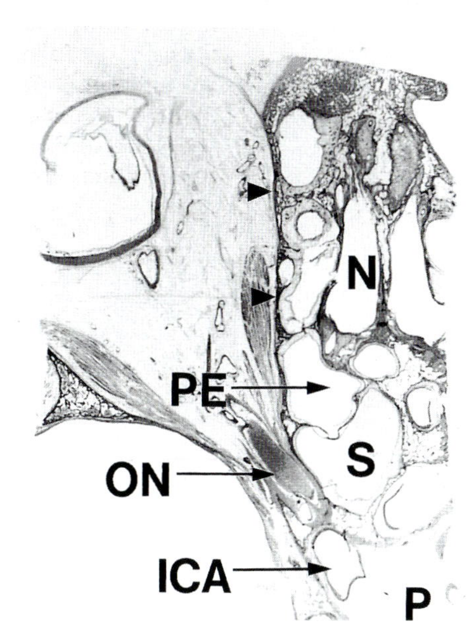

Figure 3.3 *Axial section at the level of the roof of the nasal cavity and the diaphragm sellae.* Axial section demonstrating the lamina papyracea (arrowheads), nasal cavity (N), posterior ethmoid sinus (PE), optic nerve (ON), sphenoid sinus (S), pituitary fossa (P), and internal carotid artery (ICA). From: Studying whole-mounted sections of the paranasal sinuses to understand the complications of endoscopic sinus surgery, by Michael and Eugene Rontal, The Laryngoscope 101, April 1991, reproduced by kind permission of The Laryngoscope and the authors.

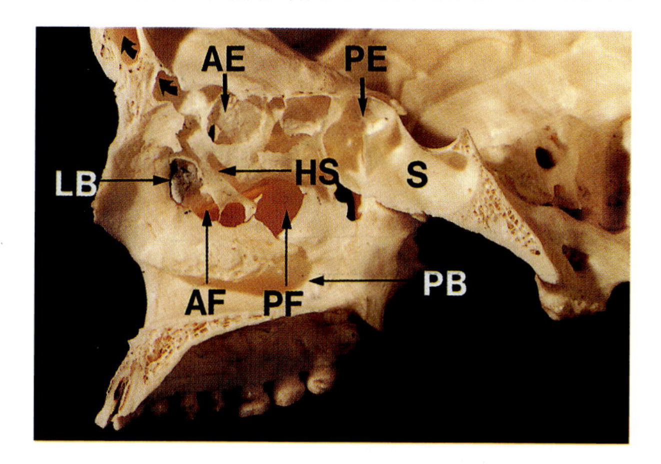

Figure 3.5 *Lateral wall of nose.* Half-skull showing the bony features of the lateral wall of the nose. The middle turbinate and superior turbinate have been removed, opening the anterior (AE) and posterior (PE) ethmoid air cells. The small curved arrows lie within the frontal recess and the frontal sinus, respectively. Other features demonstrated include the sphenoid sinus (S), perpendicular plate of the palatine bone (PB), anterior (AF) and posterior (PF) fontanelles, lacrimal bone (LB), and hiatus semilunaris (HS).

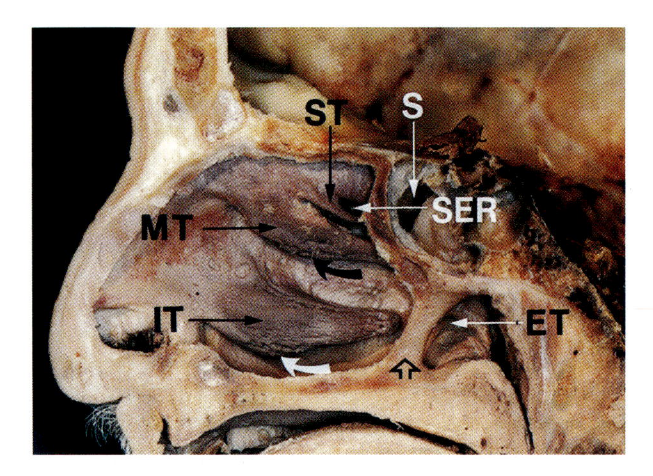

Figure 3.6 *Lateral wall of nose.* Cadaver dissection revealing the lateral wall of the nose following removal of the nasal septum. The posterior portion of the nasal septum remains at the level of the choana (open arrow). Features demonstrated include the inferior turbinate (IT), the inferior meatus (white curved arrow), the middle turbinate (MT), the middle meatus (black curved arrow), the superior turbinate (ST), the sphenoethmoid recess (SER) above it, the sphenoid sinus (S), and the Eustachian tube orifice (ET).

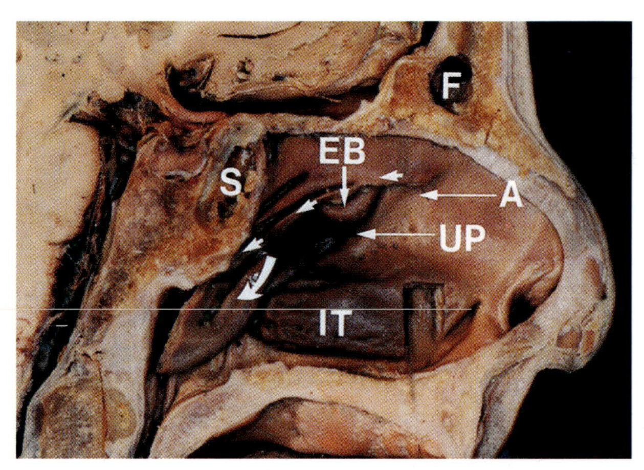

Figure 3.7 *Lateral wall of nose.* Cadaver dissection revealing more detail of the lateral wall of the nose following removal of the nasal septum and reflection of the middle turbinate posteroinferiorly (curved arrow). The cut edge of the middle turbinate is emphasized with small white arrows. Other features demonstrated include the frontal sinus (F), sphenoid sinus (S), ethmoid bulla (bulla ethmoidalis) (EB), uncinate process (UP), and agger nasi (A). Part of the inferior turbinate (IT) has been resected, and a fine polyethylene tube is shown protruding from the opening of the nasolacrimal duct. The cleft seen between the ethmoid bulla and the uncinate process is the hiatus semilunaris.

plate of the sphenoid bone, and medially by the posterior border of the vomer.

Nasal septum (Figure 3.8)

The nasal septum forms the medial wall of each nasal cavity and passes from the roof of the nasal cavity to the floor. It is composed of three separate structures, two bony and one cartilaginous. The quadrilateral cartilage is attached anteriorly to the upper and lower lateral nasal cartilages superiorly and the maxillary crest inferiorly. An accessory cartilage of Huschke may lie along this latter articulation and narrow the nasal cavity.

The bony septum is composed of the perpendicular plate of the ethmoid superiorly and the vomer posteroinferiorly. The bony septum is attached posteriorly to the face of the sphenoid and anteriorly to both the nasal bones and the spine of the frontal bone.

Up to 25% of the population has some deviation of the nasal septum without any cause or symptoms. Such deviations may occur in either the cartilaginous septum, the bony septum or in both. It may be caused by asymmetrical growth or trauma occurring either during parturition or at a later date.

The quadrilateral cartilage may be dislocated from the maxillary crest. Sometimes there is an

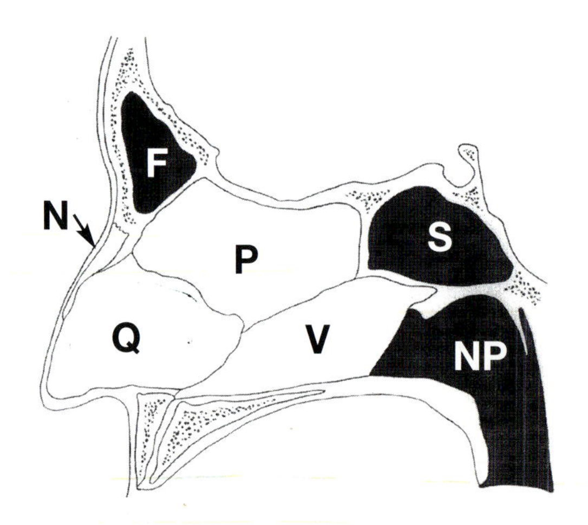

Figure 3.8 *Nasal septum.* Diagram illustrating the various components of the nasal septum – the perpendicular plate of the ethmoid bone (P), vomer (V), and quadrilateral cartilage (Q) together with the sphenoid sinus (S), frontal sinus (F), nasal bone (N), and nasopharynx (NP).

apparent thickening of the cartilaginous nasal septum in its anterior third known as the tuberculum septi or nasal septal swell body as described by Zuckerkandl. This is an area of rudimentary erectile tissue found on each side of the septum.

This swell body often overlies a thickening of the cartilaginous septum.

Superior turbinate (Figures 3.9, 3.12 and 3.14)

The superior turbinate is an integral part of the ethmoid bone and is represented as a thin curved plate of bone lying above the posterior third of the middle turbinate.

Middle turbinate and ground lamella (Figures 3.6 and 3.9–3.15)

The middle turbinate is an integral part of the ethmoid bone. It has a vertical, anterior free border, which may be slender or bulbous. Occasionally, this free border is lobulated. The posterior margin is attached to the lateral nasal wall and to the perpendicular plate of the palatine bone. Immediately posterior to this attachment lies the sphenopalatine foramen, which transmits the sphenopalatine vessels and the posterior superior nasal nerves. The middle turbinate may be pneumatized in both its vertical or horizontal anterior segments. Such a middle turbinate air cell is called a 'concha bullosa'.

The middle turbinate attaches to the skull base superiorly and to the lateral wall of the nasal cavity in a diverse manner. This attachment can be divided into three parts:

- The anterior portion of the middle turbinate lies in a paramedian sagittal plane. The vertical lamella of the middle turbinate inserts into the lateral border of the cribriform plate and is covered medially by olfactory epithelium containing fibers of the olfactory nerve in the superior portion. Careless dissection leading to avulsion of this medial lamella may lead to leakage of cerebrospinal fluid and the risk of intracranial sepsis.
- The vertical plate of the central portion of the middle turbinate rotates to lie in the coronal plane between the anterior portion medially and the lamina papyracea laterally. This part is known as the ground or basal lamella of the middle turbinate. This lamella is anatomically

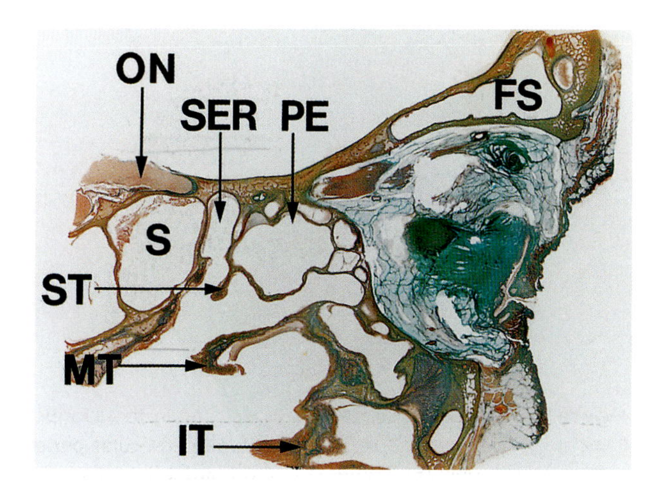

Figure 3.9 *Parasagittal section through orbital canal.* Parasagittal section demonstrating the frontal sinus (FS) extending into the orbital roof, posterior ethmoid sinus (PE), sphenoethmoid recess (SER), optic nerve (ON), superior turbinate (ST), sphenoid sinus (S), middle turbinate (MT), and inferior turbinate (IT) (Masson trichrome stain). From: Studying whole-mounted sections of the paranasal sinuses to understand the complications of endoscopic sinus surgery, by Michael and Eugene Rontal, The Laryngoscope 101, April 1991, reproduced by kind permission of The Laryngoscope and the authors.

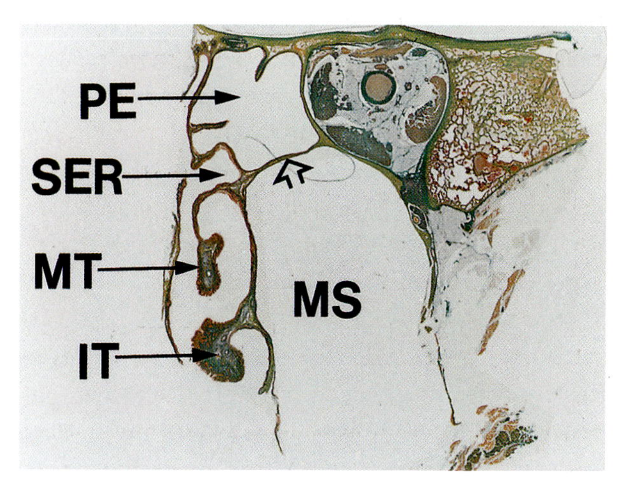

Figure 3.10 *Coronal section through posterior ethmoid sinus.* Coronal section demonstrating the posterior ethmoid sinus (PE), sphenoethmoid recess (SER), middle turbinate (MT), inferior turbinate (IT), maxillary sinus (MS), and ethmomaxillary plate (open arrow) (Masson trichrome stain). From: Studying whole-mounted sections of the paranasal sinuses to understand the complications of endoscopic sinus surgery, by Michael and Eugene Rontal, The Laryngoscope 101, April 1991, reproduced by kind permission of The Laryngoscope and the authors.

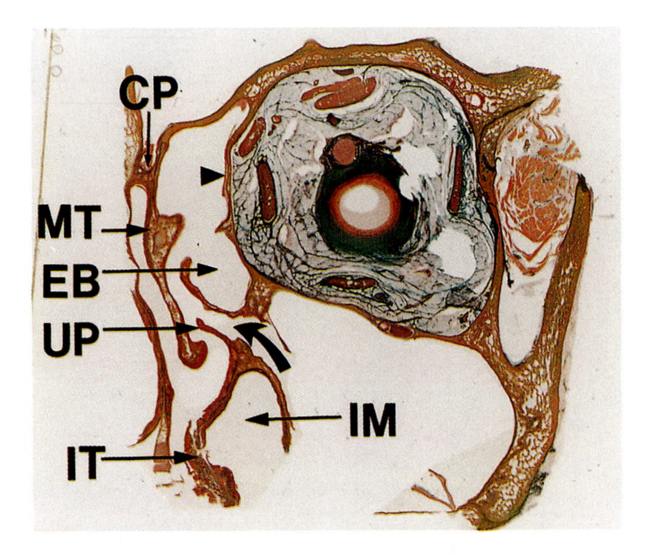

Figure 3.11 *Cross-section through ethmoid infundibulum and maxillary sinus ostium.* Cross-section demonstrating the cribriform plate (CP), lamina papyracea (arrowhead), middle turbinate (MT), ethmoid bulla (bulla ethmoidalis) (EB), uncinate process (UP), inferior turbinate (IT), and inferior meatus (IM); the curved arrow passes through the maxillary sinus ostium into the ethmoid infundibulum (Masson trichrome stain). From: Studying whole-mounted sections of the paranasal sinuses to understand the complications of endoscopic sinus surgery, by Michael and Eugene Rontal, The Laryngoscope 101, April 1991, reproduced by kind permission of The Laryngoscope and the authors.

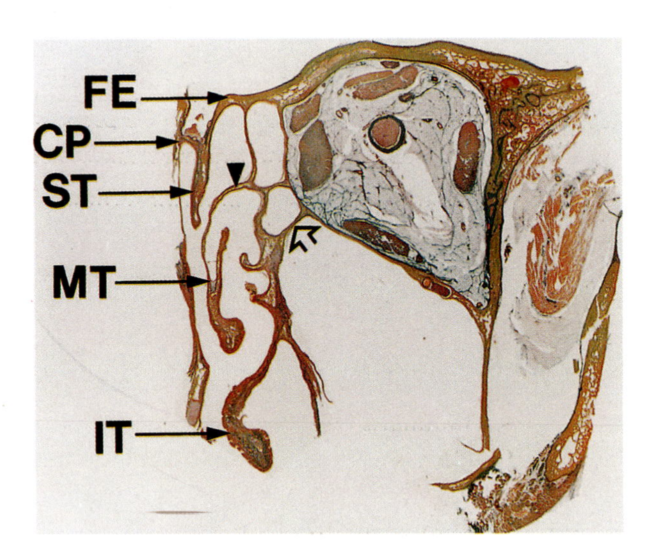

Figure 3.12 *Coronal section through posterior ethmoid sinus.* Coronal section demonstrating the superior turbinate (ST), middle turbinate (MT) with its horizontal insertion (arrowhead), inferior turbinate (IT), and ethmomaxillary plate (open arrow); note how the fovea ethmoidalis (FE), which roofs the ethmoid air cells, lies at a much higher plane than the cribriform plate (CP) (Masson trichrome stain). From: Studying whole-mounted sections of the paranasal sinuses to understand the complications of endoscopic sinus surgery, by Michael and Eugene Rontal, The Laryngoscope 101, April 1991, reproduced by kind permission of The Laryngoscope and the authors.

3.13a

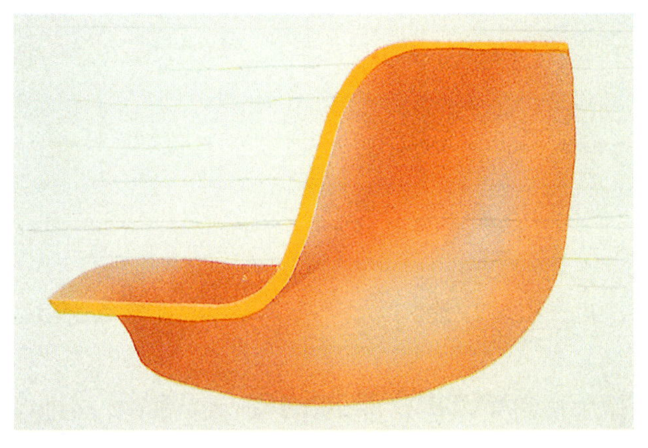

3.13b

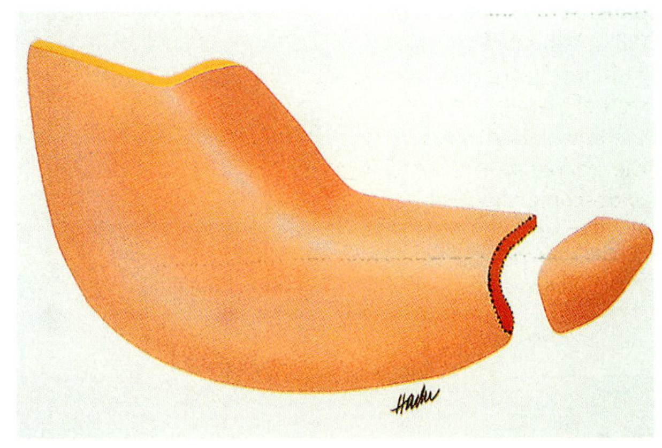

Figure 3.13 *Middle turbinate.* Diagrams showing the ground lamella of the middle turbinate from (a) medially and (b) laterally. The posterior tip of the lateral view (b) has been divided to demonstrate the vertical and horizontal plates of the turbinate. From: Functional Endoscopic Sinus Surgery: The Messerklinger Technique, by Professor Heinz Stammberger, with kind permission of the publisher Mosby-Year Book.

important because it divides the anterior ethmoid air cells from the posterior ethmoid air cells. All of the air cells anterior to the ground lamella have their ostia located in the anterior ethmoid, whereas all of the ethmoid air cells posterior to the ground lamella have their ostia located in the superior meatus. The sphenoid sinus ostia open into the sphenoethmoid recess.

- The posterior portion of the insertion of the middle turbinate runs in a horizontal plane, forming the roof of the posterior middle meatus. The bone inserts into the lamina papyracea or medial wall of the maxilla.

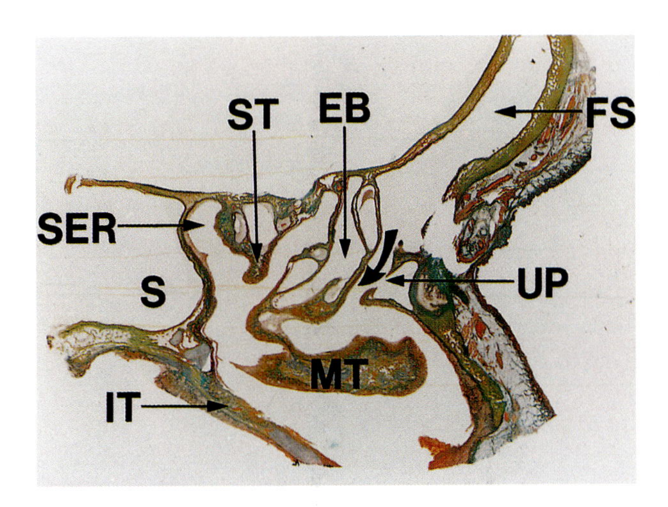

Figure 3.14 *Parasagittal section through the cribriform plate.* Parasagittal section demonstrating the frontal sinus (FS), uncinate process (UP), ethmoid bulla (bulla ethmoidatis) (EB), superior turbinate (ST), sphenoethmoid recess (SER), sphenoid sinus (S), inferior turbinate (IT), and middle turbinate (MT); the curved arrow shows the path from the frontal recess into the ethmoid infundibulum (Masson trichrome stain). From: Studying whole-mounted sections of the paranasal sinuses to understand the complications of endoscopic sinus surgery, by Michael and Eugene Rontal, The Laryngoscope 101, April 1991, reproduced by kind permission of The Laryngoscope and the authors.

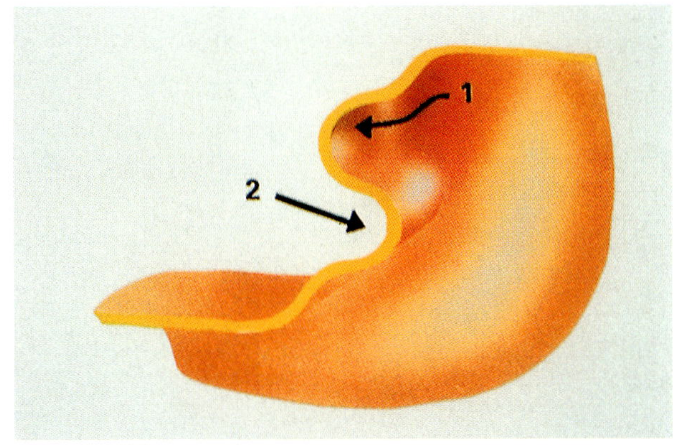

Figure 3.15 *Lateral sinus.* Diagram of the middle turbinate demonstrating how the ground lamella may be distorted by the lateral sinus (1) and the posterior ethmoid (2). Reproduced from: Functional Endoscopic Sinus Surgery: The Messerklinger Technique, by Professor Heinz Stammberger, with the kind permission of the publisher Mosby-Year Book.

Inferior turbinate (Figures 3.1, 3.4, 3.6, 3.7, and 3.10)

The inferior turbinate is a thin, curved, independent bone that articulates with the nasal surface of the maxilla and the perpendicular plate of the palatine bone. Its lower free border is gently curved. Three bony prominences project from the superior free border of the inferior turbinate. The most anterior is the lacrimal process, which attaches to the lacrimal bone and the nasolacrimal groove of the maxilla, thereby helping to form the medial wall of the nasolacrimal duct. The ethmoid process of the inferior turbinate attaches to the uncinate process and separates the anterior fontanelle from the posterior fontanelle. The third prominence, the maxillary process, projects inferiorly and laterally to attach to the maxilla and the maxillary process of the palatine bone, thus forming part of the medial wall of the maxillary sinus. Inferolateral to the inferior turbinate lies the inferior meatus, which is deepest at the junction of its anterior and middle thirds.

STRUCTURES OF LATERAL NASAL WALL

Ostiomeatal complex (Figures 3.4, 3.5, 3.7, 3.12, and 3.16)

The term 'ostiomeatal complex' is used to refer collectively to the maxillary sinus ostium, ethmoid infundibulum, hiatus semilunaris, middle meatus, frontal recess, ethmoid bulla, and uncinate process, and describes the final common drainage pathways of the frontal, maxillary, and anterior ethmoid sinuses.

The lateral wall of the middle meatus houses several key anatomical features:

- Uncinate process
- Hiatus semilunaris
- Ethmoid infundibulum
- Ethmoid bulla (bulla ethmoidalis)
- Lateral sinus
- Frontal recess

Uncinate process (Figures 3.4, 3.7, 3.11, 3.16, and 3.17)

The uncinate process is a fine, bony leaflet lying immediately posterior to the agger nasi. This thin bony prominence is usually found posterior to the

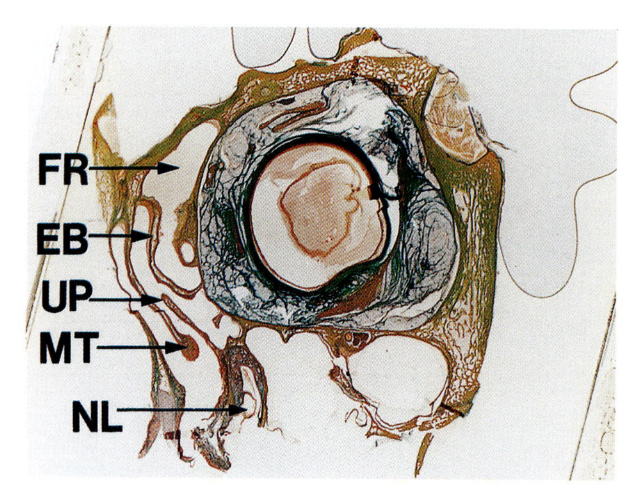

Figure 3.16 *Coronal section through ethmoid infundibulum anterior to maxillary sinus ostium.* Coronal section demonstrating the frontal recess (FR), ethmoid bulla (bulla ethmoidalis) (EB), uncinate process (UP), middle turbinate (MT), ethmoid infundibulum (EI), and nasolacrimal duct (NL) (Masson trichrome stain). From: Studying whole-mounted sections of the paranasal sinuses to understand the complications of endoscopic sinus surgery, by Michael and Eugene Rontal, The Laryngoscope 101, April 1991, reproduced by kind permission of The Laryngoscope and the authors.

leading vertical edge of the middle turbinate on the lateral wall of the nasal cavity. It can be exposed by gentle medial retraction of the middle turbinate. The superior origin of the uncinate process from the lateral bony nasal wall is variable. It may insert onto the lamina papyracea, the lacrimal bone, or the skull base, and it may even swing medially to insert into the lateral surface of the middle turbinate. Its upper extremity is usually concealed by the anterior insertion of the middle turbinate. The uncinate process then sweeps down in a posteroinferior direction, curving more posteriorly in its lower portion. The uncinate process forms the medial wall of the ethmoid infundibulum and its posterior free margin forms the anteroinferior margin of the hiatus semilunaris.

Pneumatization of infundibular cells, agger nasi cells, or the uncinate process may occur, distorting the anatomy and sometimes causing the uncinate process to bend medially and anteriorly.

At the posterior inferior insertion of the uncinate process, fine bony spicules attach the process to the perpendicular plate of the palatine bone. Bony spicules also arise from the inferior margin of the uncinate process and articulate with the ethmoid process of the inferior turbinate. It is this latter bony attachment that separates the anterior and posterior fontanelles. The fontanelles are bony dehiscences of variable size and number in the medial wall of the maxillary sinus. They are closed by mucoperiosteum. Deficiencies can sometimes be found in both the anterior and posterior fontanelles, and are known as accessory maxillary ostia.

The natural ostium of the maxillary sinus is hidden deep in the inferior portion of the infundibulum and cannot be seen with an endoscope in the middle meatus in the unoperated nose, unlike accessory maxillary ostia, which may be readily seen perforating the anterior and posterior fontanelles.

Ethmoid infundibulum (Figure 3.11)

The ethmoid infundibulum is a three-dimensional space lying lateral to the uncinate process. The medial wall of the ethmoid infundibulum is formed by the uncinate process, whereas its lateral wall is formed by the lamina papyracea, with variable contributions from the frontal process of the maxilla and from the lacrimal bone.

The anatomy of the superior part of the infundibulum varies, depending on the bony insertion of the uncinate process. Knowledge of this anatomy is of great importance to the endoscopic sinus surgeon when identifying the frontal recess.

The superior part of the uncinate process can insert laterally onto the lamina papyracea, superiorly onto the skull base or, medially onto the middle turbinate. If the uncinate process inserts laterally onto the lamina papyracea, the ethmoid infundibulum ends superiorly as a blind pit known as the terminal recess. The frontal sinus drains into the frontal recess, which in this situation is separated from the ethmoid infundibulum. This configuration limits the spread of infection from the ethmoid infundibulum and maxillary sinus to the frontal sinus. If the uncinate process inserts into the roof of the ethmoid, or passes medially to insert into the middle turbinate, then the frontal sinus and the frontal recess will open directly into the infundibulum, and disease in the ethmoid infundibulum or the maxillary sinus may affect frontal sinus drainage.

The infundibulum usually terminates posteriorly at the anterior wall of the bulla ethmoidalis,

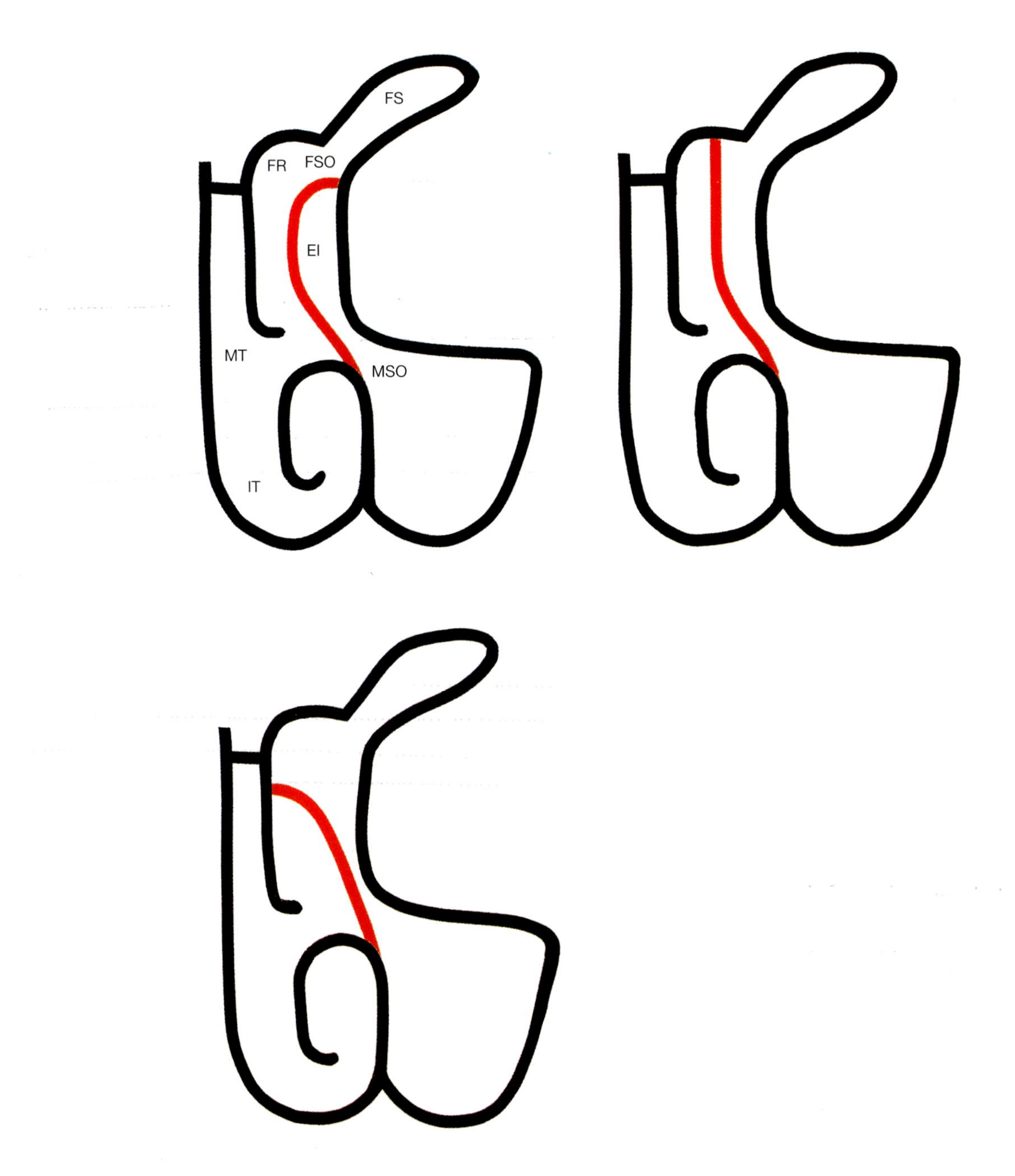

Figure 3.17 *Insertion of uncinate process.* Diagram showing a simplified version of the variations of the insertion of the uncinate process and its effect upon the drainage pattern of the frontal recess. EI, ethmoid infundibulum; FR ,frontal recess; FSO, frontal sinus ostium; FS, frontal sinus; MSO, maxillary sinus ostium; MT, middle turbinate; IT, inferior turbinate. Reproduced from: Functional Endoscopic Sinus Surgery: The Messerklinger Technique, by Professor Heinz Stammberger, with the kind permission of the publisher Mosby-Year Book.

where it communicates with the middle meatus via the hiatus semilunaris.

The lateral margin of the infundibulum is rarely farther than 1–1.5 mm from the lamina papyracea. It may be further collapsed if there are anatomical variations such as concha bullosa, or pathological conditions that compress the uncinate process against the lateral nasal wall.

Hiatus semilunaris (Figures 3.4, 3.5, and 3.7)

The hiatus semilunaris is a two-dimensional space that lies between the posterior free margin of the uncinate process and the anterior wall of the ethmoid bulla. It is usually 1–2 mm wide and forms the entrance into the ethmoid infundibulum, which lies lateral to the uncinate process.

Lateral sinus (Figure 3.15)

The lateral sinus is a variable cleft found superior and posterior to the ethmoid bulla. The lateral sinus lies between the lamina papyracea laterally and the middle turbinate medially. The roof of the ethmoid is found superiorly and the ethmoid bulla inferiorly. Posteriorly, the cleft may be extensive between the bulla and the ground lamella of the middle turbinate. Anteriorly, the lateral sinus may communicate with the frontal recess or it may be separated by the bulla inserting into the roof of the ethmoid.

Superior meatus and sphenoethmoid recess (Figures 3.6, 3.9, and 3.10)

The superior meatus lies inferolateral to the superior turbinate. It overlies the posterior ethmoid air cells, which communicate with the superior meatus. Posterior to the superior meatus lies the sphenoethmoid recess, which is related to the sphenoid ostium, which in turn ventilates the sphenoid sinus.

Middle meatus

The middle meatus is inferior and lateral to the middle turbinate and houses the anterior ethmoid sinuses. It is the final common pathway for drainage of secretions from the frontal, maxillary, and anterior ethmoid sinuses.

Inferior meatus (Figure 3.11)

The inferior meatus lies inferior and lateral to the inferior turbinate. The nasolacrimal duct opens into the inferior meatus at the junction of the anterior and middle third. The duct is protected by Hasner's valve.

Lacrimal apparatus and nasolacrimal duct (Figures 3.18 and 3.19)

The lacrimal gland produces tears. It is a serous gland situated in a shallow fossa in the superolateral aspect of the orbit. It has an orbital lobe and a smaller palpebral lobe. Twelve or more ducts release tears to moisten the conjunctiva. Excessive tears drain through the superior and inferior lacrimal canaliculi into the lacrimal sac which lies in the lacrimal fossa, anterior to the posterior lacrimal crest.

Behind the lacrimal sac, arising from the posterior lacrimal crest, is the medial palpebral ligament of the orbit. Between this and the laterally placed Whitnall's tubercle is the suspensory ligament of Lockwood, which plays an important role in suspending the globe in the orbit. The lacrimal sac drains inferiorly into the nasolacrimal duct, which passes through the medial wall of the maxilla, finally opening into the inferior meatus through Hasner's valve.

PARANASAL SINUSES

The major paranasal sinuses consist of the maxillary, ethmoid, frontal, and sphenoid sinuses. The size and shape of each of these paired sinuses are highly variable, but it is the anatomy of the ethmoid bone and its attendant air cells that is the most challenging to comprehend. Understanding the anatomy of the middle meatus and the lateral nasal wall, with their significant anatomical variations and abnormalities, is of paramount importance for both the endoscopic sinus surgeon and the radiologist who interprets the CT scan.

Frontal bone and frontal sinus (Figures 3.4, 3.5, and 3.9; Table 3.2)

The frontal bone is one of the unpaired skull bones and forms the anterior portion of the calvarium. It articulates with the ethmoid, the sphenoid, the parietal, and the nasal bones, as well as with the zygoma and the maxilla.

The frontal bone is occasionally divided in the midline by a persistent metopic suture. The frontal bone contains marrow and consequently is susceptible to osteomyelitis.

The frontal bone makes a major contribution to the floor of the anterior cranial fossa and in so doing also forms the roof of the orbits. The inferior surface of the frontal bone is notched by the foveolae ethmoidales, which close the open roof of the ethmoid labyrinths.

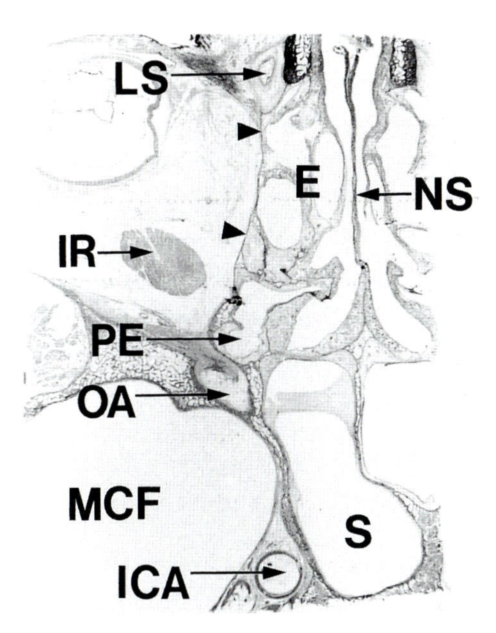

Figure 3.18 *Axial section at the level of the lacrimal sac and orbital apex.* Axial section demonstrating the lacrimal sac (LS), anterior ethmoid air cells (E), nasal septum (NS), inferior rectus (IR), lamina papyracea (arrowheads), posterior ethmoid sinus with an Onodi cell (PE), orbital apex (OA), sphenoid sinus (S), middle cranial fossa (MCF), and internal carotid artery (ICA). From: Studying whole-mounted sections of the paranasal sinuses to understand the complications of endoscopic sinus surgery, by Michael and Eugene Rontal, The Laryngoscope 101, April 1991, reproduced by kind permission of The Laryngoscope and the authors.

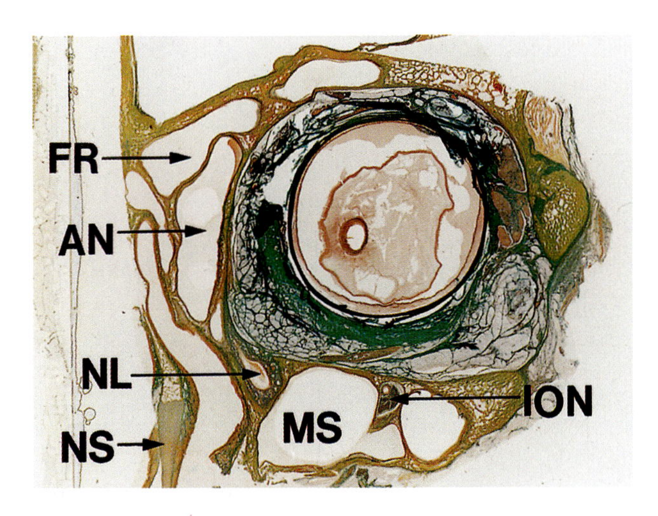

Figure 3.19 *Coronal section through anterior ethmoid sinuses.* Coronal section demonstrating the frontal recess (FR), agger nasi (AN), nasolacrimal duct (NL), nasal septum (NS), maxillary sinus (MS), and infraorbital nerve (ION) (Masson trichrome stain). From: Studying whole-mounted sections of the paranasal sinuses to understand the complications of endoscopic sinus surgery, by Michael and Eugene Rontal, The Laryngoscope 101, April 1991, reproduced by kind permission of The Laryngoscope and the authors.

Table 3.2 Important relations of the frontal sinus

Inferior
• Frontal recess opening into middle meatus
• The orbital roof
Posterior
• Anterior cranial fossa

The frontal sinus develops from pneumatization of the anterior part of the frontal recess. It is undeveloped at birth, appearing in the second year as an outgrowth of the frontal recess. On average, the top of the frontal sinus lies at the level of the mid-vertical height of the orbit by 4 years of age and reaches the height of the supraorbital rim by 8 years of age. It extends above the orbit by 10 years of age.

The extent of pneumatization of the frontal sinus is highly variable. Aplasia is seen in about 4% of the population. The two frontal sinuses are usually unequal in size and separated by a bony septum that does not lie in the midline.

The frontal sinus may extend superiorly into the superciliary region and posteriorly above the medial part of the roof of the orbit.

There may be numerous incomplete septa, giving the sinus its characteristic scalloped outline.

The thin posterior wall of the frontal sinus overlies the dura of the anterior cranial fossa, and consequently infections within the frontal sinus may spread through its posterior wall, resulting in an extradural abscess.

Frontal recess (Figures 3.5, 3.10, 3.12, 3.14, 3.16, 3.19, and 3.20; Table 3.3)

The large paranasal sinuses are connected to the nasal cavity by prechambers, which are small conduits through which ventilation of the paranasal sinus occurs and out of which mucus is propelled by the mucociliary clearence system.

Ventilation and mucociliary clearance of the frontal sinus occurs through the frontal recess into the middle meatus. The anatomy and drainage of the frontal recess is variable and depends primarily on the insertion of the ethmoid bulla and the superior portion of the uncinate process.

When the anterior wall of the ethmoid bulla inserts into the roof of the ethmoid gallery it will

Table 3.3 Possible drainage pathways from the frontal recess

Premeatal chambers: when the uncinate process inserts into the roof
Ethmoid infundibulum: when the anterior wall of the ethmoid bulla reaches the roof
Suprabullar space and lateral sinus: when the bulla is separated from the roof by the suprabullar space

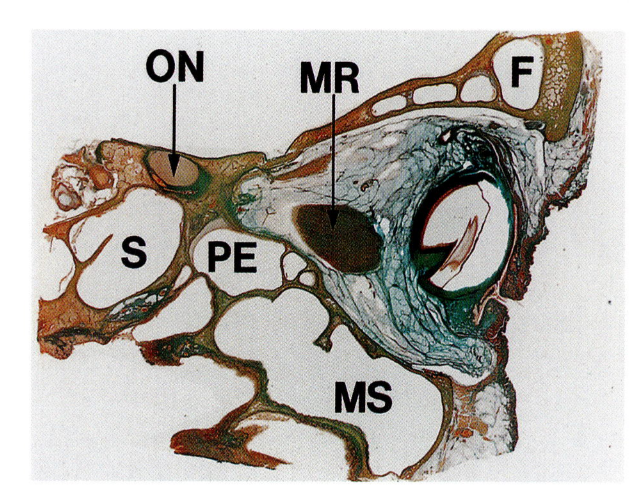

Figure 3.20 *Parasagittal section through sphenoid sinus.* Parasagittal section demonstrating the frontal sinus (F), medial rectus (MR), optic nerve (ON), sphenoid sinus (S), posterior ethmoid sinus (PE), and maxillary sinus (MS) (Masson trichrome stain). From: Studying whole-mounted sections of the paranasal sinuses to understand the complications of endoscopic sinus surgery, by Michael and Eugene Rontal, The Laryngoscope 101, April 1991, reproduced by kind permission of The Laryngoscope and the authors.

form the posterior wall of the frontal recess, thus separating it from the lateral sinus. However, this wall is often incomplete or absent, allowing the frontal recess to communicate with the lateral sinus. Depending on the anterosuperior insertion of the uncinate process, the frontal recess may open directly into the middle meatus or into the ethmoid infundibulum. The frontal recess may be constricted by surrounding structures such as a prominent ethmoid bulla or prominent agger nasi cells.

The frontonasal duct is a misnomer, and this prechamber is more appropriately named the frontal recess. It is rarely ductlike, consisting instead of a waisted bony recess communicating between the frontal sinus and the nasal cavity.

The shape of the frontal recess depends primarily on its surrounding structures. The medial border of the frontal recess usually consists of the lateral lamella of the most anterior portion of the middle turbinate. The lateral border of the frontal recess consists mainly of lamina papyracea and may have a small contribution from the uncinate process.

Superiorly, the frontal bone forms the roof with its anterior foveolae ethmoidales. Further anteriorly, the frontal bone curves upwards to form the posterior wall of the frontal sinus. The frontal ostium, which lies between the frontal sinus and the frontal recess, is usually found in the most anterosuperior part of the frontal recess, but this cannot be seen directly with the endoscope during a routine diagnostic nasal examination.

Maxilla and maxillary sinus (Figures 3.4 and 3.11; Table 3.4)

The maxilla consists of a body together with several processes, named the zygomatic process, frontal process, palatine process, and alveolar process. The maxilla articulates with the frontal bone, palatine bone, zygoma, ethmoid bone, nasal bone, and lacrimal bones.

The maxillary sinus is a space within the body of the maxilla, which is usually present at birth as a slitlike cavity. The maxillary sinus extends laterally under the infraorbital canal by 2 years of age and into the zygoma by 9 years. The lateral growth stops around 15 years of age, while the vertical growth continues until the last molar teeth erupt.

The maxillary sinus is pyramidal in shape, with the base forming the medial wall of the sinus and the apex pointing into the zygomatic process of the maxilla. The maxillary sinus may be compartmentalized by incomplete bony septa.

The anterior and posterior walls of the maxillary sinus consist of the anterior and posterior walls of the maxilla. The roof of the maxillary sinus is the floor of the orbit, which exhibits a ridge occupied by the infraorbital nerve. The floor of the maxillary sinus is formed by the alveolar recess, which lies at a lower level than the floor of the nasal cavity. This area bears the upper teeth, with the roots of the first molar and second premolar lying in close proximity to the floor of the sinus. Later in life, these roots may project through the floor, although they are still

Table 3.4 Important relations of the maxillary sinus

Superior
- Orbit and contents
- Infraorbital nerve and canal

Inferior
- Alveolar ridge and molar teeth

Posterior
- Pterygopalatine fossa pterygoid process
- Medial and lateral

Lateral
- Soft tissue of cheek

Medial
- Nasal cavity
- Anterior and posterior fontanelle
- Sinus ostium opening into ethmoid infundibulum

usually covered by a thin layer of bone and mucosa. Occasionally, during extraction of these teeth, this thin layer of bone and mucosa will be removed, thus establishing a direct connection between the lumen of the maxillary sinus and the oral cavity. This connection may persist as an 'oro–antral fistula'.

Superomedially, the ethmo-maxillary plate separates the maxillary sinus from the posterior ethmoid air cells.

The bony medial wall of the maxillary sinus is dehiscent in two areas. These areas, which are closed by periosteum and mucous membrane, are the anterior and posterior nasal fontanelles.

Accessory maxillary sinus ostia are found in both the anterior and posterior fontanelles. When present, these accessory maxillary sinus ostia can usually be seen on diagnostic endoscopy, whereas it is not possible to see the maxillary ostium which is concealed by the uncinate process.

The ostium of the maxillary sinus is superiorly placed in the medial wall of the maxilla. It opens into the inferior part of the ethmoid infundibulum at a point that transects the midpoint between the anterior and posterior insertions of the inferior turbinate.

Ethmoid bone (Figures 3.2, 3.3, and 3.21)

The ethmoid bone contributes to the medial wall of the orbit, the nasal septum, the floor of the anterior cranial fossa, and the lateral wall of the nasal cavity. It is another of the unpaired skull bones and is composed of five parts: a perpendicular plate (which comprises a portion of the bony nasal septum), a horizontal plate (the cribriform plate), a superior prominence (the crista galli), and two multicellular labyrinths, containing the anterior and posterior ethmoid air cells, suspended laterally. The ethmoid labyrinths are narrow anteriorly and expand as they pass posteriorly and follow the natural lateral curve of the medial wall of the orbit.

Ethmoid sinuses (Figures 3.3, 3.9, 3.12, 3.18, and 3.19; Table 3.5)

The ethmoid sinuses are present at birth and may or may not be aerated. They continue to enlarge until puberty. The anatomy of the ethmoid sinuses is challenging. These bony chambers are bounded by the ethmoid bone only in the lateral and medial planes. Anteriorly, the ethmoid air cells are enclosed by the lacrimal bone laterally. Superiorly, the labyrinthine cells are closed by the indentations in the thicker inferior surface of the frontal bone known as the foveolae ethmoidales. Posteriorly, the ethmoid air cells are closed by the anterolateral walls of the sphenoid sinus.

The lateral bony plate of the ethmoid, which is named the lamina papyracea, forms the medial wall of the orbit. The lamina papyracea is extremely thin and may be dehiscent in part, allowing disease to track through into the orbit. It is the most common site for inadvertent entry into the orbit during endoscopic sinus surgery.

The medial wall of the ethmoid labyrinth is composed of the middle turbinate, the superior turbinate, and, if present, the supreme turbinate. Inferior and lateral to the middle turbinate lies the middle meatus and inferolateral to the superior turbinate lies the superior meatus.

The roof of the ethmoid bone is formed by the cribriform plate. It lies medial to the vertical insertion of the middle turbinate. The olfactory nerve fibers pass through tiny foramina to supply the medial aspect of the middle turbinate and the lateral aspect of the superior part of the septum. The cribriform plate lies at a lower level than the roofs of the adjacent ethmoid air cells and tends to dip inferiorly as it passes posteriorly. The attendant dura, olfactory bulb, and frontal lobe should always be considered to be at risk during ethmoid surgery.

Injury to the cribriform plate may cause a cerebrospinal fluid leak and/or permanent anosmia. Behind the cribriform plate, the nasal cavity is roofed by the thicker horizontal plate of sphenoid bone (the planum sphenoidale).

The ethmoid clefts open medially into the nasal cavity and posteriorly into the choanae.

The sphenoethmoid recess is located posterosuperior to the superior turbinate.

The ethmoid air cells are divided into an anterior and a posterior group by the ground lamella.

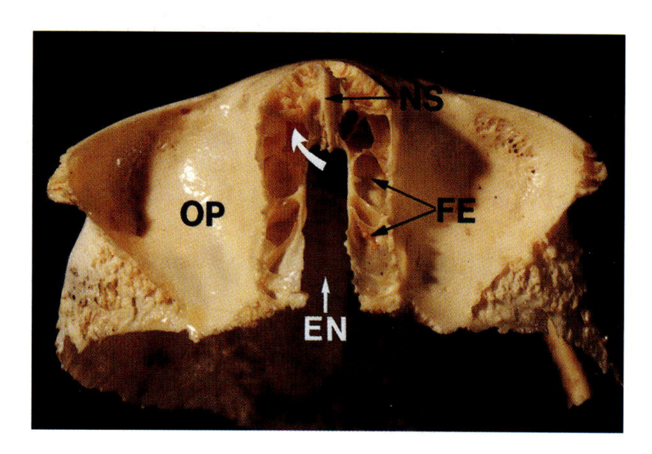

Figure 3.21 *Inferior aspect of frontal bone.* Inferior view of a disarticulated frontal bone demonstrating the ethmoid notch (EN), which receives the crista galli and cribriform plate, the nasal spine (NS), and the foveolae ethmoidales, which roof the anterior and posterior ethmoid air cells (FE). The curved arrow is directed into the frontal recess and frontal sinus. The orbital plate (OP), forming the roof of the orbit, is also shown.

Table 3.5 Important structures related to the ethmoid air cells

Superior
• Cribriform plate, olfactory bulb, and olfactory nerves
• Gyrus recti of frontal lobe
Inferomedial
• Nasal cavity
Posterior
• Sphenoid sinus
Lateral
• Orbits separated by lamina papyracea
• Lacrimal sac
• Optic nerves

Anterior ethmoid sinus (Figures 3.5, 3.18, and 3.19)

The anterior ethmoid air cells open into the middle meatus. The largest and most constant anterior ethmoid air cell is termed the ethmoid bulla (bulla ethmoidalis). The most anterior of the anterior ethmoid air cells are the agger nasi cells.

Agger nasi (Figure 3.19)

The agger nasi (the agger mound) is a smooth bony swelling or eminence in the frontal process of the maxilla that lies in front of the anterior insertion of the middle turbinate. Agger cells are identified on CT scan by their location anterior to the vertical insertion of the middle turbinate into the lateral border of the cribriform plate.

The agger mound may be pneumatized in a variable manner by the agger nasi air cells of the anterior ethmoid, and its bony wall may therefore be either thick or thin. Both the lacrimal sac and the frontal recess lie lateral to the agger nasi when the agger is not pneumatized. Anterolateral to the agger nasi and running parallel to it is the nasolacrimal duct. The frontal sinus, the nasolacrimal duct, and the agger nasi all lie in a similar coronal plane.

Ethmoid bulla (bulla ethmoidalis) (Figures 3.4, 3.7, and 3.14)

The ethmoid bulla is the most constant and largest of the anterior ethmoid air cells. It is pneumatized in a variable manner and, in some individuals, a bony lateral torus is found in the same position. The lateral wall of the ethmoid bulla consists of the lamina papyracea. Posteriorly, the bulla may attach to the ground lamella of the middle turbinate or be separated from it by a posterior extension of the lateral sinus, if present. Superiorly, the bulla may fuse with the roof of the ethmoid and form the posterior wall of the frontal recess, or it may be separated from the ethmoid roof by the suprabullar space that allows communication between the frontal recess and the lateral sinus.

Posterior ethmoid sinus (Figures 3.2, 3.3, 3.9, 3.11, and 3.20)

The posterior ethmoid air cells open into the superior meatus. The most posterior and largest of the posterior ethmoid air cells are called the Onodi cells. Onodi cells may extend posterolaterally to embrace or even surround the optic nerve. These cells may invade the body of the sphenoid and reach the anterior wall of the sella turcica.

Sphenoid bone and sphenoid sinus

(Figures 3.3, 3.6, 3.7, 3.9, 3.14, 3.18, 3.20, 3.22, and 3.23; Table 3.6)

The sphenoid bone is another of the unpaired skull bones. The sphenoid bone consists of a body that gives origin to the lesser wings superiorly and the greater wings and pterygoid processes inferiorly. The sphenoid bone articulates with the basi-occiput, the petrous and the squamous parts of the temporal bone, the parietal bone, the frontal bone, the vomer, and the perpendicular plate of the palatine bone. The sphenoid bone is traversed by five main canals: the foramen rotundum, the foramen ovale, the pterygoid canal (Vidian canal), the optic canal, and the superior orbital fissure.

The sphenoid sinus lies within the body of the sphenoid bone. The sphenoid sinus is present at birth but is not aerated. Its subsequent pneumatization continues until adulthood in a variable and asymmetrical manner.

The front of the body of the sphenoid bone is ridged by the rostrum, which articulates with the perpendicular plate of the ethmoid and the nasal septum. This ridge projects into the sinus as the intersinus septum, which rarely lies in the midline. The sphenoid sinus may lie solely anterior to the pituitary fossa and gland or it may extend posteriorly into the basi-occiput and laterally into the roots of the pterygoid process.

The pterygoid canal transmitting the Vidian nerve lies along the floor of the sphenoid sinus.

The optic nerve has an intimate relationship to the internal carotid artery. The latter courses through the petrous temporal bone to emerge medially at the petrous apex above the foramen lacerum. It deeply grooves the body of the sphenoid in an 'S' shape before turning back upon itself medial to the anterior clinoid process. Above the body of the sphenoid lies the pituitary fossa containing the pituitary gland surrounded by the cavernous sinus.

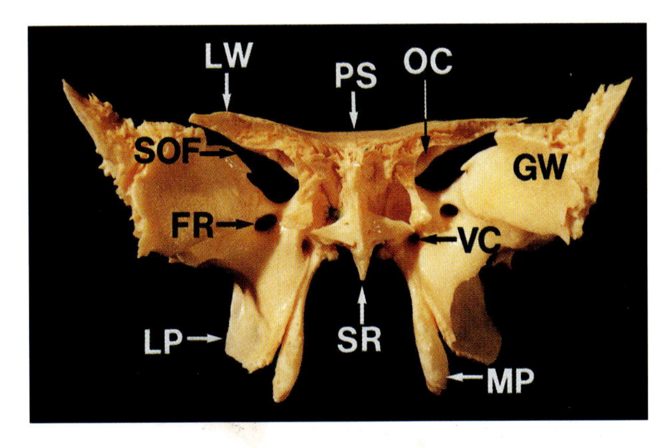

Figure 3.22 *Anterior aspect of the sphenoid bone.* This view of the sphenoid bone demonstrating the greater (GW) and lesser wings (LW), planum sphenoidale (PS), superior orbital fissure (SOF), Vidian (pterygoid) canal (VC), foramen rotundum (FR), optic canal (OC), medial (MP) and lateral (LP) pterygoid plates and the sphenoid rostrum (SR). The lateral and medial pterygoid plates are separated from the maxillary sinus by the pterygopalatine fossa, which receives the nerves from the foramen rotundum and the Vidian canal.

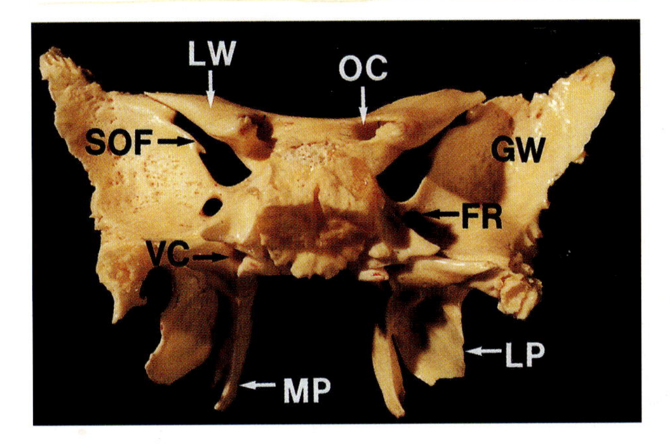

Figure 3.23 *Posterior aspect of sphenoid bone.* A view of the sphenoid bone demonstrating the greater (GW) and lesser (LW) wings, Vidian (pterygoid) canal (VC), foramen rotundum (FR), optic canal (OC), medial (MP) and lateral (LP) pterygoid plates, and superior orbital fissure (SOF).

The optic chiasma lies above the pituitary gland. From it extends the two optic nerves surrounded by the meninges and accompanied by the ophthalmic arteries as they pass through the optic canals.

The sphenoid sinus ostia are located on the anterior wall of the sinus and open into the sphenoethmoid recess, which is located posterior to the superior turbinate.

Table 3.6 Important relations of the sphenoid sinus

Superior
- Pituitary fossa with pituitary gland
- Optic chiasma and optic nerves
- Optic foramen
- Optic canal

Inferior
- Nasopharynx

Posterior
- Basi-occiput

Lateral
- Cavernous sinus and contents
- Superior orbital fissure

Anterior
- Sphenoid sinus ostium
- Posterior ethmoid sinus

IMPORTANT STRUCTURES RELATED TO THE PARANASAL SINUSES

Pterygopalatine fossa (Figures 3.6 and 3.9; Table 3.7)

The pterygopalatine fossa is an inverted pyramidal space located between the posterior wall of the maxillary sinus and the anterior face of the pterygoid plates. The pterygopalatine fossa should not be mistaken for the pterygoid fossa, which lies between the medial and lateral laminae of the pterygoid processes and the posterior wall of the maxillary sinus.

The principal contents of the pterygopalatine fossa are the sphenopalatine ganglion, the maxillary nerve, the maxillary artery and its accompanying veins. The sphenopalatine ganglion relays the parasympathetic nerve supply to the lacrimal gland, the mucous glands of the nose, the nasopharynx, the paranasal sinuses, and the palate. The maxillary nerve is the second division of the trigeminal nerve, which supplies sensation to the middle third of the face.

The pterygopalatine fossa connects through fissures and foramina with several important spaces:

- Laterally to the infratemporal fossa through the pterygomaxillary fissure
- Anteriorly to the orbit through the infraorbital fissure
- Posteriorly to the middle cranial fossa through the foramen rotundum and the pterygoid canal
- Medially to the inferior portion of the sphenoethmoid recess through the spheno-palatine foramen
- Inferior to the oral cavity through the greater and lesser palatine foramina

Orbital apex (Figures 3.7, 3.22, and 3.23)

Structures in the orbital apex are in close proximity to the posterior ethmoid and sphenoid sinuses, and must be considered at risk from disease or surgery in the vicinity.

The bony orbital apex accommodates one bony canal and two fissures:

Table 3.7 Pterygopalatine fossa

Contents
- Sphenopalatine ganglion
- Maxillary nerve (second division of trigeminal nerve)
- Maxillary artery and veins

Communications
- *Laterally* through pterygomaxillary fissure with pterygopalatine fossa
- *Medially* through sphenopalatine foramen with sphenoethmoid recess; through the greater and lesser palatine foramina with the oral cavity
- *Anteriorly* through the infraorbital fissure with the orbit
- *Posteriorly* through the foramen rotundum and the pterygoid canal with the middle cranial fossa

- The optic canal, transmitting the optic nerve and the ophthalmic artery and veins
- The superior orbital fissure, transmitting the lacrimal, frontal, and nasociliary nerves of the ophthalmic division of the trigeminal nerve, and the oculomotor, trochlear, and abducent cranial nerves
- The inferior orbital fissure, transmitting the infraorbital nerve and artery

A tendinous ring surrounds the medial aspect of the superior orbital fissure and the optic canal. From this ring arise the medial, lateral, superior, and inferior recti muscles. The levator palpebrae superioris and superior oblique muscles arise from bone just superior to the tendinous ring. In this way, the optic nerve and globe are surrounded by a cone of muscle. The lacrimal, frontal, and trochlear nerves pass anteriorly within the ring.

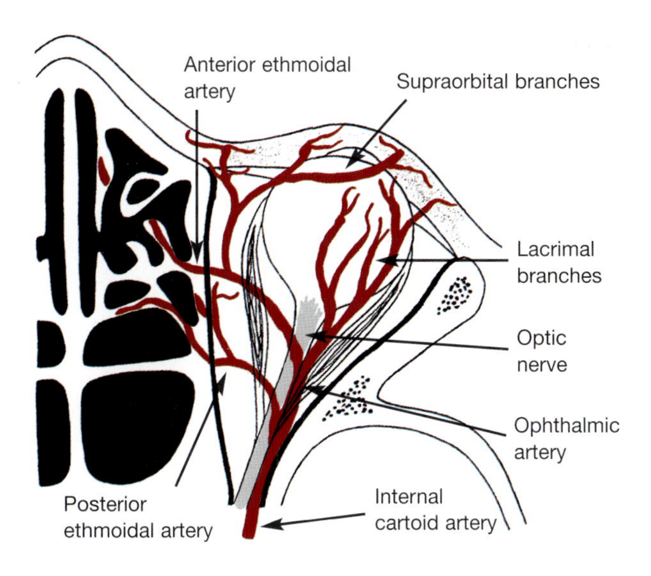

Figure 3.24 *Vascular and nerve supply of the paranasal sinuses.* Axial diagram illustrating the anterior and posterior ethmoidal arteries, ophthalmic artery, supraorbital branches, lacrimal branches, internal carotid artery, and optic nerve. The anterior and posterior ethmoid nerves accompany the arteries (not drawn).

VASCULAR SUPPLY OF NASAL CAVITY AND PARANASAL SINUSES (Figure 3.24; Table 3.8)

The vascular supply to the paranasal sinuses and the nasal cavity is from the branches of the maxillary and ophthalmic arteries.

The branches of the maxillary artery include:

- The posterior superior alveolar artery and infraorbital artery, which are branches of the maxillary artery as it enters the pterygopalatine fossa
- The greater palatine branch of the maxillary artery
- The sphenopalatine artery, which is a terminal branch of the maxillary artery and passes through the sphenopalatine foramen into the nasal cavity

Three branches of the ophthalmic artery supply the paranasal sinuses and nasal cavity: the anterior and posterior ethmoidal arteries and the supraorbital artery.

Anterior and posterior ethmoidal arteries

The anterior and posterior ethmoidal arteries are important to the endoscopic sinus surgeon because transection of either of these arteries may cause a retro-orbital hematoma and visual loss.

The anterior ethmoidal artery arises in the orbit from the ophthalmic artery, which in turn arises from the internal carotid artery. It passes through the anterior ethmoid foramen, running obliquely through the frontoethmoid suture, approximately 2–4 mm posterior to the lacrimal crest. The anterior ethmoidal artery is surrounded by thin bone and lies above the anterior face of the ethmoid bulla. This bony canal may be embedded in the roof of the ethmoid or suspended from it by a bony mesentery. The artery passes through the lateral lamina of the cribriform plate posterior to the crista galli and enters the anterior cranial fossa through the lateral margin of the cribriform plate. It should be noted that this is the thinnest and weakest portion of the skull base. The anterior ethmoidal artery supplies the anterior ethmoid air cells and the frontal sinus and sends intracranial branches to supply the dura.

Table 3.8 Neurovascular supply and lymphatic drainage of the paranasal sinuses

	Frontal sinus	*Ethmoid sinus*	*Maxillary sinus*	*Sphenoid sinus*
Arterial supply	Anterior ethmoidal artery; supraorbital artery	Anterior and posterior ethmoidal arteries; sphenopalatine artery	Facial, infraorbital, greater palatine and ethmoidal arteries	Posterior ethmoidal artery; sphenopalatine artery
Venous drainage	Communicating veins between supraorbital vein and superior ophthalmic vein	Anterior and posterior ethmoidal veins; sphenopalatine veins	Facial, infraorbital, greater palatine, and ethmoidal veins	Posterior ethmoidal veins; sphenopalatine artery
Lymphatic drainage	Submandibular lymph nodes	Submandibular lymph nodes (anterior ethmoid sinus); retropharyngeal (posterior ethmoid sinus)	Submandibular lymph nodes	Retropharyngeal lymph nodes
Nerve supply	Supraorbital nerve (branch of V2)	Anterior and posterior ethmoid nerves, and orbital branches of pterygopalatine ganglion (V2)	Infraorbital nerve; anterior, middle, and posterior branches of superior alveolar nerve (V2)	Posterior ethmoidal nerve and orbital branches of pterygopalatine ganglion (V2)

Further terminal branches pass down through the cribriform plate to supply the superior part of the medial and lateral wall of the nasal cavity and part of the external nose.

The posterior ethmoid artery is also a branch of the ophthalmic artery. It passes through the posterior ethmoid foramen in the frontoethmoid suture approximately 12 mm posterior to the anterior ethmoid foramen and passes behind the cribriform plate. It also supplies dura, and further terminal branches pass inferiorly through the cribriform plate to supply the posterosuperior aspects of the lateral and medial nasal wall.

NERVE SUPPLY OF PARANASAL SINUSES (Figure 3.24; Table 3.8)

The supraorbital nerve (a branch of the ophthalmic division of the trigeminal nerve) and the maxillary division of the trigeminal nerve carry the majority of the sensory innervation of the paranasal sinuses and the nasal cavity. The anterior and posterior ethmoid nerves are branches of the supraorbital nerve and accompany the vessels of the same names in the anterior and posterior ethmoid canals. The posterior ethmoid nerve supplies the ethmoid and sphenoid sinuses but is often absent.

4

Computed tomography of the paranasal sinuses

INTRODUCTION

For many years, rhinologists and radiologists have had to rely upon conventional radiographs for the evaluation of paranasal sinus disease. The information gleaned from such studies is mainly relevant to the general condition of the larger paranasal sinuses, especially the frontal, maxillary, and sphenoid sinuses, and yields minimal information about the delicate bony anatomical or mucosal changes that may be present in the ethmoid air cells of the lateral wall of the nose. With the development of functional endoscopic sinus surgery (FESS), such imaging has proved inadequate. Today, computed tomography (CT) scanning and magnetic resonance imaging (MRI) are the standard means by which to image the paranasal sinuses and nasal cavity. CT is the preferred method of imaging when investigating benign inflammatory disease of the paranasal sinuses. This chapter provides a basic overview of CT scanning and its application to the imaging of the sinuses.

OVERVIEW OF CT

CT scanning has come to the forefront in the routine evaluation of the sinuses. With its increasing availability and ability to provide excellent bony and soft tissue resolution, it has become the imaging modality of choice in the evaluation of sinus inflammatory disease.

With the patient placed supine in the scanner, the CT machine employs a rotating X-ray beam and a detector array. With the advent of slip-ring technology, modern-generation CT scanners employ a stationary ring of detectors while the X-ray source rotates continuously to acquire a volume of data. The projected X-ray beams pass through the subject and reach detectors, which then analyze the variably attenuated rays. The degree of beam attenuation is a direct function of the various tissue densities making up the subject. The image produced is a reflection of these densities.

CT is able to differentiate up to 4000 grades of density from air to metal. This ability allows the differentiation of all clinically relevant tissues. These density grades are measured in Hounsfield units (HU), which range from –1000 to +3000 HU. These different densities are projected as different shades of gray on an electronic screen. The CT computer is also able to manipulate the electronic raw data to provide different so-called 'windows'. Each window is centered at a specific Hounsfield value and has a selected range of values. Only those density values within the specified window will be shown as different shades of gray. Those tissues with a value outside the range will be shown as white if greater than the upper range of the window, while those with a lower value will be projected as black. With this technology, the data can be manipulated to provide windows that will optimize the depiction of soft tissue ('soft tissue or narrow window') or bone structures ('bony or wide window') (Figure 4.1). For imaging of the paranasal sinuses, a window centered at 90 HU with a window range of 350 HU is optimal to depict soft tissue pathology. Bony detail can be achieved with a level centered at 450 HU with a width of 2500 HU.

Other CT imaging parameters are also of importance in generating satisfactory images of the sinuses. In CT imaging, there is a linear relationship between the X-ray dose and the milliamperes (mA) used in image acquisition, i.e. the dose increases as mA increases. The dosage to the patient is also dependent upon the voltage, filters, and collimators used, as well as upon the slice thickness. The mA setting will vary depending on the noise level, kilovoltage (kVp), patient size, and scan slice thickness. For imaging of the paranasal sinuses, the kVp is usually set at 120 and the mA at 80.

One of the most recent developments in CT technology is the multidetector row CT scanner (MDCT). These scanners utilize a multiple linearly arranged array of detectors as opposed to just one. The newer models use up to 16 rows of detectors and acquire up to eight contiguous slices per gantry rotation. This results in a tremendous improvement in scanning time. Faster image acquisition is associated with a decrease in motion artifact. The dataset acquired is also a true isotropic volume of data that can be manipulated with minimal image degradation. This can allow for the generation of 'reformatted' images in the sagittal and/or coronal planes. These data can still be manipulated to show soft tissue or bone detail. In addition, the slice thickness of the images can be varied to provide the improved spatial resolution necessary to define the detail of the bony microanatomy and show subtle bony erosions and fractures.

CT OF THE PARANASAL SINUSES

CT is currently regarded as the imaging modality of choice for the paranasal sinuses and is used to complement diagnostic endoscopy in patient assessment.

This is especially true in the preoperative assessment of sinus inflammatory disease. Endoscopic examination and visualization of the small clefts of the ostiomeatal complex are not possible. CT examination in the coronal plane is preferred as it displays the anatomy in a perspective that is useful to the rhinologist. It precisely defines the site of inflammation and clearly identifies the bony details and any anatomical variations, such as the proximity of the orbital floor to the site of a middle meatal antrostomy, the extent of pneumatization of the ethmoid air cells, the location of the natural maxillary sinus ostium, septations of the sphenoid sinus, the positions of the internal carotid artery and the optic nerve. CT is the preferred technique for visualizing the ostiomeatal complex.

There are some limitations with CT in that it is not possible to differentiate between benign and

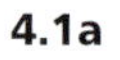

4.1a

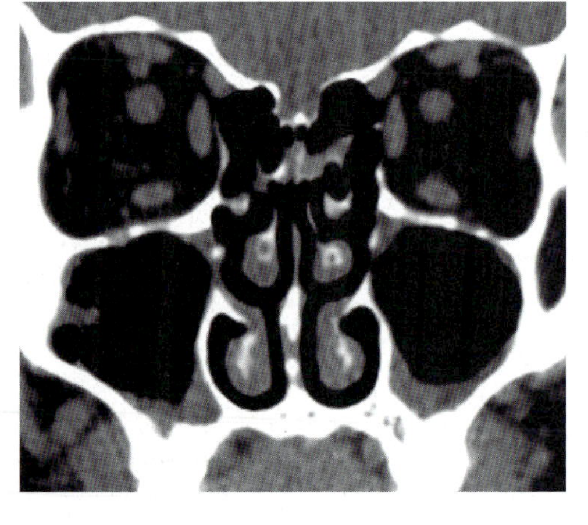

4.1b

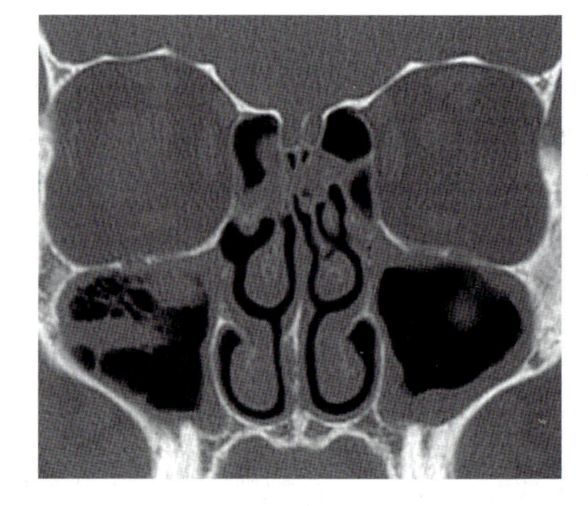

Figure 4.1 Coronal CT images through the maxillary and ethmoid sinuses. (a) Image optimized with a window (window level 90 HU, window length 350 HU) to best depict the soft tissue structures within the sinus lumen, and surrounding the sinuses. (b) Image windowed (window level 450 HU, window width 2500 HU) to demonstrate bony detail.

malignant disease. In such instances, MRI with its superior soft tissue resolution is a valuable complementary modality.

Other limitations of CT include image degradation due to various artifacts that can arise during scanning. These artifacts include the following:

- Image noise – a grainy appearance of the image is called noise. This is caused by slight variations of the density value measured by the scanner for substances of a fixed density. This effect may be limited by increasing the mA or the scan thickness in areas composed of soft tissue, but will have little effect in areas of high density contrast.
- Ring artifacts may be caused when individual detector channels show slight differences in signal output. This may result from infrequent unit calibration and may be corrected by a balancing algorithm.
- Some of the volume elements, or voxels, will contain both bone and soft tissue. The resulting grayscale value displayed in the image for that area of tissue will be based upon the average absorption value for that voxel. If there is a very large difference between the tissue densities within a voxel, streak artifacts will appear on the image. This is also known as the partial volume effect. Dental amalgam (Figure 4.2) is a common source of such artifacts. These artifacts may be limited by the use of an extended balancing algorithm at the raw data stage or by reducing the scan slice thickness. Careful patient positioning and gantry angulation may also be performed to try to avoid areas of such density change (e.g. dental fillings).
- X-ray tubes produce radiation of varying energies. Lower-energy radiation will be attenuated to a greater degree by the subject. Higher-energy radiation will be more likely to pass through the patient and reach the detector. This effect is known as beam hardening and also results in a streaklike artifact across the image. The effect may be reduced by beam filtering and the addition of a correcting algorithm. The artifacts produced are most pronounced in areas where high-density structures are in close proximity to low-density structures. Again dental amalgam is a common source of such unwanted artifacts. Careful patient positioning and filtering the beam before entry into the subject may lead to a reduction in these artifacts.
- Patient motion during scanning will result in image blurring. Patients need to be aware of the importance of remaining motionless during scanning. They should also be comfortably positioned and well supported in the CT gantry. Patients should be asked to refrain from swallowing and breathing during the short time it takes to obtain the scan.

4.2a

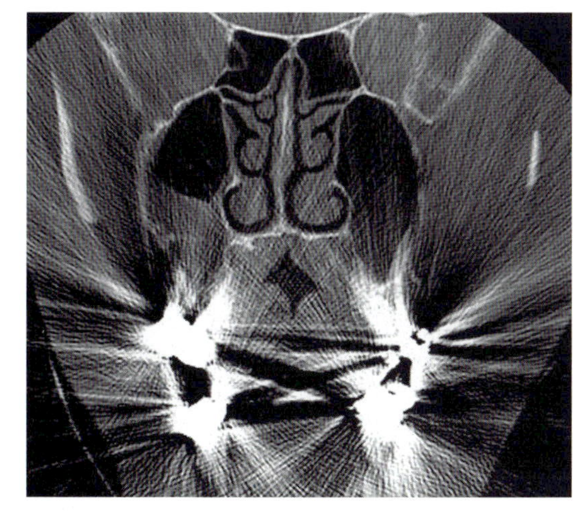

4.2b

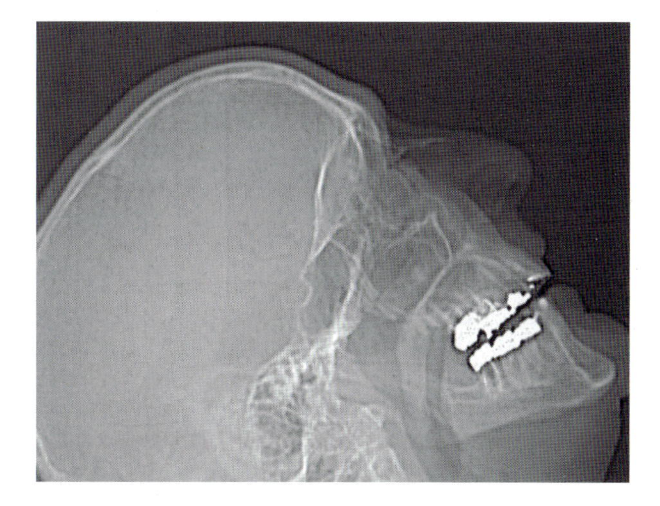

Figure 4.2 (a) A coronal CT scan through the maxillary sinuses shows significant streak artifact due to the presence of dental amalgam. (b) A CT scan scout image also depicts the metal from the amalgam.

CT imaging planes

One of the benefits of CT is the ability to obtain coronal scans of the paranasal sinuses (Figure 4.3). The scans are taken perpendicular to Reid's line, which runs between the infraorbital margin and the external auditory meatus. The perpendicular line is known as Alexander's line. The coronal view allows accurate visualization of structures that lie parallel to the infraorbitomeatal line, such as the orbital roof, the roof of the nasal cavity, and the ethmoid and sphenoid sinuses. It is also the best plane in which to assess the ostiomeatal complex. The coronal plane is also valuable in assessing intra-orbital and intracranial complications of disease.

Axial scans (Figure 4.4) are excellent at demonstrating the anterior and posterior walls of the sinuses and pterygopalatine fossa. They also demonstrate the relationship of the optic nerve to the posterior ethmoid and sphenoid sinuses. Visualization of the sphenoethmoid recess is also best in this plane.

Sagittal scans are helpful in assessing the floor of the orbit (Figure 4.5). They also provide an overview of the nearby bony and soft tissue structures such as the clivus, palate, and naso-pharynx.

Table 4.1 lists the scan planes that best evaluate the individual components of the paranasal sinus complex. Table 4.2 lists the ideal scanning planes for the evaluation of certain common disease conditions.

CT imaging parameters

With the availability of helical and now MDCT, a typical scanning protocol includes the following:

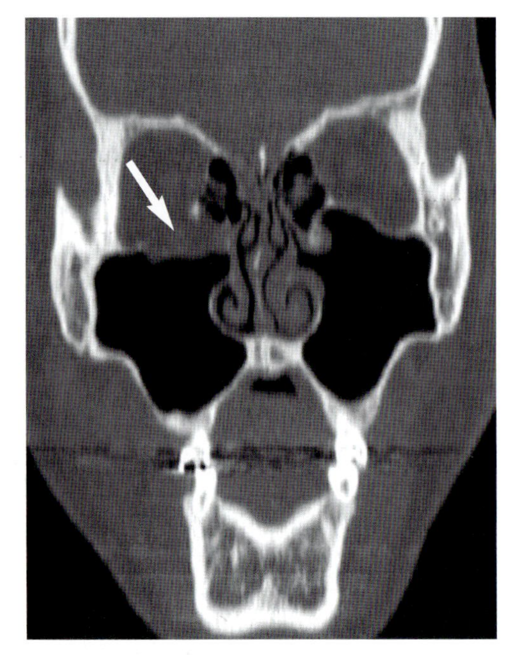

Figure 4.3 Coronal image of the facial bones including the sinuses. This was reconstructed from data from an axial CT scan. There is an orbital blowout fracture with disruption of the floor of the right orbit. Note the herniation of orbital fat and inferior displacement of the inferior rectus musculature (arrow).

4.4a

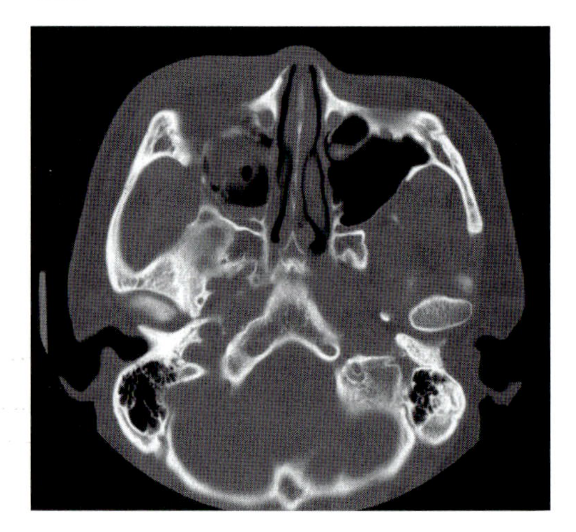

4.4b

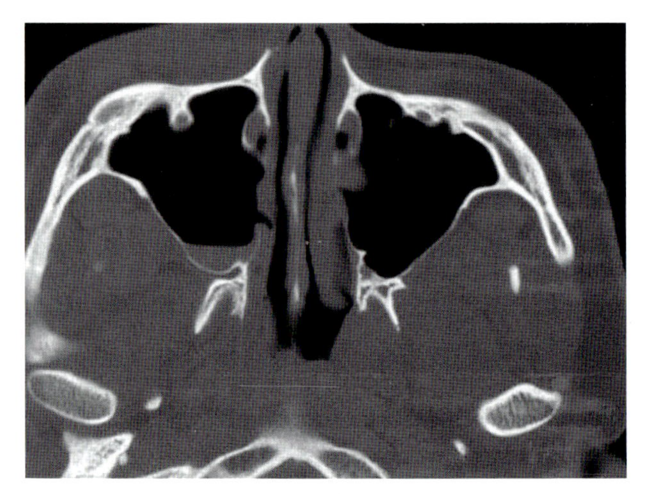

Figure 4.4 (a, b) Axial CT images of the same patient as in Figure 4.3. Right periorbital soft tissue swelling can be seen. The air–fluid level in the right antrum is compatible with blood. Axial scans best depict the status of the posterolateral antral wall.

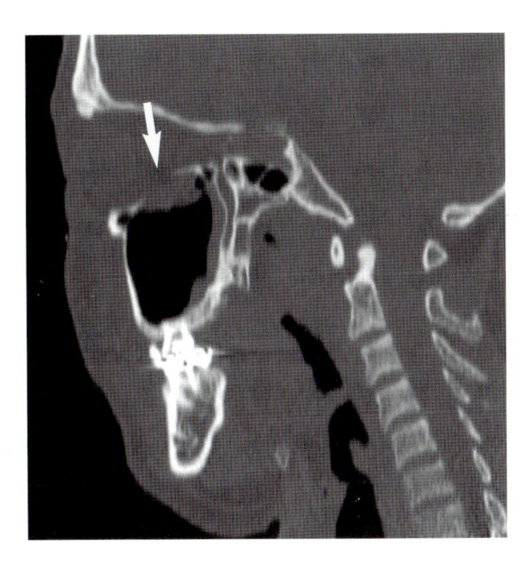

Figure 4.5 Reconstructed oblique-sagittal image of the same patient as in Figures 4.3 and 4.4. Disruption of the orbital floor is shown (arrow). This image plane also depicts the upper cervical vertebrae and the clivus, as well as the orbital roof.

Table 4.1 Scanning planes affording the most information about individual structures

Structure	*Axial scan*	*Coronal scan*
Maxillary sinus:		
Anterior wall	✓	
Posterior wall	✓	
Medial wall		✓
Roof/orbital floor		✓
Frontal sinus:		
Anterior wall	✓	
Posterior wall	✓	
Floor		✓
Sphenoid sinus:		
Anterior	✓	
Posterior	✓	
Lateral		✓
Floor		✓
Ethmoid sinus:		
Lateral wall	✓	✓
Roof		✓
Ostiomeatal complex		✓
Pterygopalatine fossa	✓	
Superior orbital fissure		✓
Optic nerve	✓	✓[a]
Cribriform plate		✓
Turbinates		✓

[a]Parasagittal scans of this region provide particularly good visualization of the optic nerve canal

(1) An axial scan is obtained with the patient supine. The CT gantry is placed parallel to the orbitomeatal line. Initially, a lateral 'scout' scan is taken which covers the anatomy inferiorly from the alveolar ridge of the maxilla to the superior aspect of the frontal sinus. If necessary, the gantry angulation is modified to take into account special problems such as limited extension of the neck or dental fillings, which may degrade the image. The kVp is 120, and the mA is 80, with a total scan time of 4.8 s.

(2) Reformatted sagittal and coronal images are then obtained. In addition, a 3D shaded surface display program for reconstructed images demonstrating the pathology (Figure 4.6) is gaining in popularity among clinicians because it can provide an overview of the anatomy of the facial bones. This may be helpful in the assessment of facial trauma.

(3) Specific areas of interest may be enlarged by one of two methods. Magnification involves the expansion of each picture element. With this technique, there is no increase in detail and

Table 4.2 Ideal scanning planes for the common disease conditions

Disorder	*Axial*	*Coronal*	*Sagittal*	*3D CT*
Trauma	✓	✓	✓	✓
Benign polyposis		✓		
Inflammatory disease		✓		
Malignancy	✓	✓	✓	✓
Mucocele/pyocele	✓	✓	±	±
Congenital anomalies	✓	✓		✓

± May or may not require sagittal or 3D CT reconstruction

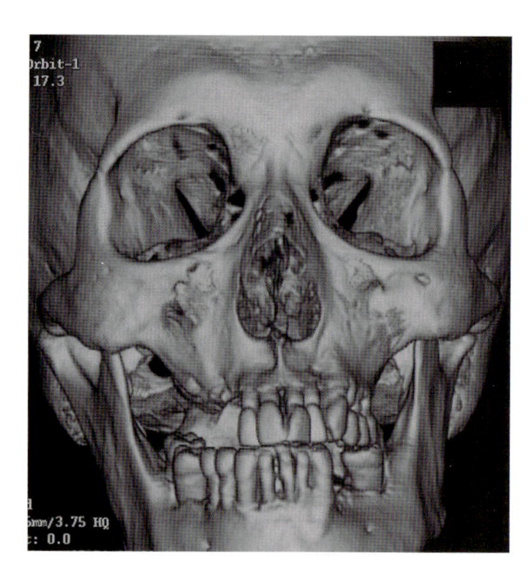

Figure 4.6 A 3D shaded surface display of the facial bones in frontal projection.

the tissue interfaces may become stepped. Zooming involves coning the field of view of a specific anatomical region to produce increased resolution. The zoom factors vary between 1 and 10. Zooming is more appropriate when studying the paranasal sinuses, and factors between 4 and 6 are generally applied.

Intravenous contrast administration

Intravenous contrast is not used routinely during the investigation of benign inflammatory disease. Intravenous contrast enhancement is indicated in those cases where neoplasms, vascular lesions, or complications of paranasal sinus disease are suspected from either the history or diagnostic examination. The vascularity of the lesion as well as its relationship to the major vessels can be assessed preoperatively. Intravenous contrast is also valuable in assessing inflammatory sinus disease that has been complicated by abscess formation, thrombosis, or intracranial or intraorbital spread of infection. The administration of contrast may help to distinguish between acute and chronic inflammatory disease, as mucosal enhancement is visible in cases of acute inflammation. Distinction between allergic and inflammatory polyps may also be aided by contrast administration, because inflammatory polyps have been noted to enhance whereas allergic polyps do not.

Contrast is administered with an automatic injector. Approximately 80–100 cm^3 of non-ionic contrast is given at a rate of 1 cm^3/s. Abnormalities will enhance if there is increased vascularity, and the degree of enhancement can be estimated by comparison with the enhancement of the great vessels.

The major potential disadvantage of contrast administration is the rare occurrence of potentially fatal anaphylactic reaction to the agent. The major non-medical disadvantage is the expense of non-ionic intravenous contrast.

REPORTING SCHEME

Due to the complex anatomy of the paranasal sinuses, it would be wise to develop a systematic approach to image interpretation and reporting. We provide here an example of such a scheme that we believe allows a thorough and accurate examination of the region (Figure 4.7).

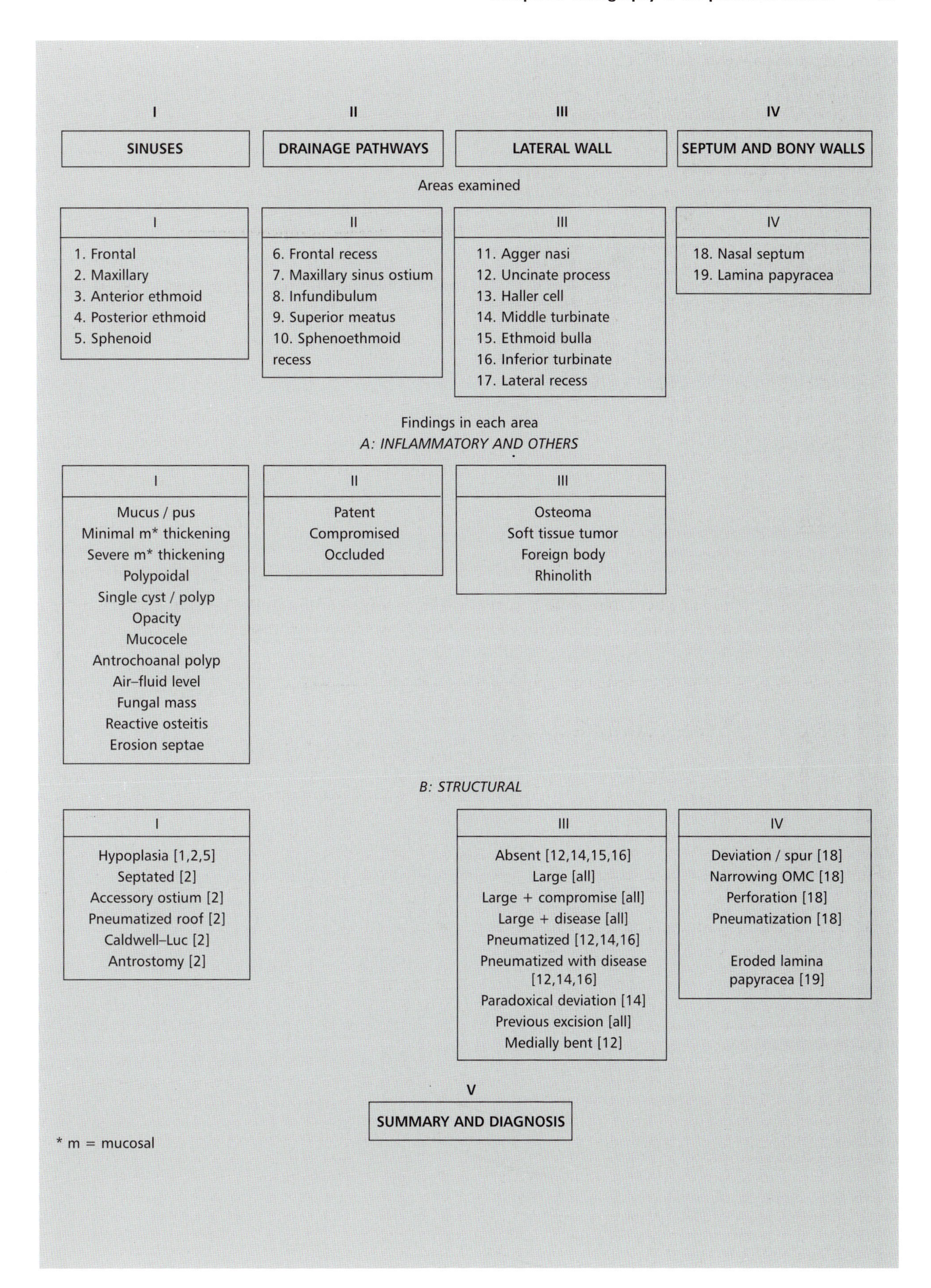

Figure 4.7 Sinus CT reporting scheme.

5

The normal anatomy of the paranasal sinuses as demonstrated by computed tomography and magnetic resonance imaging

The radiologist must be familiar with the anatomy of the ethmoid labyrinth, the larger paranasal sinuses, and their associated ventilation and drainage channels in the lateral nasal wall. The relevant anatomy is described in sequence in this chapter in the axial, sagittal, and coronal planes, with additional information about the more commonly occurring anatomical variants. Each radiologist will need to develop their own scheme for the systematic reporting of computed tomography (CT) scans of this challenging anatomical area (see Chapter 4, Table 4.3).

EXTERNAL NOSE AND NASAL BONES (Figure 5.1)

The external nose and the nasal bones are the first structures to be visualized in coronal scans. If the frontal sinuses are prominent, they will also appear in the most anterior scans.

The nasal cavity communicates anteriorly through the nares with the exterior and posteriorly through the choanae with the nasopharynx. It also communicates through the lateral nasal wall with the ethmoid, maxillary, and frontal sinuses, and more posteriorly with the sphenoid sinus.

NASAL SEPTUM (Figures 5.2–5.4)

The nasal septum, which is rarely found perfectly in the midline, is formed partly by the perpendicular plate of the ethmoid, the vomer, the palatine bones, and the quadrilateral cartilage. Most septal deviations are the result of developmental anomalies and asymmetric growth of the facial skeleton, although the nasal septum may be deviated from trauma. There may be a deviation of the bony nasal septum, the cartilaginous septum, or a combination of both.

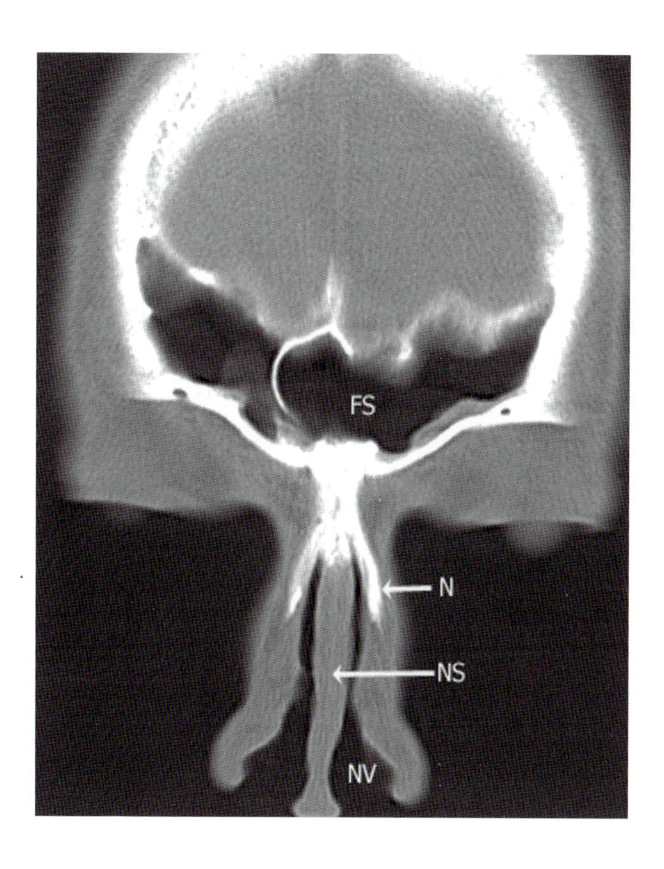

Figure 5.1 *The nasal pyramid.* Anterior coronal scan cutting through the external nose and the most anterior portion of the frontal sinus (FS), the frontal process of the maxilla (N), the nasal bones, the cartilaginous portion of the nasal septum (NS), and the nasal vestibule (NV).

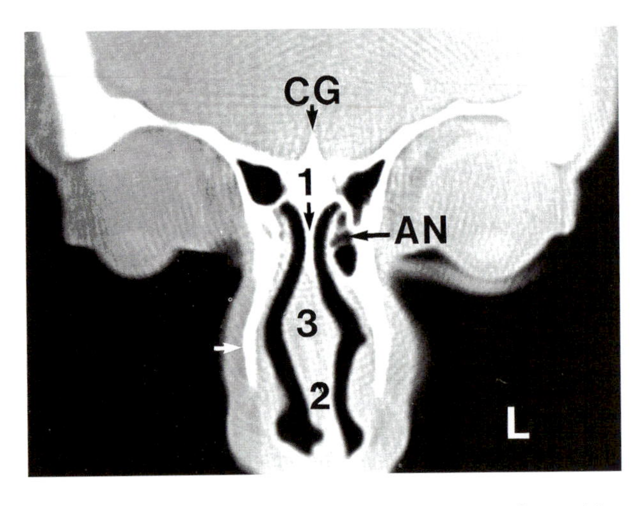

Figure 5.2 *Nasal septum.* The nasal septum is formed by the perpendicular plate of the ethmoid bone (1) and the quadrilateral cartilage (2). The localized expansion is the organ of Zuckerkandl (3), which represents the vestigial remains of erectile tissue. The nasal bones (white arrow) and the crista galli (CG) are also shown. AN, agger nasi cells.

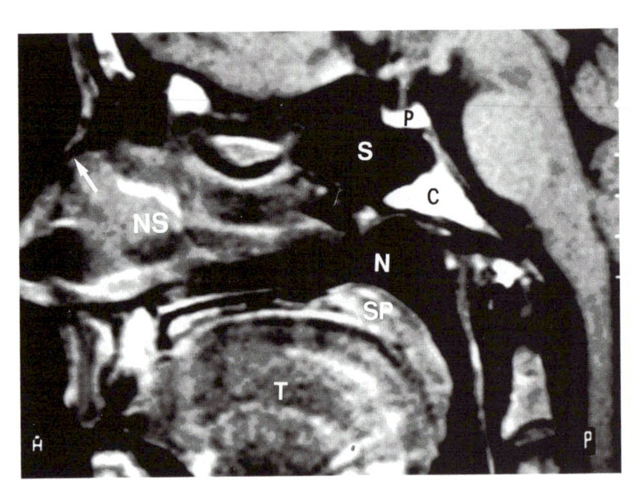

Figure 5.4 *Normal sphenoid sinus and nasal septum.* T1-weighted sagittal MRI scan demonstrating the sphenoid sinus (S), nasal septum (NS), pituitary gland and its stalk (P), nasal bone (arrow), soft palate (SP), tongue (T), nasopharynx (N), and clivus (C), which is hyperintense due to fatty marrow content.

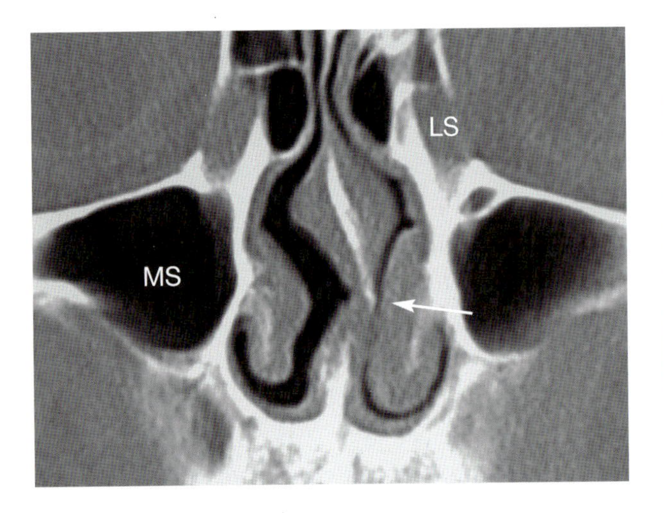

Figure 5.3 *Nasal septum.* A deviation of the nasal septum to the left is noted (arrow). MS, maxillary sinus; LS, lacrimal sac.

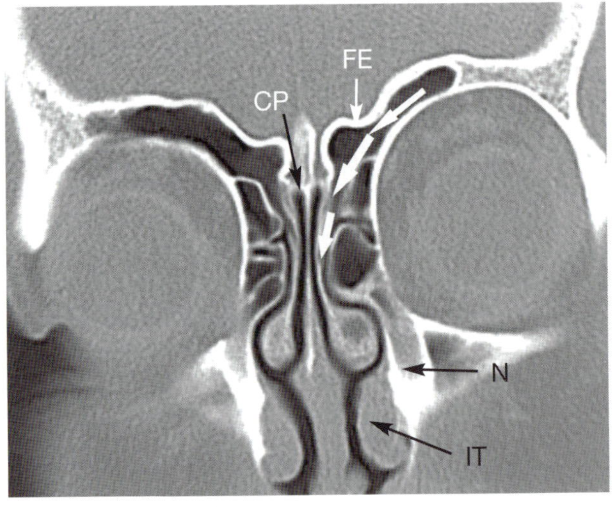

Figure 5.5 *Normal frontal recess.* A wide frontal recess is seen (arrows). The other labeled structures are: the cribriform plate (CP), fovea ethmoidalis (FE), inferior turbinates (IT), and nasolacrimal duct (N).

Defects of the cartilaginous or bony septum with intact mucosa are usually the result of a previous submucous resection or septoplasty. Small perforations seen in the septum are most commonly the result of a previous septoplasty. Causes of larger cartilaginous nasal septal perforation include previous septoplasty, untreated traumatic septal hematomas, repeated local trauma, excessive cautery for epistaxis, midline granulomas (Stewart's or Wegener's), cocaine abuse, tuberculosis, and leprosy. Atraumatic bony septal perforations are usually secondary to syphilis.

CRISTA GALLI (Figures 5.2 and 5.5–5.8)

The crista galli is the vertical extension of the perpendicular plate of the ethmoid bone above the cribriform plate into the anterior cranial cavity to which the dura mater is attached. The crista galli may be filled with fatty marrow. It may be pneumatized (usually from the frontal recess), and a large air cell may replace the entire body. If the lumen of the air cell is narrow, it may become obstructed by minimal mucosal swelling. When the ostium of an

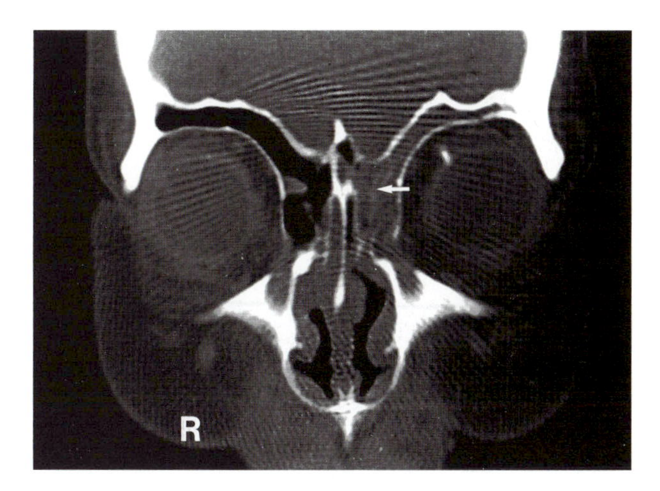

Figure 5.6 *Pneumatized crista galli.* The pneumatized crista galli is draining into a diseased frontal recess (arrow).

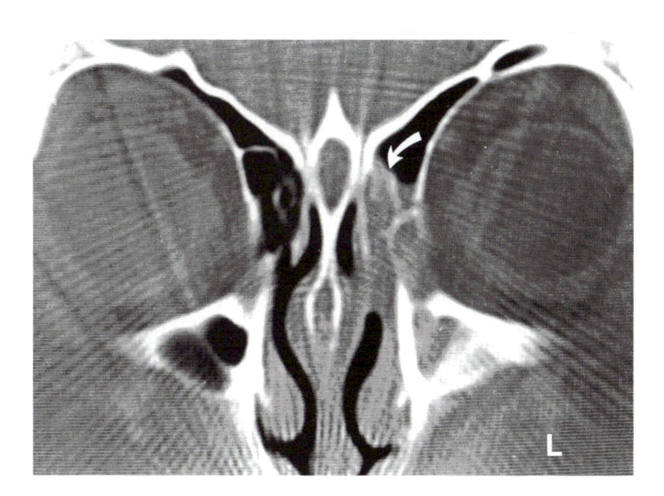

Figure 5.7 *Inflammatory disease in a pneumatized crista galli.* In this patient, there is a mucocele of the crista galli. This air cell usually drains into the frontal recess and both of these regions are usually involved simultaneously with inflammatory disease (arrow).

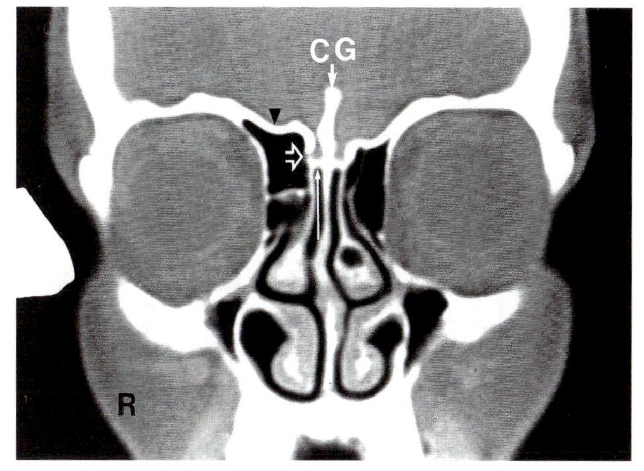

Figure 5.8 *Cribriform plate and fovea ethmoidalis.* The fovea ethmoidalis can clearly be seen to be both higher (arrowhead) and thicker than the cribriform plate (arrow). This demonstrates the hazards of surgery in this area. Note the bony channel for the anterior ethmoidal artery on the right (open arrow). The crista galli is also demonstrated (CG). Other findings include bilateral bony hypertrophy of the middle turbinates and a small air cell in the left middle turbinate (concha bullosa).

air cell is occluded, a mucocele may develop. Patients with such an anomaly may present with headaches. Isolated frontal recess disease with secondary infection of a crista galli air cell may have normal endoscopy.

FRONTAL SINUS (Figures 5.9–5.12)

The frontal sinuses are asymmetrical paired cavities located between the anterior and posterior tables of the frontal bone. They are frequently divided by numerous incomplete bony septi into several intercommunicating air cells. The frontal air cells usually lie in the same coronal plane, but occasionally one sinus lies behind the other, in which case it is referred to as a supernumerary frontal sinus. The frontal sinus is connected to the nasal cavity by the frontal recess.

The shape and size of the frontal sinus is highly variable and it may be hypoplastic or even absent. CT evaluation of the sinuses with narrow window settings alone may also lead to misinterpretation of the underdeveloped sinus as a sinus exhibiting pathology. A wide or bone window setting will identify this as hypoplasia and exclude the possibility of a well-developed sinus with pathology affecting its lumen. Asymmetry of the frontal sinuses is more common in those races with dolicho-cephalic heads, such as the Mongoloid race.

Extensive pneumatization of the superciliary portion of the frontal bone or a giant multiseptate frontal sinus is a common variant in both normal individuals and acromegalics. It is not uncommon for this to be the only part of the frontal bone that is pneumatized, and the normal supraorbital extension of the frontal sinus may be absent.

Variations in frontal sinus anatomy

- Aplasia
- Hypoplasia

5.9a

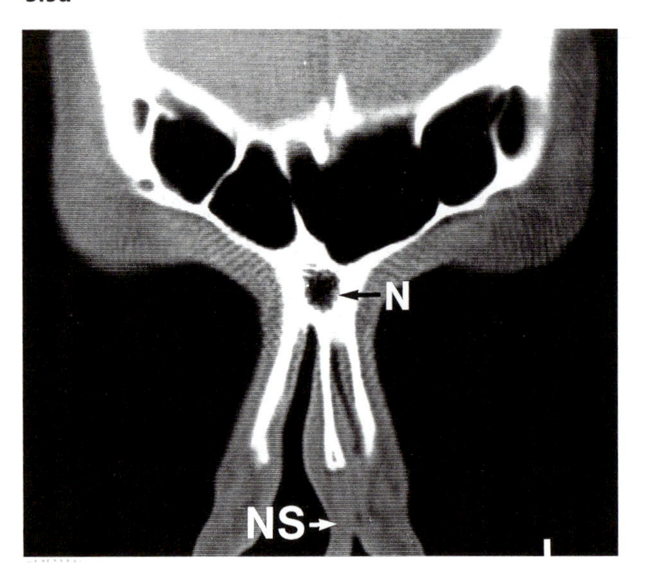

5.9b

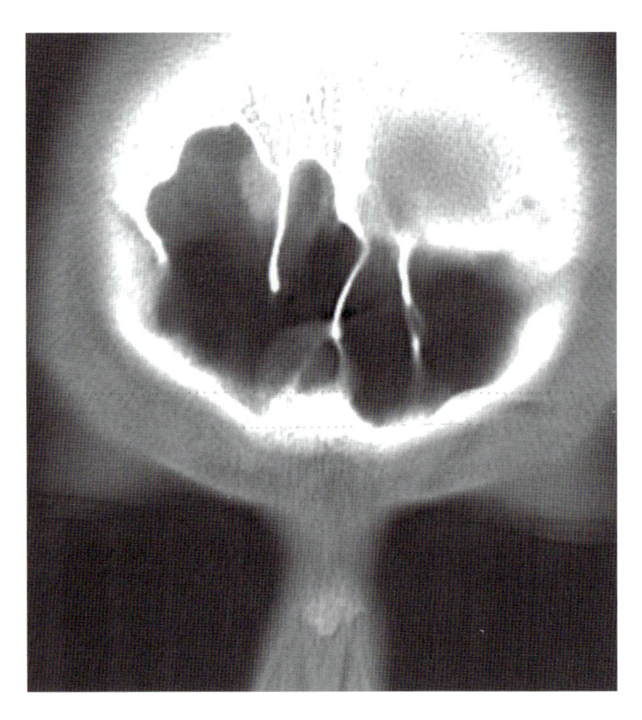

Figure 5.9 *Septation of a normal frontal sinus.* (a) Coronal scan of the frontal sinuses demonstrating a multiseptated frontal sinus, normal nasal bones, and an anterior deviation of the cartilaginous nasal septum (NS) to the left. Note the nasal cell (N), which, if extensive, may compromise the frontal recess. (b) Multiple incomplete septations can be seen in the frontal sinuses.

- Giant multiseptated sinus
- Supernumerary sinus
- Asymmetry

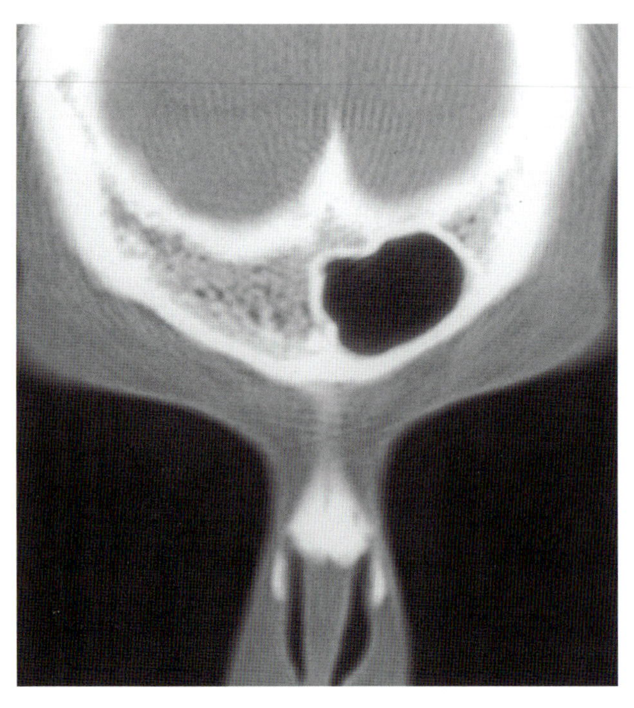

Figure 5.10 *Aplasia of the right frontal sinus.* This is a common anomaly where one of the frontal sinuses is partially or completely undeveloped.

FRONTAL BULLA (Figure 5.13)

The anterior ethmoid air cells may encroach upon the frontal sinuses. These cells become clinically significant when they are so closely related to the frontal recess that they obstruct ventilation and drainage of the frontal sinus. This variant may be seen on the coronal scan as either a solitary air cell or a collection of air cells situated in the medial part of the floor of the frontal sinus, projecting into the lumen of the sinus. These cells, also referred to as frontal bullae, usually drain into an already-narrowed frontal recess.

FRONTAL RECESS (Figures 5.5 and 5.14–5.16)

The frontal recess is an hourglass-shaped bony channel through which the frontal sinus drains into the ostiomeatal complex. It is not visualized at the time of routine, preoperative endoscopy, and CT in the coronal and sagittal plane is ideal for assessing this region. The anatomy is extremely variable: a short, wide frontal recess may be easily visualized on a single scan, while a more tortuous and narrow frontal recess cannot usually be seen on a single

5.11a

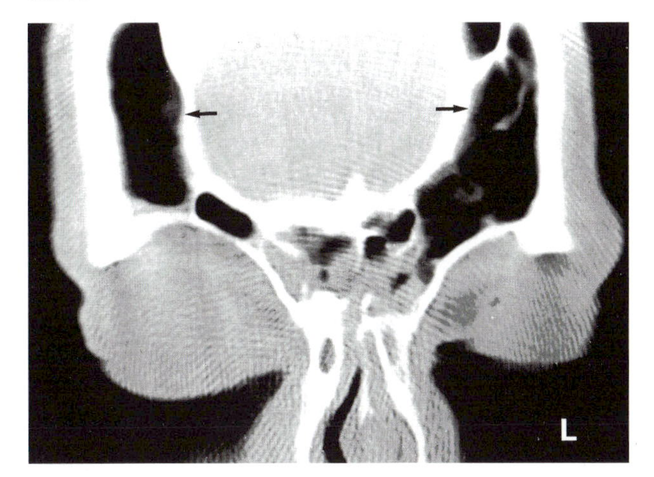

5.11b

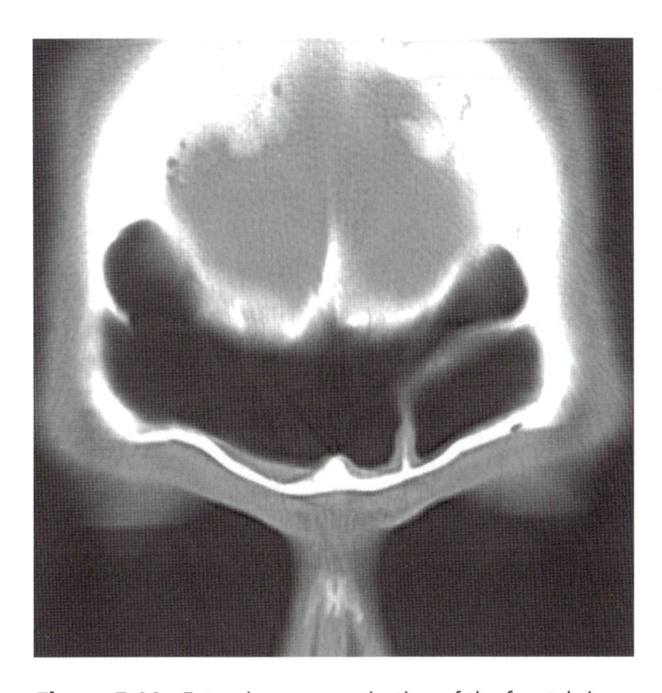

Figure 5.11 *Extensive pneumatization of the frontal sinus.* (a) Coronal scan of the frontal sinuses demonstrating extensive pneumatization of the frontal bone (arrows). In this case, the anterior ethmoid cells narrow the frontal recess and contain diseased mucosa. These anterior ethmoid cells are characteristically located along the floor of the frontal sinus, close to the midline. (b) Another example of large frontal sinuses occupying a large part of the frontal bone.

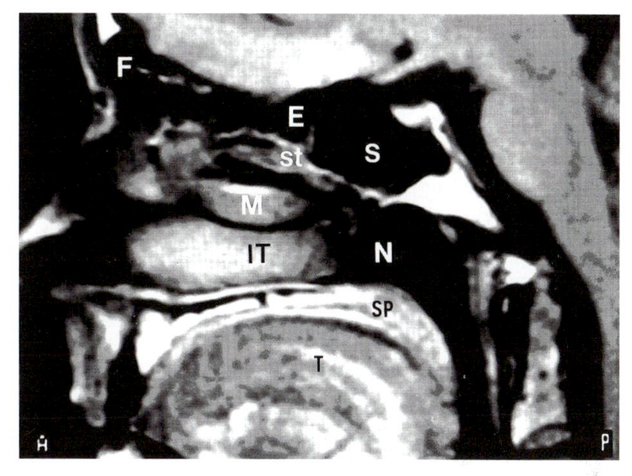

Figure 5.12 *Normal sagittal MRI scan.* T1-weighted MRI scan demonstrating the frontal sinus (F), ethmoid sinus (E), sphenoid sinus (S), and superior (st), middle (M), and inferior (IT) turbinates, as well as the nasopharynx (N), soft palate (SP), and tongue (T). Note that the posterior ethmoid cells are larger than the anterior cells.

coronal slice because the frontal recess runs obliquely with its distal (inferior) end more posterior than its proximal (superior) end.

The route of ventilation and drainage of the frontal sinus through the frontal recess depends upon embryological development. The frontal recess may open into:

- The premeatal groove when the uncinate process attaches to the lamina papyracea – this passes anterior to the hiatus semilunaris and therefore drains independently of the ethmoid infundibulum and the maxillary and ethmoid sinuses;
- The ethmoid infundibulum – in this situation, inflammation affecting the maxillary sinus may spread along the infundibulum to affect the frontal sinus.

The dimensions of the frontal recess are variable. If it is wide and short, the sinus is easily ventilated. However, if the frontal recess is long, tortuous, and narrow, and runs between crowded anterior ethmoid air cells, then minimal swelling can impede the drainage of the frontal sinus and predispose it to recurrent infection.

The frontal recess may be localized on coronal CT scans by identifying the superior insertion of the uncinate process. This insertion is variable and determines whether the frontal recess drains into the ethmoid infundibulum or the premeatal groove. When the uncinate process inserts laterally into the lamina papyracea, the ethmoid infundibulum forms a blind recess – the recessus terminalis (terminal recess) – and the frontal recess drains medially into the premeatal chamber of the ethmoid sinus. When

5.13a

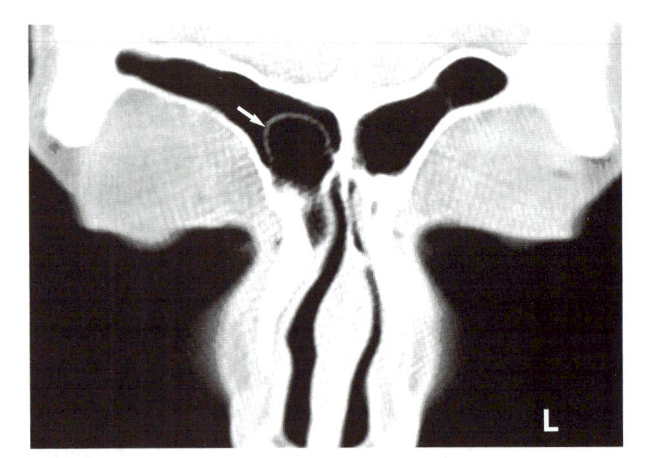

5.13b

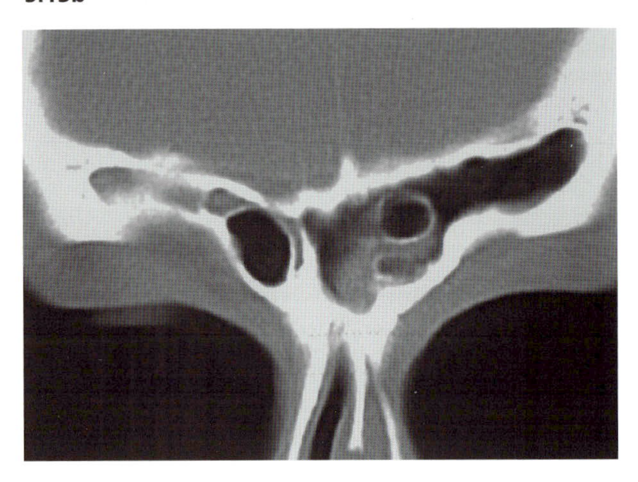

Figure 5.13 *Frontal bulla.* (a) Anterior scan through the frontal sinus demonstrating a small, anteriorly placed ethmoid air cell projecting into the floor of the frontal sinus (arrow). This is called a frontal bulla. (b) Anterior scan through the frontal sinus demonstrating a frontal bulla associated with inflammatory disease in the frontal recess and floor of the frontal sinus.

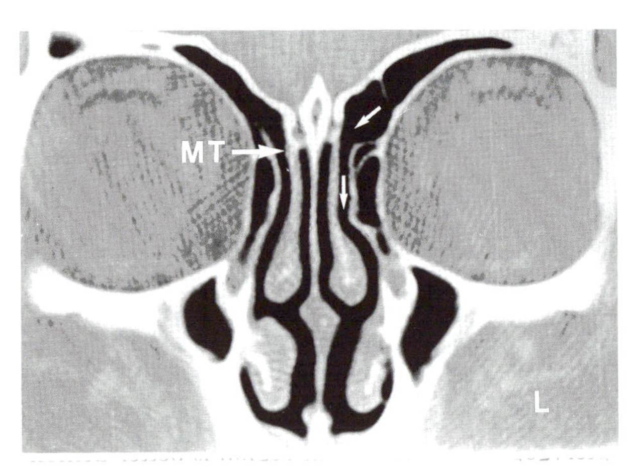

Figure 5.14 *Normal frontal recess.* Scan demonstrating a normal, wide, patent frontal recess (upper arrow). In this patient, the frontal recess drains directly into the middle meatus (lower arrow). The vertical insertion of the middle turbinate (MT) can be clearly seen.

5.15a

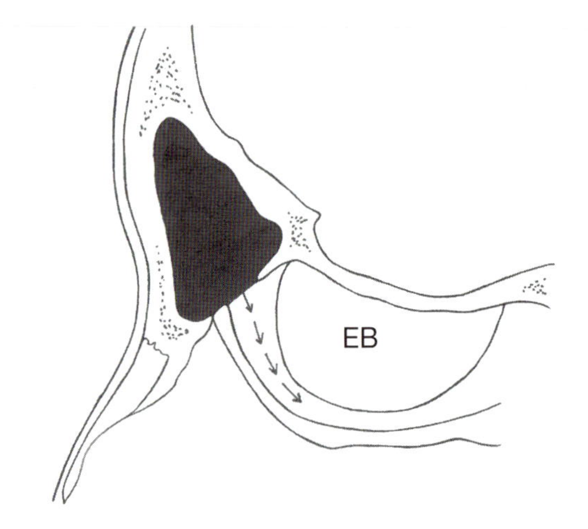

5.15b

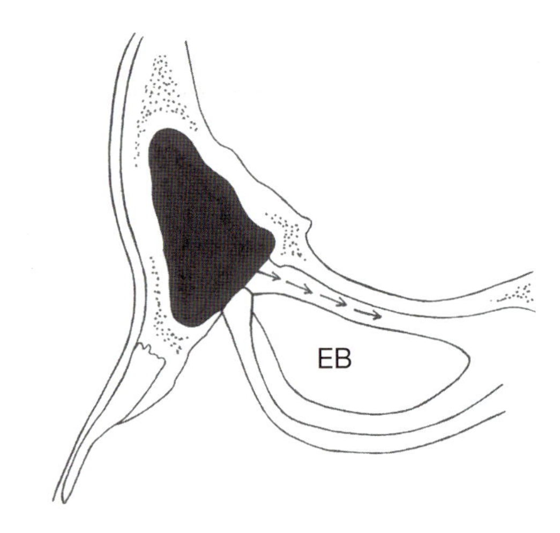

5.15c

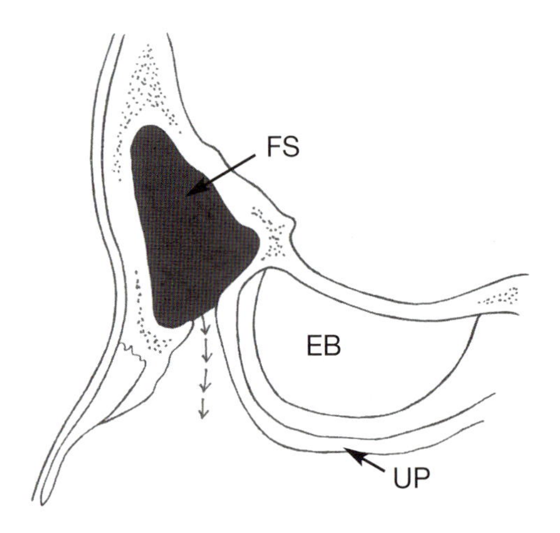

Figure 5.15 *Variations in drainage of the frontal recess.* (a) Frontal recess drainage (arrows) into the ethmoid infundibulum. (b) Frontal recess drainage (arrows) into the suprabullar (EB), which drains into the lateral recess. (c) Frontal recess drainage (arrows) into the middle meatus as the uncinate process (UP) insertion is into the lateral wall. FS, frontal sinus.

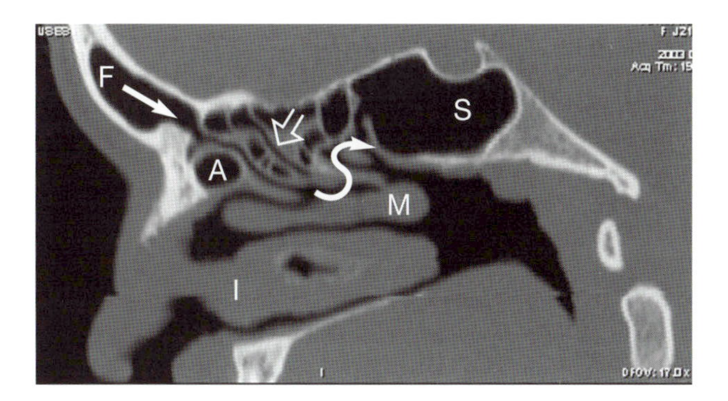

Figure 5.16 *Sagittal CT scan through the frontal sinus.* CT scan demonstrating a normal frontal sinus (F) draining into the frontal recess (arrow). The other structures seen are the inferior turbinate (I), middle turbinate (M), agger nasi air cell (A) and uncinate process attached inferiorly, ground lamella (open arrow), ethmoid labyrinth, sphenoid sinus (S), and sphenoethmoid recess (curved arrow).

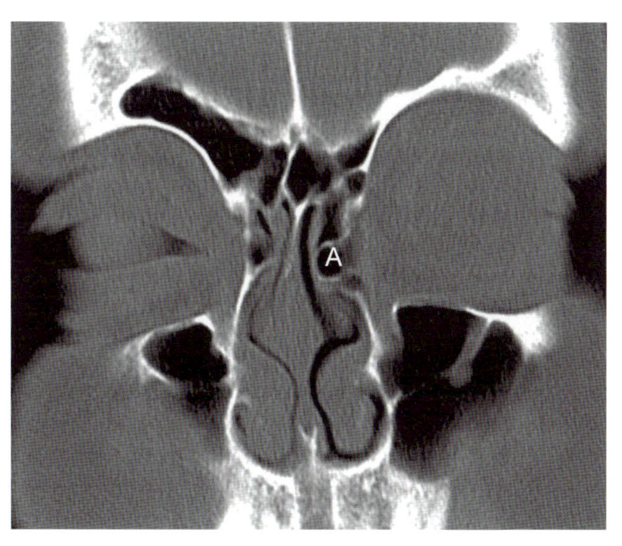

Figure 5.17 *Agger nasi cell.* Scan demonstrating an agger nasi cell (A) close to the frontal recess.

the uncinate process inserts into the roof of the ethmoid sinus, or medially onto the middle turbinate, the frontal sinus drains directly into the ethmoid infundibulum. The frontal recess may pneumatize the crista galli, middle turbinate, or the agger nasi and can thus both influence and be influenced by disease in these adjacent air cells.

Anatomical variants that compromise the frontal recess

- Enlarged agger nasi air cells
- Hypertrophied middle turbinates
- Concha bullosa
- Large anterior protruding ethmoid bulla
- Deviation of the nasal septum

AGGER NASI CELLS (Figures 5.17–5.19)

The agger mound is a prominence seen anterior and superior to the insertion of the vertical plate of the middle turbinate. When present, the agger nasi air cells are situated within the agger mound and are usually part of the anterior ethmoid sinuses. The agger mound may be acellular, unicellular, or multicellular.

MAXILLARY SINUS (Figures 5.20–5.27)

The maxillary sinuses are the largest of the paranasal sinuses. They are pyramid-shaped cavities with the apex pointing towards the zygoma and the base forming the medial wall of the maxillary sinus. Most maxillary sinuses are symmetrical. CT in the coronal plane demonstrates the maxillary sinus to be narrow anteriorly (i.e. in the same plane as the vertical plate of the middle turbinate), widest in its mid-portion (i.e. in the same plane as the ground lamella of the middle turbinate), and narrow again posteriorly.

The roof of the maxillary sinus forms the orbital floor, which is narrow posteriorly and wider anteriorly. The inferior surface of the orbital floor is grooved by the infraorbital canal, containing the infraorbital nerve and its accompanying vessels. This nerve passes through the infraorbital fissure, traverses the infraorbital canal, and exits through the infraorbital foramen, which is situated below the inferior margin of the orbital rim. The bone surrounding the infraorbital nerve is usually thin and may be affected by erosion and reactive osteitis with new bone formation in cases of chronic inflammatory sinus disease.

The posterior wall of the maxillary sinus is narrow and forms the anterior boundary of the pterygopalatine fossa. This region is better demonstrated by CT in the axial plane.

The medial wall of the maxillary sinus forms part of the lateral wall of the nasal cavity. The bone of the medial wall is usually deficient over a large

5.18a

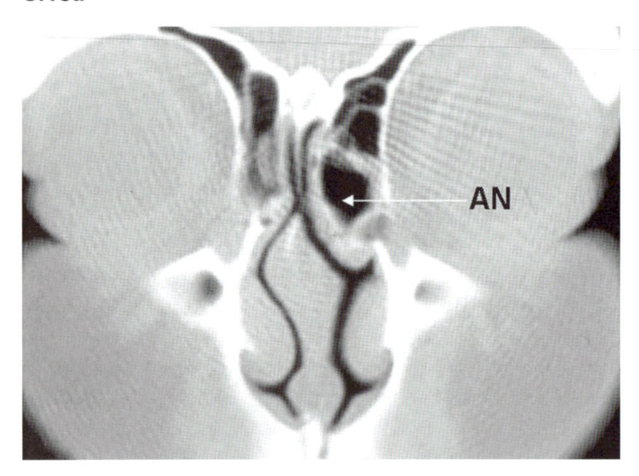

5.18b

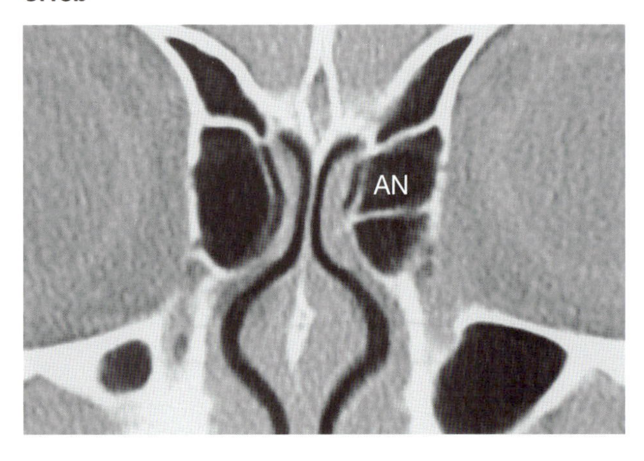

Figure 5.18 *Agger nasi cell.* (a, b) Two examples of a large agger nasi cell (AN) occluding the frontal recess.

area, and the dehiscence is closed by the mucosa of both the nasal cavity and the maxillary sinus, covering a thin fibrous layer in continuation with the periosteum. This area is divided into the anterior and posterior nasal fontanelles. These latter two sections are separated by the ethmoid process of the inferior turbinate. These fontanelles should not be misinterpreted as bony erosion associated with disease. Small defects are frequently found in the membranous fontanelles, which are the accessory maxillary sinus ostia. These are usually situated immediately above the inferior turbinate and open directly into the middle meatus.

The maxillary sinus has several recesses: the alveolar recess, lateral recess, and superior recess. The most frequently encountered recess is the alveolar recess, which is an inferior extension of the sinus into the alveolar ridge. The extension of the maxillary sinus into the zygoma is called the lateral recess of the maxillary sinus. The superior recess is the superomedial extension of the sinus, which can have a variable relationship with the orbit. The superior recess is well demonstrated by CT in the axial plane and may be mistaken for a large ethmoid air cell. The ethmoid sinus should be noted to be lying medially.

The maxillary sinus is separated from the posterior ethmoid sinus by the ethmo-maxillary

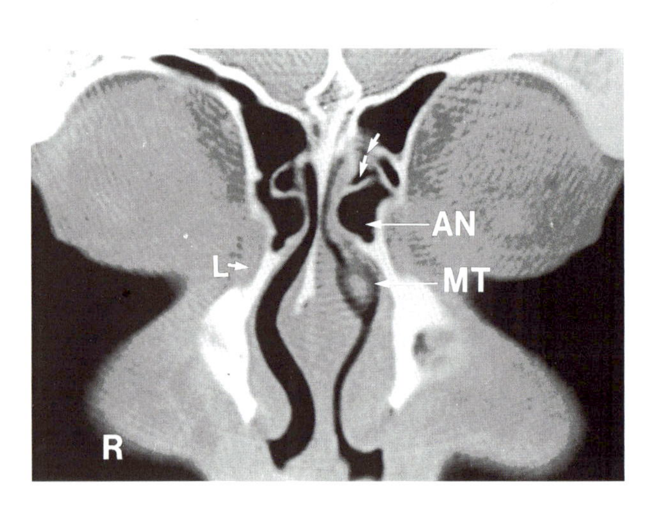

Figure 5.19 *Agger nasi cell.* Scan demonstrating a large agger nasi cell (AN) occluding the frontal recess (arrows). The larger the agger nasi cell, the greater the encroachment on the neck of the middle turbinate (MT), resulting in a restricted frontal recess. The normal lacrimal fossa (L) is seen on the right side.

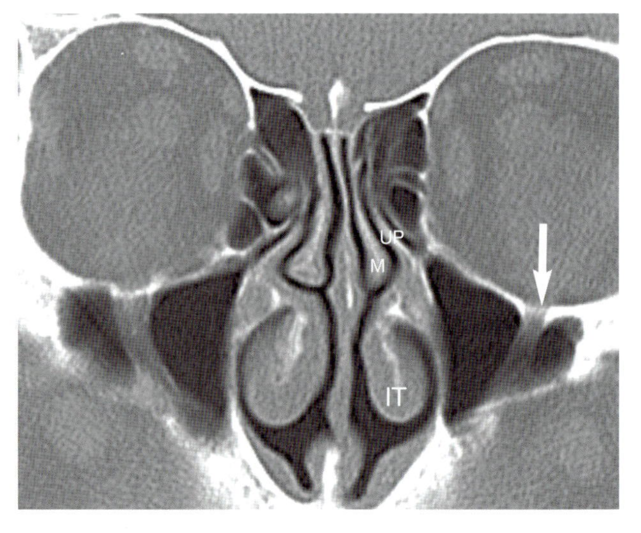

Figure 5.20 *Maxillary sinus.* Anterior scan of the maxillary sinus demonstrating the infraorbital nerve (arrow) traversing through the roof of the maxillary sinus. The other structures to note are the inferior turbinate (IT), middle turbinate (M), and uncinate process (UP).

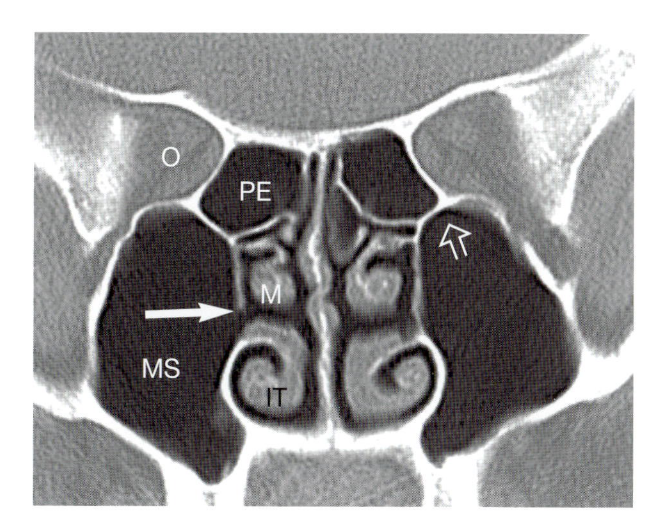

Figure 5.21 *Maxillary sinus.* Scan through the middle of the maxillary sinus (MS) showing an accessory sinus ostium (arrow), posterior ethmoid sinus (PE), orbit (O) and ethmomaxillary plate (open arrow), middle turbinate (M), and inferior turbinate (IT).

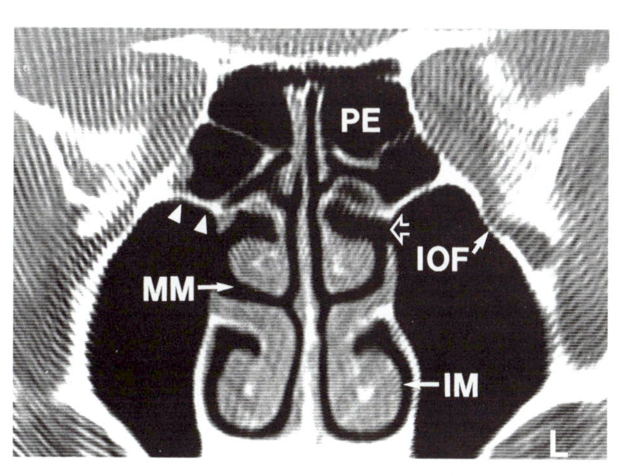

Figure 5.23 *Accessory maxillary ostia.* Coronal scan of the posterior ethmoid air cells (PE) and maxillary sinus demonstrating a large accessory maxillary sinus ostium on the right just lateral to the middle turbinate and a smaller one on the left (open arrow) close to the posterior part of the middle meatus (MM). The thin plate of bone separating the superomedial margin of the maxillary sinus from the posterior ethmoid air cells is the ethmomaxillary plate (arrowheads). Note the inferior orbital fissure (IOF) and the inferior meatus (IM).

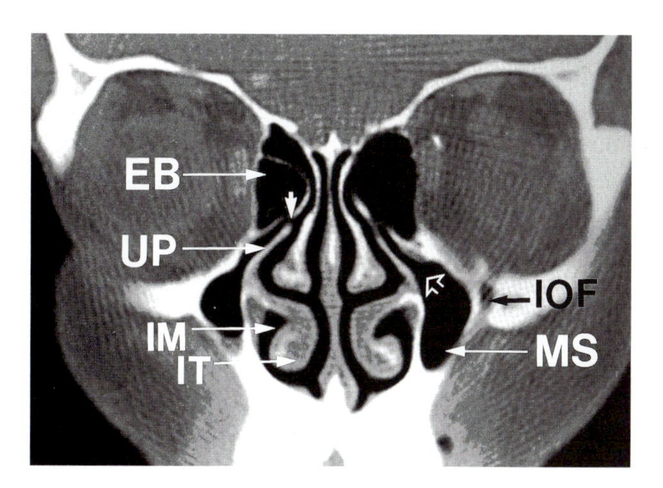

Figure 5.22 *Normal maxillary sinus.* Scan demonstrating the anterior portion of the maxillary sinus (MS) draining through the maxillary ostia into the ethmoid infundibulum (open arrow). The infundibulum channel is bounded superolaterally by the ethmoid bulla (EB) and inferomedially by the uncinate process (UP). The ethmoid infundibulum opens into the hiatus semilunaris. The latter is a two-dimensional slit-like opening that connects the infundibulum to the middle meatus (short white arrow). The infraorbital foramen (IOF), inferior turbinate (IT), and inferior meatus (IM) are also shown.

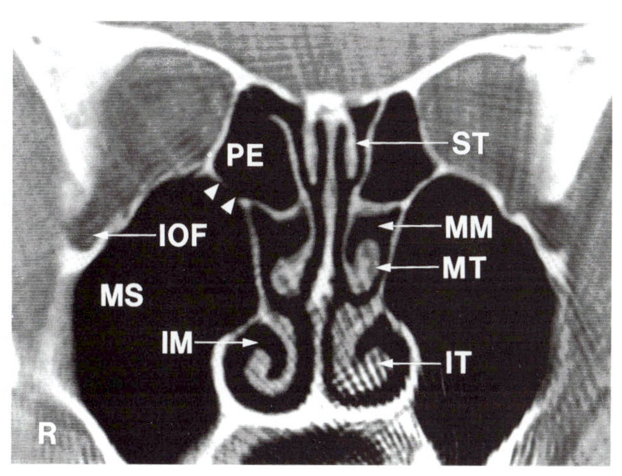

Figure 5.24 *Turbinates.* Coronal scan through the middle portion of a normal maxillary sinus (MS) clearly showing the superior (ST), middle (MT), and inferior (IT) turbinates with their corresponding superior, middle (MM), and inferior (IM) meatus. The posterior ethmoid sinus (PE) is separated from the maxillary sinus by the ethmomaxillary plate (arrowheads). The inferior orbital fissure (IOF) is also shown.

plate. Defects secondary to a previous transantral ethmoidectomy will be seen in this plate.

Maxillary sinus ostium (Figure 5.22)

The natural ostium of the maxillary sinus is located in the superomedial aspect of the medial sinus wall. This natural ostium is located at the inferolateral end of the ethmoid infundibulum, which is the narrow channel lying between the lateral surface of the uncinate process, the lamina papyracea, and the anterior surface of the ethmoid bulla. The ethmoid infundibulum opens through the hiatus semilunaris into the middle meatus.

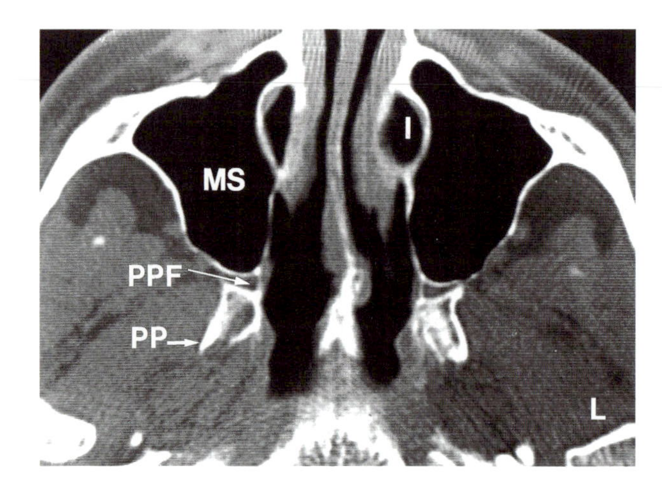

Figure 5.25 *Normal axial scan.* This demonstrates the maxillary sinus (MS), the pterygopalatine fossa (PPF), and the pterygoid process (PP). The superior aspect of the inferior meatus (I) is transected in this view.

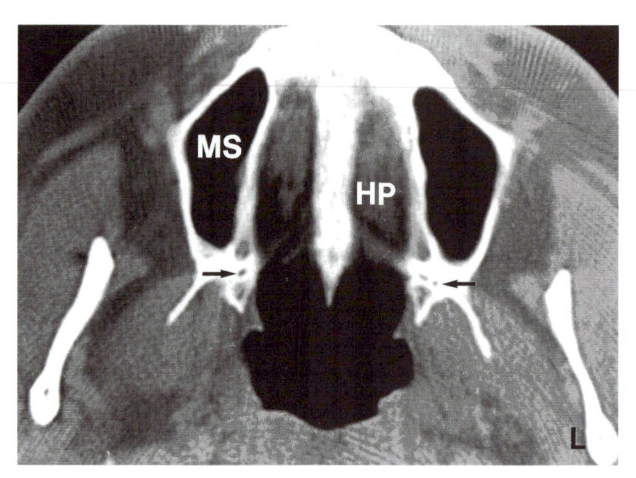

Figure 5.26 *Normal axial scan.* This demonstrates a section through the hard palate (HP) and the alveolar recesses of the maxillary sinuses (MS). The palatine foramina, which transmit the greater and lesser palatine nerves, are also shown (arrows).

The maxillary sinus ostium is not seen during routine office endoscopy in the unoperated nose, and it is rarely possible to identify any anatomical variations that may be compromising the ventilation of this sinus and therefore possibly predisposing the sinus to recurrent infections. The common anomalies that may compromise the natural ostium include Haller's cells, lateral deviations of the uncinate process, and a large ethmoid bulla. Each of these anomalies are best demonstrated by coronal CT.

Accessory maxillary sinus ostia (Figure 5.23)

The accessory maxillary sinus ostia are small defects frequently found in the membranous anterior or posterior nasal fontanelles. These are situated immediately above the inferior turbinate and usually open directly into the anterior or posterior portions of the middle meatus. Accessory maxillary sinus ostia do not normally assist in drainage of the maxillary sinus. They may be readily identified on endoscopy and may be misinterpreted as the true maxillary sinus ostium. The latter, which opens into the depths of the ethmoid infundibulum, is not visualized without resection of the uncinate process.

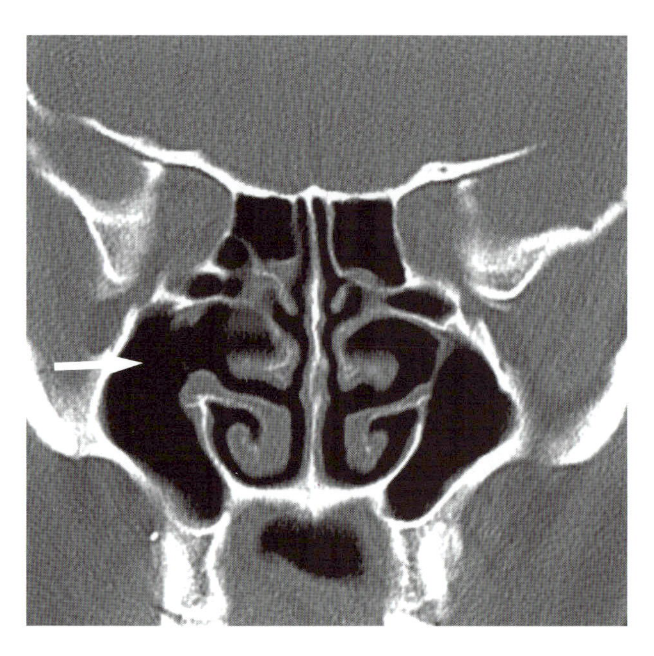

Figure 5.27 *Accessory ostium.* The medial wall of the maxillary sinus may have a small or large accessory sinus ostium. In this individual, there is a large defect in the medial wall of the right maxillary sinus (arrow).

ETHMOID SINUS (Figures 5.28–5.39)

The ethmoid bone lies between the orbits. It comprises a horizontal plate, a vertical plate, and, on either side of the latter, the ethmoid labyrinths. The ethmoid labyrinth is separated from the orbit by the delicate lamina papyracea.

The vertical plate of the ethmoid bone extends above the horizontal cribriform plate into the anterior cranial fossa as the crista galli. The horizontal plate of the cribriform plate is perforated for transmission of the olfactory nerve fibers from the roof of the nasal cavity. On either side of the crista galli, the gyrus rectus of the frontal lobe and the olfactory bulb rest upon the olfactory fossa.

The cribriform plate lies at a variable level in relation to the foveolae ethmoidales. It may lie well below the roof of the ethmoid or in some cases in the same plane as the foveolae ethmoidales. This is well demonstrated on CT in the coronal plane.

The ethmoid labyrinths are divided into an anterior and a posterior group of air cells. The ground lamella or basal lamella of the middle turbinate is the dividing line between the anterior and posterior ethmoid cells. The anterior ethmoid air cells are usually smaller and more numerous than the posterior group. The anterior ethmoid air cells drain into the middle meatus, whereas the posterior cells drain into the superior meatus.

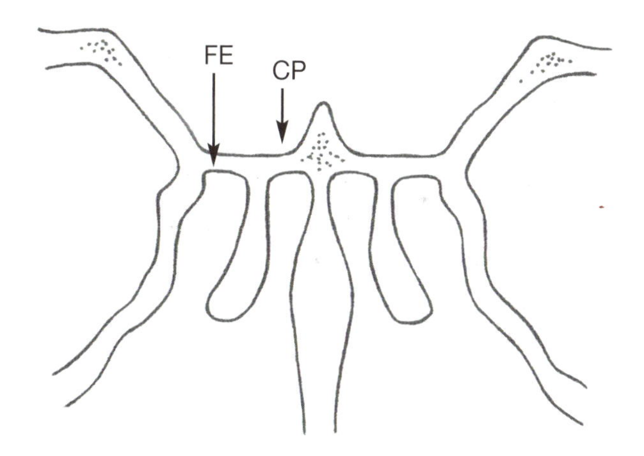

Figure 5.28 *Cribriform plate type 1.* In this type of cribriform plate (CP), the plate and the fovea ethmoidalis (FE) are in the same plane.

ANTERIOR ETHMOID SINUSES (Figures 5.5, 5.22, 5.36, 5.37, and 5.40)

The anatomy of the anterior ethmoid sinus is variable. These variations are of clinical interest when they cause obstruction of the ostiomeatal complex. The ostiomeatal complex is the key to the development of most inflammatory diseases of the frontal, maxillary, and ethmoid sinuses.

The ostiomeatal complex is a term used to describe collectively that area of the anterior ethmoid into which the frontal, maxillary, and anterior ethmoid sinuses drain. The ostiomeatal complex comprises the frontal recess, the infundibulum, the hiatus semilunaris, and the adjacent portion of the middle meatus. Anatomically, this area is bounded by the medial wall of the maxillary sinus and the lamina papyracea laterally, the lateral surface of the uncinate process anteriorly and medially, and the anterior wall of the ethmoid bulla posteriorly.

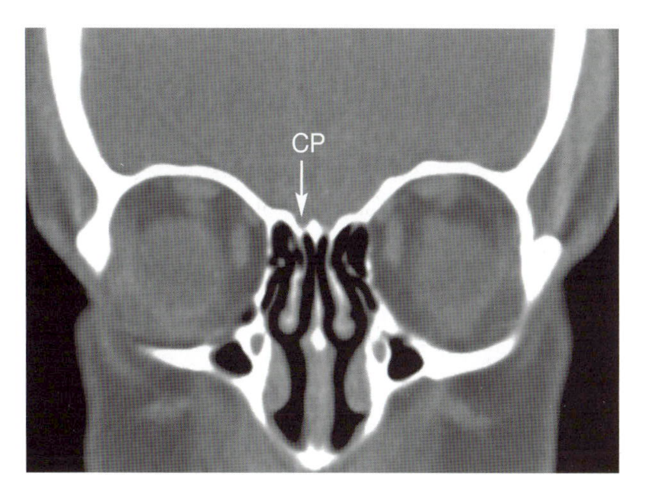

Figure 5.29 *Cribriform plate type 1.* Scan demonstrating a cribriform plate (CP) and fovea ethmoidalis in the same plane.

ETHMOID BULLA (BULLA ETHMOIDALIS) (Figure 5.22)

The largest and most constantly present anterior ethmoid air cell is the ethmoid bulla. It is the most prominent structure seen clinically when the middle turbinate is retracted medially. The anterior wall of the ethmoid bulla forms the posterior margin of the ethmoid infundibulum. The roof of the ethmoid

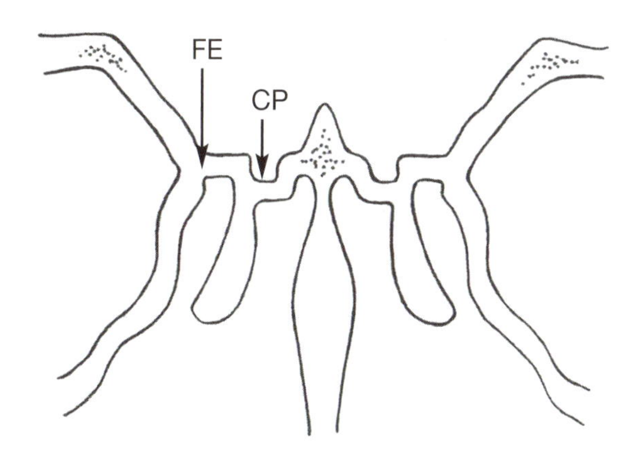

Figure 5.30 *Cribriform plate type 2.* In this type of cribriform plate (CP), the plate is in a slightly lower plane than the fovea ethmoidalis (FE).

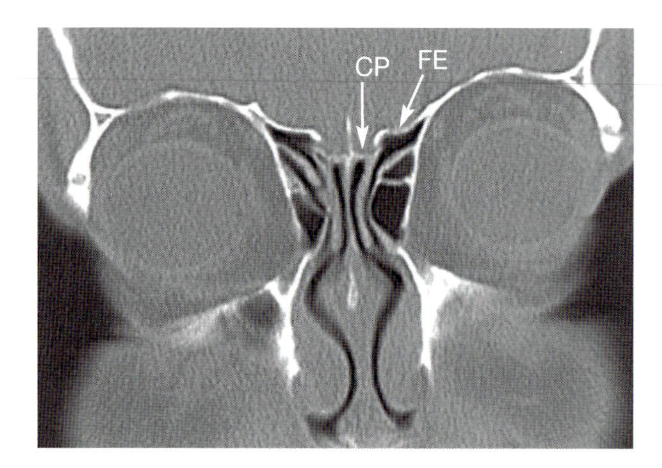

Figure 5.31 *Cribriform plate type 2.* Scan demonstrating a cribriform plate (CP) in a slightly lower plane than the fovea ethmoidalis (FE).

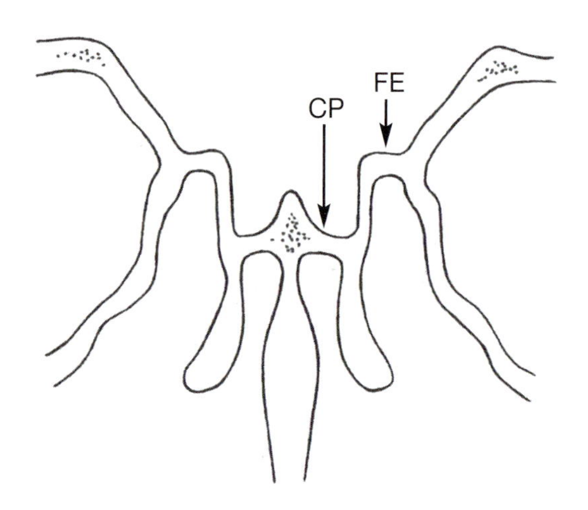

Figure 5.32 *Cribriform plate type 3.* In this type of cribriform plate (CP), the plate is in a lower plane than the fovea ethmoidalis (FE), and is at risk of injury during surgery.

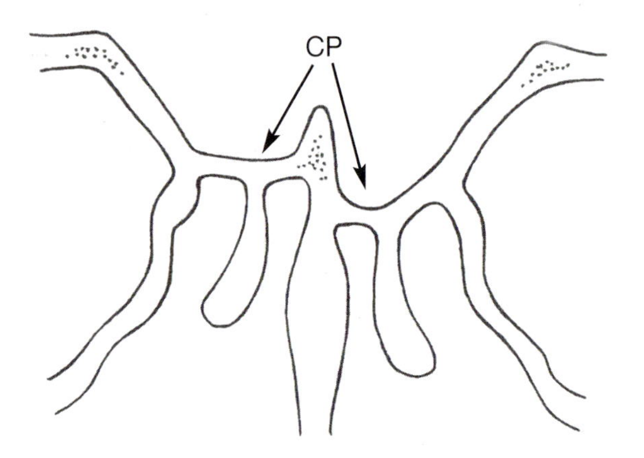

Figure 5.33 *Asymmetry of cribriform plate.* Asymmetry in the position of the cribriform plate (CP) is important to assess before surgery, as there is a higher risk of anterior cranial fossa and cribriform plate injury.

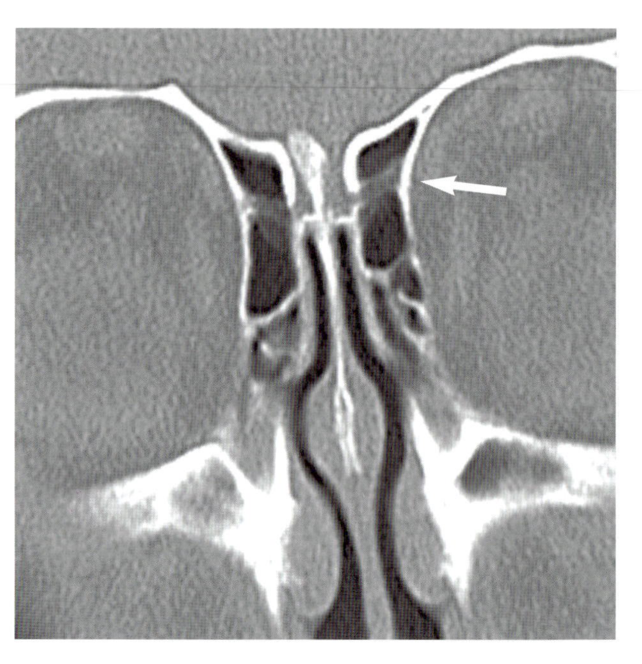

Figure 5.34 *Anterior ethmoidal artery.* Anterior scan demonstrating the anterior ethmoidal artery (arrow), the lamina lateralis, and a type 3 cribriform plate.

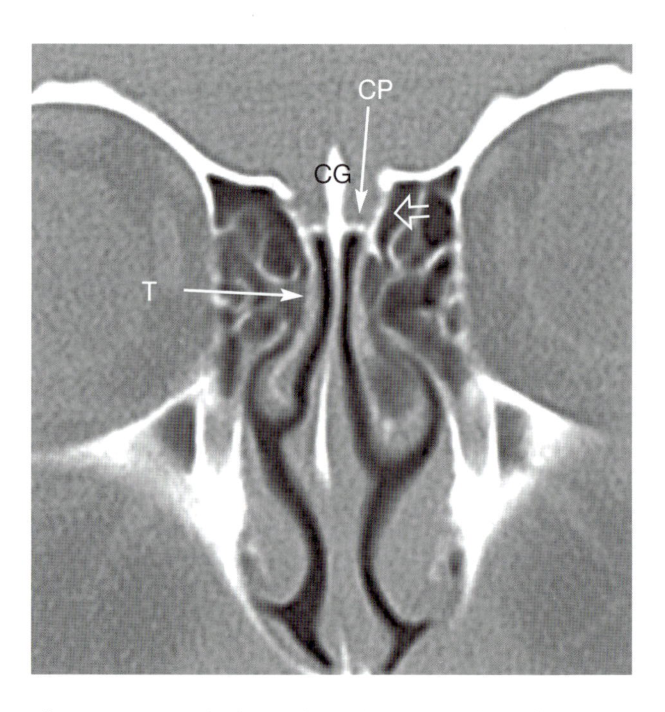

Figure 5.35 *Cribriform plate.* The crista galli (CG) projects intracranially and offers attachment to the falx cerebri. On either side is the cribriform plate (CP), through which the olfactory nerves enter the nasal cavity. The lamina lateralis (open arrow) is the thinnest part of the fovea ethmoidalis. The vertical plate (T) of the middle turbinate is attached to the roof of the ethmoid bone close to the lamina, which can easily be injured during endoscopic sinus surgery.

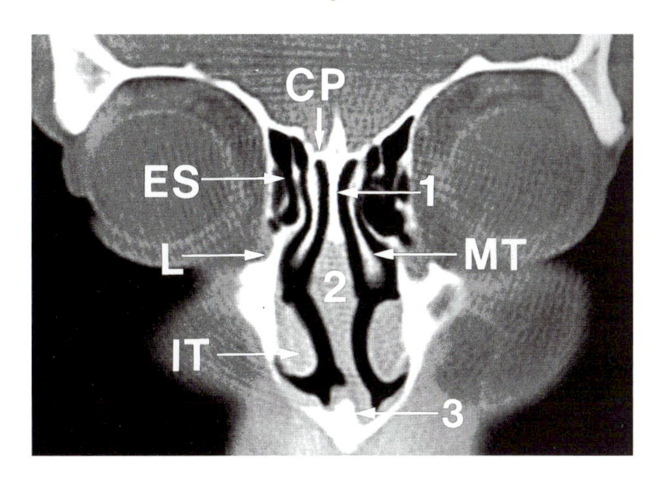

Figure 5.36 *Anterior ethmoid sinuses and nasal septum.* The nasal septum is formed by the perpendicular plate of the ethmoid bone (1), the cartilaginous septum (2), and the vomer inferiorly (3). The anterior ethmoid cells (ES) are located lateral to the vertical insertion of the middle turbinate (MT). Note the lacrimal fossa (L), which contains the lacrimal sac, the cribriform plate (CP), and the anterior end of the inferior turbinate (IT).

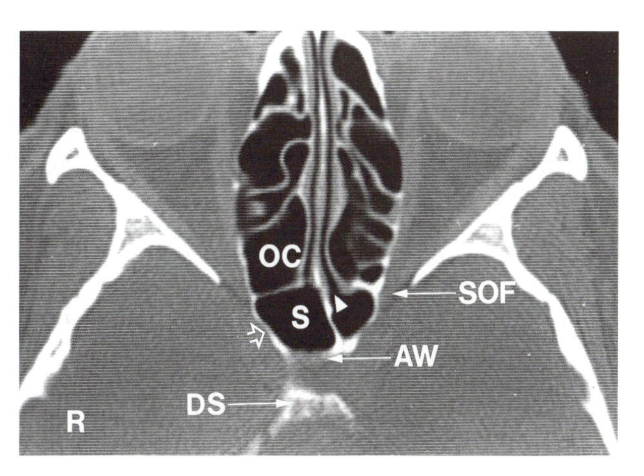

Figure 5.38 *Normal axial scan.* This demonstrates the posterior ethmoid Onodi cell (OC), the superior orbital fissure (SOF), the sphenoid sinus (S), the sphenoid sinus ostium (arrowhead), the impression of the internal carotid artery (open arrow), and the anterior wall (AW) and posterior bone (DS) of the dorsum sella.

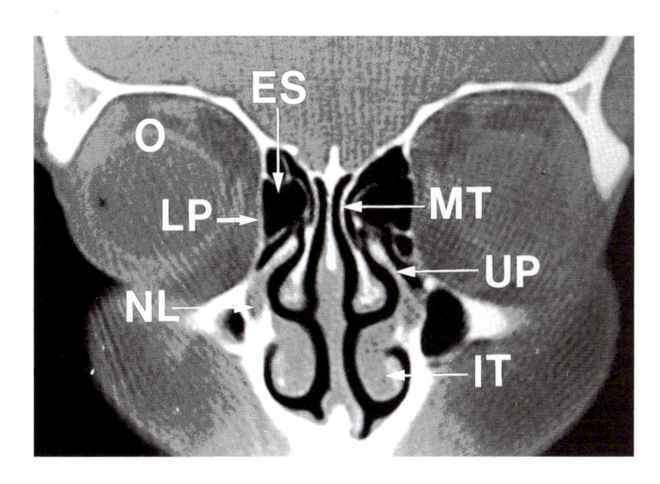

Figure 5.37 *Anterior ethmoid sinuses.* Anterior coronal scan, more posterior than Figure 5.36. The lamina papyracea (LP) separates the anterior ethmoid cells (ES) from the orbit (O). The nasolacrimal duct (NL), the uncinate process (UP), the inferior turbinate (IT), and the vertical insertion of the middle turbinate (MT) are also demonstrated.

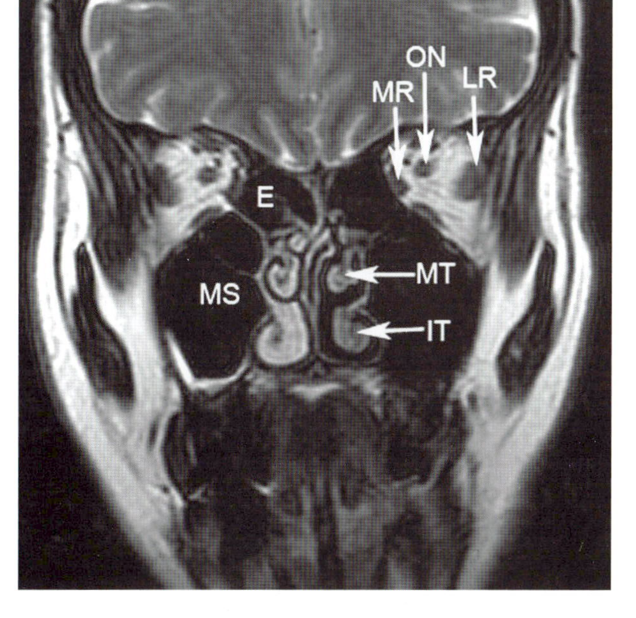

Figure 5.39 *Ethmoid sinus.* Coronal MR scan demonstrating the ethmoid sinus (E), Maxillary sinus (MS), middle turbinate (MT), inferior turbinate (IT), optic nerve (ON), medial rectus muscle (MR), and lateral rectus muscle (LR).

bulla may be continuous with the roof of the ethmoid sinus or it may be separated by a suprabullar extension of the lateral sinus.

The ethmoid bulla may be the site of inflammatory disease or may predispose the patient to inflammatory disease by obstructing the ostiomeatal complex. It is unusual to find isolated ethmoid bullitis, and the ethmoid bulla is more commonly involved in generalized inflammatory disease of the ethmoid sinus.

If the ethmoid bulla is large, it may obstruct the middle meatus by impinging on the middle turbinate and cause headaches and nasal obstruction without any inflammatory changes in the adjacent paranasal sinuses. However, the ethmoid bulla may also predispose to recurrent or chronic inflammation in the adjacent sinus if its configuration causes obstruction of the ostiomeatal complex. A large ethmoid bulla may overhang the hiatus semilunaris, or it may reduce the lumen of the ethmoid infundibulum, decreasing the ventilation and drainage of the adjacent sinuses.

UNCINATE PROCESS
(Figures 5.22, 5.37, 5.41, and 5.42)

The uncinate process forms the anterior and medial walls of the ethmoid infundibulum. The posterior free margin of the uncinate process forms the anterior border of the hiatus semilunaris. The uncinate process of the ethmoid bone extends inferiorly to fuse with the ethmoid process of the inferior turbinate. This fusion is usually at least 1 cm posterior to the distal end of the nasolacrimal duct. However, it is not uncommon to see this area of fusion quite close to the nasolacrimal duct. This observation should alert the surgeon to the risk of injury to the nasolacrimal apparatus, because a generous uncinate resection may result in chronic epiphora if the nasolacrimal duct is transected. With such an anomaly, the ethmoid infundibulum extends more anteriorly, and disease in this area may affect the nasolacrimal apparatus – especially the more distal duct, which has a membranous wall. The superior insertion of the uncinate process is variable. It may turn laterally to insert into the lamina papyracea or it may insert superiorly into the roof of the ethmoid. On occasion, the uncinate process turns medially and inserts into the vertical plate of the middle turbinate, as discussed above under anatomical variations of the frontal recess.

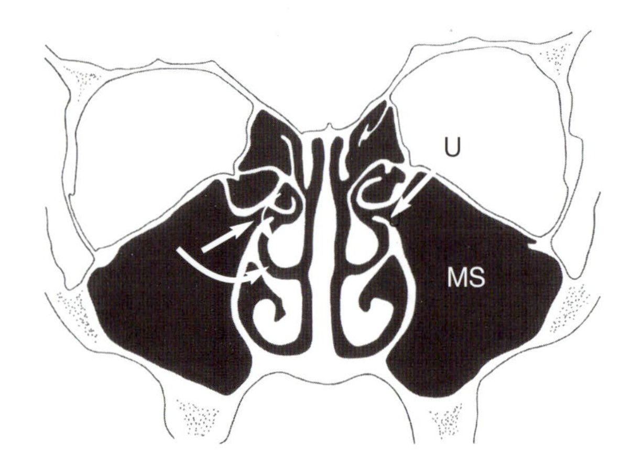

Figure 5.40 *Ostiomeatal complex.* Diagram showing the various components of the ostiomeatal complex: the ethmoid infundibulum (arrow), and middle meatus (curved arrow), into which the frontal recess, maxillary sinus (MS), and anterior ethmoid sinus drain. U, uncinate process.

ETHMOID INFUNDIBULUM
(Figures 5.22 and 5.42)

This critical drainage channel is bordered by the uncinate process anteromedially, the anterior surface of the ethmoid bulla posteriorly, and the lamina papyracea laterally. The ethmoid infundibulum connects the natural ostium of the maxillary sinus to the middle meatus via the hiatus semilunaris. Variations in the anatomy of the related structures that border the ethmoid infundibulum, namely the uncinate process and the ethmoid bulla, can result in permanent narrowing or intermittent obstruction of this channel. The ethmoid infundibulum may also be compromised by anomalies of the middle turbinate. Anteriorly and superiorly, the frontal recess may open into the ethmoid infundibulum. Posteriorly, when present, the lateral sinus, which lies between the ethmoid bulla and the basal lamella, also opens via the hiatus semilunaris into the ethmoid infundibulum.

HIATUS SEMILUNARIS (Figure 5.22)

The hiatus semilunaris is a semilunar two-dimensional aperture bounded posteriorly by the anterior surface of the ethmoid bulla and anteriorly by the posterior free margin of the uncinate process. The hiatus semilunaris is the opening through which the ethmoid infundibulum drains into the middle meatus.

LATERAL OR GROUND SINUS (RECESS) AND BASAL LAMELLA
(Figures 5.43 and 5.44)

The basal or ground lamella of the middle turbinate is the septum that divides the anterior from the

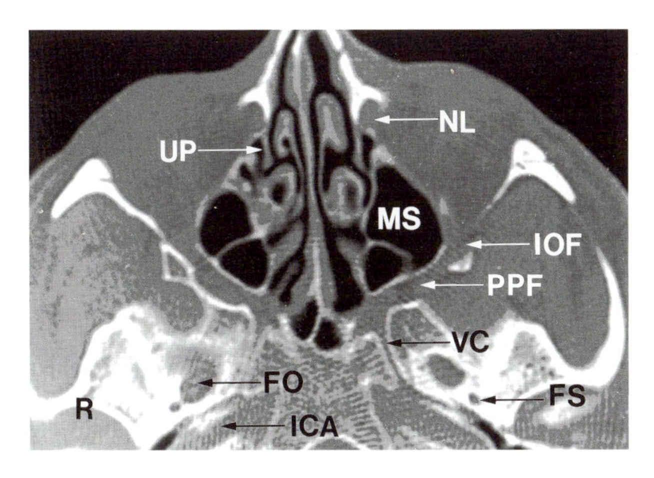

Figure 5.41 *Normal axial scan.* This scan demonstrates the uncinate process (UP) arising close to the wall of the nasolacrimal duct (NL). Also demonstrated are the Vidian canal (VC), foramen ovale (FO), foramen spinosum (FS), pterygopalatine fossa (PPF), infraorbital fissure (IOF), maxillary sinus (MS), and internal carotid artery (ICA).

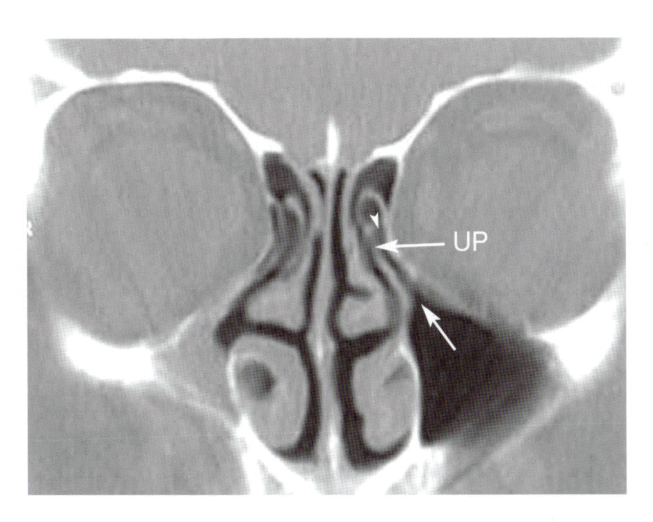

Figure 5.42 *Uncinate process.* Coronal scan demonstrating the uncinate process (UP) inserting high into the lamina papyracea. The frontal recess (arrowhead) drains medial to the ethmoid infundibulum (arrow).

posterior ethmoid sinuses. The lateral sinus is an inconstant space located posterior to the ethmoid bulla and anterior to the basal lamella. It may extend above the ethmoid bulla as the suprabullar space. If the lateral sinus communicates with the frontal recess, then inflammatory disease may spread along this route.

The lateral recess opens directly into the posterosuperior part of the hiatus semilunaris and is sometimes referred to as the superior recess of the hiatus semilunaris. A large ethmoid bulla overhanging this aperture, a concha bullosa, or a swollen medially bent uncinate process can impede the drainage of the lateral recess into the middle meatus. The radiologist must be able to identify the lateral sinus, as inflammatory disease may be confined to the lateral sinus and only identifiable on CT scan.

MIDDLE MEATUS
(Figures 5.22, 5.23, and 5.37)

The middle meatus is the space inferolateral to the middle turbinate, into which the anterior ethmoid, frontal, and maxillary sinuses eventually drain. The middle meatus can be more clearly seen by medial retraction of the middle turbinate during endoscopy. The most prominent structure within the middle meatus is usually the ethmoid bulla. The uncinate process lies anterior to the ethmoid bulla. The size of the middle meatus can vary – for example, it may be deep when the maxillary sinus is atelectatic and the posterior fontanelle is retracted laterally. The middle meatus and the nasal cavities are small when the sinuses are well developed.

Anatomical variants of the middle meatus

The middle meatus may be compromised by a large ethmoid bulla, a deviated nasal septum, a bony septal spur, or one of the many variants of the middle turbinates, such as an abnormally aerated middle turbinate (a concha bullosa), a secondary middle turbinate, or an accessory middle turbinate. These anatomical variants are discussed in detail in Chapter 6.

MIDDLE TURBINATE
(Figures 5.22–5.24 and 5.37)

The middle turbinate arises from the medial aspect of the ethmoid labyrinth. Anteriorly, the middle turbinate is suspended from the roof of the ethmoid by a vertical bony plate. The vertical plate of the middle turbinate serves as an important anatomical landmark for the cribriform plate during intranasal surgery and should not be resected, in case revision surgery is required in the future. The head of the

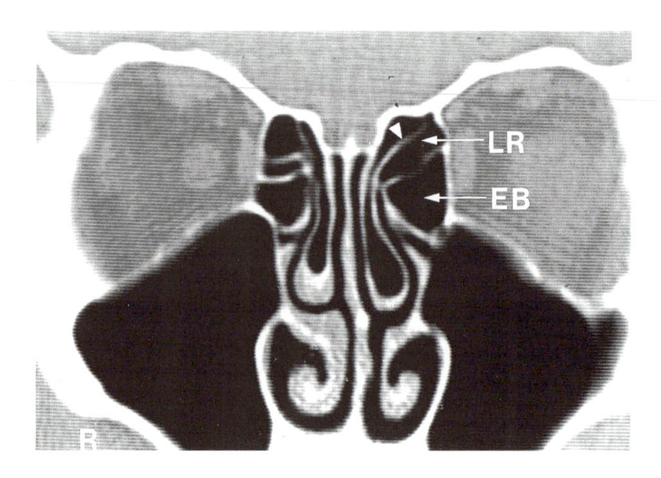

Figure 5.43 *Lateral sinus.* Coronal scan demonstrating bilateral conchae bullosae. The horizontal insertion of the left middle turbinate (arrowhead) is seen. The space between the posterior margin of the ethmoid bulla (EB) and the horizontal insertion of the middle turbinate is the lateral recess (LR).

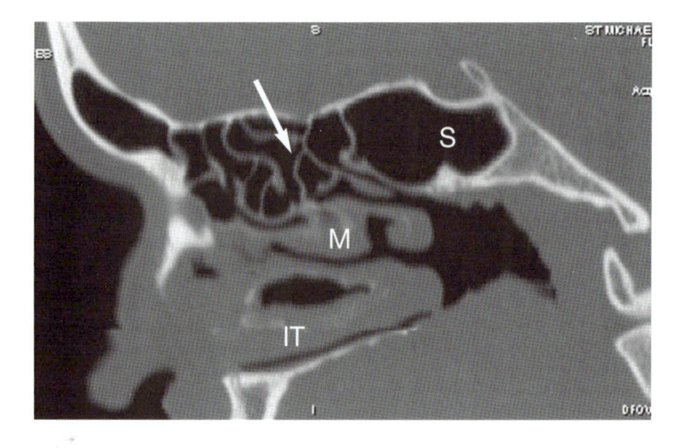

Figure 5.44 *Basal lamella.* Sagittal scan demonstrating the basal lamella (arrow), middle turbinate (M), inferior turbinate (IT), and sphenoid sinus (S).

middle turbinate is slightly bulbous in shape and is continuous posteriorly with the free margin of the middle turbinate. The head usually protrudes anterior to the vertical plate by 1–2 mm, although occasionally it may protrude by over 1 cm. It is therefore an unreliable landmark for the uncinate process.

Several thin inconstant plates that insert laterally onto the lamina papyracea may be seen arising from the middle turbinate. The largest and most constant of these horizontal plates curves laterally to insert onto the lamina papyracea and forms the roof of the middle meatus. This is referred to as the basal or ground lamella, and separates the anterior ethmoid sinuses from the posterior ethmoid sinuses.

The free margin of the middle turbinate is usually bulbous, but on occasion it may be triangular or bifid or have a sagittal groove that divides it incompletely into unequal parts.

INFERIOR TURBINATE AND INFERIOR MEATUS

(Figures 5.5, 5.12, 5.22–5.24, 5.35–5.37, and 5.45–5.56)

The anterior end of the inferior turbinate and the inferior meatus are the first structures to be seen on clinical examination of the nasal cavity. The inferior turbinate is an independent bone that articulates laterally with the conchal ridge of the medial process of the maxilla. The inferior meatus lies inferolateral to the inferior turbinate, and the nasolacrimal duct is the only structure that opens into this meatus.

The mucous membrane of the inferior turbinate contains erectile tissue, the dilatation of which may be responsible for much of the soft tissue hypertrophy. A marked reduction in the size of the inferior turbinate may be noted following the application of a topical vasoconstrictor such as xylometazoline, thus indicating that such patients may benefit from cauterization or a limited turbinectomy. Irreversible hypertrophy of the inferior turbinates may be indicative of vasomotor or allergic rhinitis.

Preoperative CT is rarely indicated to assess hypertrophy of the inferior turbinates. However, if there is suspicion of ethmoid sinus disease causing secondary inferior turbinate vasodilatation, or of the presence of a large bony inferior turbinate causing obstruction, then this can be well demonstrated by CT. Submucosal resection of the enlarged bony portion of the inferior turbinate bone may be curative. Soft tissue hypertrophy of the inferior turbinate is much more common than bony hypertrophy, and is also well demonstrated by CT. An uncommon cause of enlargement of the inferior turbinate is pneumatization of the turbinate bone. This unusual finding is associated with the pneumatization being derived from the maxillary sinus.

POSTERIOR ETHMOID SINUSES (Figures 5.24 and 5.38)

The posterior ethmoid air cells are larger in size than the anterior cells, but are fewer in number. They drain into the superior meatus, which is situated inferolateral to the superior turbinate. An inconstant additional turbinate may be situated above the superior turbinate, and is called the supreme turbinate. The largest and most posterior of the posterior ethmoid air cells is called the Onodi cell, after the anatomist who first described it. It exposes a lateral bulging of the optic canal, a so-called 'tuberculum opticum'. The Onodi cell shares a common wall with the adjacent sphenoid sinus, and is best demonstrated by CT in the axial plane.

Onodi cells are of great clinical importance, as they have an intimate relationship with the optic nerve, from which they are separated by a thin delicate bony septum. It is not uncommon for the bone to be dehiscent in this region, and it is critical to identify the relationship of the optic nerve to the posterior ethmoid in order to avoid injury to the nerve and consequent blindness.

The pneumatization of the posterior ethmoid is variable, and it is not uncommon for the posterior ethmoid sinuses to extend beyond the confines of the ethmoid bone. The posterior ethmoid may expand superiorly into the orbit forming supra-orbital cells, or it may expand laterally to encompass the optic nerve. These variants, if not identified preoperatively, pose extreme hazards to the patient's vision.

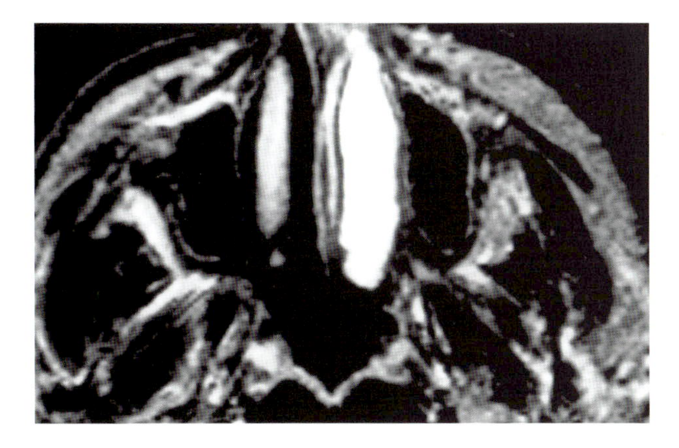

Figure 5.45 *Normal nasal cycle.* This MR scan shows the inferior turbinate is hyperintense on the left side, showing changes from normal preferential airflow through one nasal passage. This should not be mistaken for an abnormality in the turbinate.

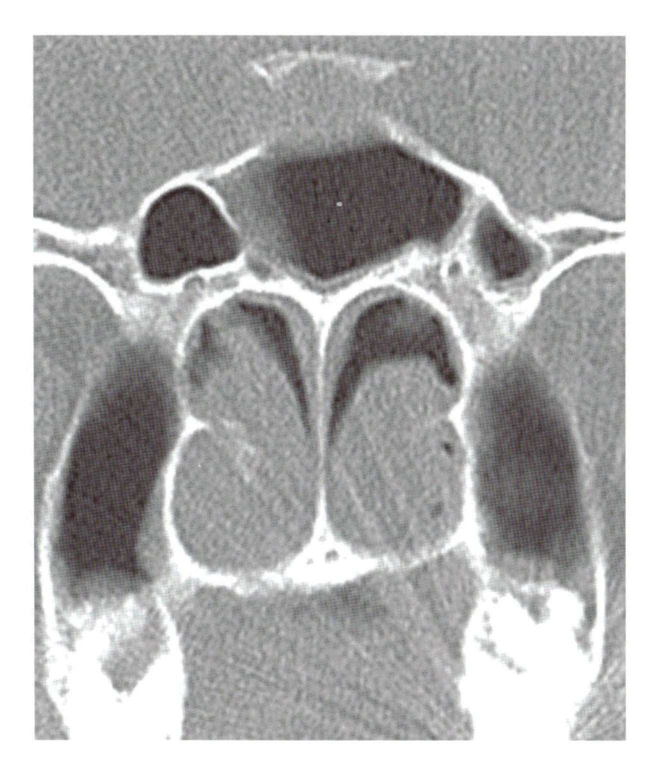

Figure 5.46 *Inferior turbinate hypertrophy.* Bilateral large inferior turbinates are occluding the posterior nares.

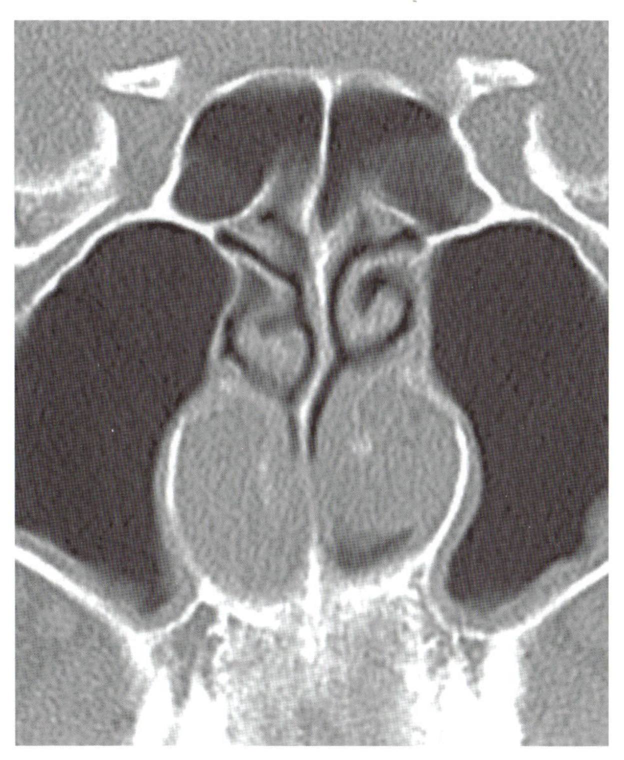

Figure 5.47 *Inferior turbinate hypertrophy.* Bilateral large inferior turbinates are noted.

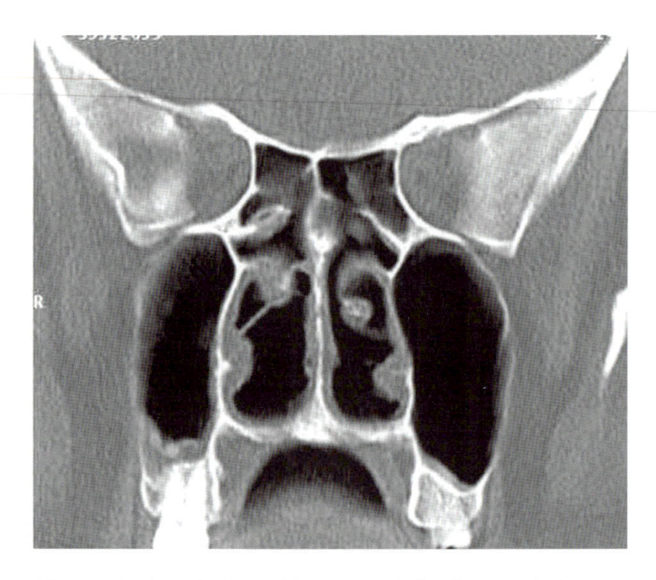

Figure 5.48 *Inferior turbinectomy.* Following surgical resection the remains of the inferior turbinates are seen as a small protrusion on the lateral wall of the nasal cavity.

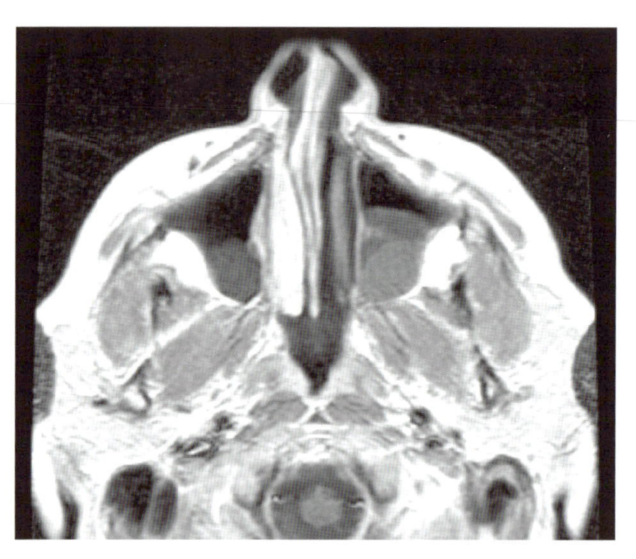

Figure 5.50 *MRI of inferior turbinates.* Axial T1-weighted image post Gd-DTPA administration showing enhancement of the inferior turbinates.

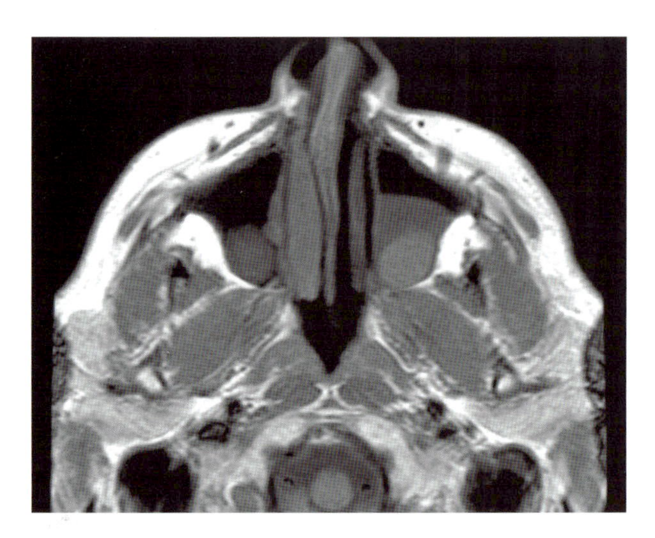

Figure 5.49 *MRI of inferior turbinates.* Axial T1-weighted image of the inferior turbinates demonstrating the normal isointense appearance of the turbinates pre Gd-DTPA administration.

SPHENOID SINUS

(Figures 5.4, 5.12, 5.57–5.67)

The sphenoid is a complex bone with several processes. The lesser wing and the anterior clinoid process are attached anteriorly to the planum sphenoidale. The anterior clinoid process houses the canal of the optic nerve and also forms the superior margin of the superior orbital fissure. The superomedial aspect of the superior orbital fissure is separated from the optic canal by a thin piece of bone called the optic strut. The greater wing of the sphenoid is situated more inferiorly and forms part of the orbital wall and the inferior margin of the superior orbital fissure. The pterygoid processes arise from the greater wing of the sphenoid and form the posterior border of the pterygopalatine fossa. The greater wing of the sphenoid makes a major contribution to the anteromedial part of the middle cranial fossa. The foramen rotundum and the Vidian canal traverse the body of the sphenoid and are lateral relations of the sphenoid sinus. Posteriorly, the foramen ovale and foramen spinosum perforate the greater wing close to the petrous apex.

The sphenoid sinuses are asymmetrical and vary in their degree of pneumatization. Superiorly, the sphenoid sinus is related to the pituitary fossa and the pituitary gland. On either side of the sinus lie the cavernous sinuses, which transmit the internal carotid artery and the third, fourth, and sixth cranial nerves. The intracavernous portion of the internal carotid artery passes superiorly alongside the body of the sphenoid sinus. It comes to lie medial to the anterior clinoid process before perforating the dura, which roofs the cavernous sinus, and then becomes the terminal or cerebral part of the artery. The internal carotid artery may sometimes lie within the lumen of the sphenoid sinus. It is usually separated by a thin plate of bone, but this may be dehiscent. Inferiorly, the sphenoid sinus is related to the

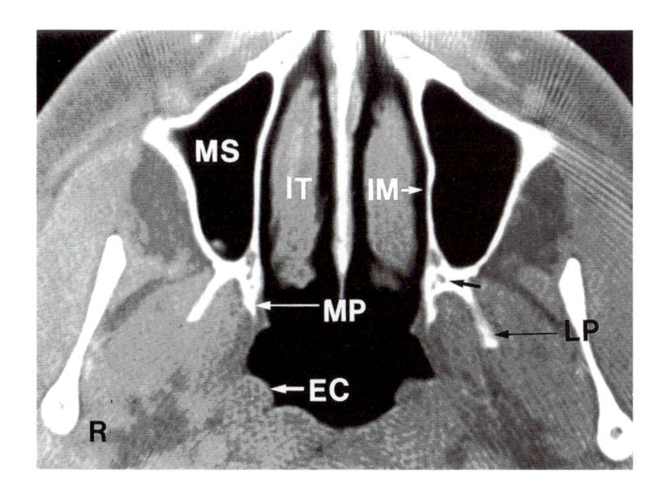

Figure 5.51 *Normal axial scan.* This scan demonstrates the maxillary sinuses (MS), inferior turbinate (IT), and inferior meatus (IM). Posterior to the maxillary sinus lie the medial (MP) and lateral pterygoid (LP) plates, which enclose the pterygoid fossa. The palatine canals are shown (arrow). The eustachian cushion (EC) is shown protruding into the nasopharynx.

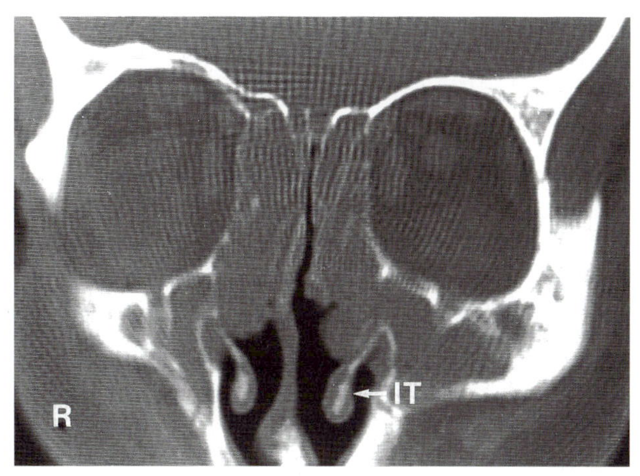

Figure 5.53 *Decongested inferior turbinates.* Coronal scan demonstrating extensive polypoidal soft tissue densities in the maxillary and ethmoid sinuses. As a consequence of chronic abuse of topical decongestants, the inferior turbinates (IT) are small and shrunken. There has been little effect on the middle turbinates. This is probably due to erectile tissue, which is abundant on the inferior turbinate but limited in its distribution on the middle turbinate.

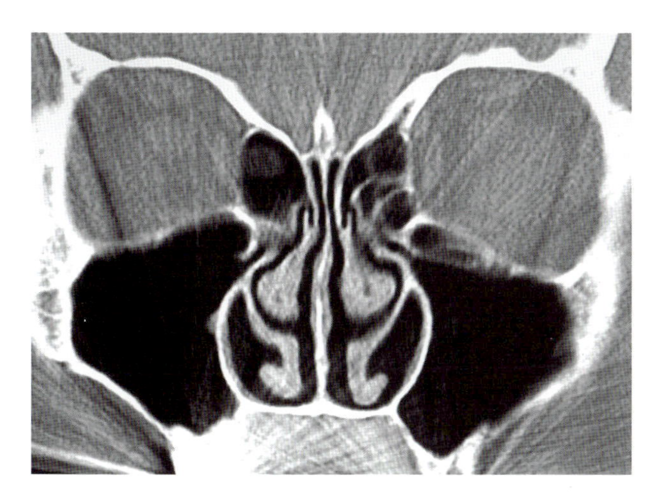

Figure 5.52 *Decongested inferior turbinates.* Coronal scan showing the inferior turbinates to be small within a roomy nasal cavity.

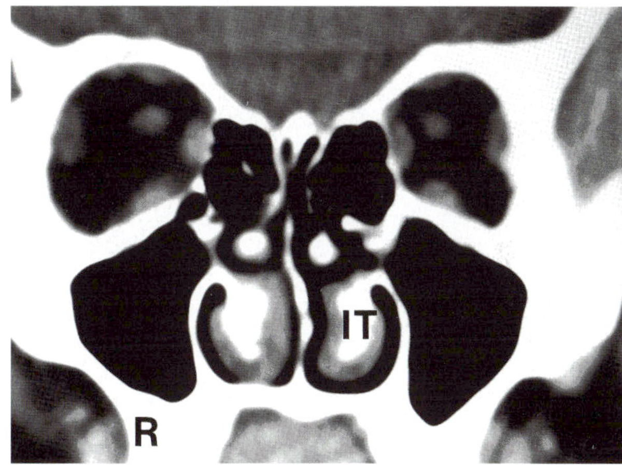

Figure 5.54 *Bony hypertrophy of the inferior turbinates.* Narrow-window scan demonstrating bony hypertrophy of the inferior turbinates (IT). The uncinate process is deviated medially, leading to disease in the ethmoid infundibulum (arrow). The orbital apex is also well demonstrated.

nasopharynx, the Eustachian tubes and Eustachian cushions.

It is not uncommon to find a multiseptate sinus. Several pneumatized recesses extend from the sinus into the surrounding structures. The commonest is the lateral recess, which when present passes between the Vidian canal and the foramen rotundum. On occasion, the entire greater wing of the sphenoid bone, which makes a major contribution to the floor of the middle cranial fossa, is pneumatized. The anterior clinoid, the lesser wing of the sphenoid, the dorsum sella, and sometimes the posterior clinoid process may be pneumatized. The sinus may also extend into the pterygoid processes. The floor of the sphenoid sinus may be dehiscent. This finding should not be misinterpreted as the natural ostium of the sinus. The dehiscence may be further eroded by benign or malignant disease. This is well demonstrated by CT in the coronal plane.

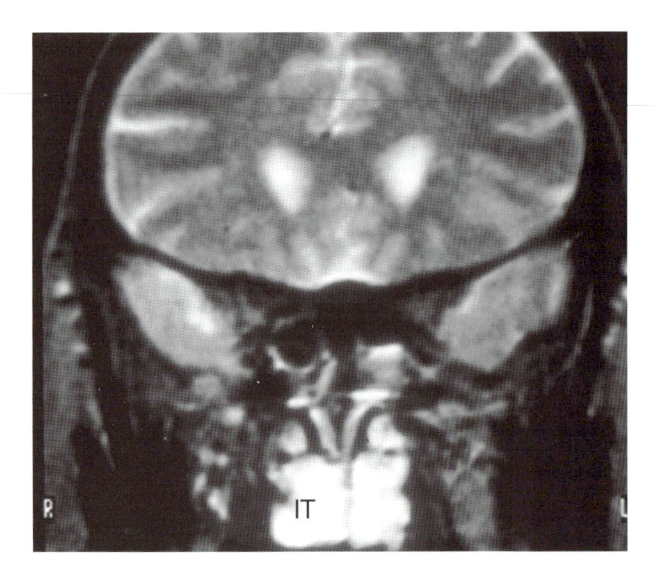

Figure 5.55 *Inferior turbinate hypertrophy.* This patient has such extensive soft tissue hypertrophy of the posterior ends of the inferior turbinates (IT) that the choanae are almost totally occluded. The turbinates are hyperintense in this T2-weighted MRI scan.

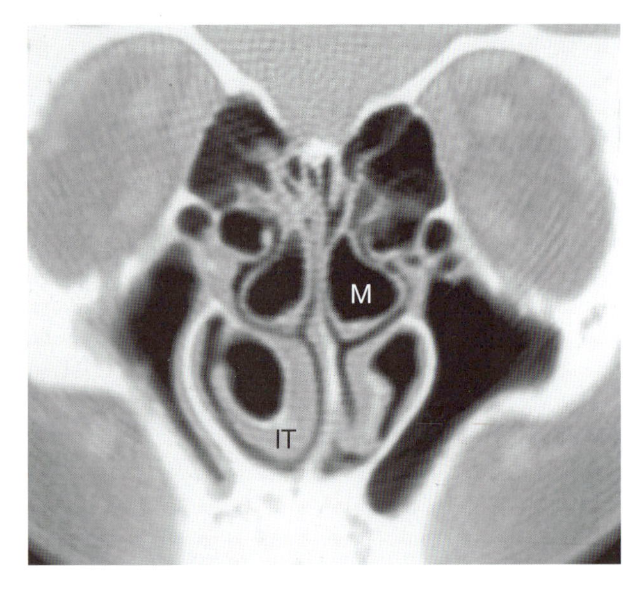

Figure 5.56 *Pneumatized inferior turbinate.* The inferior turbinate is an independent bone articulating with a ridge on the medial aspect of the maxilla. Rarely, it is incorporated into the maxilla, and pneumatization of the inferior turbinate (IT) from the adjacent maxillary sinus may occur. This is seen on the right side. Bilateral conchae bullosae are also noted (M).

The sphenoid sinus drains through a small ostium in the anterior wall, close to the roof of the sinus, into the sphenoethmoid recess. This is poorly demonstrated by CT in the coronal plane, but is well demonstrated on scans taken in the axial plane or following sagittal reformation of images taken in the axial plane.

PTERYGOPALATINE FOSSA
(Figures 5.25, 5.26, 5.41, and 5.68–5.70)

The pterygopalatine fossa is shaped like an inverted pyramid bounded anteriorly by the maxillary sinus, medially by the palatine bone, and posteriorly by the pterygoid plates of the sphenoid bone. It communicates with the orbit, the nasopharynx, the paranasal sinuses, the infratemporal fossa, and the middle cranial fossa, and may form a major channel for the spread of infection or tumor. The contents of the fossa are surrounded by loose connective tissue and fat, which allows for CT assessment of the fossa. CT does not clearly demonstrate the contents of the pterygopalatine fossa, but, following the administration of intravenous contrast, the terminal branches of the maxillary artery may be seen as small enhancing structures. Obliteration of the fat spaces in the pterygopalatine fossa is indicative of disease, the commonest being malignancy invading the space.

The pterygopalatine fossa communicates directly with many of the surrounding anatomical regions, and these channels may be identified by CT. Posteriorly, the pterygopalatine fossa communicates with the middle cranial fossa via the foramen rotundum, which transmits the maxillary nerve. Inferiorly, the pterygopalatine fossa tapers to its apex and receives the Vidian or pterygoid canal. This canal passes anteriorly through the body of the sphenoid from the foramen lacerum and transmits the Vidian nerve. The pterygopalatine fossa communicates with the oral cavity through the greater and lesser palatine canals, and laterally with the infratemporal fossa, containing the medial and lateral pterygoid muscles, via the pterygomaxillary fissure. Medially, it communicates through the sphenopalatine foramen with the sphenoethmoid recess and the nasal cavity. Anterosuperiorly, it communicates with the orbit through the infraorbital fissure. Perineural transmission of tumor can occur along the nerves traversing through the pterygopalatine fossa.

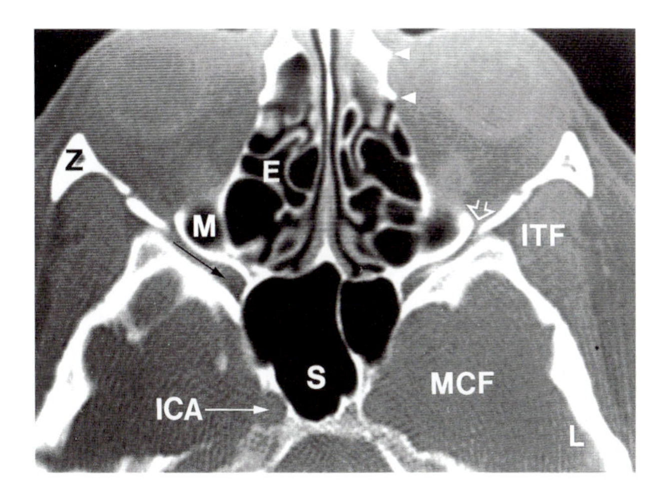

Figure 5.57 *Normal axial scan.* This scan demonstrates the anterior and posterior lacrimal crests (arrowheads), ethmoid labyrinth (E), superior recess of the maxillary sinus (M), zygoma (Z), pterygopalatine fossa (black arrow), inferior orbital foramen (open arrow), infratemporal fossa (ITF), middle cranial fossa (MCF), sphenoid sinus (S), and internal carotid artery (ICA).

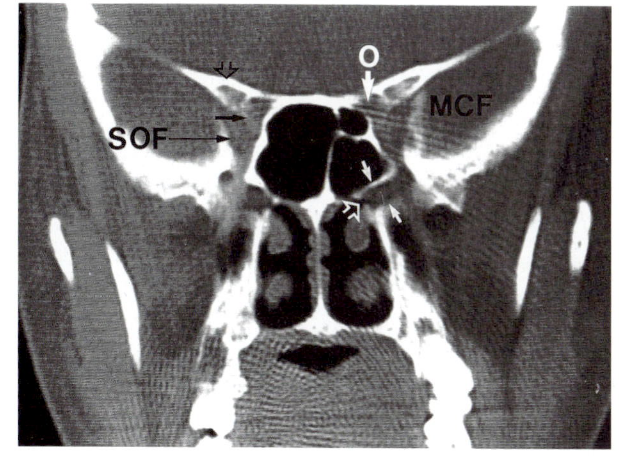

Figure 5.59 *Sphenoid sinus.* The sphenoethmoid recess (open white arrow) communicates with the pterygopalatine fossa through the sphenopalatine foramen (between white arrows). The optic foramen (O) is separated from the superior orbital fissure (SOF) by the optic strut (black arrow). The planum sphenoidale of the lesser wing of the sphenoid is demonstrated (open black arrow); the middle cranial fossa (MCF) can also be seen.

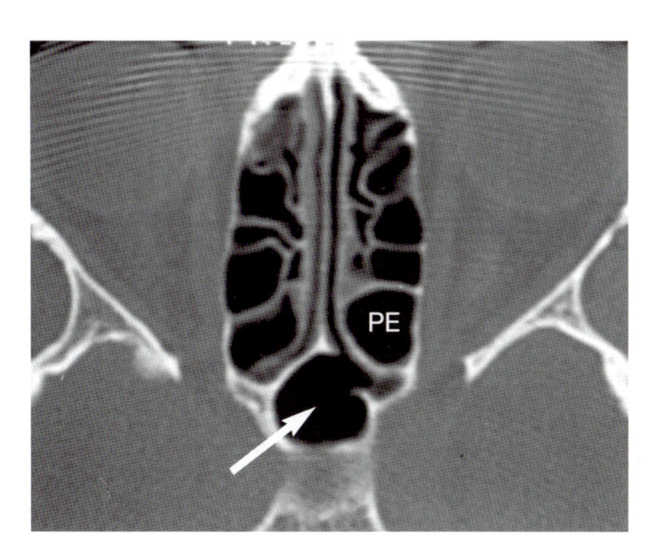

Figure 5.58 *Normal sphenoid sinus.* In this individual, there is a single normal sphenoid sinus draining into the left side (arrow). PE, posterior ethmoid sinus.

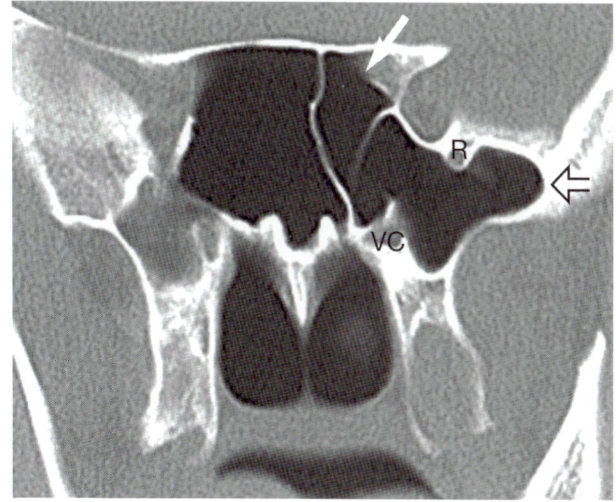

Figure 5.60 *Sphenoid sinus.* The lateral recesses of the sphenoid sinus (open arrow) and dehiscence of the roof of the sphenoid close to the optic nerve (arrow) on the left side can be seen, as can the foramen rotundum (R) and Vidian canal (VC).

ORBITAL APEX

(Figures 5.59–5.61 and 5.71–5.75)

The orbit is the bony cavity that houses the eyeball, the extraocular muscles, and neurovascular structures, including the optic nerve. The apex of the orbit communicates through the optic canal, the superior orbital fissure, and the inferior orbital fissure with the middle cranial fossa, the pterygopalatine fossa, and the inferior temporal fossa, respectively.

Medially, the optic canal and nerve are separated from the posterior ethmoid and sphenoid sinuses by the lamina papyracea and a small part of the lesser wing of the sphenoid. Inferolaterally, the optic canal and nerve are separated from the superior orbital fissure by a spicule of bone called the optic strut, which is the root of the lesser wing of the sphenoid.

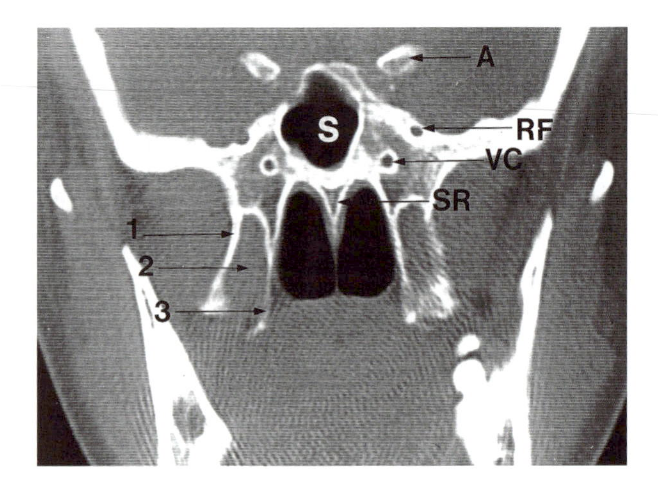

Figure 5.61 *Sphenoid sinus.* Scan demonstrating the sphenoid sinus (S), foramen rotundum (RF), Vidian canal (VC), anterior clinoid process (A), and sphenoid rostrum (SR), as well as the lateral (1) and medial (2) pterygoid plates and the pterygoid fossa (3).

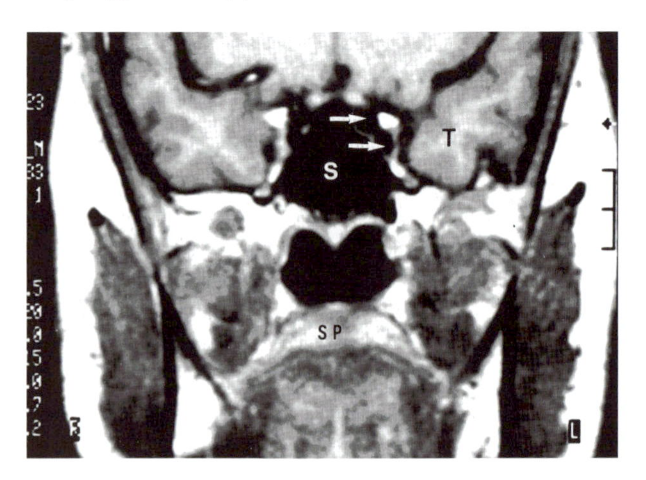

Figure 5.62 *Sphenoid sinus.* T1-weighted MRI scan demonstrating the sphenoid sinus (S) and internal carotid artery (arrows) located on the lateral wall of the sinus. The other normal structures shown include the soft palate (SP) and the temporal lobes (T) in the middle cranial fossa.

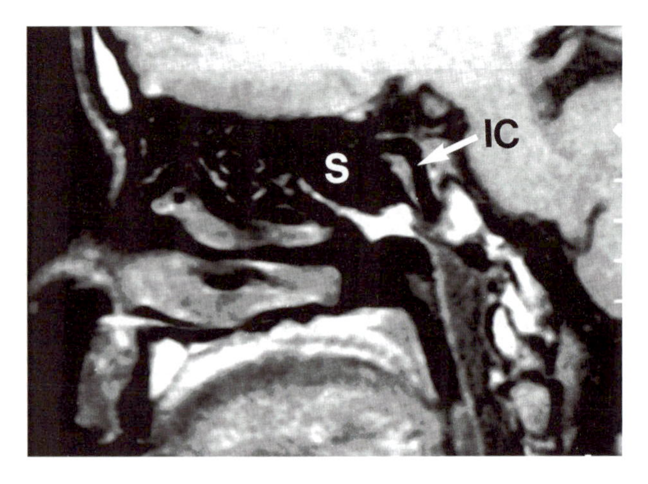

Figure 5.63 *Sphenoid sinus.* Sagittal T1-weighted MRI scan demonstrating the signal-void internal carotid artery (IC), which is located close to the roof of the sinus (S).

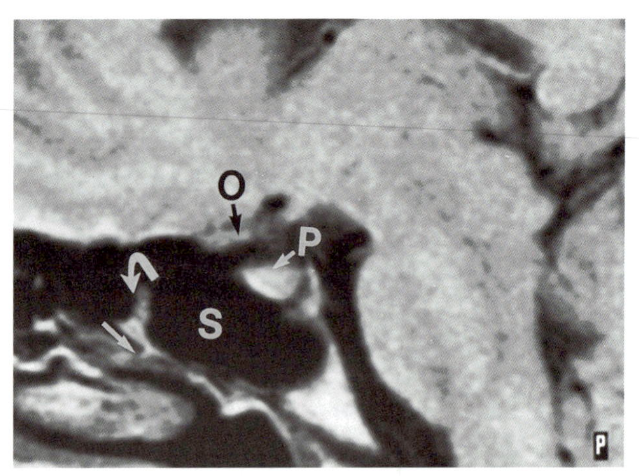

Figure 5.64 *Sphenoid sinus.* Sagittal T1-weighted MRI scan demonstrating the normal sphenoid sinus (S) draining through an anterior-placed opening close to the roof of the nasal vault (curved arrow). The small space (straight arrow) above the superior turbinate is the sphenoethmoid recess. The optic nerve (O) lies above and lateral to the sphenoid sinus, and the pituitary gland (P) lies above the sinus.

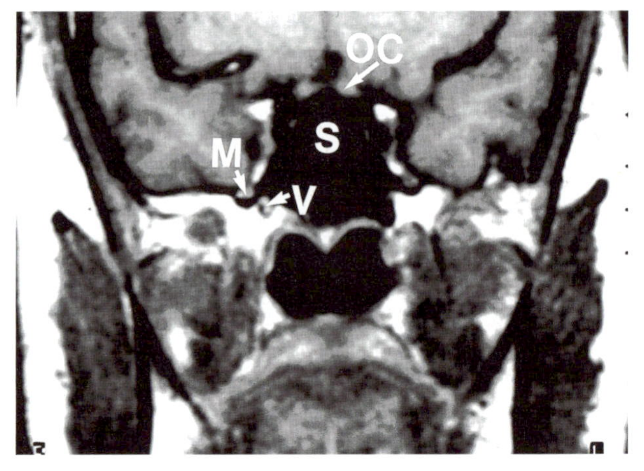

Figure 5.65 *Sphenoid sinus.* Coronal T1-weighted MRI scan demonstrating the sphenoid sinus (S), the maxillary division of the trigeminal nerve running through the foramen rotundum (M), the Vidian nerve within the Vidian canal (V), and the optic chiasm (OC).

The optic nerve is surrounded by a prolongation of the meninges. The ophthalmic artery usually lies inferior to the optic nerve.

The superior orbital fissure lies obliquely between the greater and the lesser wings of the sphenoid. The tendinous ring that surrounds the medial aspect of the superior orbital fissure shows enhancement following the administration of

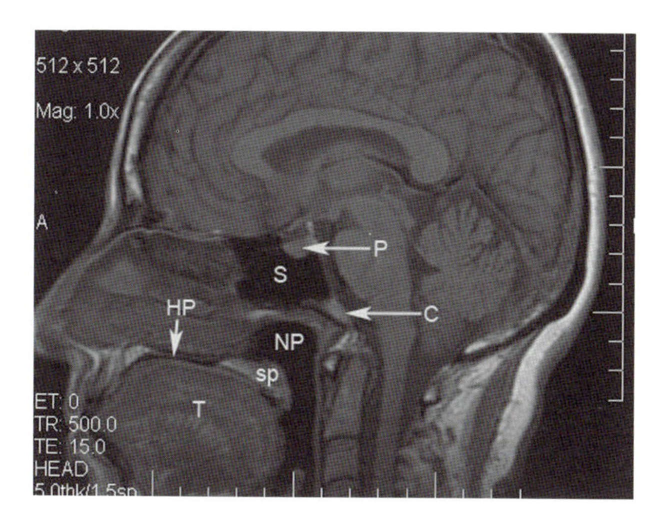

Figure 5.66 *Sphenoid sinus.* Sagittal T1-weighted MRI scan demonstrating the sphenoid sinus (S), pituitary gland (P), nasopharynx (NP), soft palate (sp), tongue (T), hard palate (HP), and clivus (C).

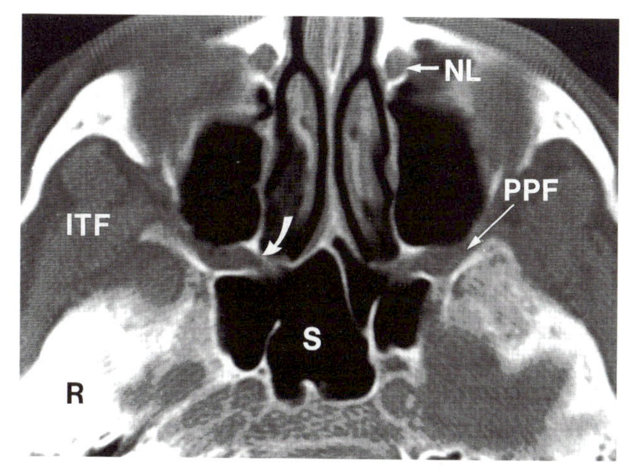

Figure 5.68 *Normal axial scan*. This scan demonstrates the nasolacrimal duct (NL), the sphenopalatine foramen (curved arrow) entering the pterygopalatine fossa (PPF), the sphenoid sinus (S), and the infratemporal fossa (ITF).

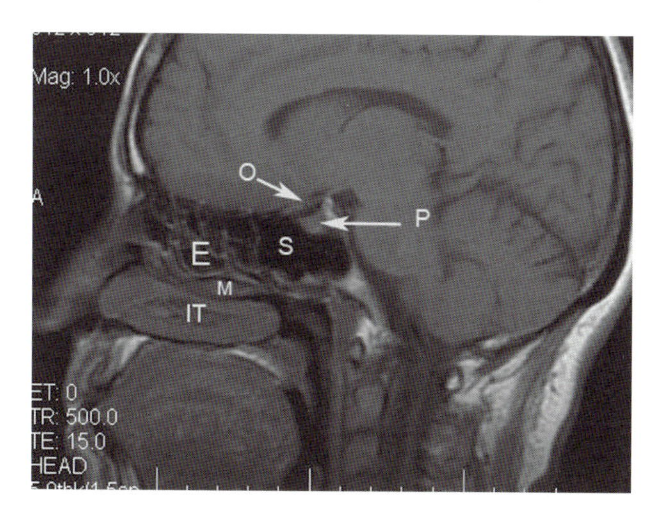

Figure 5.67 *Sphenoid sinus.* Sagittal T1-weighted MRI scan demonstrating the sphenoid sinus (S), pituitary gland (P), optic nerve (O), ethmoid sinuses (E), middle turbinate (M), and inferior turbinate (IT).

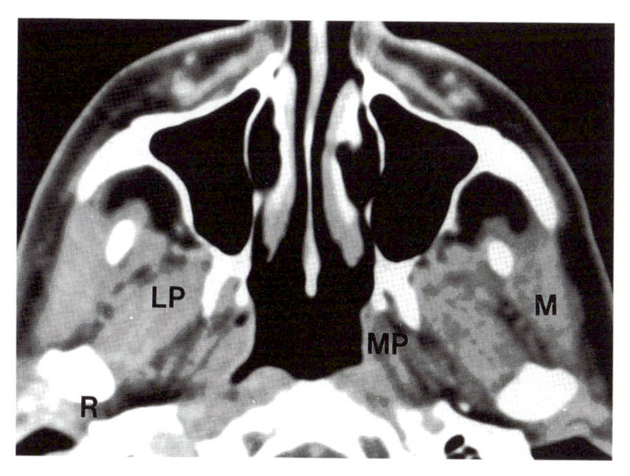

Figure 5.69 *Normal axial scan.* This narrow-window scan demonstrates the muscles of mastication, namely the lateral pterygoid (LP), medial pterygoid (MP), and masseter (M). The muscles are clearly separated by fat planes.

intravenous contrast, and should not be mistaken for tumor.

The infraorbital fissure transmits the infraorbital nerve, and is the main communication between the orbit and both the pterygopalatine fossa and the infratemporal fossa.

CT of the orbital apex usually demonstrates these anatomical features clearly separated by fat. If the fat planes are obscured, this may indicate early infiltration with tumor or aggressive infection.

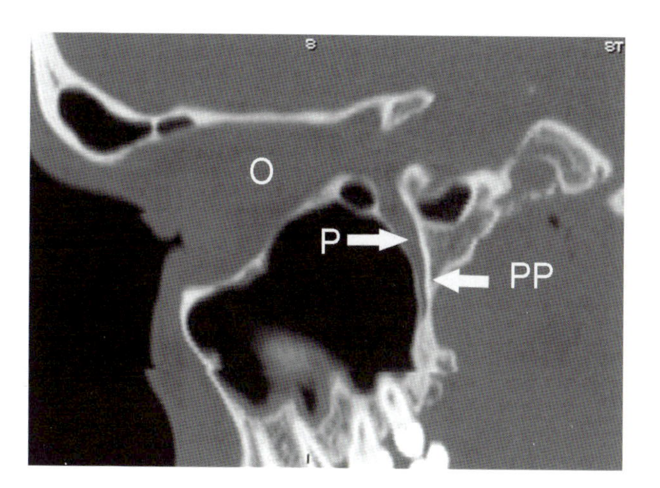

Figure 5.70 *Pterygopalatine fossa.* This space (P) is seen on this sagittal CT scan to lie between the maxillary sinus anteriorly and the pterygoid plates (PP) posteriorly. O, orbit.

LACRIMAL SAC AND NASOLACRIMAL DUCT
(Figures 5.57, 5.68, 5.76, and 5.77)

The nasolacrimal apparatus consists of the lacrimal gland situated in the superolateral aspect of the orbit, the lacrimal sac, and the nasolacrimal duct. The sac and the duct are the final drainage pathways for the tears produced by the lacrimal gland. The lacrimal sac is a membranous sac situated in the lacrimal fossa inferolateral to the medial canthus. The lacrimal fossa is bounded anteriorly by the anterior lacrimal crest of the frontal process of the maxilla and posteriorly by the posterior lacrimal crest, which is a ridge on the lacrimal bone. The lacrimal sac has a bulbous fundus superiorly. Inferiorly, it tapers to become continuous with the nasolacrimal duct.

The nasolacrimal duct has two parts: an intraosseous part and a membranous part. The duct is directed inferiorly, posteriorly, and slightly laterally. The intraosseous part is bounded by the maxilla, the lacrimal bone, and the inferior turbinate. The duct is narrowest in the middle. Inferiorly, it lies beneath the nasal mucosa and opens into the highest point of the inferior meatus, where it is protected by Hasner's valve.

The lacrimal fossa is readily identified as a small impression in the inferomedial orbital wall by CT in both the axial and the coronal planes. The lacrimal sac is usually seen as a soft tissue density in the lacrimal fossa. It may be air-filled on occasion, and should not be mistaken for orbital emphysema.

The membranous part of the nasolacrimal duct varies in its relationship to the base of the uncinate process and the ethmoid infundibulum. This relationship should be identified prior to any surgery in the region. The nasolacrimal duct may be

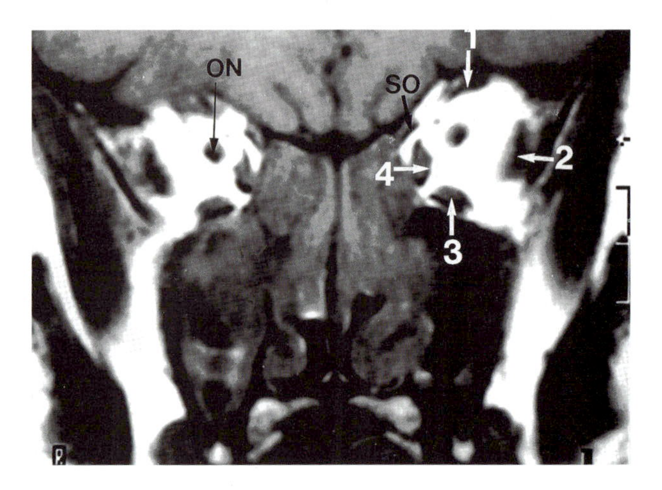

Figure 5.72 *Orbital apex.* The orbital apex is well demonstrated on this coronal T1-weighted MRI scan showing the medial rectus (4), lateral rectus (2), inferior rectus (3), superior rectus (1), and superior oblique (SO) muscles, as well as the optic nerve (ON). This scan also demonstrates inflammatory and polypoidal disease in the sinuses. The fat in the orbit is bright on this T1-weighted sequence.

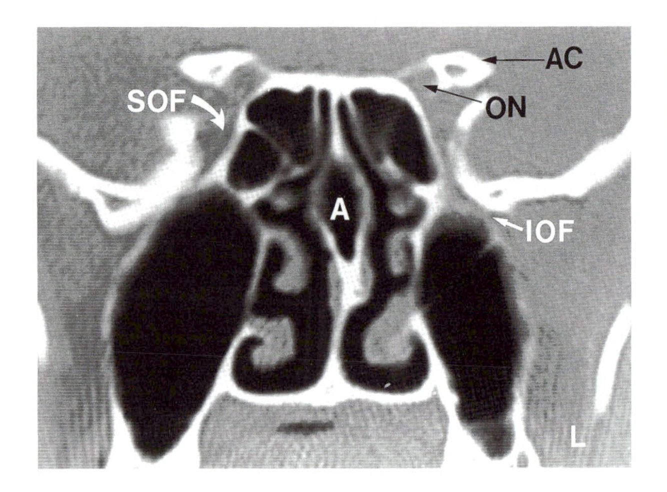

Figure 5.71 *Orbital apex.* Scan demonstrating the normal characteristics of the inferior orbital fissure (IOF), superior orbital fissure (SOF), optic nerve (ON), and anterior clinoids (AC). The nasal septum is pneumatized (A).

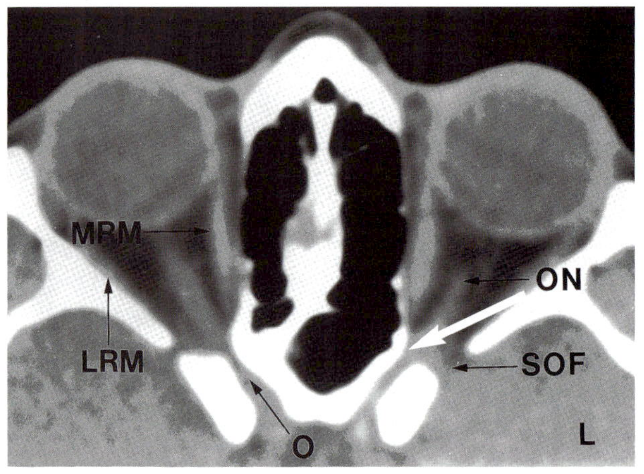

Figure 5.73 *Orbital apex and extraocular muscles.* Axial scan demonstrating the bony optic canal (O), the optic nerve (ON) passing through this canal, and the laterally placed superior orbital fissure (SOF). The medial (MRM) and lateral (LRM) rectus muscles are well demonstrated.

injured by a generous uncinectomy conducted during an endoscopic procedure, or by an excessive resection of the anterior margin of the natural ostium of the maxillary sinus. If the inferior turbinate is resected close to the base, the duct may be injured, resulting in permanent occlusion of the nasolacrimal canal and epiphora. The nasolacrimal duct may also become obstructed by inflammatory disease, trauma, or neoplastic processes.

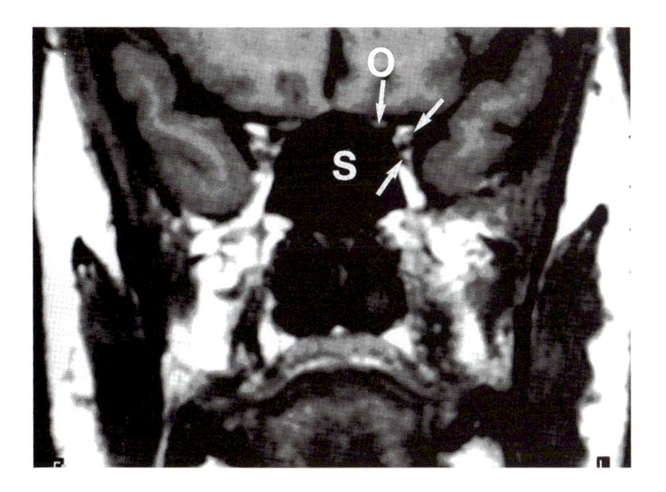

Figure 5.74 *Tendinous ring of Zinn (annulus of Zinn).* Posterior coronal T1-weighted MRI scan through the sphenoid sinus (S) demonstrating the tendinous ring of Zinn at the orbital apex, which gives origin to the rectus muscles (arrows). The optic nerve (O) is superomedial to the annulus.

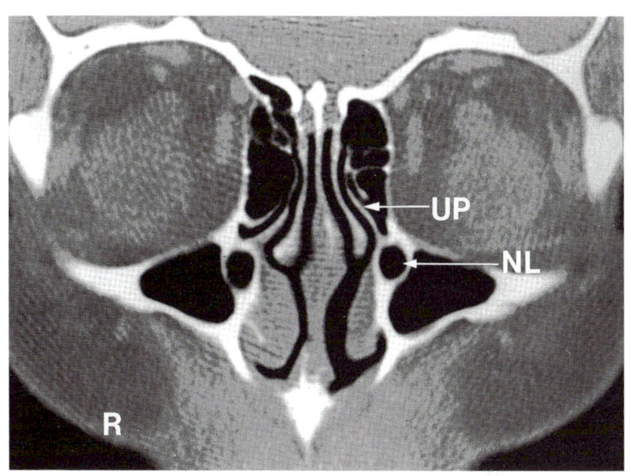

Figure 5.76 *Nasolacrimal duct.* Anterior coronal scan demonstrating air in both nasolacrimal ducts (NL). The nasolacrimal duct is bounded by the maxilla, lacrimal bone, and inferior turbinate. Both uncinate processes (UP) are elongated. Note the intimate relationship between the origin of the uncinate processes and the nasolacrimal duct.

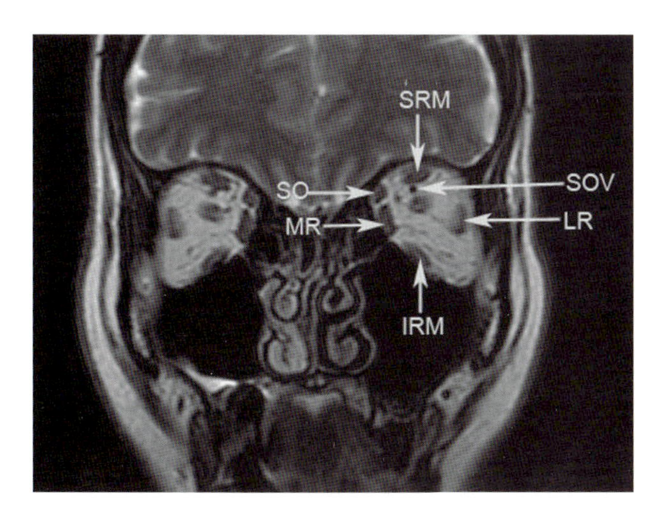

Figure 5.75 *Orbit.* Coronal MRI scan demonstrating the medial rectus muscle (MR), lateral rectus muscle (LR), superior rectus muscle (SRM), superior ophthalmic vein (SOV), superior oblique muscle (SO), and inferior rectus muscle (IRM).

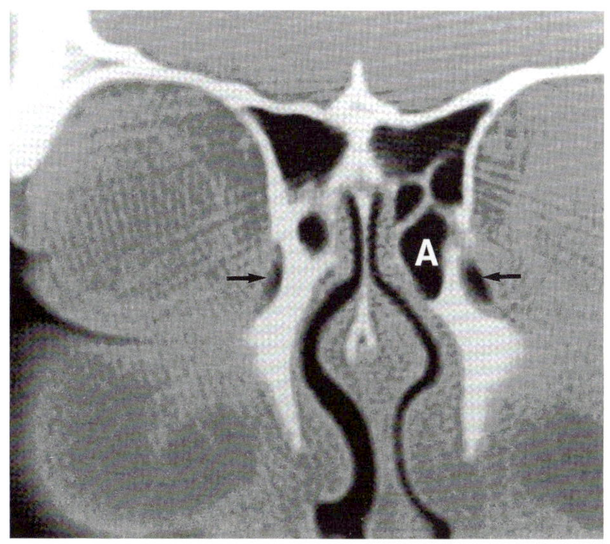

Figure 5.77 *Air in the lacrimal sac.* The small air collections seen along the inferomedial aspect of the orbits are air within the lacrimal sac (arrows). This should not be mistaken for orbital emphysema following fracture or infection. An agger nasi cell (A) is also demonstrated.

6

Anatomical variants of the ostiomeatal complex in the paranasal sinuses

Messerklinger demonstrated that ventilation and drainage of the anterior ethmoid sinus, the maxillary sinus, and the frontal sinus are dependent upon the patency of the ostiomeatal complex through which these sinuses connect into the nasal cavity.

Most sinus infections are rhinogenic in origin and spread from the ostiomeatal complex to secondarily involve the frontal and maxillary sinuses. The small clefts of the ostiomeatal complex in the lateral nasal wall are easily narrowed or occluded by mucosal edema, resulting in impaired ventilation, failure of mucociliary clearance, and the stagnation of mucus and/or pus in the larger paranasal sinuses.

This process is usually reversible, and once the ostiomeatal complex is reopened, the secondary disease within the larger maxillary and frontal sinuses usually resolves spontaneously. If, however, there is an anatomical variant that narrows these key ethmoid clefts, then a minimal amount of mucosal edema may predispose the patient to recurrent infections and may result in chronic inflammatory changes in the mucosa.

Previously, surgical procedures to alleviate recurrent or chronic inflammatory episodes have been directed at the larger paranasal sinuses. The ventilation of these sinuses was improved by creating new and theoretically effective alternative drainage pathways. The alternative drainage procedures, such as an inferior meatal antrostomy, are now known not to redirect the flow of mucus through the newly created opening (antrostomy), but only to act as 'drains' when the mucociliary system is overwhelmed by mucus and pus. The persistence of symptoms following these procedures is usually secondary to persistent disease in the anterior ethmoid affecting the natural ostia and the ostiomeatal complex. When ostiomeatal complex disease is present, recurrent sinus infections may also occur despite there being a widely patent natural accessory ostium.

Functional endoscopic sinus surgery is directed at the natural drainage pathways. The limited surgical resection of tissue that widens these natural clefts and improves sinus ventilation usually leads to a reversal of the mucosal disease in the larger paranasal sinuses. Direct endoscopic examination and visualization of the small clefts of the ostiomeatal complex are not possible, and consequently computed tomography (CT), especially in the coronal plane, is essential for the assessment of the patient with recurrent or persistent sinusitis. Coronal CT allows the radiologist to determine the site and extent of disease in the paranasal sinuses and in the surrounding soft tissues and to identify those anatomical variants that may predispose the individual to sinusitis. Although it is recognized that anatomical variations occur in individuals with no history of rhinosinusitis, variations of the size or position of the normal structures in the lateral nasal wall can impede optimal sinus drainage and occur alongside recurrent sinusitis. Important anatomical variants in the sinuses and the nasal cavity of which surgeons must be aware prior to any intervention are discussed in this chapter.

These important anatomical variants are listed in Table 6.1.

Table 6.1 Important anatomical structures of the ostiomeatal complex and their variations

I. Variations in the structures of the ostiomeatal complex

1. Large agger nasi cells
   - When present and enlarged, agger nasi cells can obstruct the frontal recess
2. Uncinate process
   - Aplasia or hypoplasia
   - Medial or lateral deflection
   - Pneumatization
   - Hypertrophy
   - Accessory middle turbinate
3. Middle turbinate
   - Paradoxically bent middle turbinate
   - Secondary middle turbinates
   - Lateralization of middle turbinate
   - Aplasia or hypoplasia
   - Hypertrophy
   - Soft tissue and bony hypertrophy of middle turbinate
   - Concha bullosa
4. Ethmoid bulla
   - Large:
     Protrudes into middle meatus
     Overhangs hiatus semilunaris
     Obstructs ethmoid infundibulum
     Obstructs frontal recess
   - Hypoplasia
5. Large Haller's cells
   - When present and enlarged, a Haller's cell can obstruct the natural ostium of the maxillary sinus and the infundibulum
6. Nasal septum
   - Deviation of nasal septum and septal spurs

II. Other variants to note before surgery

- Dehiscence of lamina papyracea
- Dehiscence of orbital floor
- Low-lying fovea ethmoidalis
- Dehiscence of optic nerve canal
- Dehiscence of internal carotid artery bony wall
- Hypoplasia of maxillary sinus
- Ethmomaxillary sinus
- Ethmosphenoid sinus
- Unilateral atresia of nasal cavity

AGGER NASI CELLS (Figures 6.1–6.5)

The extent of pneumatization of the agger mound can be clearly seen on CT scans in the coronal plane. Agger nasi cells are usually pneumatized from the frontal recess. Enlarged agger nasi cells may involve the frontal recess either by obstructing the frontal recess mechanically if they are well developed or by direct spread of inflammation.

Pneumatization of the agger mound may be so extensive that it encroaches either upon the lacrimal bone or upon the neck of the middle turbinate. Pneumatization of the agger mound can shorten the neck of the middle turbinate, resulting in a tight frontal recess. The agger nasi cells are closely related to the lacrimal sac, being separated from the latter only by the delicate lacrimal bone. This thin bony plate may be naturally dehiscent and, as a result, inflammation can spread readily into the lacrimal sac, resulting in epiphora, dacryocystitis, and sometimes preseptal or periorbital cellulitis.

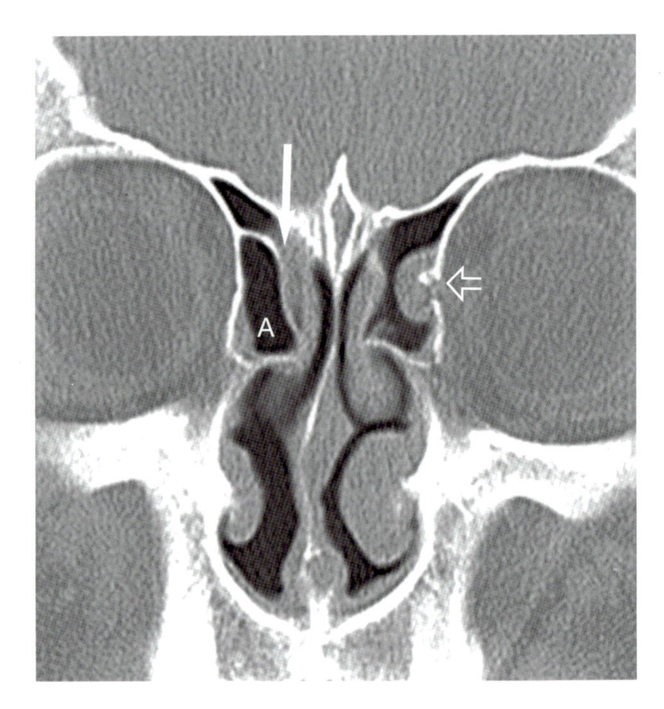

Figure 6.1 *Large agger nasi cell.* CT scan demonstrating a large right agger nasi cell (A) occluding the frontal recess (arrow) and resulting in frontal recess disease, normal lacrimal fossae. Note the erosion of the lateral wall of the orbit on the left side (open arrow).

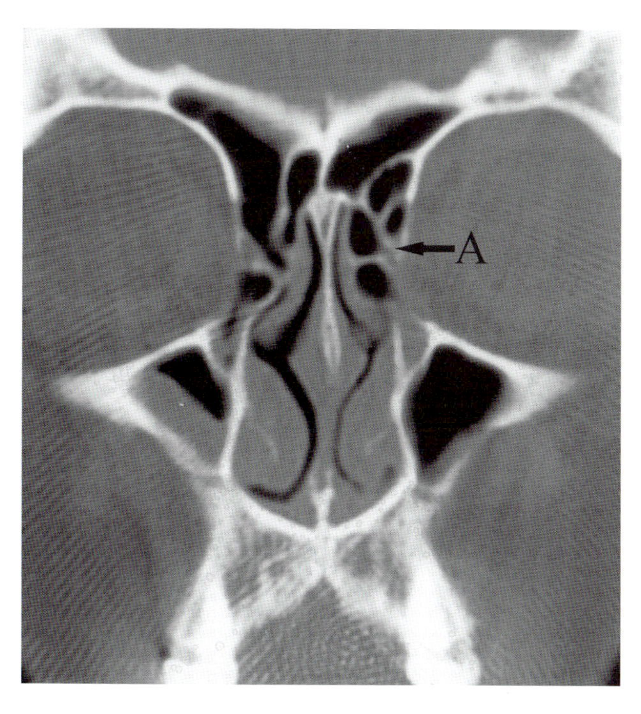

Figure 6.2 *Multiseptate agger nasi cell.* CT scan demonstrating a multiseptate agger nasi cell (A) on the left side.

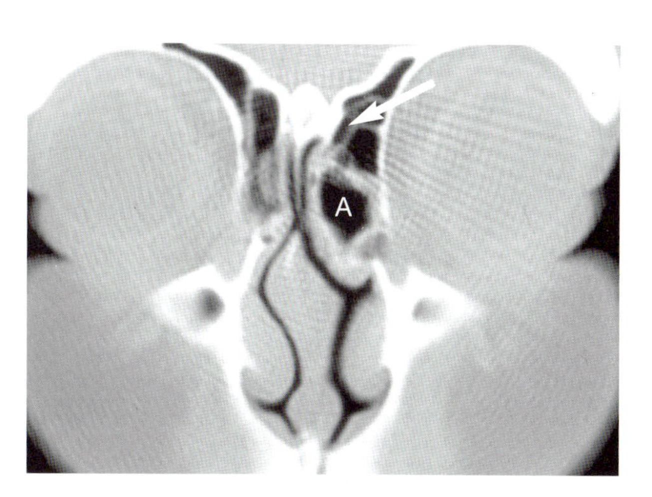

Figure 6.4 *Agger nasi cell and encroachment on neck of middle turbinate.* Anterior CT scan showing a large agger nasi (A) cell encroaching on the waist of the middle turbinate and compromising the frontal recess (arrow) on the left side.

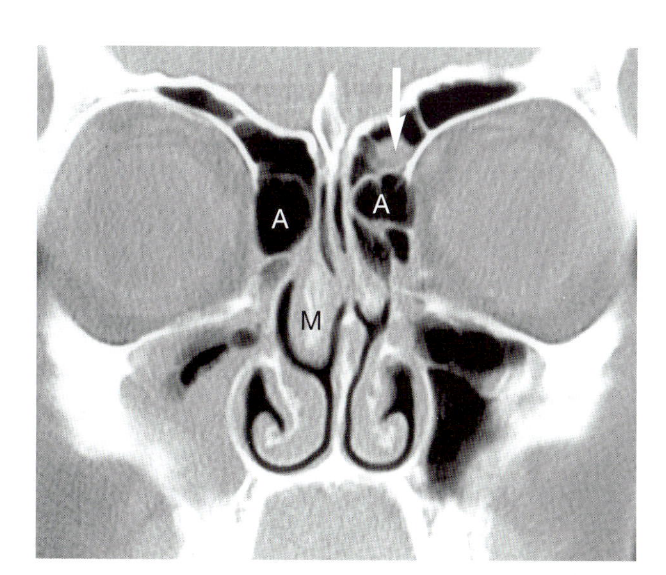

Figure 6.3 *Agger nasi cell and frontal recess disease.* Inflammatory disease can be seen in the large agger nasi cells and the left frontal recess (arrow). The large agger nasi cells (A) encroach on the neck of the middle turbinate. The larger the agger nasi cell, the greater the encroachment on the neck of the middle turbinate (M), resulting in a restricted frontal recess. The medial wall of the orbit is extremely thin and inflammation may spread through the wall to involve the orbit or the lacrimal sac.

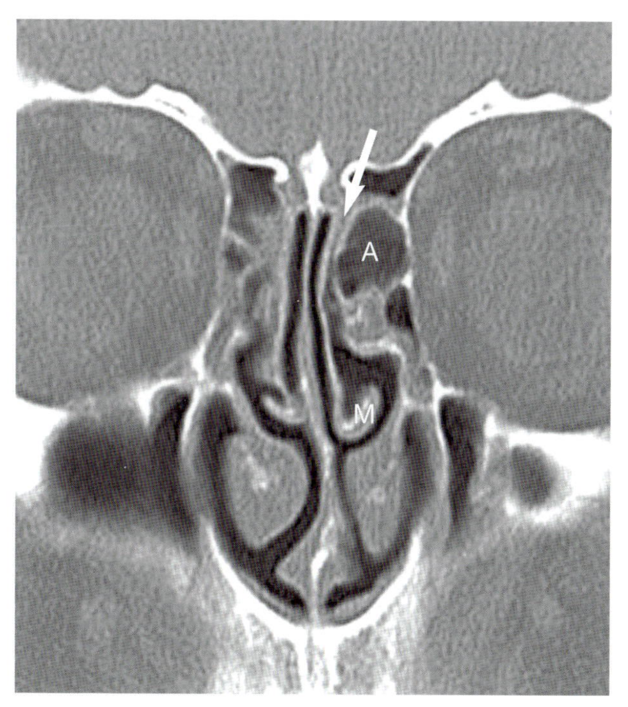

Figure 6.5 *Agger nasi cell and encroachment on neck of middle turbinate.* A large agger nasi cell (A) is against the vertical plate of the middle turbinate (M) associated with appositional changes in the frontal recess very close to the lamina lateralis of the cribriform plate (arrow) – the thinnest part of the plate, where extra precaution is necessary during endoscopic procedures.

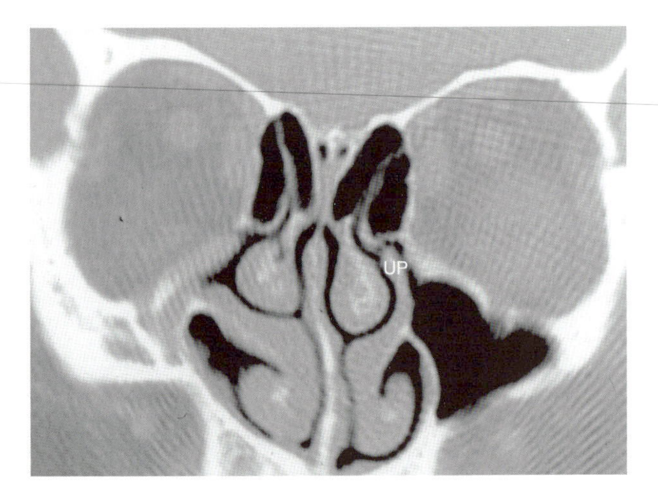

Figure 6.6 *Aplasia of uncinate process.* CT scan demonstrating a normal-appearing uncinate process (UP) on the left side. The maxillary sinus on the left side is normal. The UP is not visualized on the right side. This is associated with type III maxillary sinus hypoplasia on the right side.

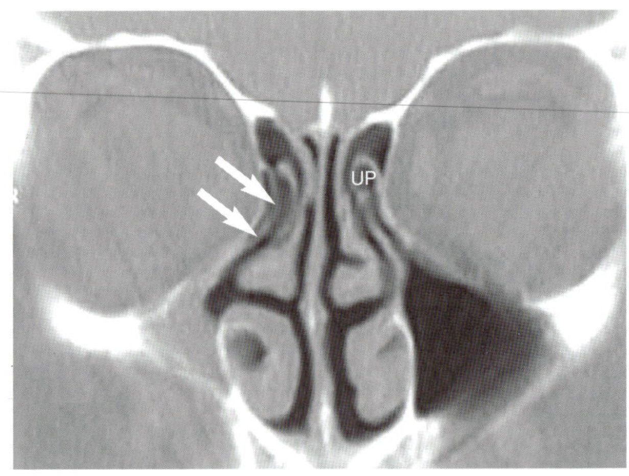

Figure 6.7 *Hypoplasia of uncinate process.* CT scan demonstrating lateral retraction of the posterior fontanelle of the maxillary sinus and right maxillary sinus hypoplasia. The uncinate process appears absent; however, on closer inspection, it can be seen adherent to the inferior orbital wall (arrows). The left uncinate process (UP) is seen to curve laterally and to insert on the lateral wall of the orbit.

UNCINATE PROCESS

Uncinate process aplasia (Figure 6.6)

Aplasia of the uncinate process is associated with type III maxillary sinus hypoplasia.

Uncinate process hypoplasia (Figure 6.7)

Various anomalies of the uncinate process can occur. Rarely, the uncinate process is hypoplastic. Hypoplasia of the uncinate process has been associated with hypoplasia of the maxillary sinus. In this condition, the middle meatus is wide and the posterior fontanelle is retracted into the cavity of the maxillary sinus. The uncinate process is plastered against the inferomedial wall of the orbit. A traditional uncinectomy can lead to orbital penetration and injury. The uncinate process has an intimate relationship with the ethmoid infundibulum and the middle meatus.

Medial deviation of the uncinate process (Figures 6.8 and 6.9)

The commonest anatomical variants associated with inflammatory disease of the adjacent paranasal sinuses are medial deviations and elongated free margins of the uncinate process. In these circumstances, the uncinate process may abut the middle turbinate, thus obstructing the middle meatus.

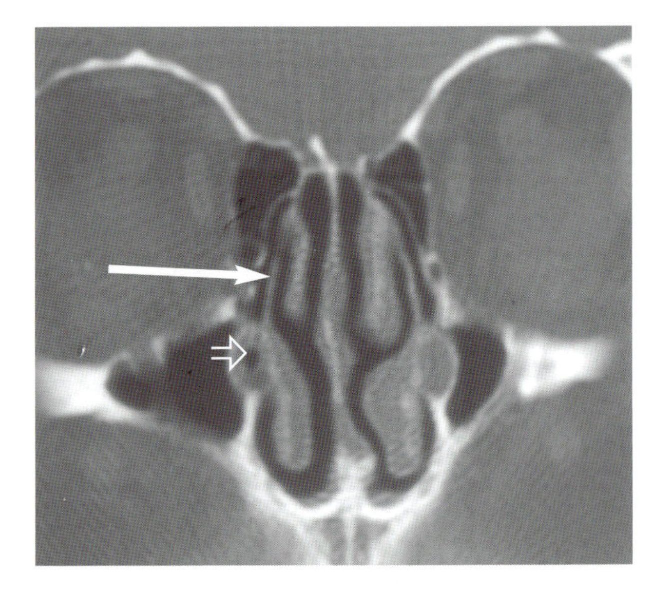

Figure 6.8 *Medially bent uncinate process.* CT scan demonstrating medial deflection of the uncinate processes (long arrow). The base of the uncinate process is close to the nasolacrimal duct (open arrow), and a generous uncinectomy can result in postoperative epiphora.

Long uncinate process (Figure 6.10)

A long uncinate process will narrow the hiatus semilunaris between its posterior margin and the ethmoid bulla, especially if the bulla is well pneumatized.

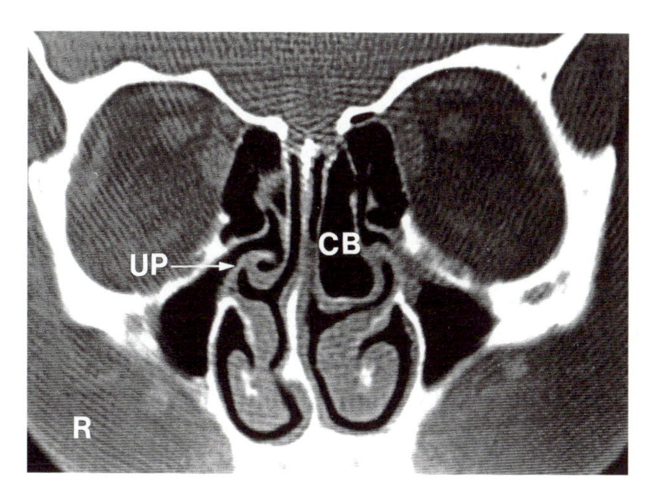

Figure 6.9 *Medially bent uncinate process*. The right uncinate process (UP) is medially rotated and has come into intimate contact with the middle turbinate. Although the hiatus semilunaris is not obstructed, the medially bent uncinate process is occluding the middle meatus. This CT scan also demonstrates a very large left-sided concha bullosa (CB), onto which the left uncinate process abuts.

Anterior protrusion of the uncinate process (Figure 6.11)

The uncinate process may also protrude anteriorly and compromise the middle meatus. The uncinate process may be rotated medially to such an extent that its posterior free margin projects anteriorly. Clinically, the anterior end of an anteriorly rotated uncinate process resembles a Mexican hat and may be incorrectly identified as an accessory or double middle turbinate. This anomaly may cause mucosal apposition that subsequently leads to inflammatory changes and polypoidal degeneration.

Inferior deflection of the uncinate process (Figures 6.10 and 6.12)

The free margin of the uncinate process may be long, deflect inferiorly, and fold upon itself, thus impeding drainage through the hiatus semilunaris.

Aerated uncinate and hypertrophy of the uncinate process (Figures 6.13–6.15)

An aerated uncinate may become large enough to occlude the ethmoid infundibulum, or it may even be the site of polyp formation. A swollen, inflamed

6.10a

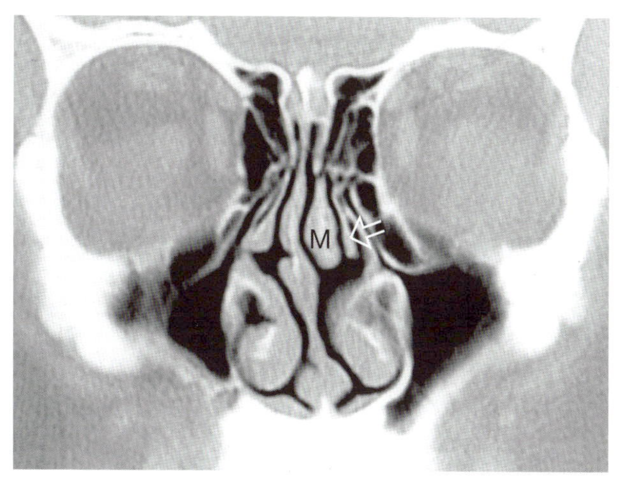

6.10b

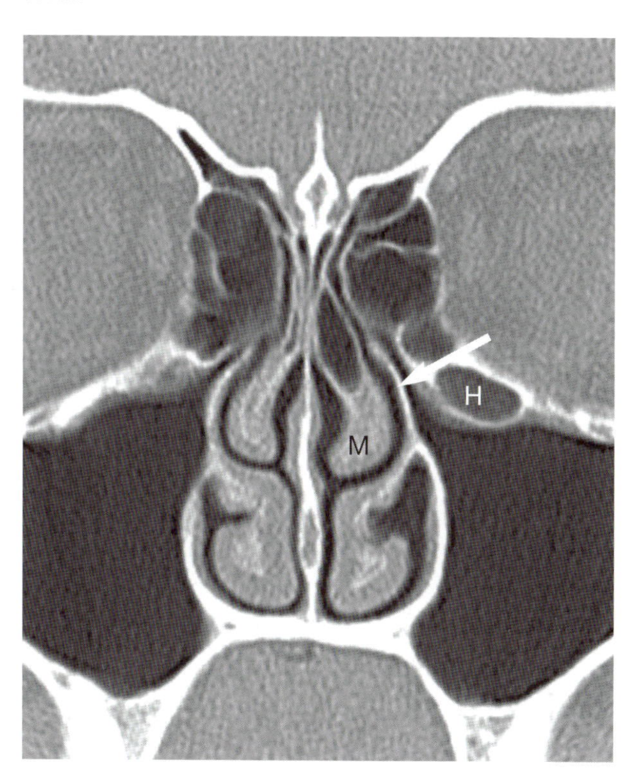

Figure 6.10 (a) *Elongated uncinate process*. An elongated uncinate process is seen turned medially on the right side, which can obstruct the hiatus semilunaris (the cleft connecting the ethmoid infundibulum to the middle meatus). The middle turbinate is small. There is a long uncinate process on the left side that has a sharp U-shaped bend and is deflected inferiorly (open arrow). M, middle turbinate. (b) *Long uncinate process*. Bilateral long uncinate processes are noted inferior and medial to the ethmoid infundibulum (arrow). The arrow shows the drainage of the maxillary sinus ostium into the ethmoid infundibulum. M, middle turbinate; H, Haller's cell.

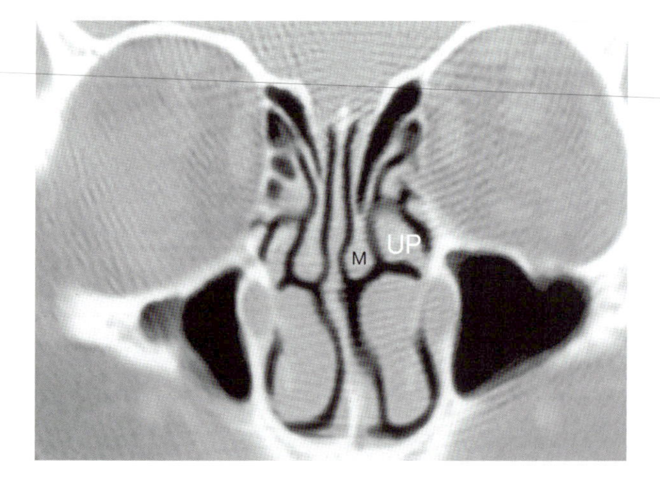

Figure 6.11 *Anteriorly bent uncinate process.* The uncinate processes (UP) in this coronal CT scan are rotated anteriorly to such an extent that they project anteriorly into the middle meatus. M, middle turbinate.

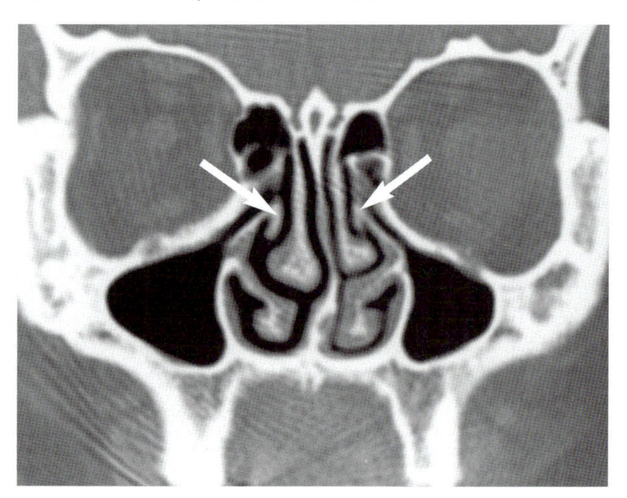

Figure 6.12 *Inferior deflection of uncinate process.* The uncinate processes (arrows) are inferiorly deflected.

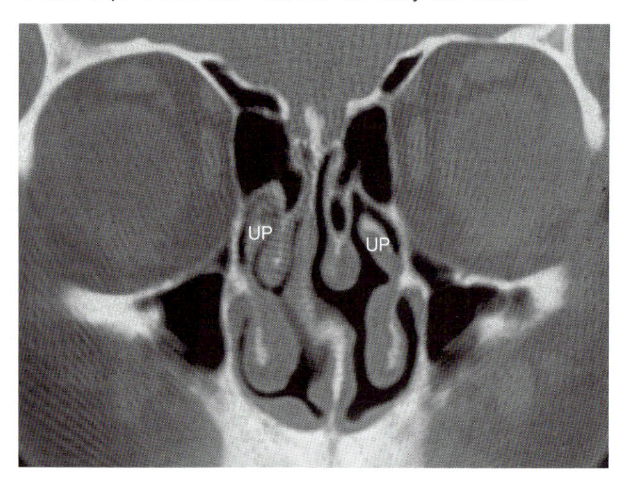

Figure 6.13 *Hypertrophied uncinate process.* Grossly enlarged uncinate processes can be seen projecting anteromedially into the middle meatus (UP). On the left side, the middle meatus appears to be almost filled by the uncinate process. The nasal septum, which is deviated to the left, shows evidence of prior trauma.

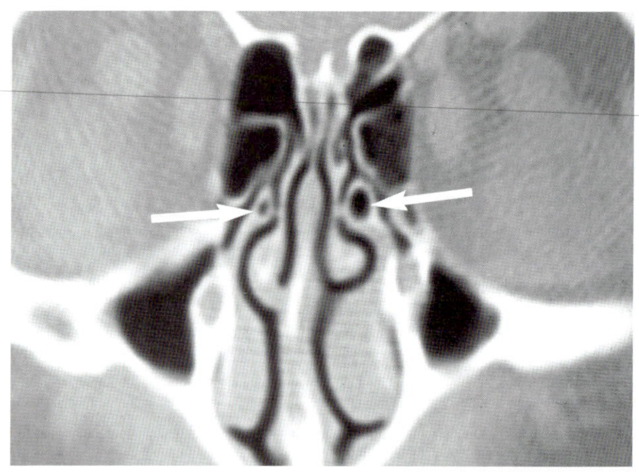

Figure 6.14 *Pneumatized uncinate process.* The tiny uncinate process may be aerated. In this CT scan, both uncinate processes are pneumatized (arrows). The enlarged aerated uncinate process on the left compromises the middle meatus and the ethmoid infundibulum. An aerated uncinate may become large enough to occlude the ethmoid infundibulum, or it may be the site of polyp formation.

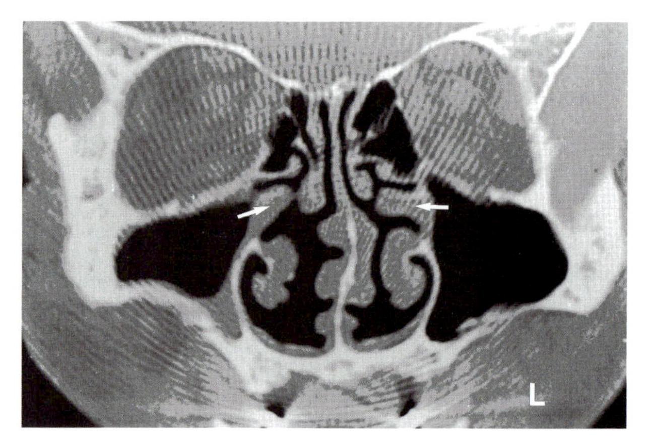

Figure 6.15 *Enlarged uncinate processes.* Coronal CT scan demonstrating bilateral enlargement and medial deviation of the uncinate processes (arrows). These enlarged uncinate processes have narrowed the infundibula.

uncinate process is clearly visualized by endoscopy, but pneumatization of the uncinate process cannot be differentiated from hypertrophy by endoscopy.

Lateral deviation of the uncinate process

The uncinate process may deviate laterally, causing obstruction of the ethmoid infundibulum and the maxillary sinus ostium. Should the posterior free margin of the uncinate process be deflected medially, it may resemble a turbinate and has been incorrectly referred to as an accessory or double middle turbinate.

Accessory middle turbinate
(Figures 6.16 and 6.17)

When the free posterior margin of the uncinate process deflects medially, it resembles a Mexican hat and may be incorrectly identified clinically as an accessory or double middle turbinate. This anomaly may cause mucosal apposition, subsequently leading to inflammatory changes and polypoidal degeneration. The accessory middle turbinate may be mistaken for a polyp on casual examination.

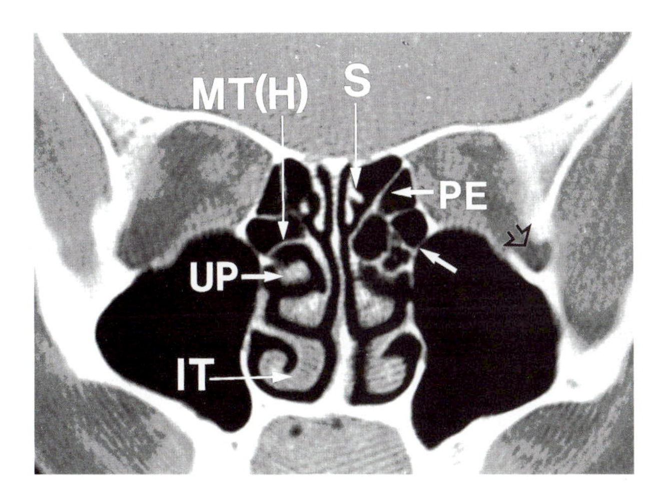

Figure 6.16 *Medially bent uncinate process.* The right uncinate process (UP) is medially bent and protrudes into the middle meatus. Note the inferior turbinate (IT), the horizontal plate of the middle turbinate (MT(H)), and the superior and supreme turbinates (S). The ethmomaxillary plate (arrow) separates the maxillary sinus from the posterior ethmoid sinus (PE). The inferior orbital fissure can also be seen.

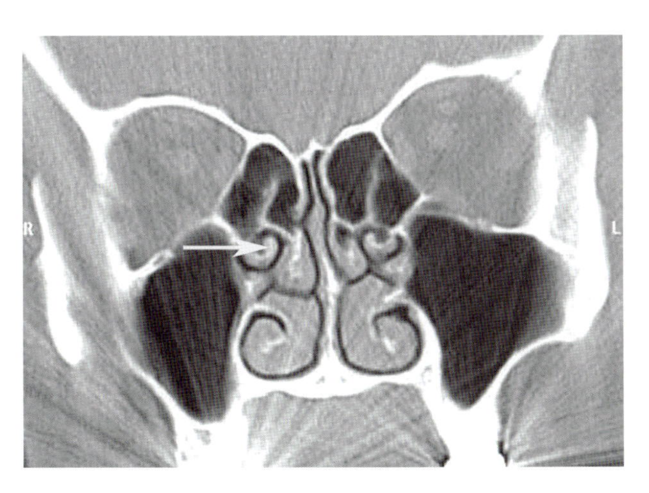

Figure 6.17 Accessory middle turbinate. When the free posterior edge of the uncinate process is deflected medially then it is misinterpreted as an accessory middle turbinate (arrow).

MIDDLE TURBINATE ANOMALIES

The advent of CT has advanced our understanding of the variations that occur of the middle turbinate. The presence and significance of middle turbinate abnormalities should be viewed in the light of the patient's symptoms. These anatomical variants are readily identified by CT; they include aeration of the middle turbinate (a concha bullosa), hypertrophy of the middle turbinate, paradoxically bent middle turbinate, lateralization of the turbinate, bony hypertrophy of the middle turbinate, and partial or complete agenesis.

Paradoxically bent middle turbinate
(Figure 6.18)

Normally, the lateral surface of the middle turbinate is concave, curving away from the lateral nasal wall to allow space for the middle meatus. When the lateral surface of the middle turbinate is convex or the turbinate appears to be bending medially, it is called a 'paradoxically bent middle turbinate'. This usually occurs bilaterally and may reduce the middle meatus considerably. A concha bullosa occurring in a paradoxically bent middle turbinate may further reduce the middle meatus and at times may contribute to the pathogenesis of sinus disease.

Lateralized middle turbinate
(Figures 6.19 and 6.20)

A lateralized middle turbinate is a middle turbinate that is laterally displaced, resulting in contact with the adjacent uncinate process. A lateralized middle turbinate may obstruct the ethmoid infundibulum.

Secondary middle turbinate and sagittal grooves in middle turbinate
(Figures 6.21–6.24)

Rarely, a small secondary middle turbinate is seen in the middle meatus. A secondary middle turbinate should not be confused with an anteriorly bent uncinate process, which is also called an 'accessory

6.18a

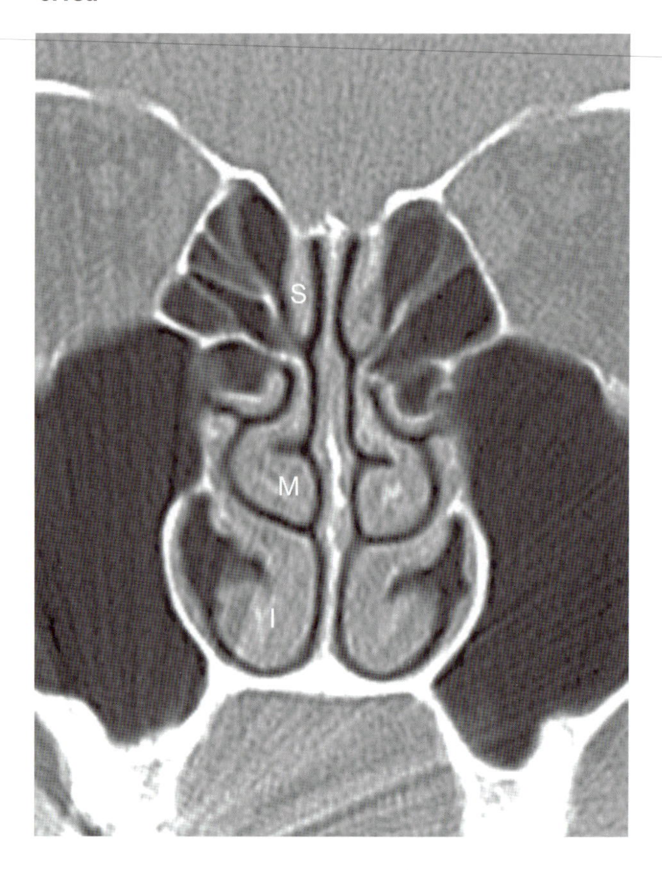

6.18b

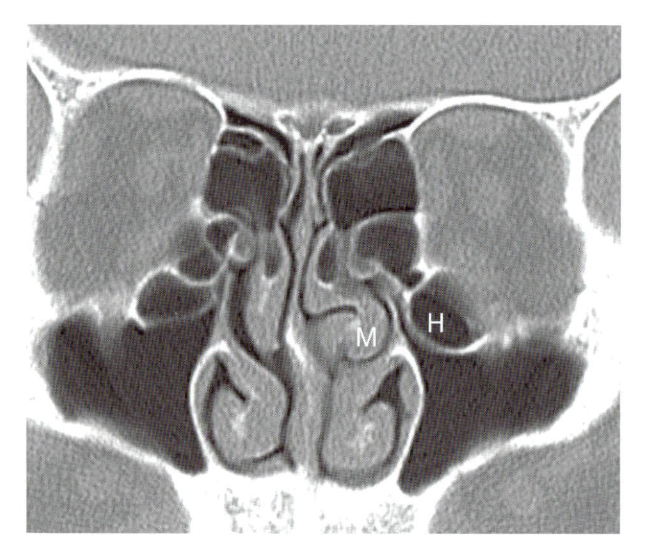

Figure 6.18 *Paradoxically bent middle turbinate*. (a) There is bilateral paradoxical curvature of the middle turbinates (M). I, inferior turbinate; S, superior turbinate. (b) There is a left paradoxical curvature of the middle turbinate (M) and a Haller's cell (H), narrowing the ostiomeatal complex.

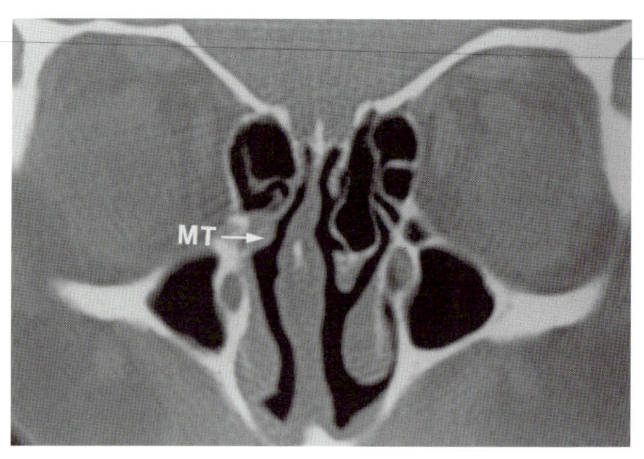

Figure 6.19 *Lateralized middle turbinate*. The middle turbinate (MT) is laterally displaced, resulting in contact with the adjacent uncinate process. A lateralized middle turbinate may obstruct the ethmoid infundibulum. In this patient, a left concha bullosa with aeration of the vertical plate is seen.

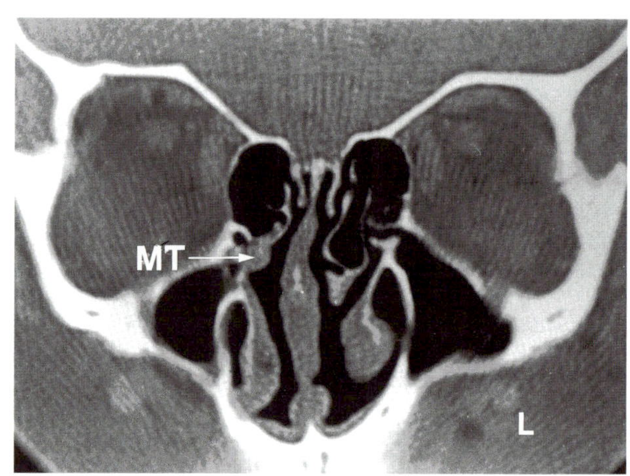

Figure 6.20 *Lateralized middle turbinate* (MT).

middle turbinate', nor should it be mistaken for a polyp. These secondary middle turbinates are composed of bone covered by soft tissue, and project medially from the lateral nasal wall into the middle meatus before turning superiorly within the meatus to appear as an inverted turbinate. This anomaly has not been noted to compromise the ostiomeatal complex. The inferior free margin of the middle turbinate may be grooved or ridged.

Hypertrophy of the middle turbinate (Figures 6.25 and 6.26)

It is not possible on routine clinical examination to differentiate between a hypertrophied and a pneumatized middle turbinate. However, the difference

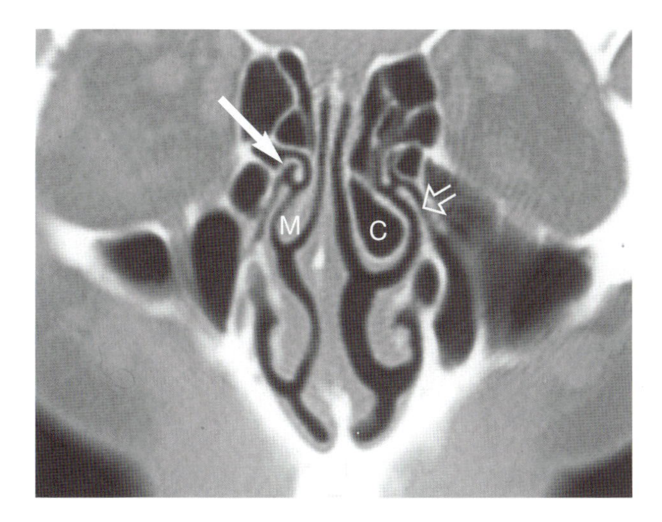

Figures 6.21 *Secondary middle turbinate*. The secondary middle turbinate (arrow) is seen protruding like a small shelf into the middle meatus. Note that the right middle turbinate (M) is hypoplastic or small and there is a concha bullosa (C) on the left side. The uncinate process is indicated by the open arrow.

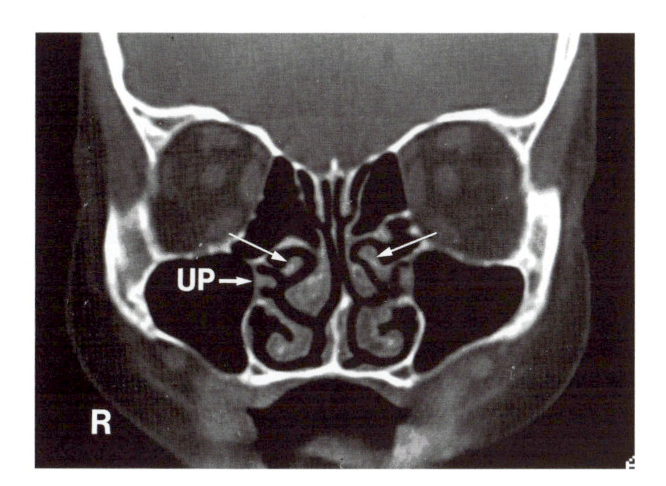

Figure 6.22 *Secondary middle turbinate*. A secondary middle turbinate (arrows) is seen bilaterally. The uncinate process (UP) is seen to be bent medially.

is readily apparent on CT scans. The hypertrophy of the middle turbinate may be bony, soft tissue, or a combination of the two.

Hypoplasia and aplasia of the middle turbinate

(Figures 6.21, 6.27, and 6.48a)

It is not uncommon to see asymmetry in the size of the middle turbinates. Deviation of the nasal septum occurs when the middle turbinate is pneumatized or hypertrophied on one side. As a result, there is contralateral hypoplasia or aplasia of the middle turbinate.

In some individuals, the middle turbinate may not develop completely. This condition is referred to as a 'rudimentary' or 'vestigial' middle turbinate.

6.23a

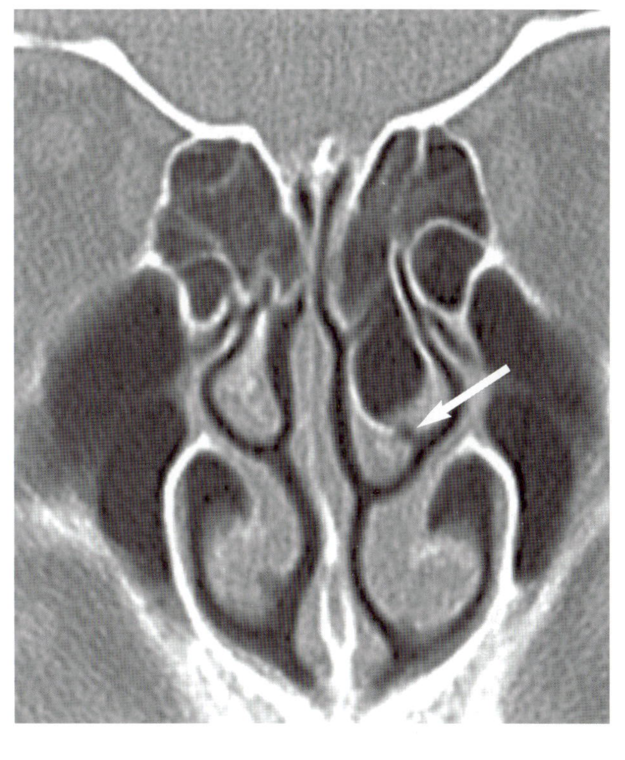

6.23b

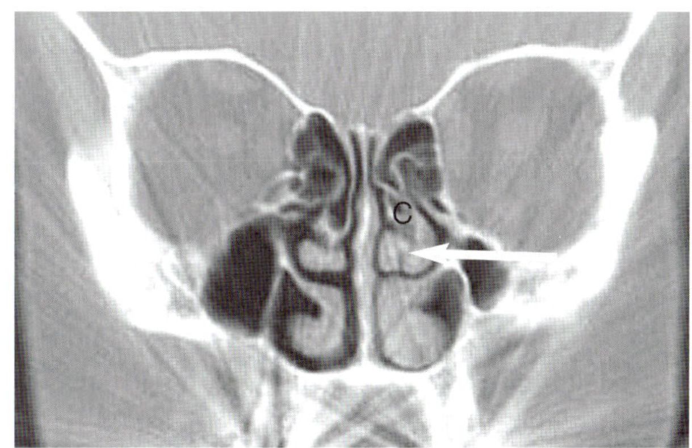

Figure 6.23 *Grooved middle turbinate*. (a) CT scan demonstrating sagittal groove (arrow) along the free margin of the left middle turbinate. (b) CT scan demonstrating a sagittal groove (arrow) along the free margin of the left middle turbinate with a concha bullosa (C).

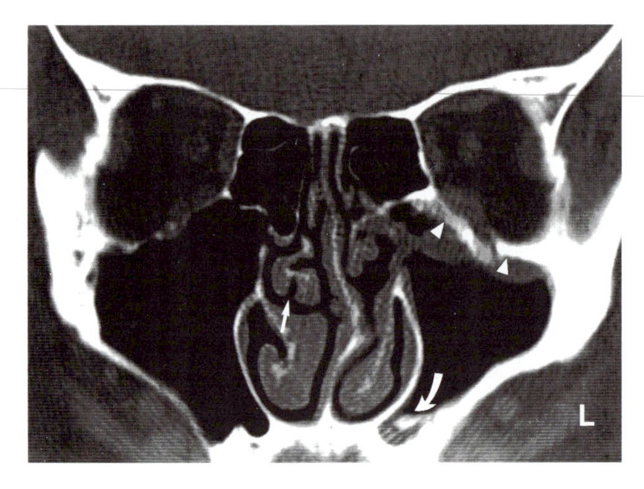

Figure 6.24 *Grooved middle turbinate.* CT scan demonstrating a sagittal groove (arrow) along the inferior free margin of the right middle turbinate. There is evidence of chronic sinusitis with reactive osteitis near the infraorbital canal (arrowheads), which is characteristic of benign disease. Note the unerupted tooth in the floor of the maxillary sinus (curved arrow).

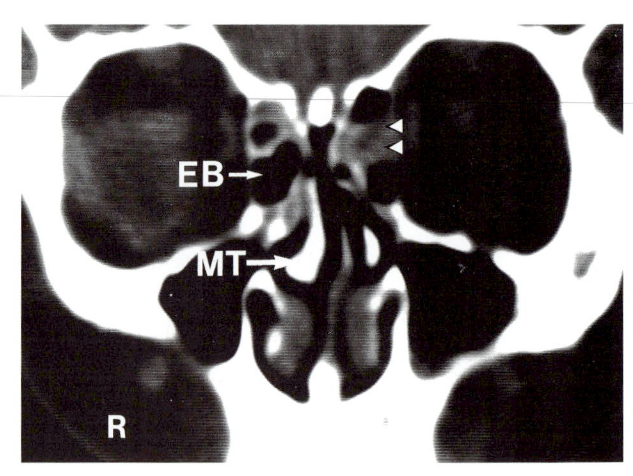

Figure 6.26 *Bony hypertrophy of the middle turbinate.* CT scan demonstrating that the right middle turbinate (MT) is predominantly bony with no soft tissue hypertrophy. This warns the surgeon that the resection may be difficult. Inflammatory disease is seen in the right ethmoid infundibulum and in the left suprabullar space (arrowheads) above the ethmoid bulla (EB).

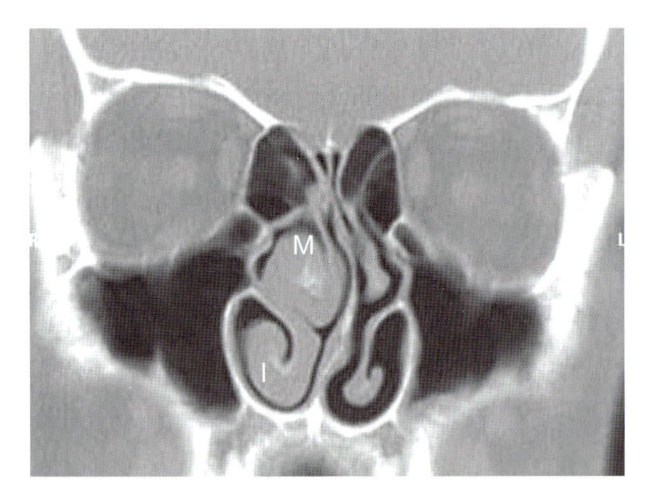

Figure 6.25 *Soft tissue hypertrophy of middle turbinates.* CT scan demonstrating that the enlargement of this right middle turbinate (M) is predominantly soft tissue hypertrophy. There is associated deviation of the adjacent nasal septum. The inferior turbinate (I) is also hypertrophied.

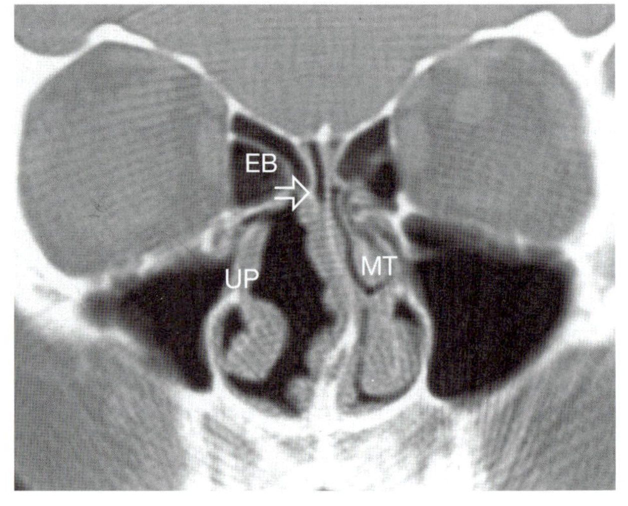

Figure 6.27 *Vestigial middle turbinate with hypertrophy of uncinate process.* There was no history of previous surgery in the patient; however, the right middle turbinate was found to be vestigial (open arrow) and the uncinate process (UP) was grossly enlarged. The right ethmoid bulla (EB) and the left middle turbinate (MT) are normal.

Concha bullosa of the middle turbinate (Figures 6.28–6.40; Table 6.2)

When a turbinate contains an air cell, it is referred to as a concha bullosa. The incidence of conchae bullosae is approximately 24%, and these may be unilateral or bilateral. Most conchae bullosae are asymptomatic and are incidental radiographic findings. A concha bullosa becomes of clinical significance when it is large enough to compress the ethmoid infundibulum or middle meatus, obstruct the nasal cavity, or cause lateral displacement of the uncinate process.

Such patients present with sinugenic headaches or recurrent sinusitis. The air cell within the middle turbinate is lined by respiratory epithelium and therefore can be affected by any of the disorders that affect the paranasal sinuses. When large, a concha bullosa may compromise the middle meatus and ostiomeatal complex.

The air cell may be confined to the free margin, the vertical plate, or the horizontal plate of the middle turbinate, or the entire middle turbinate may be pneumatized. The middle turbinates are pneumatized from the ethmoid sinuses, the frontal recess, a lateral sinus, or the agger nasi cells. Occasionally, a concha bullosa is aerated directly from

6.28a

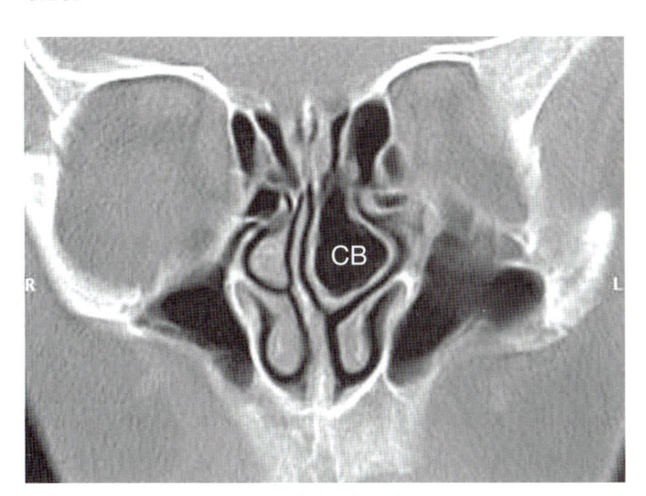

6.28b

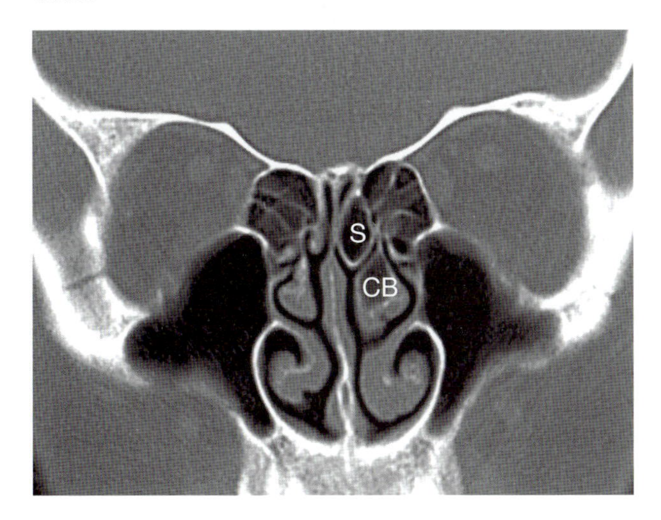

Figure 6.28 (a) *Concha bullosa with compromised ethmoid infundibulum*. This large left-sided concha bullosa (CB) also demonstrates aeration of the vertical plate of the middle turbinate. (b) *Concha bullosa of superior and middle turbinates*. Left-sided conchae bullosa (CB) of the middle and superior (S) turbinates are noted.

6.29a

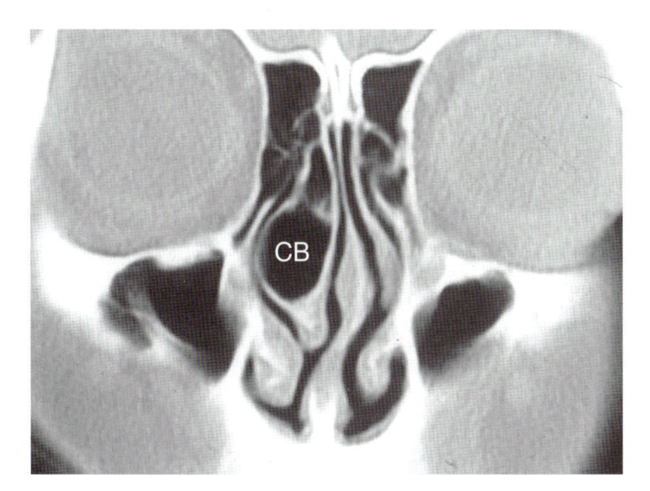

6.29b

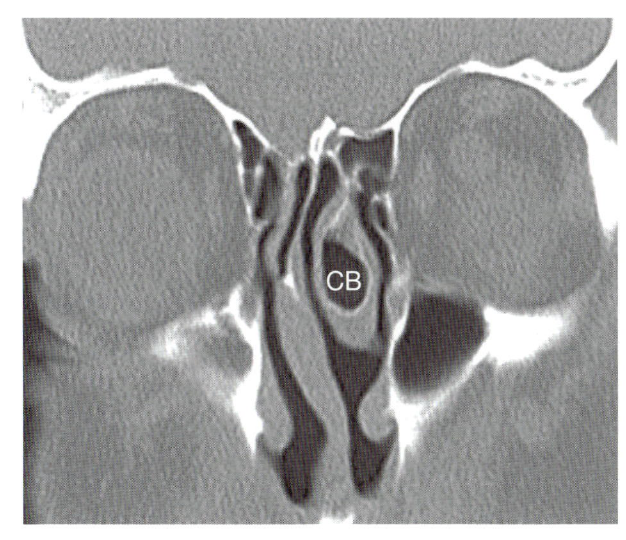

Figure 6.29 (a) *Concha bullosa with compromised ethmoid infundibulum*. This large right-sided concha bullosa (CB) has reduced the adjacent infundibulum to a narrow slit. It is protruding anteriorly and hanging inferiorly against the inferior turbinate. There is secondary deflection of the nasal septum to the opposite side, and the contralateral middle turbinate may be small and paradoxically bent, as is seen in this case. (b) *Concha bullosa protruding anteriorly*. This large concha bullosa (CB) is protruding anteriorly, compromising the frontal recess.

Table 6.2 Conditions that can occur in a concha bullosa

- Concha bullitis (an acute bacterial infection)
- Mucocele/pyocele
- Polyps arising within the concha bullosa
- Polyps arising from the conchal sinus (the lateral surface of the concha bullosa)

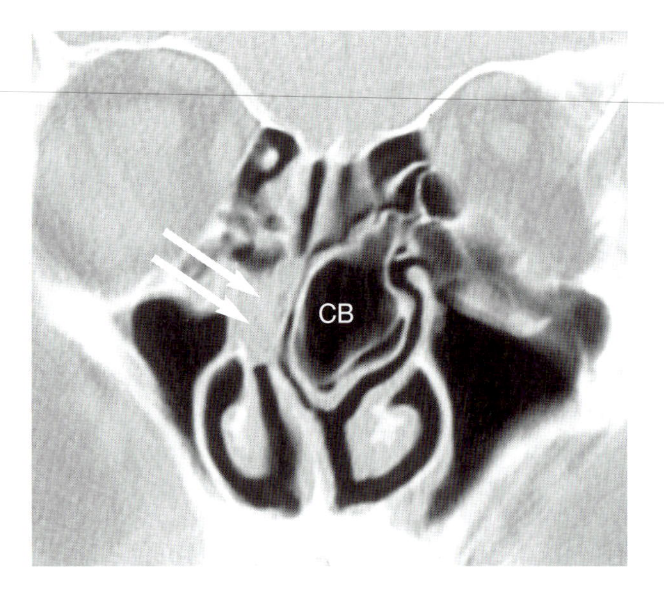

Figure 6.30 *Concha bullosa with compromised ethmoid infundibulum.* A giant concha bullosa (CB) on the left side has compromised the middle meatus on the ipsilateral side. It has deviated the nasal septum to the right and has narrowed the ostiomeatal complex on the opposite side, resulting in inflammatory disease (arrows) on the right side.

the nasal cavity or from the middle meatus. The superior meatus may extend into the vertical plate of the middle turbinate. This particular type of air cell is referred to as an interlamellar cell. In this case, the middle turbinates are pneumatized from the ethmoid bulla.

The small cleft between the ethmoid bulla laterally and the middle turbinate medially is called the conchal or turbinate sinus. The adjacent mucosa may make contact if either one of these structures is enlarged. CT scans taken in the asymptomatic phase may demonstrate early mucosal apposition between a concha bullosa and the adjacent structures. Prolonged contact between these mucosal surfaces results in inflammatory changes in the mucosa, with or without polypoidal degeneration. The turbinate sinus is one of the commonest sites for polyp formation.

A large concha bullosa may cause secondary deflection of the nasal septum to the opposite side, and the contralateral middle turbinate may be small or paradoxically bent.

The air cell within a concha bullosa is lined with respiratory epithelium and is thus predisposed to the same inflammatory disorders that can occur in

6.31a

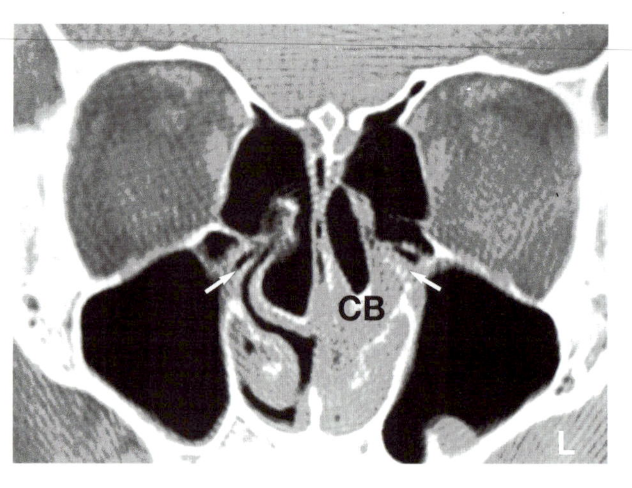

6.31b

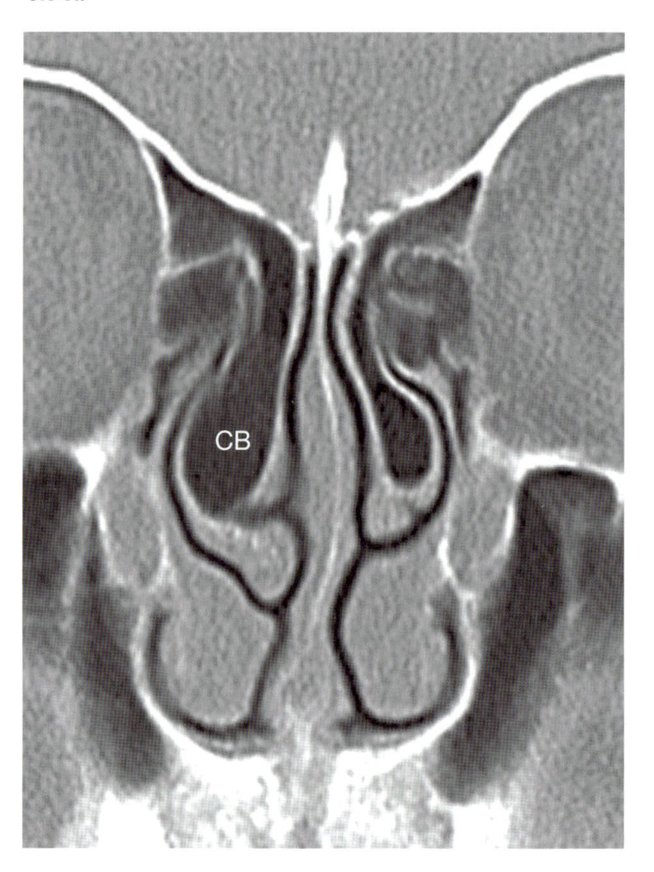

Figure 6.31 *Bilateral concha bullosa.* (a) The large air cell in this left middle turbinate (CB) has produced apposition of the middle and inferior turbinates. The large ethmoid bulla together with the concha bullosa has occluded the left middle meatus. The ethmoid infundibulum is indicated by the arrows. (b) The conchae bullosa are located in bilateral paradoxically curved middle turbinates (CB).

6.32a

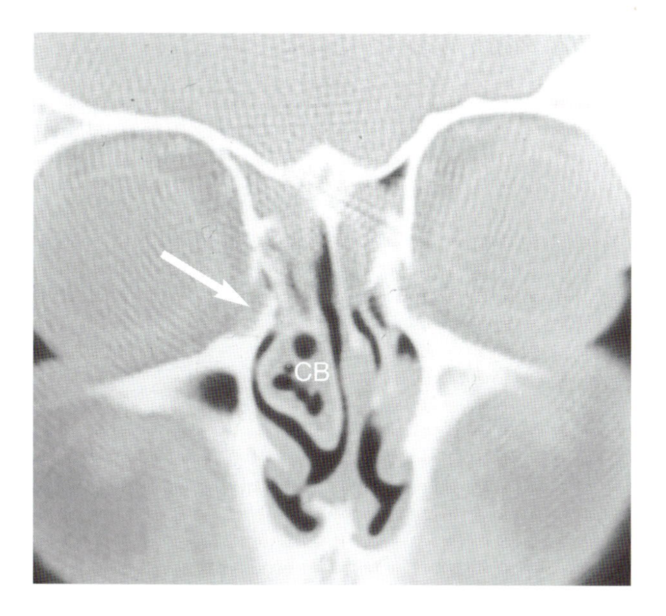

6.32b

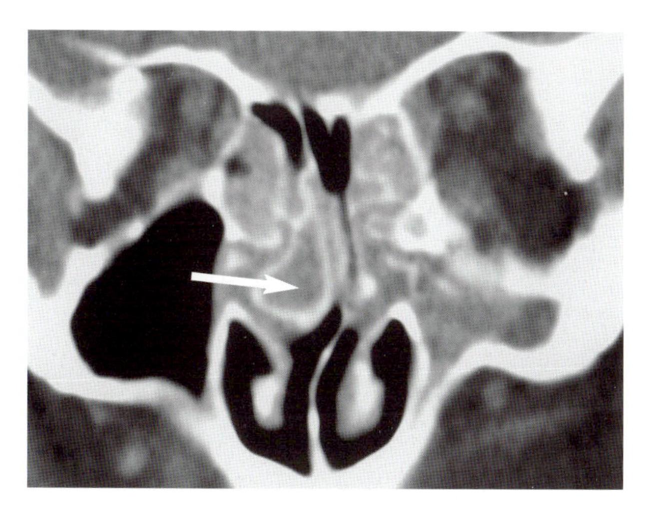

Figure 6.32 *Inflammatory disease in a concha bullosa*. (a) Coronal CT scan demonstrating a large right diseased concha bullosa (CB) protruding anteriorly and compromising the premeatal region and frontal recess. Inflammatory disease is seen in both frontal sinuses. Normally, the middle turbinate is not seen in anterior coronal CT scans, where the frontal sinus and the lacrimal fossa (arrow) are visualized. (b) *Inflammatory disease in a right concha bullosa*. Coronal CT scan demonstrating a large right diseased concha bullosa (arrow) with inflammatory disease in its lumen and in both ethmoid sinuses, ostiomeatal complex, and left maxillary sinuses.

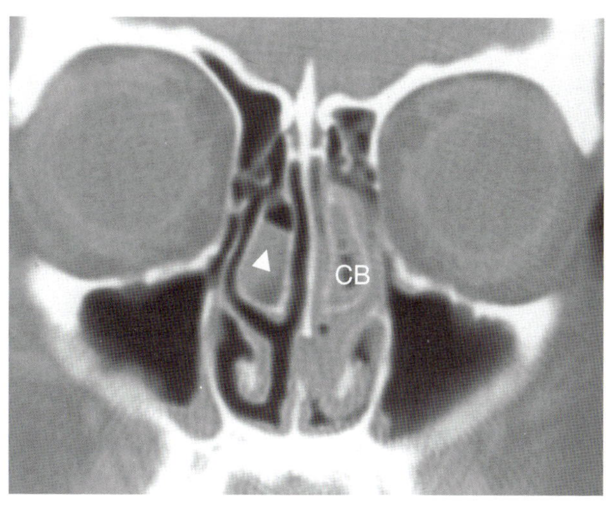

Figure 6.33 *Concha bullitis*. Note the air–fluid level in the left concha bullosa (arrowhead). There is also inflammatory disease in the left concha bullosa (CB), with significant compromise of the adjacent ostiomeatal complex.

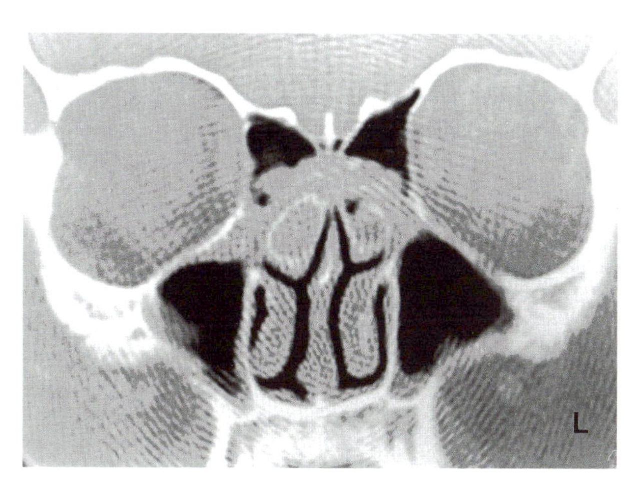

Figure 6.34 *Concha bullosa mucocele*. Coronal CT scan demonstrating a bilateral concha bullosa mucocele and extensive ostiomeatal complex disease.

any paranasal sinus. An acute sinusitis or concha bullitis may be demonstrated as an air–fluid level, or bubbles of air may be seen within the retained secretions. If the ostium of a concha bullosa becomes occluded, its lumen may become filled with mucus. This condition is termed a mucocele, the clinical features of which are nasal obstruction and headaches. Secondary infection will result in pyocele.

CT is less helpful in diagnosing a concha bullosa in the presence of extensive sinonasal polyposis. In this situation, the normal demarcation planes of air, bone, and soft tissue are obscured and detail cannot always be ascertained.

6.35a

6.35b

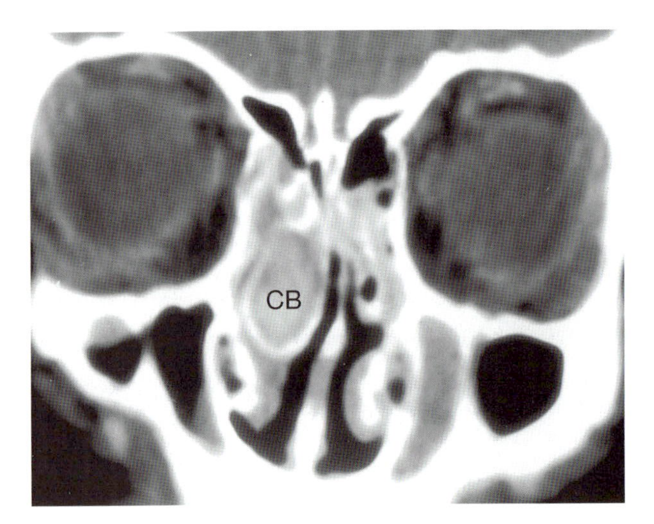

Figure 6.35 *Concha bullosa mucocele.* (a) Axial CT scan demonstrating a large mucocele of a right concha bullosa (CB) with mucosal enhancement. As with any other mucocele, secondary infection will result in a pyocele. Resection of the lateral plate of the middle turbinate is curative. This patient would have remained symptomatic if surgery aimed specifically at the middle turbinate had not been undertaken. (b) Coronal CT scan demonstrating a large mucocele of the right concha bullosa (CB).

6.36a

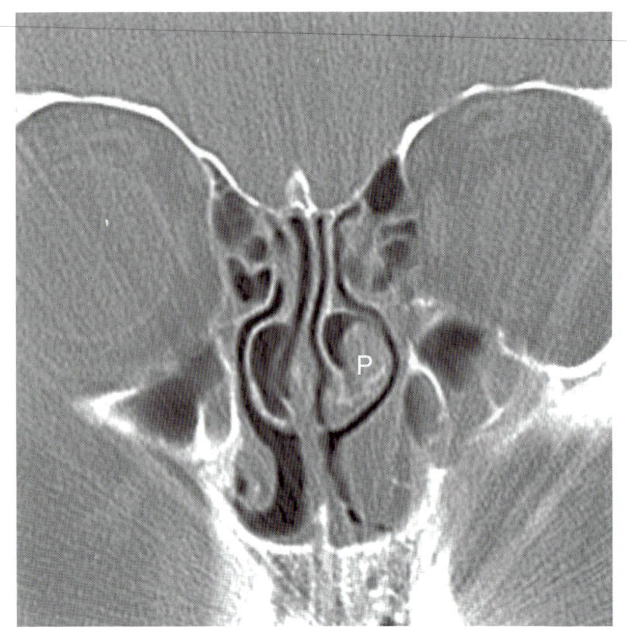

6.36b

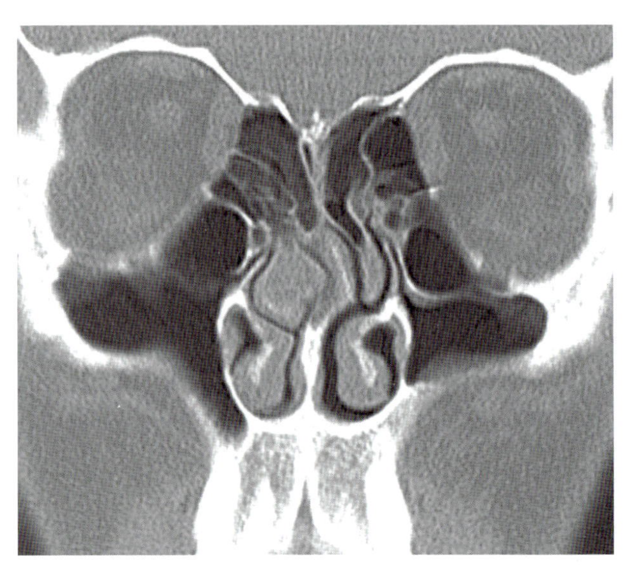

Figure 6.36 *Polyp in concha bullosa.* (a) A small polyp (P) is seen in the lumen of a left concha bullosa. (b) A polyp fills the entire lumen of a concha bullosa on the right side.

ETHMOID BULLA

(Figures 6.41–6.50)

The ethmoid bulla (bulla ethmoidalis) is variable in its pneumatization. It may be multiseptated and large, or sometimes absent. The ethmoid bulla may be the site of inflammatory disease, or it may have no mucosal disease, but its configuration may cause inflammatory disease in the neighboring larger paranasal sinuses by obstructing the ostiomeatal complex.

It is unusual to find isolated ethmoid bullitis, and the ethmoid bulla is more commonly involved in generalized inflammatory disease of the ethmoid sinus. The frontal recess may be occluded by an

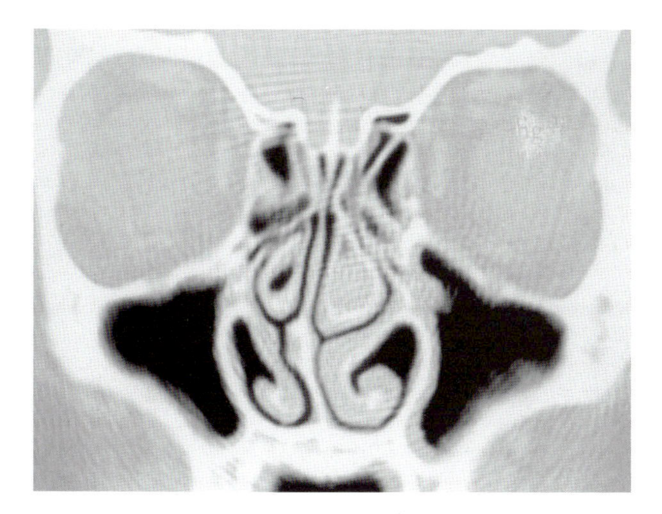

Figure 6.37 *Polyp in concha bullosa*. Polypoidal degeneration is seen in the lumen of the left concha. There is ostiomeatal complex disease on the left side.

6.38a

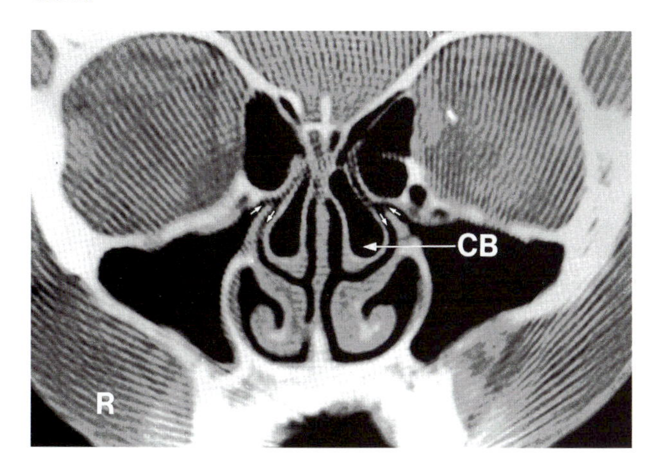

6.38b

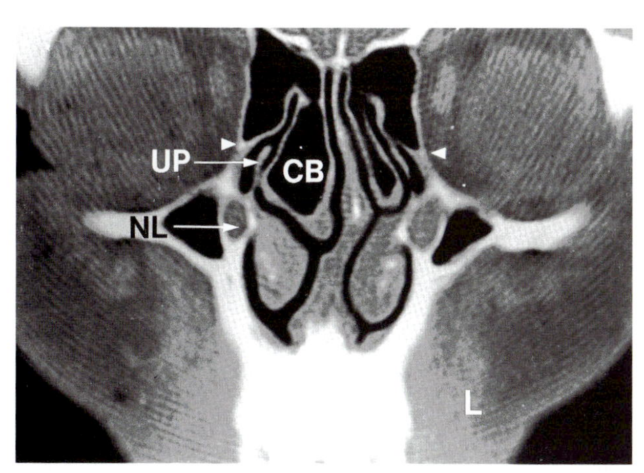

Figure 6.38 (a) *Concha bullosa*. CT scan demonstrating a bilateral large concha bullosa (CB) with narrowing of the ostiomeatal complex and the middle meati (small arrows). (b) *Bilateral concha bullosa*. The middle turbinates are pneumatized from the ethmoid bulla. The basal lamella is seen to insert onto the lamina papyracea (arrowheads). The base of the uncinate process (UP) inserts close to the nasolacrimal duct (NL).

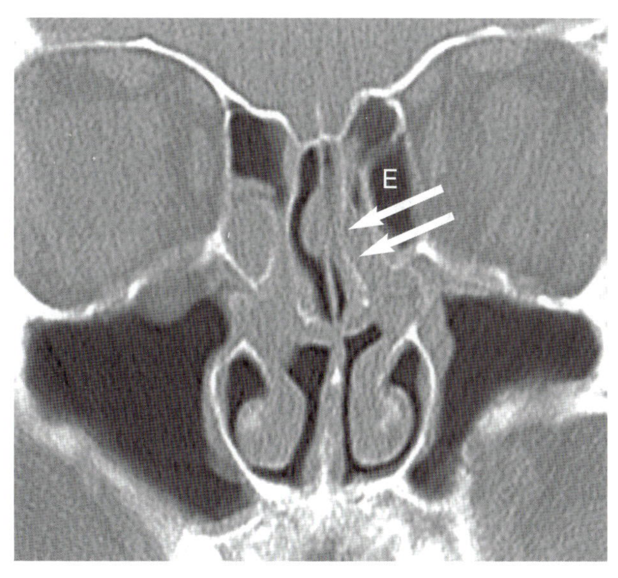

Figure 6.39 *Turbinate sinus polyps*. The small cleft between the ethmoid bulla (E) laterally and the middle turbinate medially is called the conchal or turbinate sinus (arrows). The turbinate sinus is one of the commonest sites for polyp formation. This coronal scan demonstrates multiple polyps wedged in the conchal sinus. Bilateral ostiomeatal complex disease can be seen.

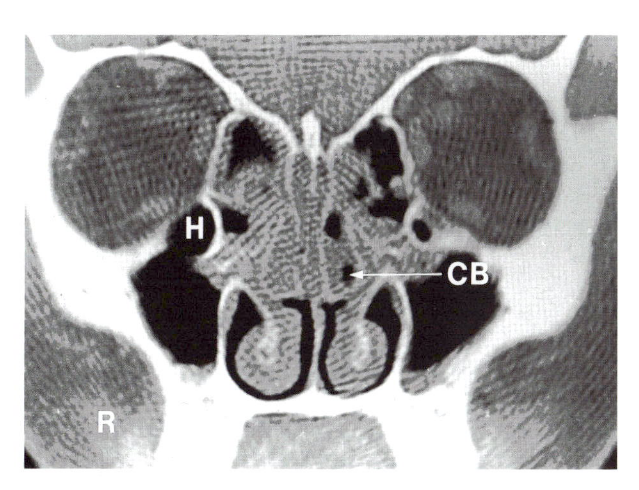

Figure 6.40 *Ostiomeatal complex disease*. CT scan demonstrating extensive ostiomeatal complex disease as well as disease in both conchae bullosa (CB). The narrowed ethmoid infundibula are further compromised by Haller's cells (H).

ethmoid bulla that expands anteriorly. If the ethmoid bulla enlarges anteroinferiorly, it may overhang the hiatus semilunaris and occlude the ethmoid infundibulum, thus obstructing its narrow drainage pathway and preventing ventilation and drainage of the adjacent sinuses. If the ethmoid bulla protrudes medially, it may make contact with the adjacent lateral surface of the middle turbinate,

6.41a

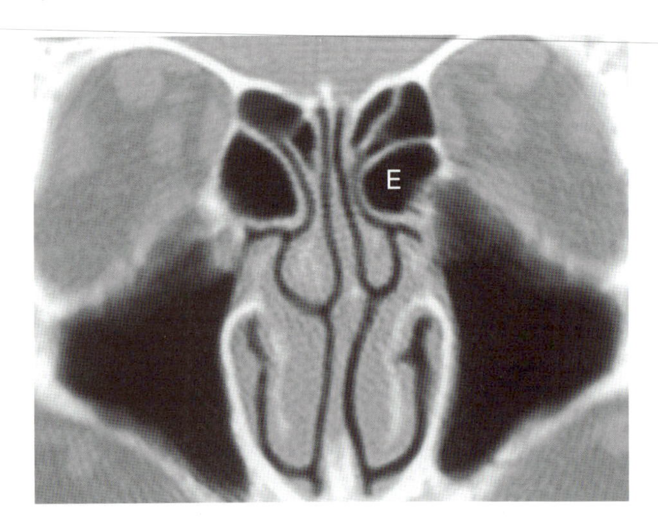

6.41b

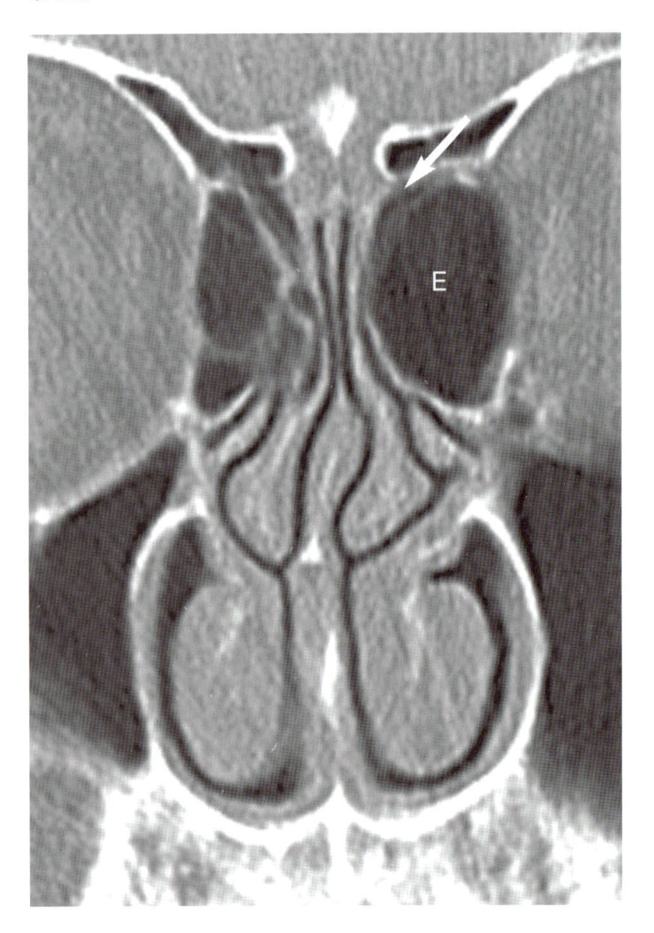

Figure 6.41 *Large ethmoid bulla*. (a) A large ethmoid bulla (E) extends medially on both sides. (b) A large ethmoid bulla (E) extends medially, obstructing the frontal recess left side (arrow).

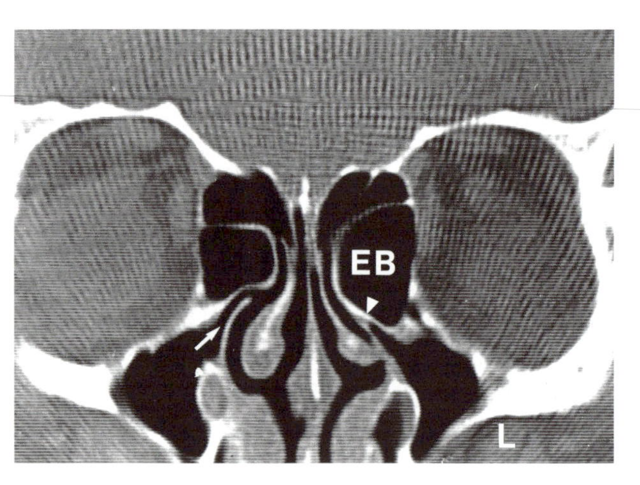

Figure 6.42 *Large ethmoid bulla*. A large ethmoid bulla (EB) is present on the left side, obstructing the hiatus semilunaris (arrowhead). The ethmoid infundibulum, hiatus semilunaris, and middle meatus on the right are normal (arrow).

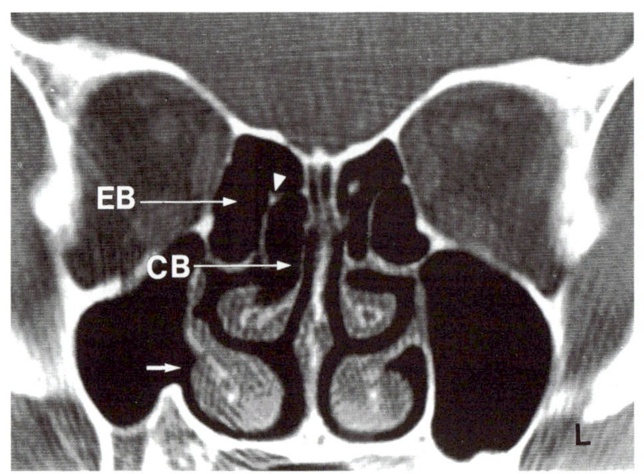

Figure 6.43 *Large ethmoid bulla and concha bullosa*. This patient presented with headaches. The coronal CT scan demonstrates a large ethmoid bulla (EB) in contact (arrowhead) with a large air cell in the vertical plate of the right middle turbinate (a concha bullosa (CB)) on the right side. This patient had previously undergone a right intranasal antrostomy (arrow), but had remained symptomatic. Following resection of the ethmoid bulla and the middle turbinate air cell her contact headaches were relieved.

resulting in facial pain, nasal obstruction, and contact headaches without any inflammatory changes in the adjacent paranasal sinuses.

HALLER'S CELLS (Figures 6.51–6.54)

Haller's cells are named after the 18th century anatomist Albert von Haller, who described this

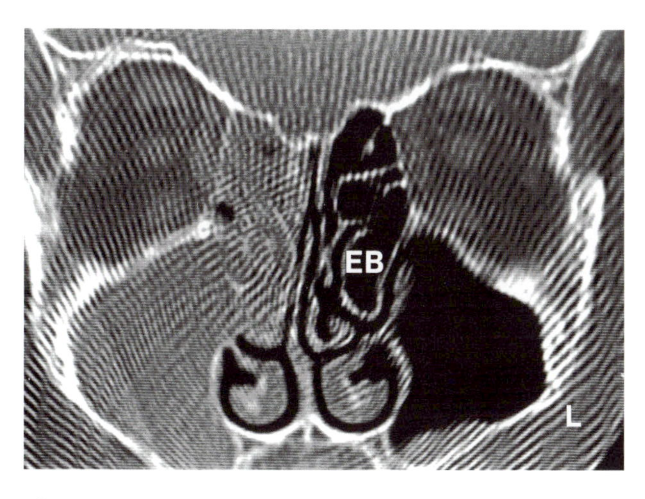

Figure 6.44 *Large ethmoid bulla overhanging the hiatus semilunaris.* An ethmoid bulla may be the site of inflammatory disease or may predispose the patient to inflammatory disease by obstructing the ostiomeatal complex. This CT scan demonstrates a large ethmoid bulla (EB) overhanging the hiatus semilunaris on the left side. Similar findings on the right side resulted in a unilateral pansinusitis.

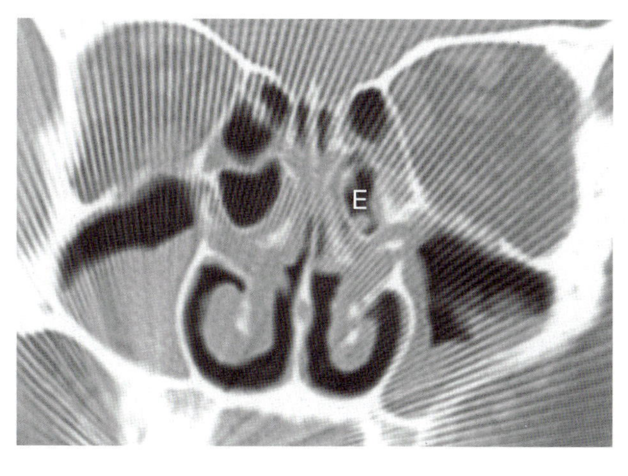

Figure 6.46 *Large ethmoid bulla overhanging the hiatus semilunaris.* Bilateral large ethmoid bullae (E) are seen overhanging the hiatus semilunaris and middle meatus, with inflammatory disease in the ostiomeatal complex. Interestingly, there is very little disease in the lumen of the bullae. There is disease in the suprabullar space.

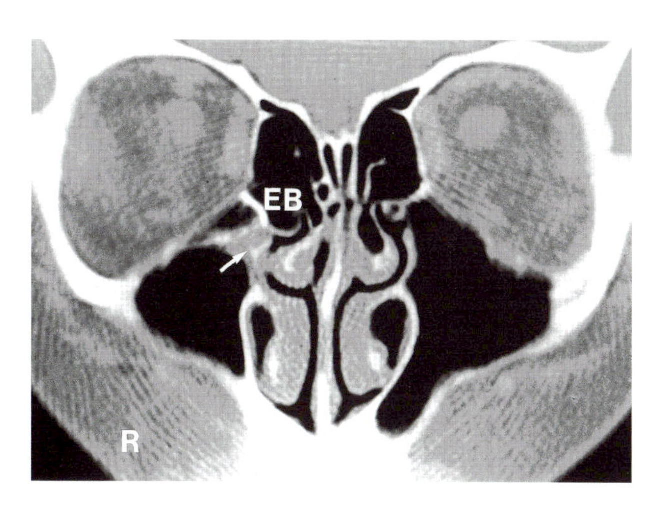

Figure 6.45 *Large ethmoid bulla overhanging the hiatus semilunaris.* CT scan showing an example of early compromise of the right maxillary sinus ostia and ethmoid infundibulum (arrow), with a large ethmoid bulla (EB) overhanging the hiatus semilunaris. The large ethmoid bulla indirectly reduces the ventilation and drainage of the adjacent sinuses. This has resulted in early infundibular disease.

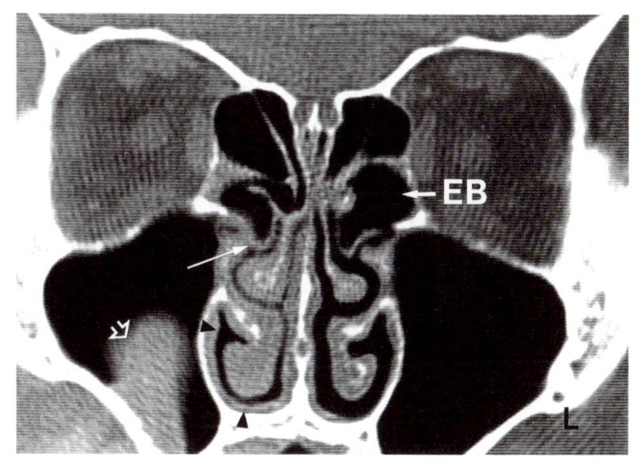

Figure 6.47 *Inferiorly extending ethmoid bullae.* Coronal CT scan through the ostiomeatal complex demonstrating large ethmoid bullae (EB) overhanging the hiatus semilunaris (arrow), with compromise of the ethmoid infundibulum and thereby compromise of ventilation and drainage of the maxillary sinus. There is retained mucus (open arrow) in the floor of the right maxillary sinus. Mucosal thickening can be seen in the inferior meatus and in the floor of the right nasal cavity (arrowheads).

particular anatomical variant. Routine office endoscopy infrequently allows identification of anatomical variations that may be compromising the ventilation of the maxillary sinus and therefore predisposing the sinus to recurrent infections. One such anomaly that may compromise the natural maxillary ostium is a Haller's cell. These cells are lateral extensions of the anterior ethmoid cells into the inferomedial margin of the floor of the orbit superior to the natural ostium of the maxillary sinus, and they are clearly demonstrated by CT in the coronal plane. A solitary large Haller's cell situated lateral to the maxillary sinus ostium may be an incidental finding. It may narrow the lumen and

6.48a

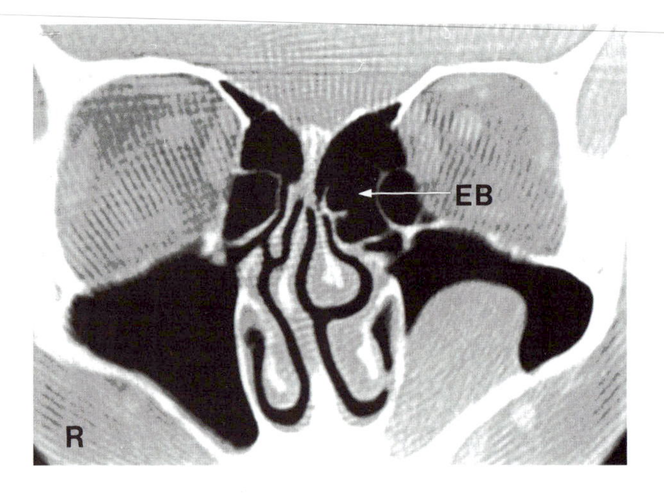

6.48b

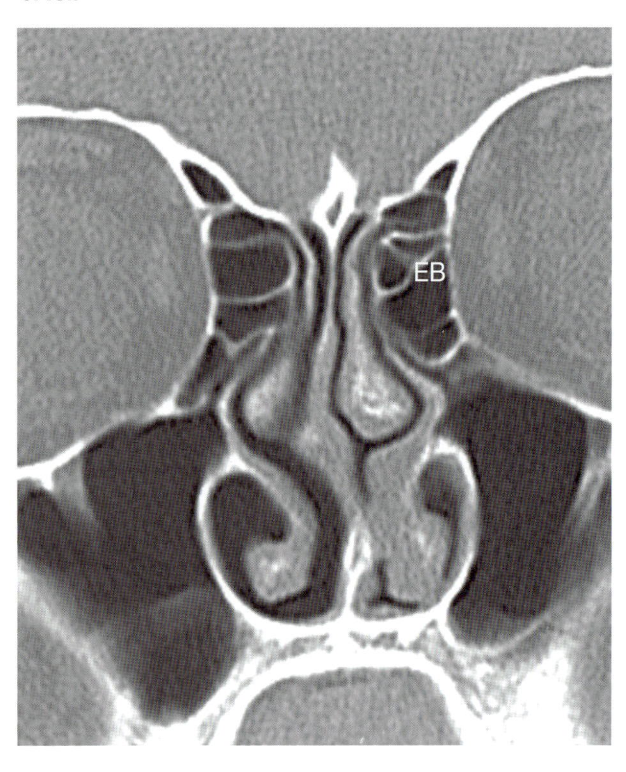

Figure 6.48 *Multiseptate ethmoid bulla.* (a) The enlarged left ethmoid bulla (EB) of this patient is divided by multiple septae. This grossly enlarged bulla has compromised the frontal recess and the hiatus semilunaris. There is a considerable amount of retained secretions in the left maxillary sinus. Note hyperplasia of the right middle turinate. (b) The ethmoid bulla (EB) of this patient is divided by multiple septae bilaterally.

6.49a

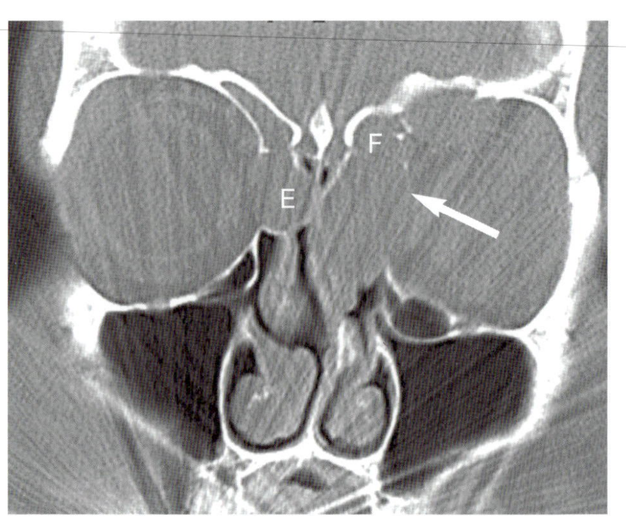

6.49b

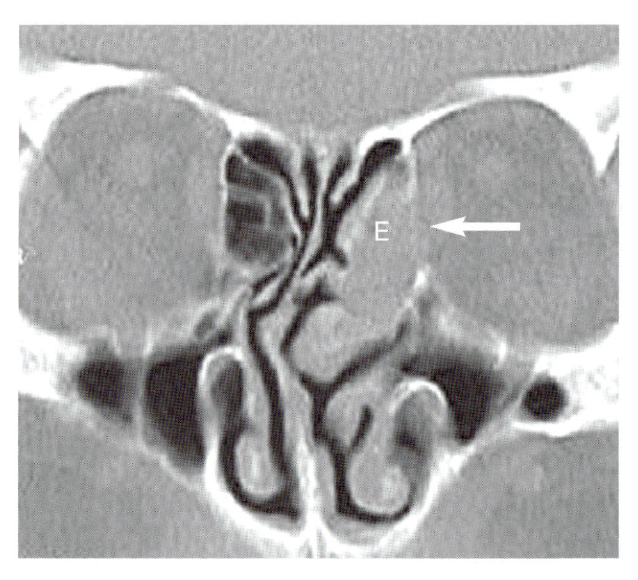

Figure 6.49 *Mucocele of ethmoid bulla.* (a) There are bilateral mucoceles of the ethmoid bulla (E); the left ethmoid bulla is large, overhanging the infundibulum. There is expansion, with mucoid material in its lumen. The lamina papyracea is eroded (arrow). The frontal recesses (F) are obstructed with disease. (b) The left ethmoid bulla (E) mucocele has expanded into the orbit, and this is associated with thinning of the lamina papyracea (arrow).

predispose to recurrent or chronic inflammatory disease in the maxillary and frontal sinuses by narrowing the ethmoid infundibulum.

Pneumatization of the floor of the orbit by Haller's cells may be extensive.

DEVIATION OF THE NASAL SEPTUM (Figures 6.55–6.62)

Deviation of the nasal septum is either develop-mental in origin as a result of asymmetric facial skeletal growth or due to trauma. There may be a deviation of the bony nasal septum, the cartilaginous nasal

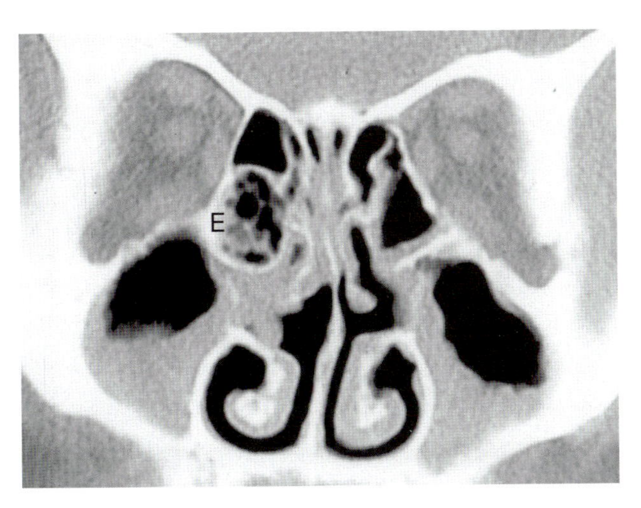

Figure 6.50 *Diseased ethmoid bulla.* There is mucopurulent material in the lumen of the bulla (E), associated with ostiomeatal complex disease and bilateral maxillary sinusitis.

6.51a

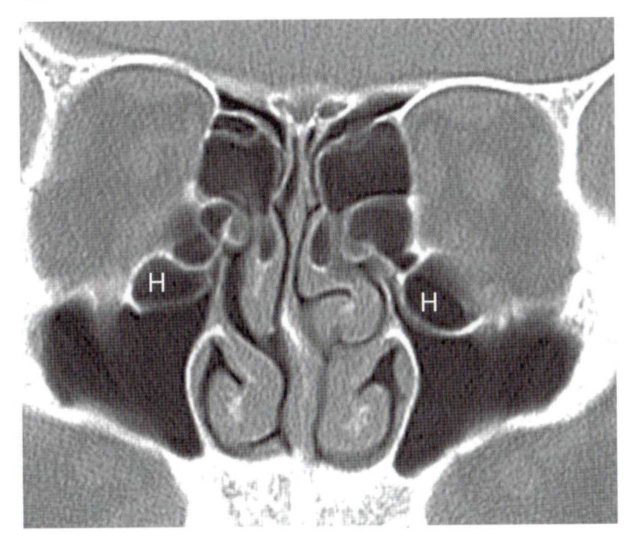

6.51b

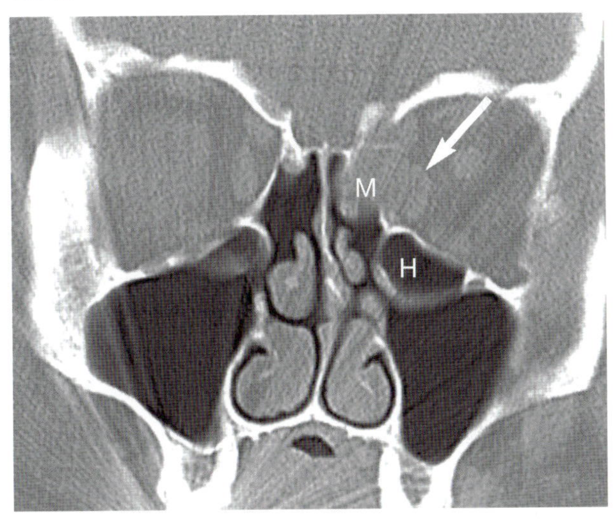

Figure 6.51 *Large Haller's cell.* (a) This patient has a large Haller's cell on both sides (H). (b) This patient has a large Haller's cell (H) and there are changes in keeping with a bilateral ethmoidectomy. There is erosion of the left lamina papyracea associated with a small mucocele (M) close to the medial rectus muscle (arrow).

septum, or a combination of both. While deviations of the nasal septum are common, not all are of clinical significance. Septal deviations may limit access into the nasal cavity and the middle meatus, and a septoplasty may be required.

Deviation of the nasal septum is associated with compensatory hypertrophy of the contralateral inferior and sometimes the middle turbinate. Bony projections may extend laterally from the nasal septum. These long septal bony spurs, which vary in size, may be large enough to push into the lateral nasal wall, coming into contact with the middle or inferior turbinates or in extreme cases curling up into the middle meatus. Such contact may lead to severe headaches as well as nasal obstruction.

The nasal septum may be pneumatized, either in continuity with an aerated crista galli or posteriorly as an extension of the rostrum of the sphenoid sinus.

DEHISCENCE OF THE LAMINA PAPYRACEA AND FLOOR OF ORBIT (Figures 6.63–6.65)

Natural dehiscence in the lamina papyracea may serve as small channels allowing the spread of infection into the orbit. These should not be misinterpreted as pathological erosions. The defects also allow easy inadvertent entrance into the orbit during endoscopic sinus surgery or increase the ease with which orbital contents can be drawn into a microdebrider. Surgeons must be aware of these defects, as unintentional entrance can injure the orbital muscles or the optic nerve.

LOW-LYING FOVEA ETHMOIDALIS AND CRIBRIFORM PLATE (Figures 6.66–6.71)

The fovea ethmoidalis and the cribriform plate form the roof of the nasal cavity. The cribriform

6.52a

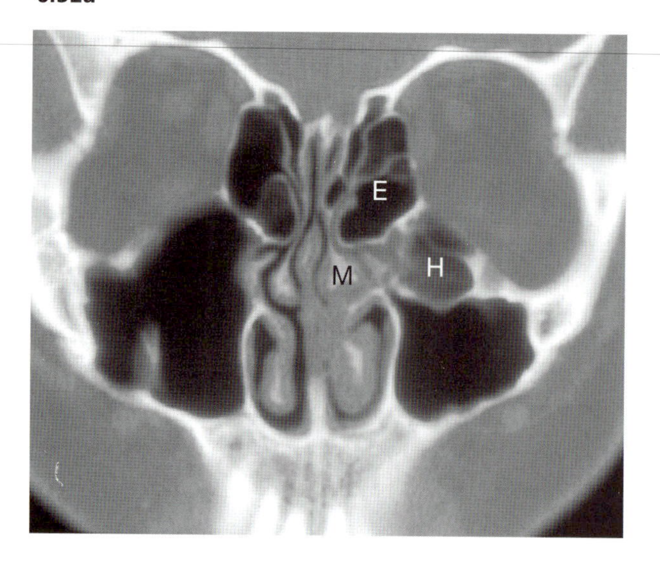

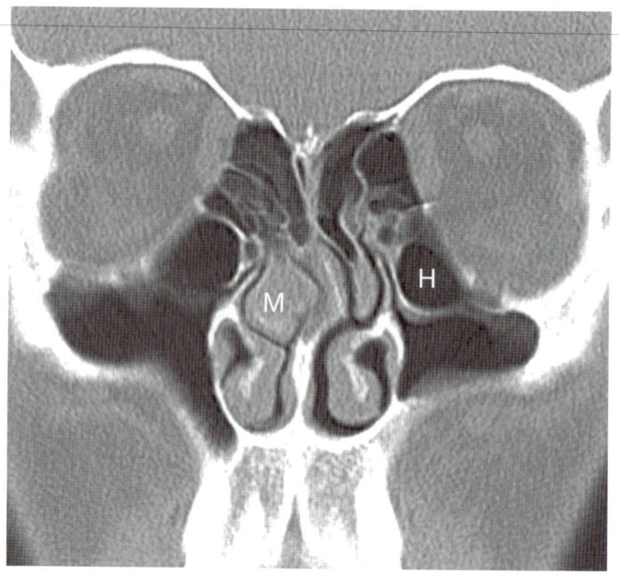

Figure 6.53 *Large Haller's cell.* CT scan demonstrating narrowing of ostiomeatal complex by Haller's cells (H). Note the hypertrophy of the middle turbinate (M) on the right side.

6.52b

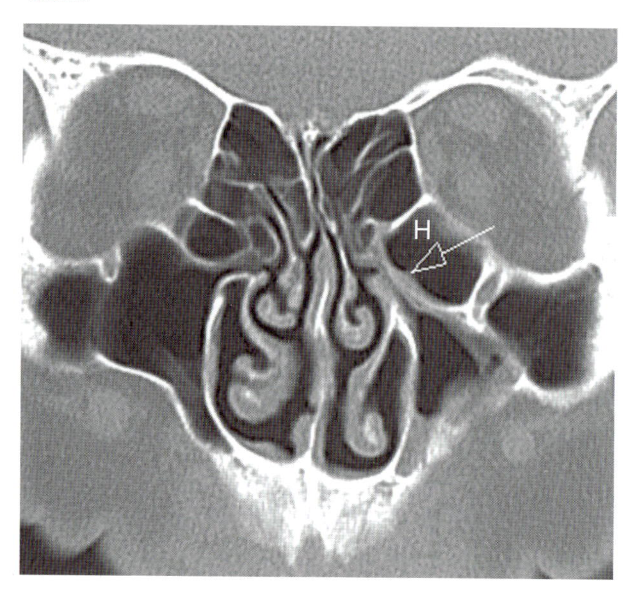

Figure 6.52 *Large Haller's cell.* (a) This patient has a large Haller's cell on the left side (H). There is compromise of the ostiomeatal complex on the left side. E, ethmoid bulla; M, middle turbinate. (b) This patient has a large Haller's cell on the left side (H) pneumatizing the entire floor of the orbit on the left side. The ethmoid infundibulum is narrowed (arrow).

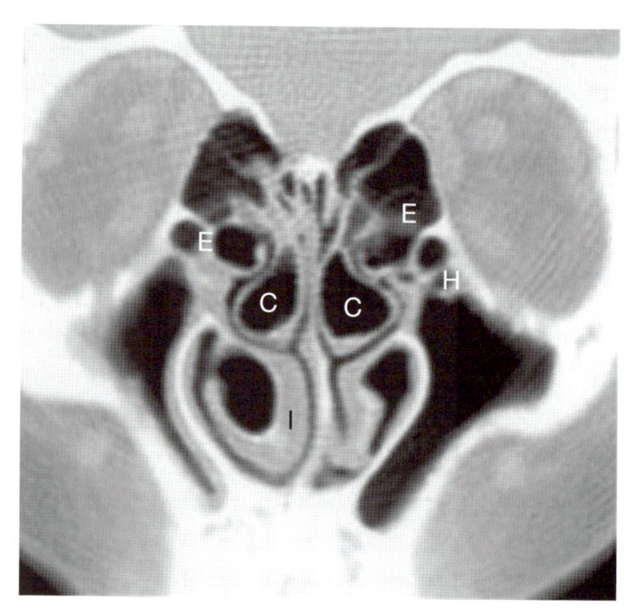

Figure 6.54 *Combination of several anatomical variants.* Middle turbinate anomalies are often seen as incidental findings, playing no role in the inflammatory process. Sometimes a combination of anatomical variations may be necessary for ostiomeatal complex disease, with middle turbinate anomalies being a cofactor. This coronal CT scan is such an example, with a bilateral concha bullosa (C), multiseptated ethmoid bullae (E), and Haller's cells (H), all of which contribute towards ostiomeatal complex compromise. In addition, the right inferior turbinate (I) appears pneumatized.

6.55a

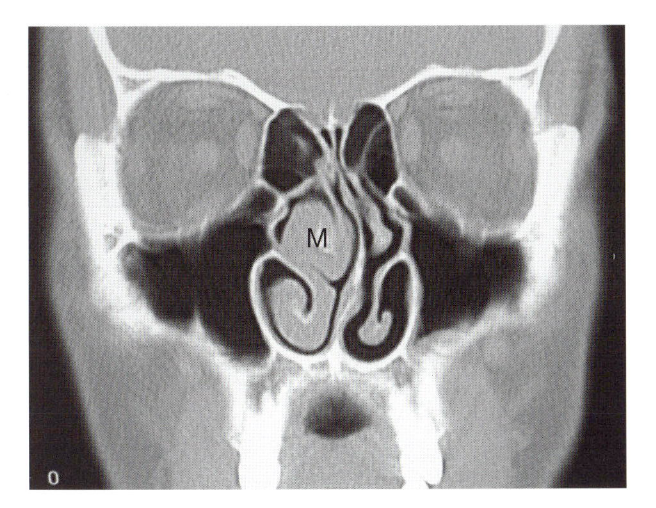

6.55b

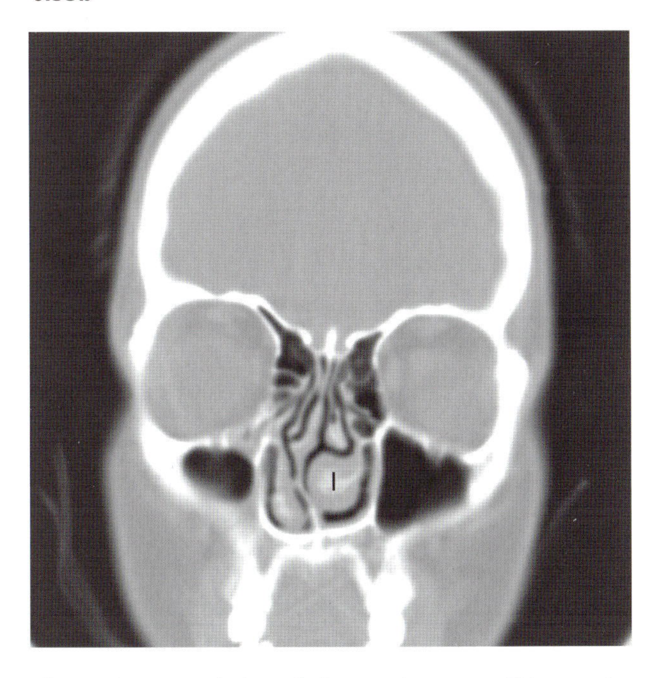

Figure 6.55 *Deviation of the nasal septum*. This may be associated with hypertrophy of the contralateral middle and inferior turbinates. (a) Deviation of the nasal septum to the left is noted with hypertrophy of the right middle turbinate (M). (b) Deviation of the nasal septum is associated with hypertrophy of the inferior turbinate (I) on the left side.

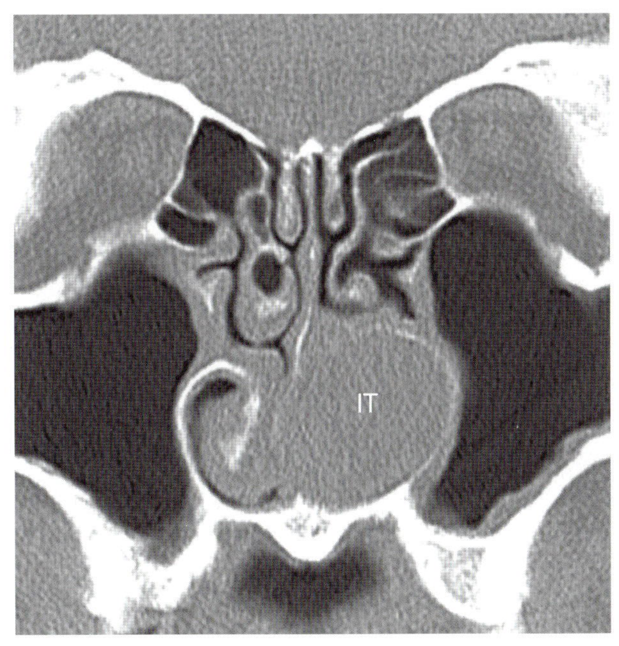

Figure 6.56 *Polypoidal hypertrophy of the inferior turbinate with nasal septal deviation*. The nasal septum is deviated to the right as a result of polypoidal degeneration of the inferior turbinate (IT).

plate is the medial part of the horizontal plate of the ethmoid bone and is only 2–3 mm wide. It supports the olfactory bulbs of the cerebrum, and is perforated by approximately 20 foramina that transmit the fibers of the olfactory nerve. At the junction between the foveola and the cribriform plate lies the lamina lateralis, which provides attachment to the middle turbinate. The lamina lateralis can easily be injured during a middle turbinate resection, which can cause cerebrospinal fluid rhinorrhea, permanent anosmia and subarachnoid hemorrhage and can increase the risk of intracranial infection. The anterior ethmoidal vessels exit through foramina between the lateral lamella and the fovea ethmoidalis. The arteries can be injured during surgery, leading to the rapid development of a retro-orbital hematoma.

The level of the cribriform plate is variable. It has been graded by Keros into three types depending upon its position with relation to the roof of the ethmoid (see Figures 5.28–5.34):

- Type 1: the fovea ethmoidalis and the cribriform plate are in the same plane
- Type 2: the cribriform plate is at an intermediate level
- Type 3: the cribriform plate is at the level of or below the optic nerve

This is well demonstrated on coronal CT scans.

6.57a

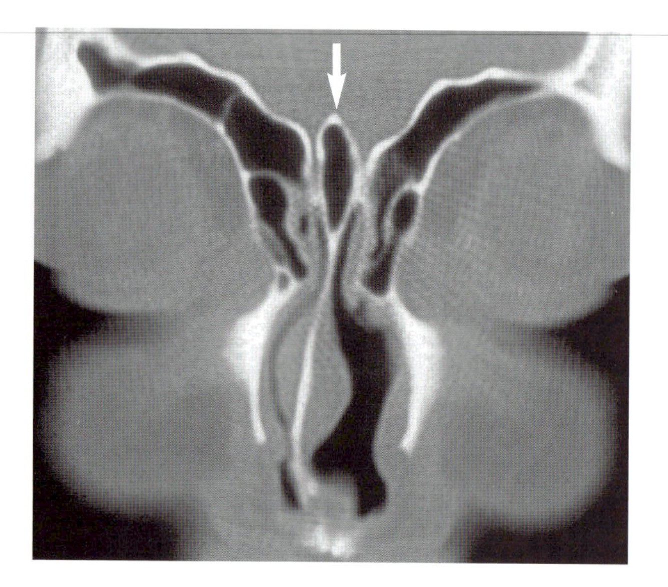

6.57b

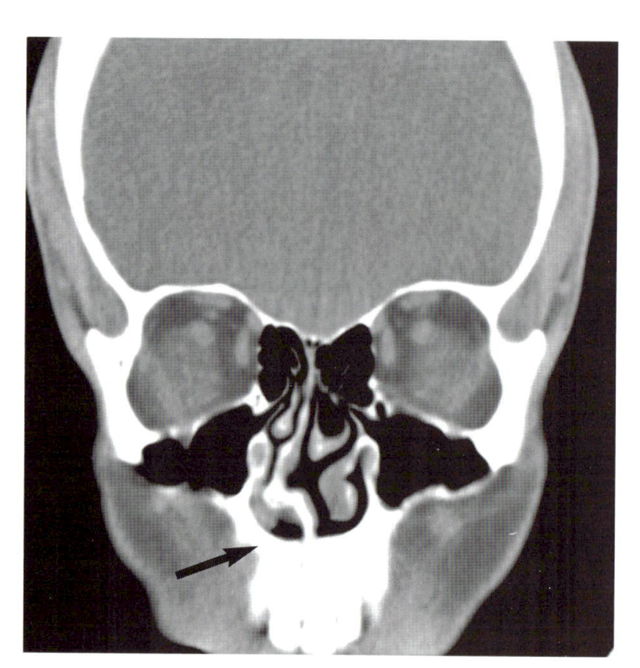

Figure 6.57 *Post-traumatic nasal septal deviation*. (a) The nasal septal deviation limits entry into the right nasal cavity. The crista galli is pneumatized (arrow). (b) The septal spur (arrow) – probably post-traumatic – is pushing against the lateral nasal wall.

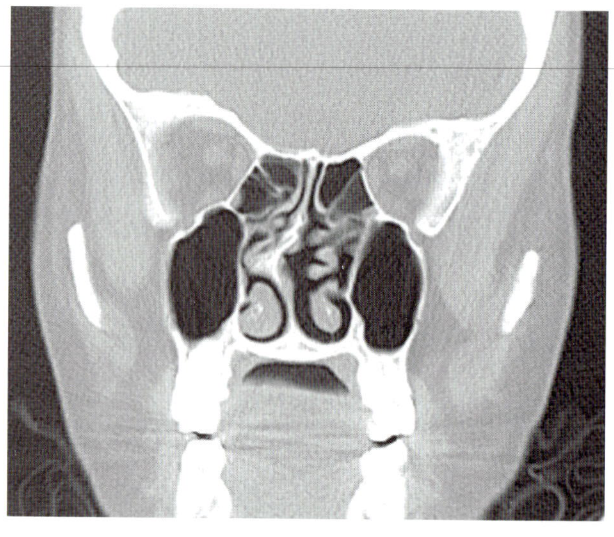

Figure 6.58 *Nasal septal spur.* The septal spur is abutting onto the posterior part of the lateral nasal wall.

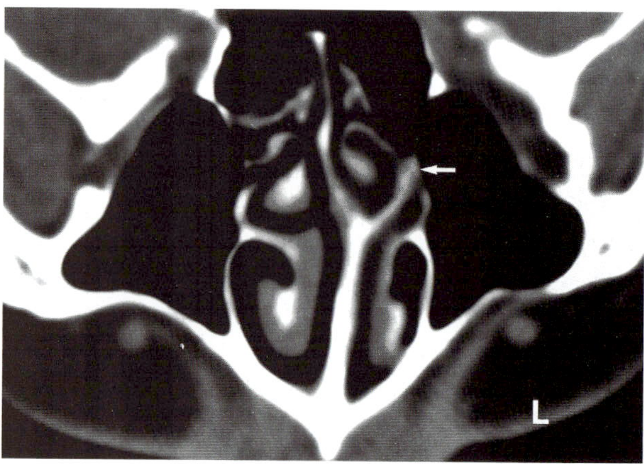

Figure 6.59 *Nasal septal spur*. The long nasal septal spur is impinging onto the lateral nasal wall in the middle meatus (arrow).

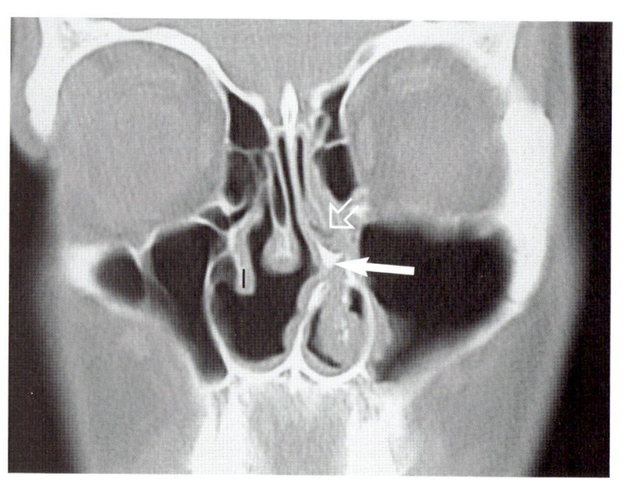

Figure 6.60 *Ostiomeatal compromise due to nasal septal deviation*. The deviation of the nasal septum (arrow) is occluding the right ostiomeatal complex. The right inferior turbinate (I) has been partially resected in the past. The left middle turbinate is wedged along with the uncinate process in the ostiomeatal complex (open arrow).

6.61a

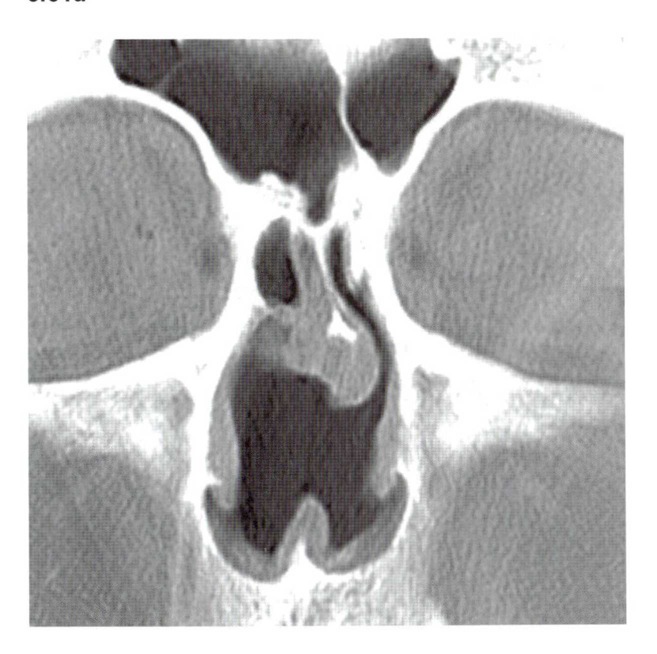

6.61b

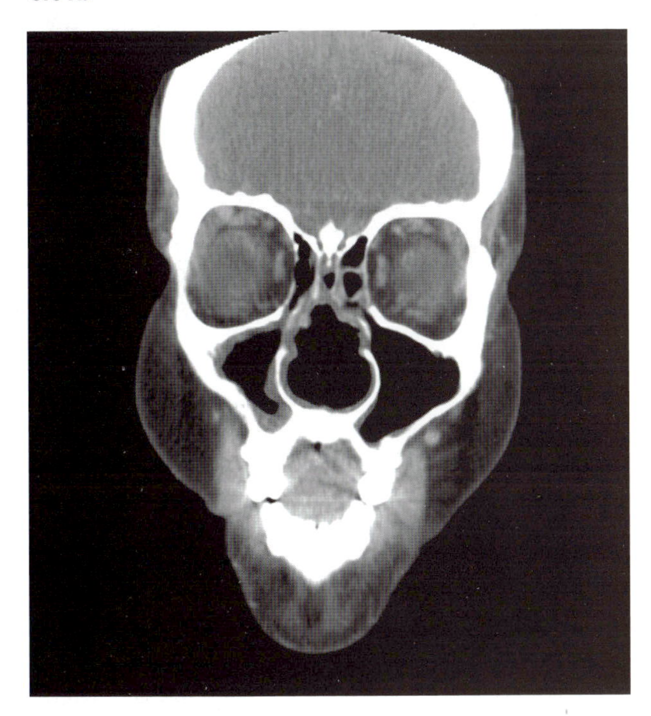

Figure 6.61 *Nasal septal perforation*. (a, b) Septal defects are often seen in patients who have undergone septoplasty. They are also known to occur in patients who pick their noses. The other causes are cocaine abuse, exposure to chromium, and granulomatous infection.

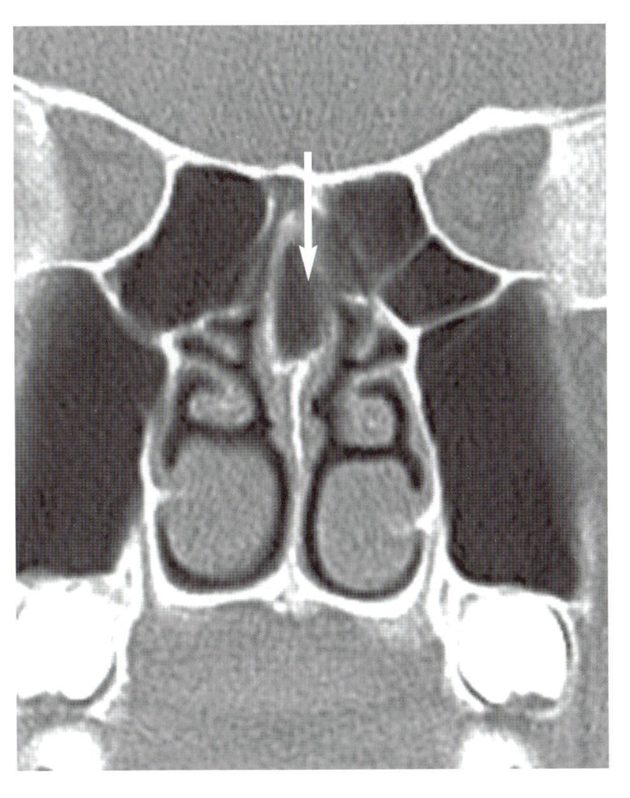

Figure 6.62 *Aerated nasal septum*. The nasal septum may be pneumatized (arrow) as a result of extension of an aerated crista galli or anterior extension of the sphenoid sinus. The posterior portion of the perpendicular plate of the ethmoid in this patient is aerated (arrow) from an anterior extension of the sphenoid sinus.

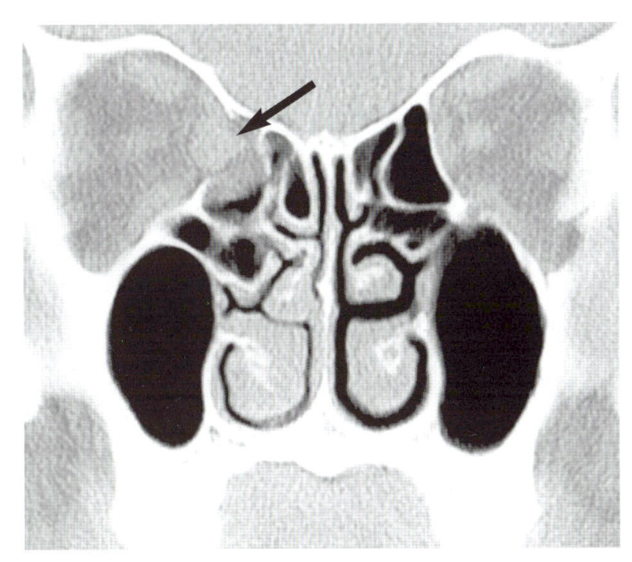

Figure 6.63 *Dehiscent lamina papyracea*. The medial rectus muscle and orbital fat are protruding into the ethmoid sinus through a congenital defect in the medial margin of the orbit (arrow). This patient has no history of previous surgery. Without prior knowledge of this anomaly, sinus surgery may involve serious complications.

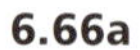

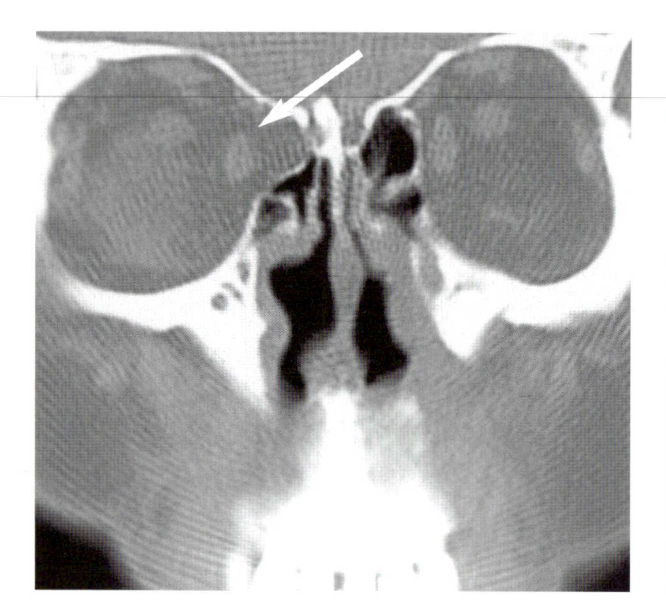

Figure 6.64 *Dehiscent lamina papyracea.* There are changes suggestive of previous surgery. Without a preoperative CT scan, it would be difficult to determine whether the defect in the lamina papyracea (arrow) is congenital or acquired.

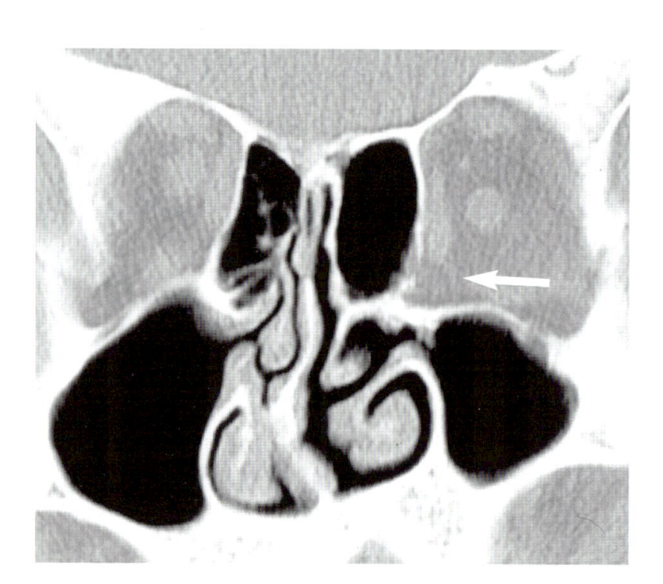

Figure 6.65 *Asymmetry and protrusion of orbital wall.* The maxillary sinus on the left side is smaller and there is asymmetry of the orbit and the lateral nasal walls. The medial margin of the orbit is protruding into the nasal cavity. There is deviation of the nasal septum to the right. The lamina papyracea is deficient inferiorly (arrow).

6.66a

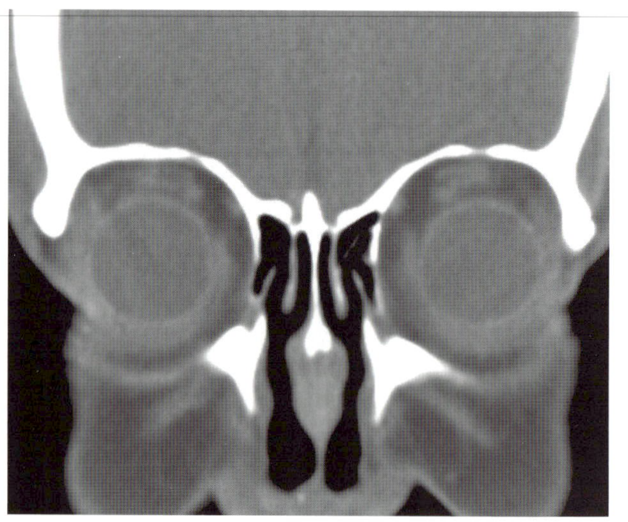

6.66b

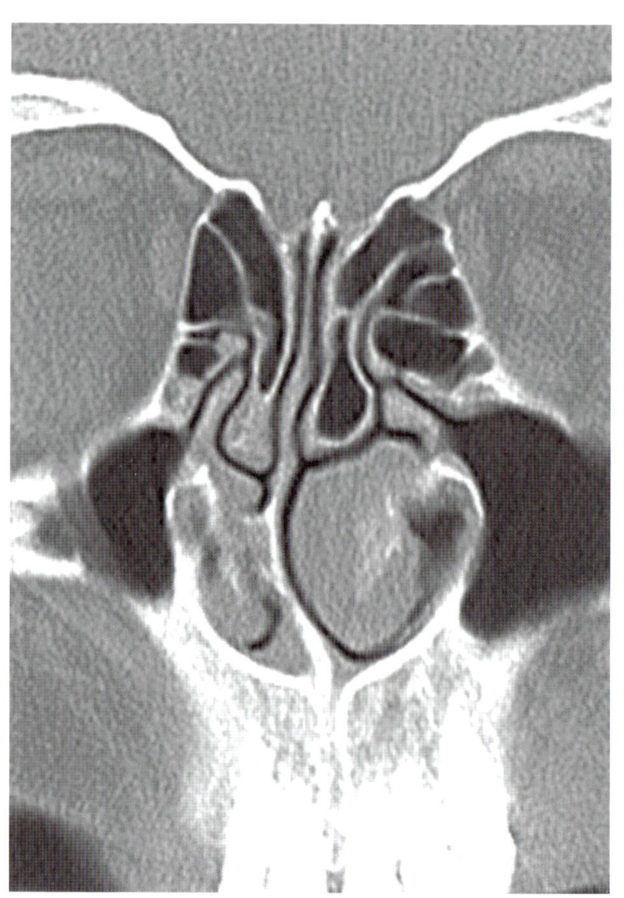

Figure 6.66 *Fovea ethmoidalis and cribriform plate type 1.* (a, b) The cribriform plate and the fovea ethmoidalis are in the same plane.

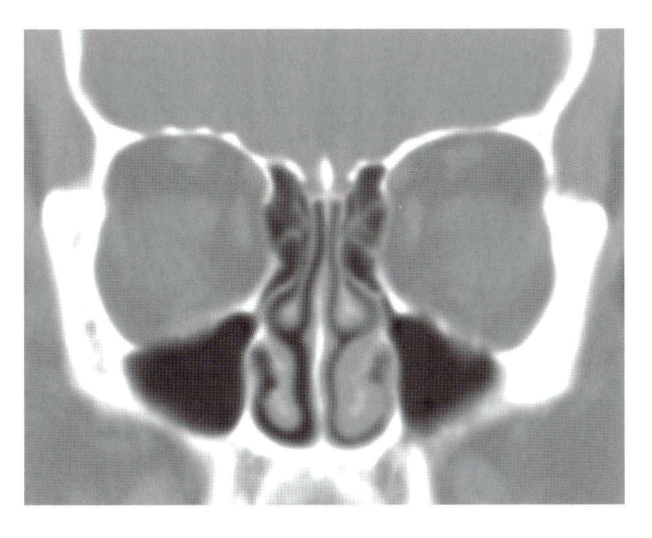

Figure 6.67 *Fovea ethmoidalis and cribriform plate type 2*. The cribriform plate is at a lower plane when seen in relation to the roof of the ethmoid.

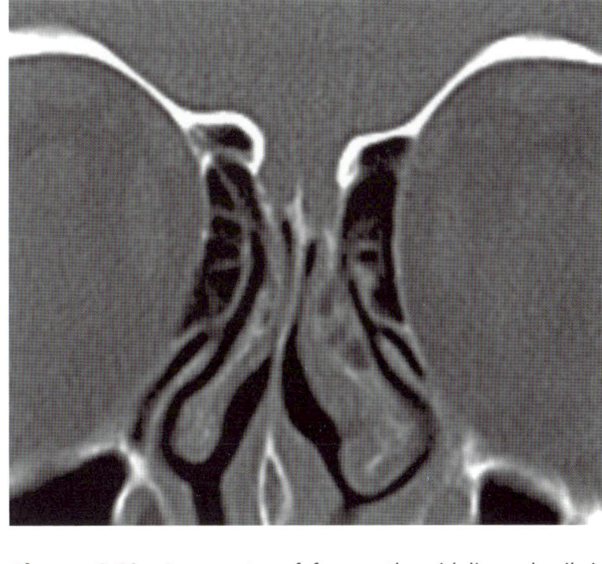

Figure 6.69 *Asymmetry of fovea ethmoidalis and cribriform plate type 3*. There is asymmetry in the roof when compared with each side. These patients have a greater risk of injury during sinus surgery.

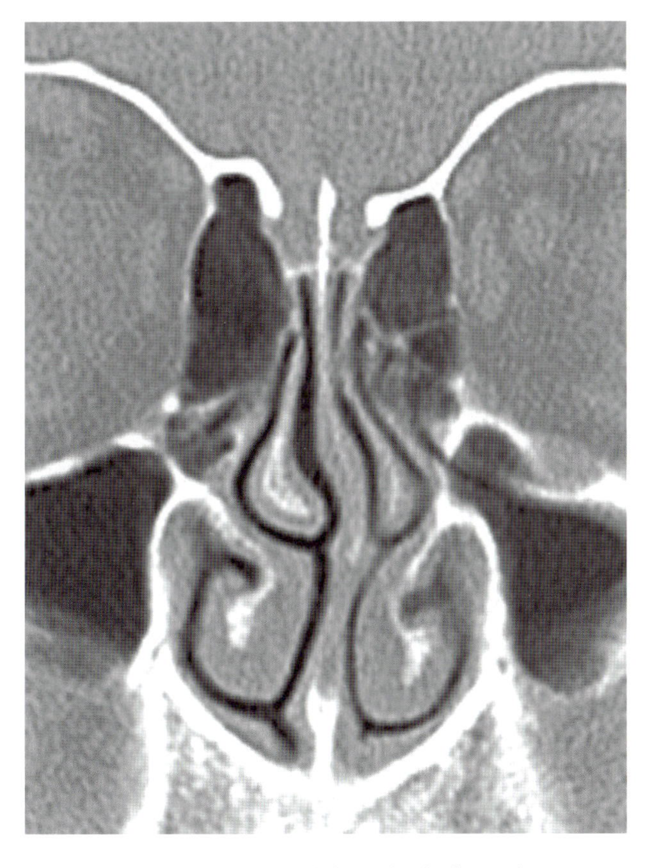

Figure 6.68 *Fovea ethmoidalis and cribriform plate type 3*. The fovea ethmoidalis is at a significantly lower plane than that of the roof of the ethmoid. This type is at a higher risk for trauma during sinus surgery.

DEHISCENCE OF THE BONY WALL AROUND THE OPTIC NERVE (Figures 6.71 and 6.72)

The optic nerve is intimately related to the lateral wall of the posterior ethmoid sinus and the roof of the sphenoid sinus. The posterior ethmoid sinus may expand superiorly into the orbit, forming supraorbital cells, or it may expand laterally to encompass the optic nerve with expanded Onodi cells. These variants, if not identified preoperatively, pose extreme hazards to the patient's vision. The bony dehiscences or thinning of the optic nerve canal pose an added greater risk of trauma to the optic nerve during surgery. If surgery is contemplated in the posterior ethmoid sinuses or sphenoid sinus, it is recommended that at least biplanar CT scans be taken to assess this area of risk, which may be poorly seen on coronal scans.

INTERNAL CAROTID ARTERY WALL DEHISCENCE (Figure 6.73)

The bony walls of the sphenoid sinus around the internal carotid artery may be deficient, making it vulnerable during surgery. An ethmosphenoid sinus anomaly is a clinically important, albeit uncommon,

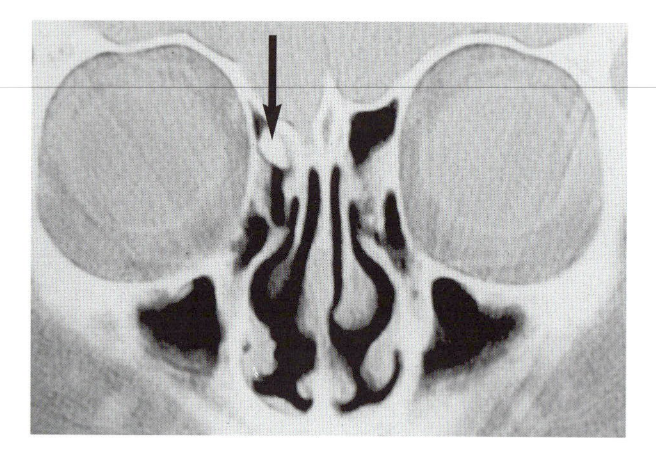

Figure 6.70 *Asymmetry of fovea ethmoidalis and cribriform plate type 3*. There is asymmetry in the roof when compared with each side. A small osteoma is seen in the frontal recess on the right side (arrow).

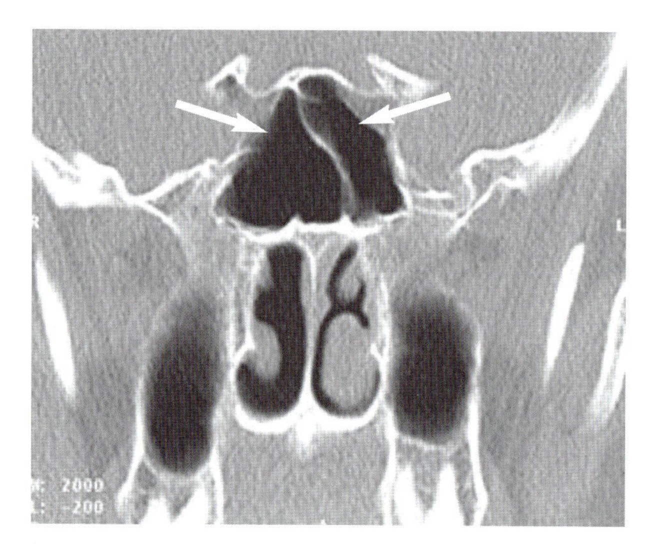

Figure 6.71 *Dehiscence of the bony wall around optic nerve*. The bony wall that surrounds the optic nerve (arrow) is deficient. The optic nerve is vulnerable during any sinus surgery in such patients.

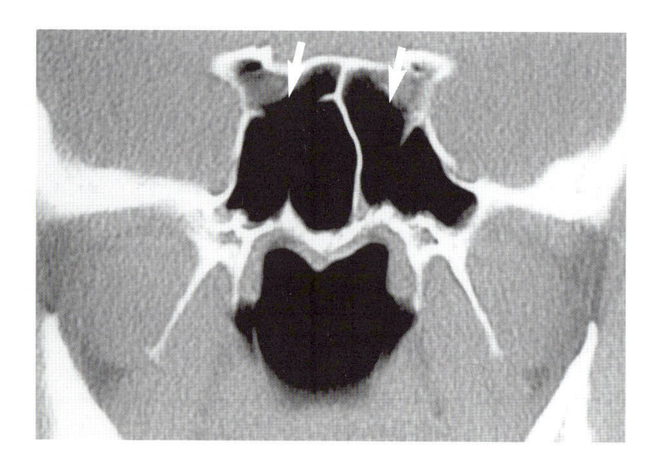

Figure 6.72 *Dehiscence of the bony wall around optic nerve*. The bony optic nerve canal (arrow) along the roof of the sphenoid sinus is absent. Only a thin periosteum and the sinus mucosa separate the nerve from the sinus.

6.73a

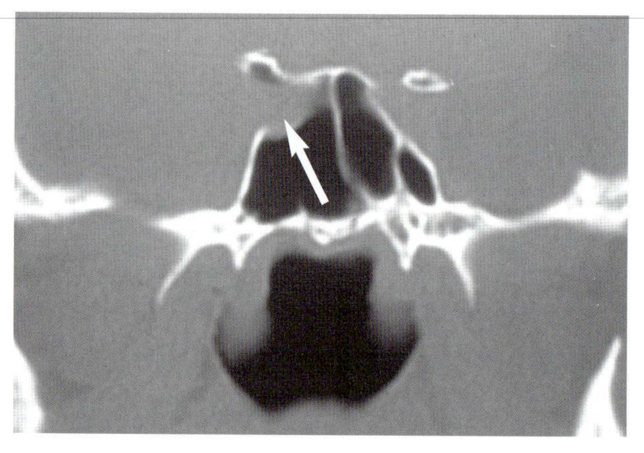

6.73b

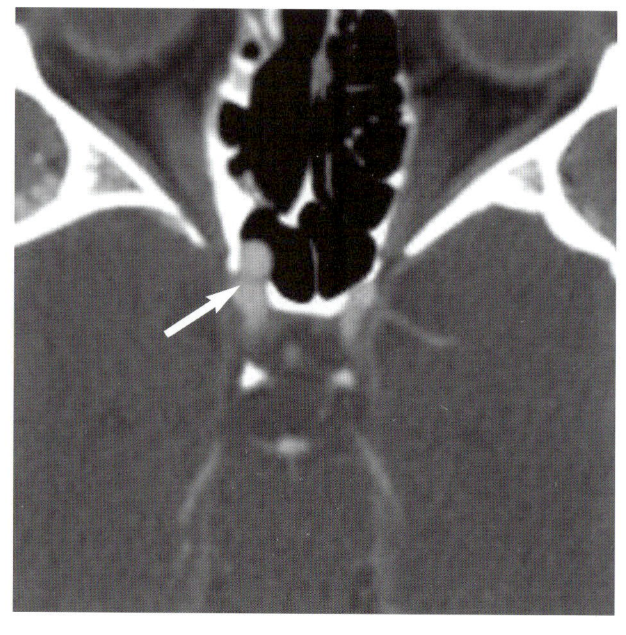

Figure 6.73 (a) *Dehiscence of the bony wall around internal carotid artery*. The bony wall around the right internal carotid artery (arrow) is deficient and the artery is protruding into the lumen of the sphenoid sinus. (b) *Protrusion of internal carotid artery into sphenoid sinus*. Contrast-enhanced axial CT scan demonstrating the right internal carotid artery (arrow) intruding into the sphenoid sinus lumen through a small defect in the wall of the sinus.

variation because of the alteration to the structures related to the lateral wall of the sphenoid and ethmoid sinuses. Normally, the internal carotid artery is in close relation to the sphenoid sinus, but with the ethmoid sinus expanding into the sphenoid bone, the internal carotid artery lies along the lateral wall of the posterior ethmoid sinus. Surgical intervention is more common in the posterior ethmoid sinus than the sphenoid sinus, and the surgeon should be made aware of the close proximity of the internal carotid artery to the posterior ethmoid when an ethmosphenoid sinus anomaly is identified.

ANATOMICAL VARIANTS OF THE MAXILLARY SINUS

Anatomical variants of the maxillary include asymmetry, hypoplasia of one or both maxillary sinuses, septated maxillary sinus, double maxillary sinus, atelectatic maxillary sinus, and ethmomaxillary sinus.

Hypoplasia of the maxillary sinus

(Figures 6.74–6.80)

Primary maxillary sinus hypoplasia

Primary hypoplasia of the maxillary sinus is a developmental abnormality that can be identified radiologically in patients with and without sinus disease (Table 6.3).

Asymmetric sinuses may be demonstrated by plain radiographs. A smaller sinus may, however, be misinterpreted as a sinus of normal dimensions with chronic maxillary sinusitis, especially in patients with a history of persistent upper respiratory tract infection. In such circumstances, these patients may be erroneously subjected to prolonged medical management and may undergo surgical exploration only to find normal sinus mucosa within the smaller sinus cavity. The superior bone, air, and soft tissue contrast resolution of CT enables the radiologist to diagnose such variants accurately and has led to the finding of the association of hypoplasia of the uncinate process with hypoplasia of the maxillary sinus. With increasing severity of the hypoplasia, a corresponding degree of hypoplasia or aplasia of the uncinate has been noted. This finding should be documented, because an attempted uncinectomy in these patients will lead to inadver-

6.74a

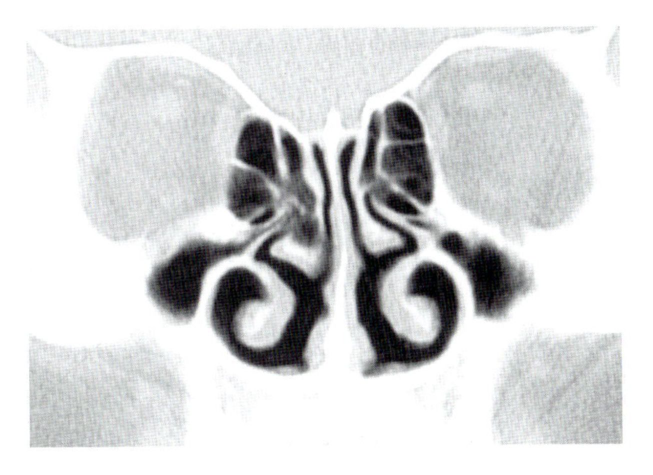

6.74b

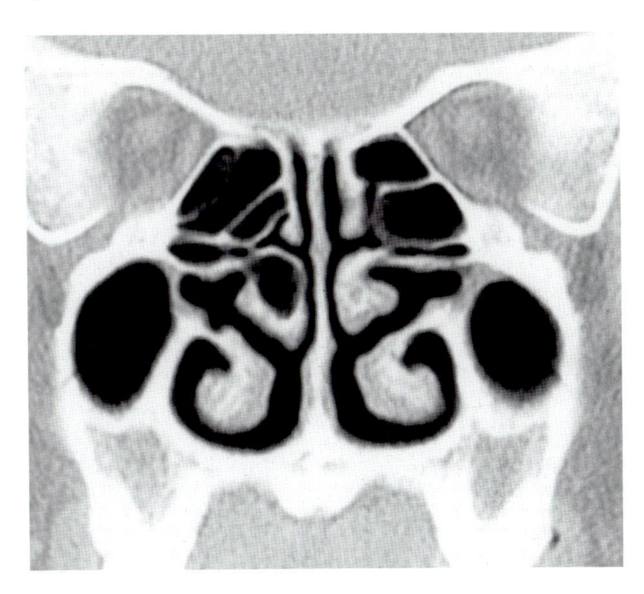

Figure 6.74 *Type I maxillary sinus hypoplasia.* (a, b) CT scans from the same patient demonstrating the maxillary sinus volume to be small. No other abnormality is seen.

Table 6.3 Imaging findings in primary maxillary sinus hypoplasia

- Enlargement of ipsilateral orbits
- Enlargement of superior and inferior orbital fissures
- Enlargement of pterygopalatine fossa
- Widening of middle meatus and retraction of fontanelles
- Elevation of canine fossa
- Lateralized infraorbital nerve
- Uncinate process hypoplasia and lateralization
- Small ethmoid bulla
- Asymmetric cribriform plate
- Low-lying fovea ethmoidalis

6.75a

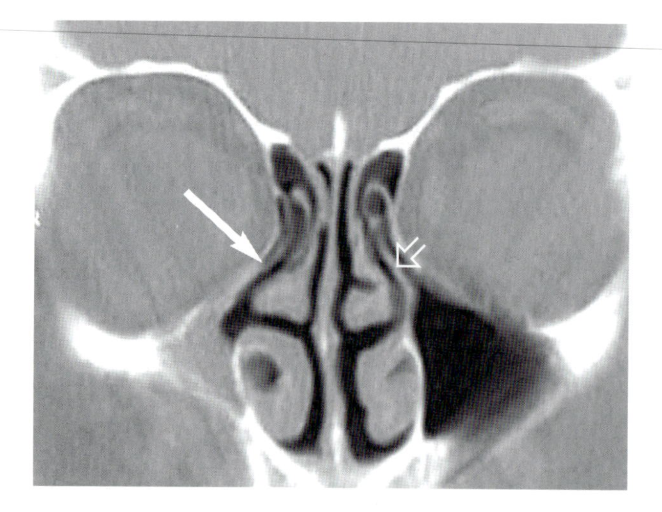

6.75b

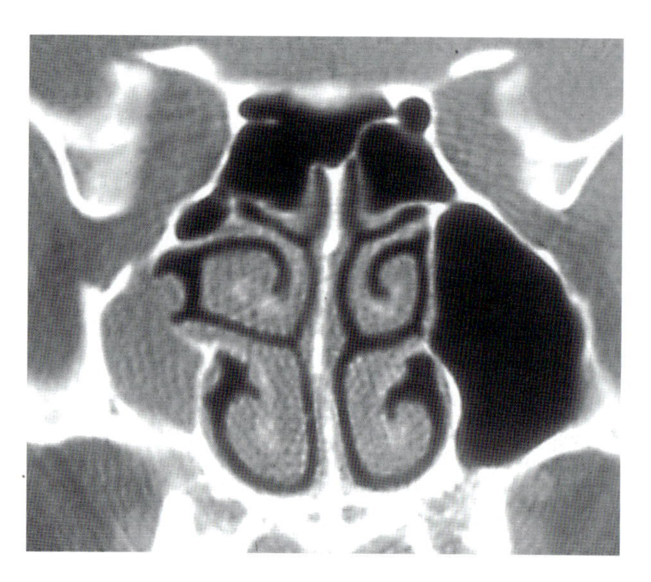

Figure 6.75 *Type II maxillary sinus hypoplasia*. (a, b) CT scans from the same patient demonstrating the maxillary sinus volume to be small on the right side. There is opacification of the sinus lumen and the uncinate process (arrow) is plastered against the lateral nasal wall. Note the normal uncinate process on the left side (open arrow).

6.76a

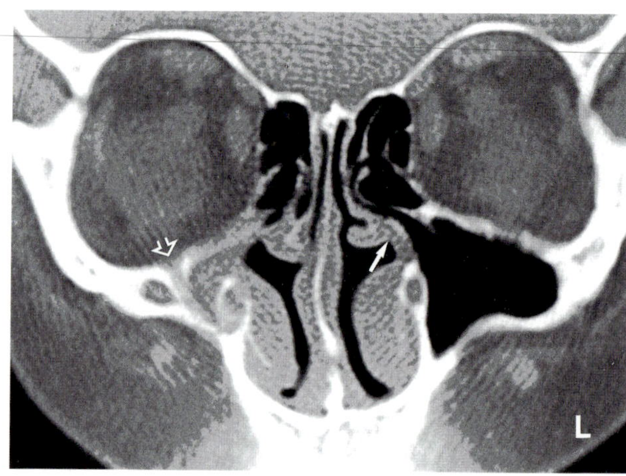

6.76b

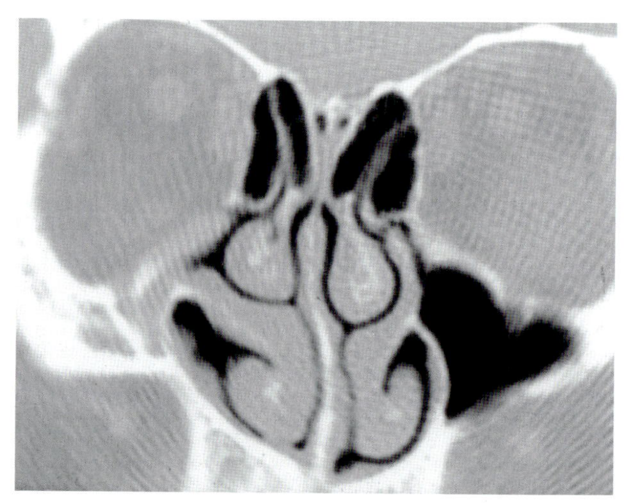

Figure 6.76 *Type III unilateral maxillary sinus hypoplasia*. (a) Coronal CT scan demonstrating a hypoplastic sinus on the right side. Consequently, the right orbital floor lies at a lower level than the left orbital floor. The right orbit is larger and the infraorbital canal (open arrow) appears more laterally placed. There is apposition of the uncinate process and a paradoxically bent middle turbinate (arrow) on the left side. (b) Coronal CT scan demonstrating a hypoplastic sinus on the right side, with elevation of the canine fossa.

tent entry into the orbit through the lamina papyracea or orbital floor.

Bolger and Parsons analyzed a series of 202 consecutive CT scans, and noted a prevalence of maxillary sinus hypoplasia in 10% of this population. They presented a classification system (types I, II, and III) based upon the radiographic features of the sinus as seen on CT.

In *type I maxillary sinus hypoplasia* (incidence 7%) there is only a mild decrease in the maxillary sinus volume, with a normal uncinate process and a normal ethmoid infundibulum.

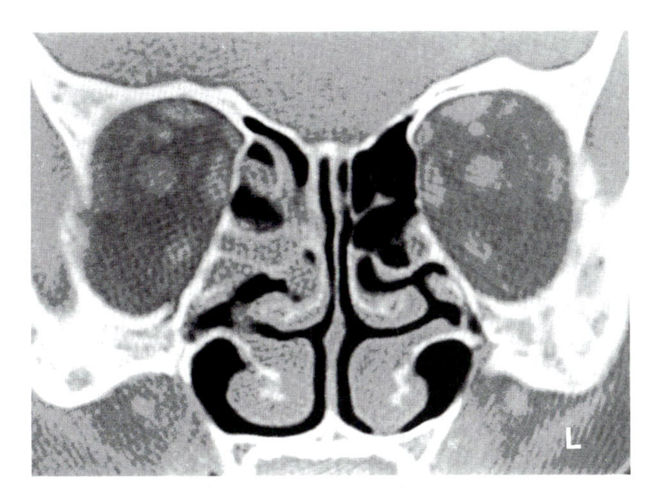

Figure 6.77 *Type III bilateral maxillary sinus hypoplasia.* Bilateral hypoplasia of the maxillary sinus with a wider nasal cavity and large orbit is noted. The canine fossa is deep.

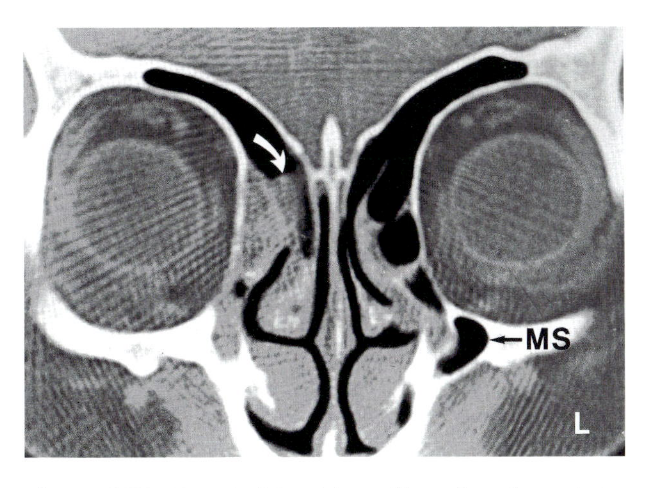

Figure 6.78 *Type III bilateral maxillary sinus hypoplasia.* There is bilateral maxillary sinus hypoplasia (MS). In addition, there is a frontal recess (curved arrow) and ethmoid sinus disease.

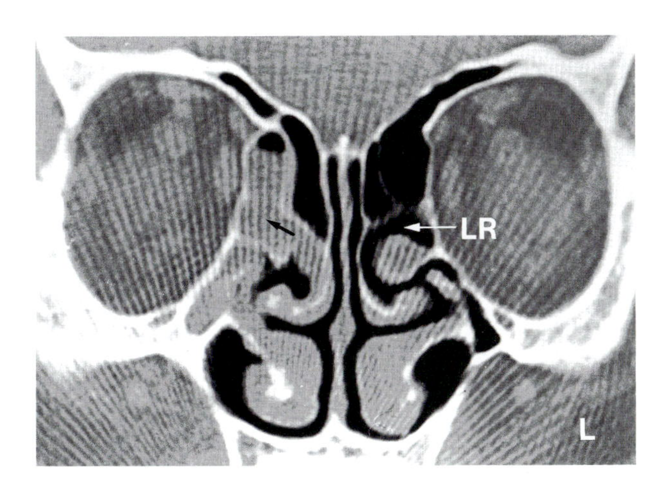

Figure 6.79 *Type III bilateral maxillary sinus hypoplasia.* The maxillary sinuses are small and the frontal recess is draining into the lateral sinus (LR).

6.80a

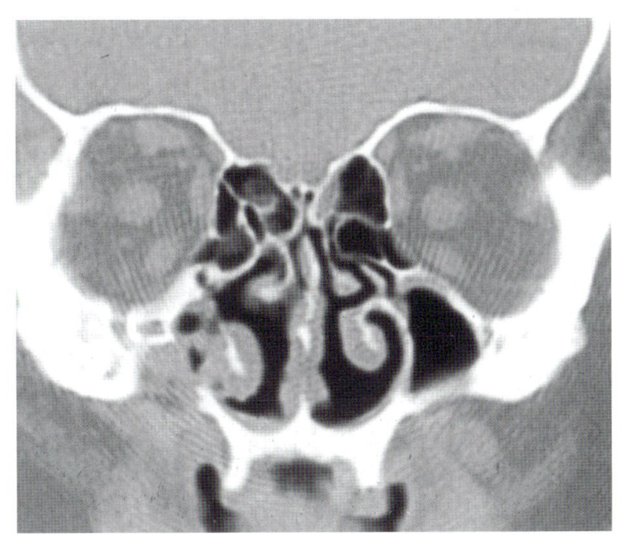

6.80b

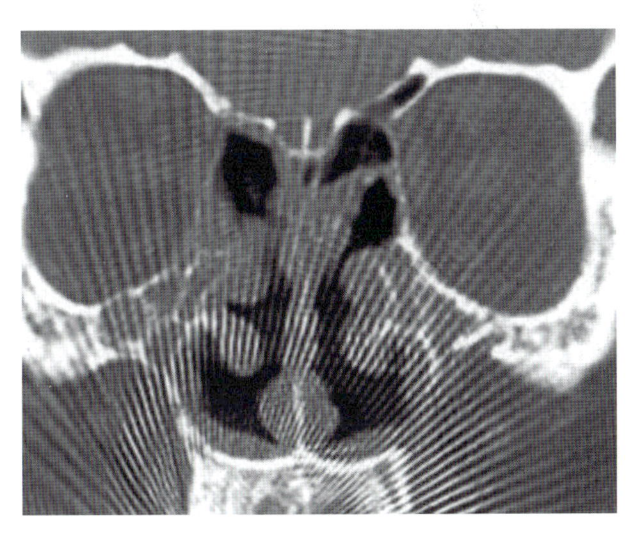

Figure 6.80 *Postoperative hypoplasia of maxillary sinus.* There are changes due to previous Caldwell–Luc surgery on the right side. As a result, there is a decrease in the size of the sinus, with mucosal thickening and scarring in the sinus. (b) This patient has changes due to previous Caldwell–Luc surgery in both maxillary sinuses. Again, there is a decrease in the size of the sinus, with mucosal thickening and scarring in the sinus.

In *type II maxillary sinus hypoplasia* (incidence 3%), there is a mild to moderate reduction in the volume of the maxillary sinus combined with CT evidence of an absent or hypoplastic uncinate process and an absent or poorly defined ethmoid infundibulum due to the uncinate process being fused with the inferomedial wall of the orbit. There is marked retraction of the posterior fontanelle into the cavity of the maxillary sinus, and the membranous fontanelle may be misdiagnosed as an air–fluid level.

In type III maxillary sinus hypoplasia (incidence 0.5%), the maxillary sinus is primarily absent and consists only of a cleft. The ethmoid infundibulum and the uncinate process are absent in type III. The nasal cavity and orbit on the involved side are usually enlarged. The maxillary sinus and the nasal cavity are inversely proportional to one another. The smaller is the maxillary sinus, the larger is the nasal cavity on the same side.

The orbital rim may be at a lower level than the normal side, with the eyeball appearing deeply placed with an apparent 'exophthalmos' on the contralateral side. The sinus does not extend laterally as expected and the infraorbital foramen appears to be more laterally placed. The pterygopalatine fossa and the superior and inferior orbital fissures are enlarged and the bony walls are thick. The natural ostium is bony.

Acquired hypoplasia of the maxillary sinus

Acquired hypoplasia of the maxillary sinus can occur as the result of a variety of factors:

- Trauma, including Caldwell–Luc surgery
- Infection
- Radiation
- Fibrous dysplasia
- Paget's disease
- Systemic disease

It is represented by a maxilla of normal size, with the inflammatory reaction producing a partial or complete obliteration and resorption of the sinus lumen.

Hyperplasia of the maxillary sinus

Maxillary sinus hyperplasia is an uncommon condition in which there has been extensive pneumatization of the maxilla, with large recesses that pneumatize the alveolar ridge and the lateral recesses of the zygoma. There is compensatory narrowing of the nasal cavity in these patients.

Septated maxillary sinus (Figure 6.81)

The maxillary sinus may be subdivided by septi that may be either fibrous or bony and that incompletely divide the sinus into two unequal halves. These septi usually extend from the infraorbital canal to the lateral wall of the sinus, thereby forming a superolateral and an inferomedial compartment. These compartments usually communicate with each other through a defect somewhere in the septum. Such anomalies should be identified to prevent incomplete drainage procedures that may result in the persistence of sinus disease. A double maxillary sinus is a rare anomaly where two independent cavities in the same maxilla drain into the middle meatus through two separate ostia.

Ethmomaxillary sinus (Figures 6.82 and 6.83)

Pneumatization of the posterior ethmoid sinuses is variable, and may extend beyond the confines of the ethmoid bone. In this condition, the posterior ethmoid sinus extends laterally into the maxilla, forming an ethmomaxillary sinus. An ethmomaxillary sinus may extend superiorly into the orbit, laterally it may surround the optic nerve, and

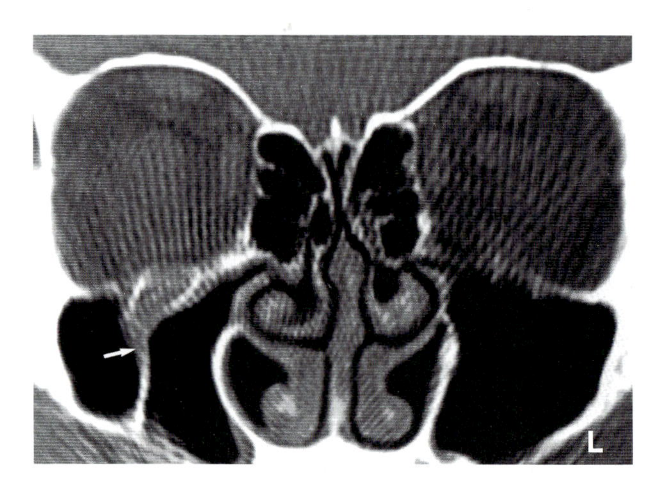

Figure 6.81 *Septated maxillary sinus.* In this CT scan, a bony septum (arrow) is seen arising from the region of the infraorbital canal, which extends to the lateral wall, dividing the right maxillary sinus into two unequal halves. These compartments usually communicate with each other through a defect somewhere in the septum.

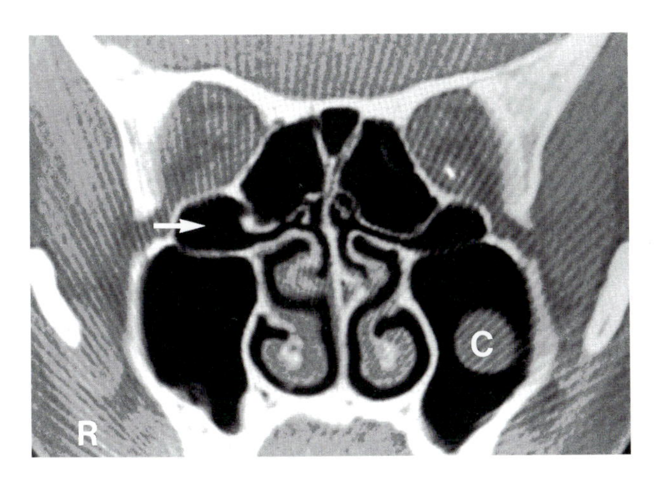

Figure 6.82 *Ethmomaxillary sinus.* The ethmomaxillary sinus (arrow) is connected to the superior meatus by a short and medially directed bony channel. A small cyst (C) can be seen in the left maxillary sinus.

posteriorly it can extend into the sphenoid bone. Irrespective of the bone that is pneumatized, all of these additional air cells drain into the superior meatus. This anomaly has the appearance of a septated sinus, but it can be differentiated by identifying the superior compartment that, having developed from the posterior ethmoid, drains into the superior meatus. The adjacent superior meatus is usually deeper and larger, whereas the related maxillary sinus is smaller or normal in size.

CHOANAL ATRESIA (Figure 6.84)

Choanal atresia is a congenital malformation associated with failure of canalization of the nasal cavity. The atretic plate may be bony, membranous, or a combination of the two.

There are several hypotheses for the cause of this malformation. According to some, failure of resorption of the mesodermal plate results in bony atresia, and membranous atresia is persistence of the buccopharyngeal membrane. Bilateral choanal atresia presents at birth with the immediate need to establish an airway.

A unilateral bony or membranous atresia usually presents later in life, with a history of lifelong unilateral nasal obstruction, nasal discharge, nasal asymmetry, deformity, and snoring.

6.83a

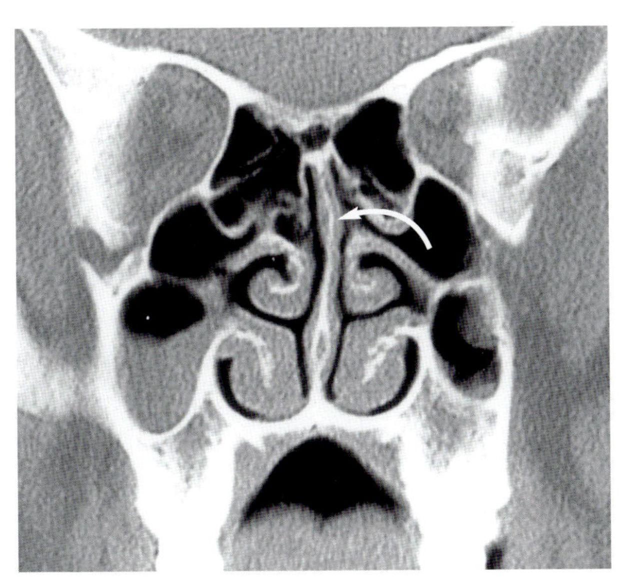

6.83b

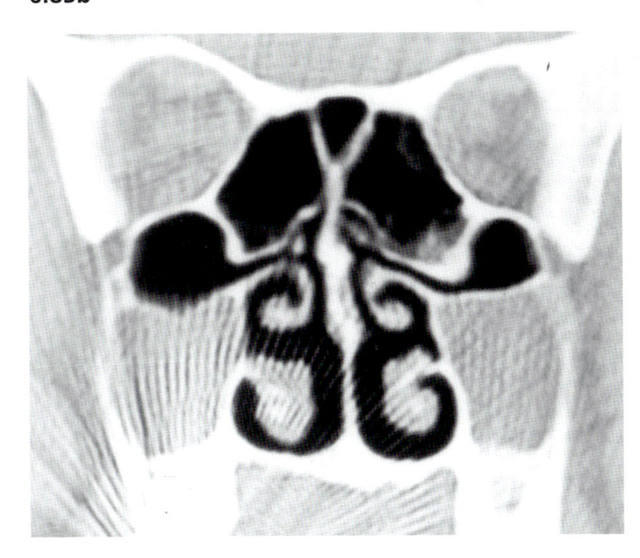

Figure 6.83 *Ethmomaxillary sinus.* (a) An ethmomaxillary sinus is an extension of the ethmoid sinus around the maxillary sinus and drains into the superior meatus (curved arrow) – as opposed to a septated sinus, where the two compartments drain into the middle meatus. (b) The ethmomaxillary sinus appears as a deep recess around the maxillary sinus, and the maxillary sinus is opacified bilaterally from sinusitis.

6.84a

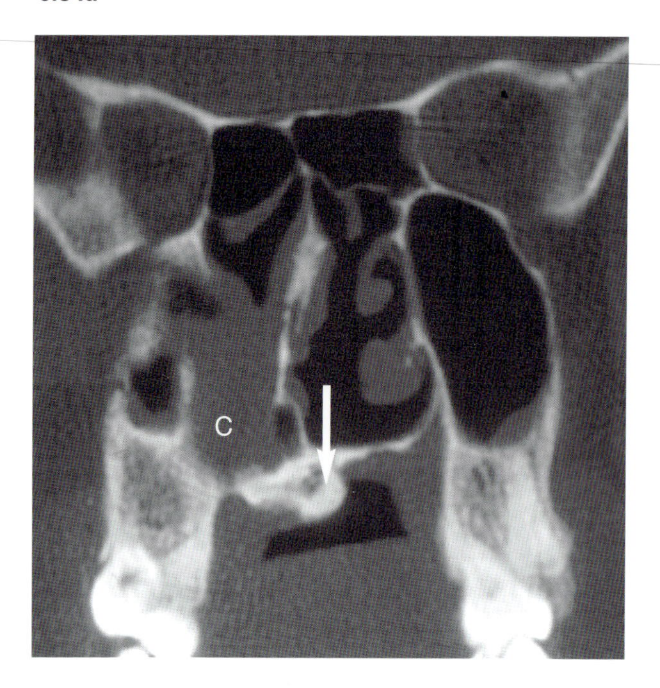

6.84b

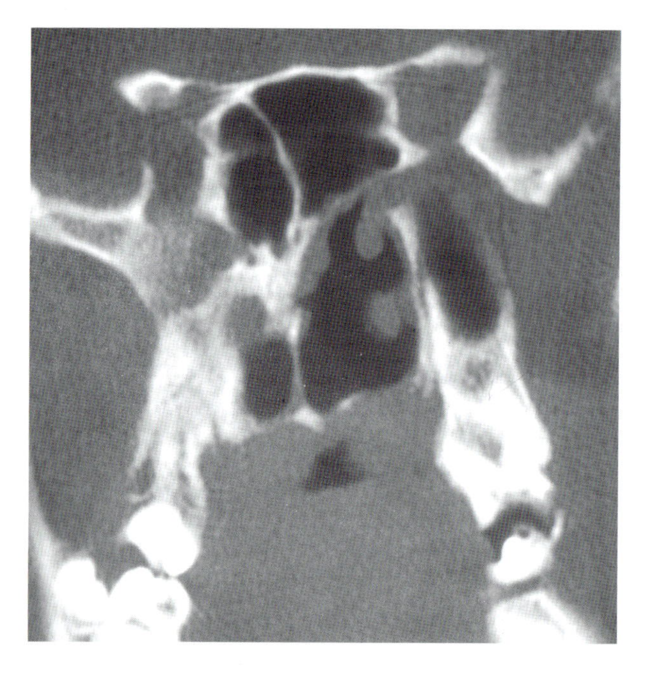

Figure 6.84 *Choanal atresia*. (a, b) This 22-year-old patient presented with unilateral nasal obstruction. She had had right-sided obstruction since childhood, and the CT scan demonstrates the presence of soft tissue in the posterior nasal cavity. In addition, the bony right posterior choanal aperture (C) is smaller when compared with the left side. As a result, there is asymmetric development of the sinus walls and the surrounding bony walls. Note the bony exostosis of the hard palate. This is a dense compact bony mass, also referred to as a torus palatinus (arrow), and is believed to be hereditary with a female predominance. Surgical removal is necessary if the patient has difficulty in swallowing, or needs orthodontic or denture fitting.

7

The radiological features of inflammatory diseases

INTRODUCTION

Historically, surgical procedures to alleviate recurrent or chronic sinusitis were directed at the larger paranasal sinuses. It was thought that the ventilation of these sinuses could be improved by creating new, and theoretically more effective, alternative drainage pathways. Alternative drainage procedures, such as the inferior meatal antrostomy, are now known not to redirect the flow of mucus through the newly created opening (the antrostomy), but only to act as a 'drain' when the mucociliary system is overwhelmed by mucus and pus. The persistence of symptoms following these procedures is usually secondary to persistent disease in the anterior ethmoid air cells affecting the natural ostia and the ostiomeatal complex. Recurrent sinus infections may also occur despite there being a widely patent natural accessory ostium when ostiomeatal complex disease is present.

Functional endoscopic sinus surgery is directed at the natural drainage pathways. The limited surgical resection of the tissue responsible for 'obstruction' of the ethmoid prechambers widens these natural clefts and improves both sinus ventilation and drainage, and can lead to reversal of the mucosal disease in the larger paranasal sinuses.

Surgical excision of the uncinate process and the uncovering of the natural maxillary sinus ostium can lead to resolution of the secondary changes seen in the larger sinuses.

Plain radiographs have in the past been used to screen for the presence of sinus infection in the frontal, maxillary, or sphenoid sinuses. The mucosal lining of the sinus may be thickened, and if mucus or pus is collecting in the sinus, an air–fluid level may be evident. In cases of severe sinusitis, the extensive mucosal edema and fluid exudate will make the sinus appear totally opaque. The infection may be confined to only one cavity – usually the maxillary or the frontal sinus – or it may involve all of the sinuses on one side causing a 'pansinusitis'. Spread of infection from the anterior ethmoid complex to the posterior ethmoid sinus is usually through a defect in the ground lamella.

ACUTE SINUSITIS

(Figures 7.1–7.3)

Acute sinusitis is characterized clinically by malaise, nasal obstruction, purulent nasal discharge, postnasal drip, and facial pain. The characteristic distribution of the pain or headache may help the clinician in determining the origin of the disease. The pain of frontal sinusitis radiates to the forehead and is usually associated with a generalized headache. In acute maxillary sinusitis, the pain usually radiates from the medial canthus to the cheek. The pain may also radiate to the alveolar region, mimicking dental disease. Acute ethmoid sinusitis is associated with pain that tends to localize to the bridge of the nose and behind the medial canthus of the eye. It is often cyclical, being worse in the morning after rising.

Sphenoid sinusitis probably occurs more frequently than is appreciated. Patients are more likely to be investigated for the cause of headache by

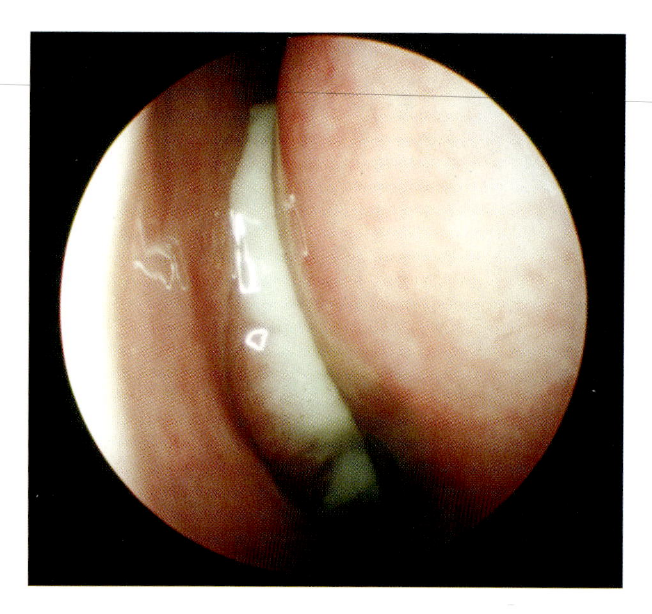

Figure 7.1 *Endoscopic view of acute sinusitis.* Pus is seen in the middle meatus due to acute maxillary and ethmoid sinusitis.

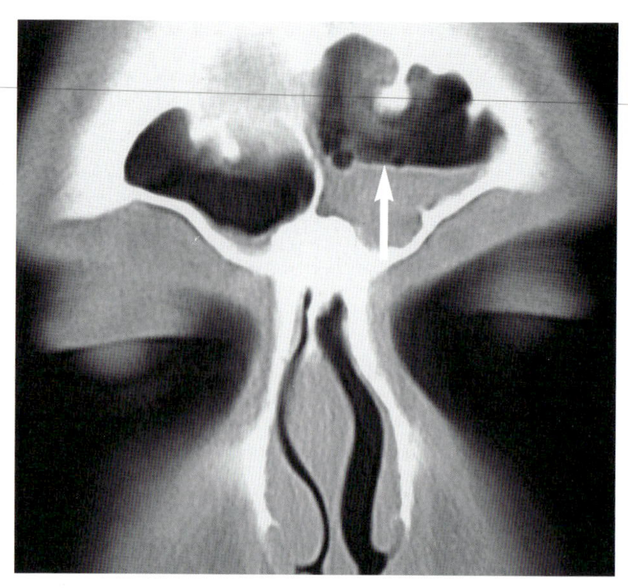

Figure 7.3 *Acute frontal sinusitis.* CT scan demonstrating the air–fluid level in the left frontal sinus (arrow).

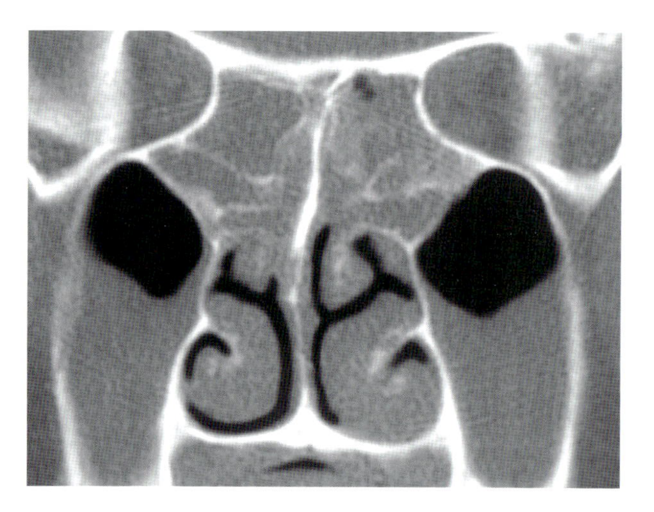

Figure 7.2 *Acute bilateral maxillary and ethmoid sinusitis.* Air–fluid levels can be identified in the maxillary sinuses. In addition, there are inflammatory changes in the ethmoid sinuses. CT scans performed during the acute phase of disease may obscure the ostiomeatal complexes and any anatomical variants.

neurologists with routine head scans. These patients present with posterior occipital or vertical headache, as well as retro-orbital pain. In all types of sinusitis, the pain is more severe if the ostium of the sinus becomes totally obstructed and an empyema forms. This situation can cause severe morbidity, as the infection can spread through the sinus walls leading to intraorbital or intracranial sepsis.

CHRONIC SINUSITIS (Figures 7.4–7.8)

The symptoms of chronic sinusitis are variable, and generally mild. These patients frequently present with recurrent headaches and facial pain. There is usually a combination of nasal obstruction, rhinorrhea and postnasal drip. Multiple episodes of acute (recurrent) sinusitis or a prolonged episode of persistent (subacute) infection are classified as 'chronic sinusitis'. Epistaxis, anosmia or cacosmia, and nasal vestibulitis may be caused by chronic sinusitis.

The radiological features of chronic sinusitis are similar to those of acute sinusitis when there is an acute process superimposed upon the chronic disease.

The computed tomography (CT) features of chronic sinusitis are as follows:

- There is mucosal thickening or retained secretion in the lumen of the involved sinus. Over time, the mucoperiosteum becomes thickened, and chronic fibrosis with polypoid proliferation and retained secretions contribute to the opacification of the involved sinuses.
- Recurrent or chronic sinusitis will produce osteitis with new bone formation along the contours of the sinus cavity. The extent of the osteitis is proportionate to the frequency of infection and the length of the clinical history.

7.4a

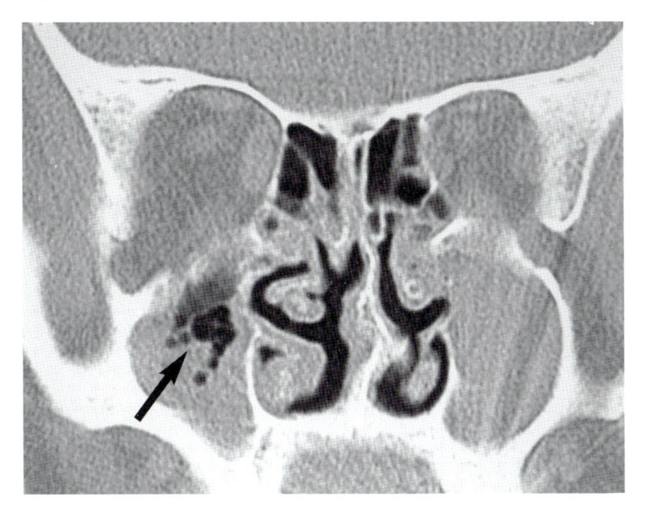

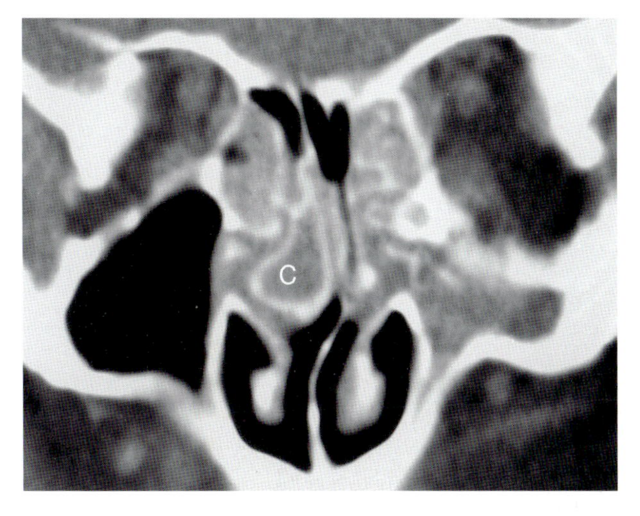

Figure 7.5 *Chronic ethmoid sinusitis*. CT scan demonstrating opacification of the ethmoid sinuses with the septum being coarse and thickened as a result of recurrent sinus infection. Fluid and inflammatory changes can be seen in the lumen of the right concha bullosa (C).

7.4b

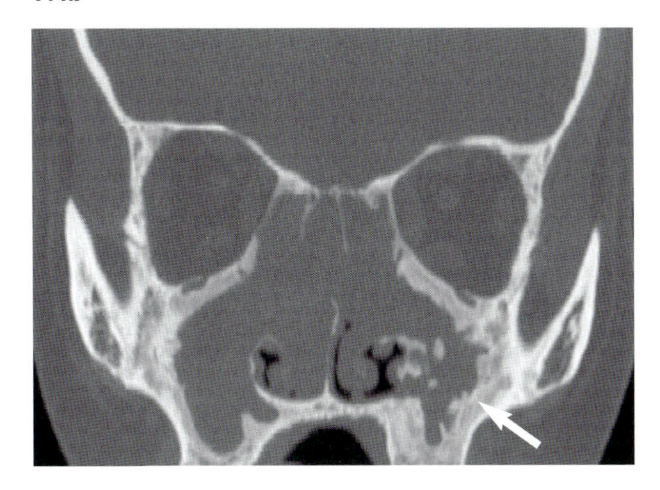

Figure 7.4 *Chronic maxillary sinusitis*. (a) CT scan demonstrating mucosal disease with fluid in the right maxillary sinus and a loculated air and mucus discharge (arrow) in the lumen. There is fluid in the left maxillary sinus, and reactive osteitis is seen in the walls of the maxillary sinuses bilaterally. (b) CT scan demonstrating reactive osteitis (arrow) involving the left maxillary sinus walls as a result of chronic recurrent sinusitis.

- The resulting sclerosis can lead to thickening of the sinus wall and a diminished volume of the sinus cavity.
- The sinus walls may be eroded by chronic benign inflammation, usually occurring along the medial wall of the maxillary sinus and around the infraorbital canal.
- If chronic infections occur during childhood, the sinus may remain small and hypoplastic.

MAGNETIC RESONANCE IMAGING (MRI) FEATURES OF SINUSITIS

Normal sinonasal mucus is a combination of secretions from the submucosal glands and the proteinaceous secretion from the goblet cells. Transudates are serous collections with hydrogen protons in abundance. The free mobile hydrogen protons in fluids cause long T1 and T2 relaxation times. Consequently, the classic appearance of low signal intensity on T1-weighted scans and hyperintensity (brighter) on T2-weighted scans will be evident. The other factors that influence the T1 and T2 relaxation times of sinus fluid are the presence of proteinaceous material, hemorrhage, and the viscosity of the fluid.

Unlike serous collections, inflammatory fluid is a protein-rich fluid with a variable amount of hydrogen protons, and is brighter on T1-weighted scans. This makes inflammatory fluid appear either bright on T1-weighted and T2-weighted scans or as a combination of low and high signal intensity.

The classic MRI appearance of benign inflammatory sinusitis is thickened mucosa of low to intermediate signal intensity on T1-weighted scans. On proton density-weighted and T2-weighted scans, the thickened mucosa is hyperintense (brighter) in

7.6a

7.6b

7.6c

7.6d

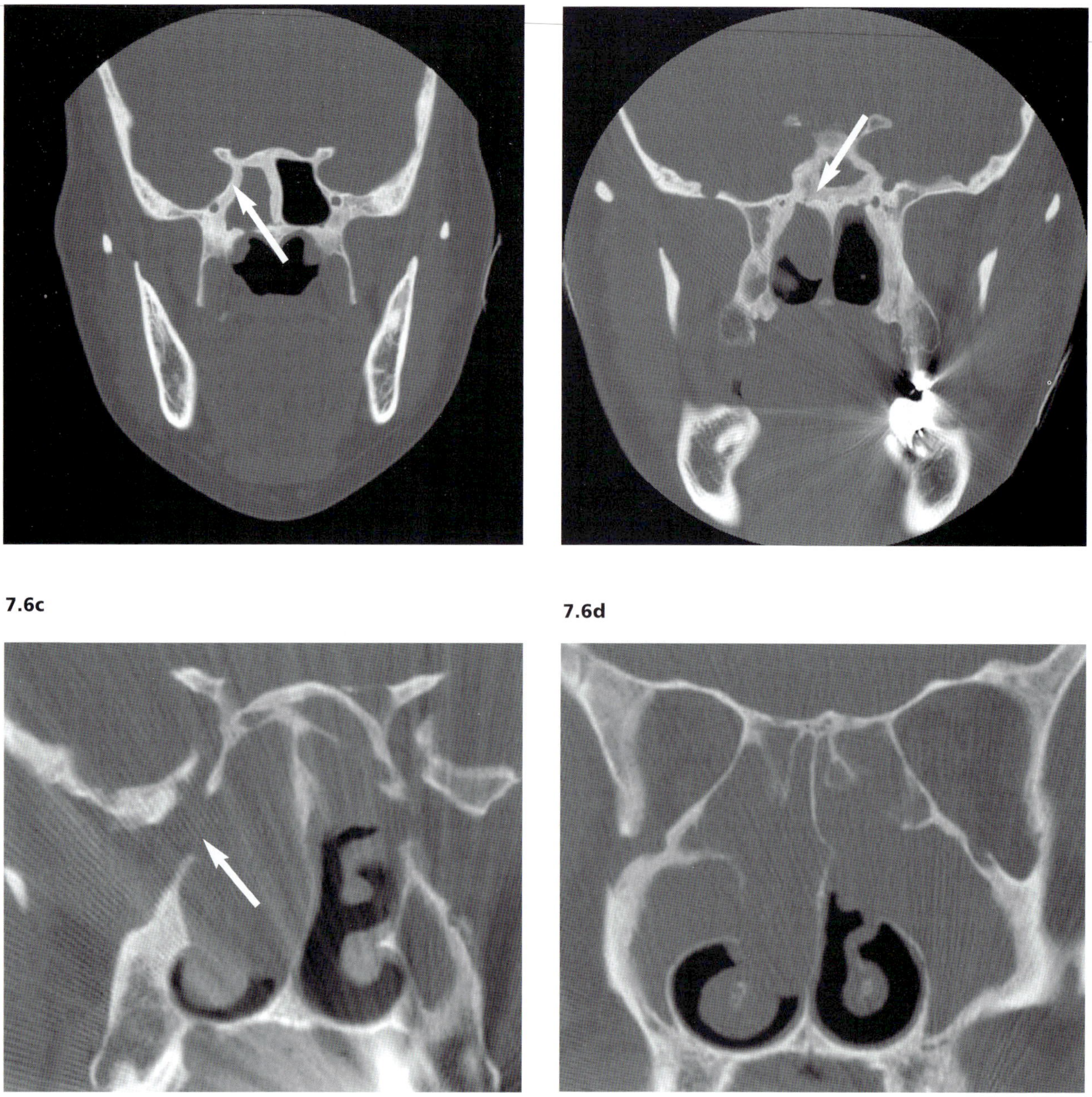

Figure 7.6 *Chronic sphenoid sinusitis*. (a) CT scan demonstrating chronic sphenoid sinusitis, with reactive thickening of the bony wall in the right side (arrow). There is erosion of the floor of the sinus. (b) This patient with a history of cystic fibrosis demonstrates hypertrophic reactive changes in the wall of the sphenoid sinus (arrow). (c, d) The sinonasal mucosa is thickened and polyps are present. There is erosion of the lateral wall of the maxillary sinus in the posterior scans (arrow).

signal intensity. Following the administration of the gadolinium-based contrast agent Gd-DTPA, there is intense enhancement of the inflamed mucosa.

The high signal intensity of inflamed mucosa on T2-weighted scans helps to differentiate active inflammation from fibrosis or scarring, which is of intermediate or low signal intensity on all imaging sequences. Tumors are also intermediate in signal intensity, and consequently differentiation between tumor and fibrosis may be difficult.

Most malignant lesions evoke an inflammatory reaction in the sinonasal mucosa, thus making a carcinoma appear larger than its actual size on CT scans. With MRI scans, it is possible to differentiate the tumor from these benign secondary inflammatory changes, due to the wide differences in their

7.7a

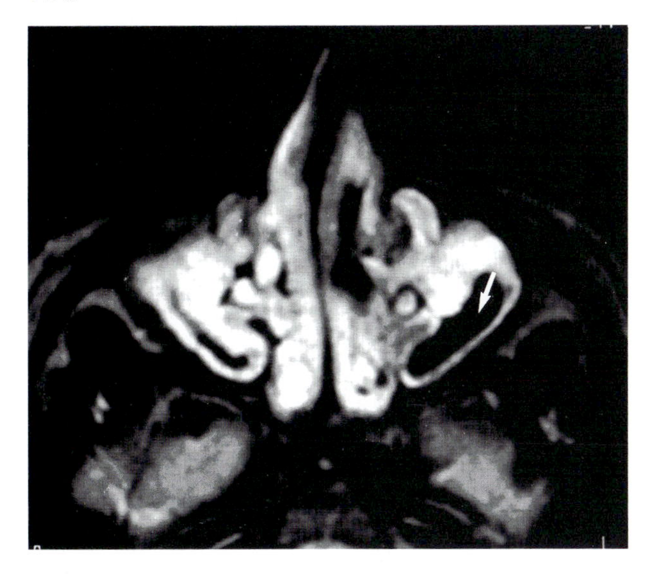

7.7b

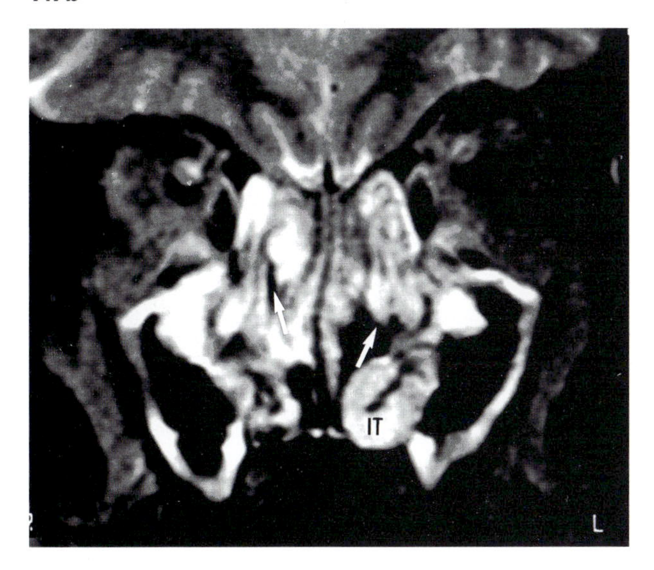

Figure 7.7 (a) *Chronic sinusitis*. T2-weighted MRI scan demonstrating thickened hyperintense mucosa in the maxillary and ethmoid sinuses bilaterally. The dark area is an area of residual air in the left maxillary sinus (arrow). (b) *Postoperative recurrent sinusitis*. In this patient, a T1-weighted MRI scan (not shown) demonstrated densities in the ethmoid and maxillary sinuses that were of intermediate signal. This T2-weighted axial MRI scan shows hyperintensity of the thickened mucosa in the postoperative ethmoid cavity and in the maxillary sinus (arrows). These are non-specific inflammatory changes seen in the ostiomeatal complex bilaterally. A large swollen inferior turbinate (IT) is seen on the left side.

signal intensities. The precise size and margins of the tumor are more clearly delineated on MRI scans, as the signal intensities for inflammation and tumor vary.

MUCOUS RETENTION CYSTS OF THE PARANASAL SINUSES

(Figures 7.9–7.13)

These benign cysts can arise secondary to trauma, infection, or allergy. They occur following obstruction of either a minor salivary gland or a mucus-secreting gland. Mucous retention cysts seen in the floor of the maxillary sinus are most frequently the result of occlusion of the submucosal mucinous glands. These are often seen in perfectly healthy and asymptomatic patients. Serous retention cysts arise due to the accumulation of serous fluid in the submucosal.

Mucous retention cysts are lined with respiratory epithelium, whereas serous cysts have no definable epithelial lining. Retention cysts are usually asymptomatic and can be seen as an incidental finding on 2–5% of sinus radiographs. Retention cysts may be situated along the infraorbital nerve as it passes through the roof of the maxillary sinus, and give rise to paresthesia. Retention cysts rarely require treatment. It is important, however, to rule out the presence of imaging features which may suggest underlying aggressive disease.

The radiological features of retention cysts are as follows:

- There is a dome-shaped density, usually arising along a wall of the sinus. These cysts are of fluid density on CT scans and are hypointense onT1-weighted and hyperintense onT2-weighted MRI scans.
- The surrounding anatomy is usually normal. Large cysts may cause bony remodeling. If the cyst fills the sinus cavity, a crescentic rim of air above the cyst usually allows one to differentiate the cyst from a mucocele.
- Retention cysts cannot be differentiated from polyps. Such differentiation is clinically irrelevant, as both of these entities are benign, and the treatment of the two conditions is identical.

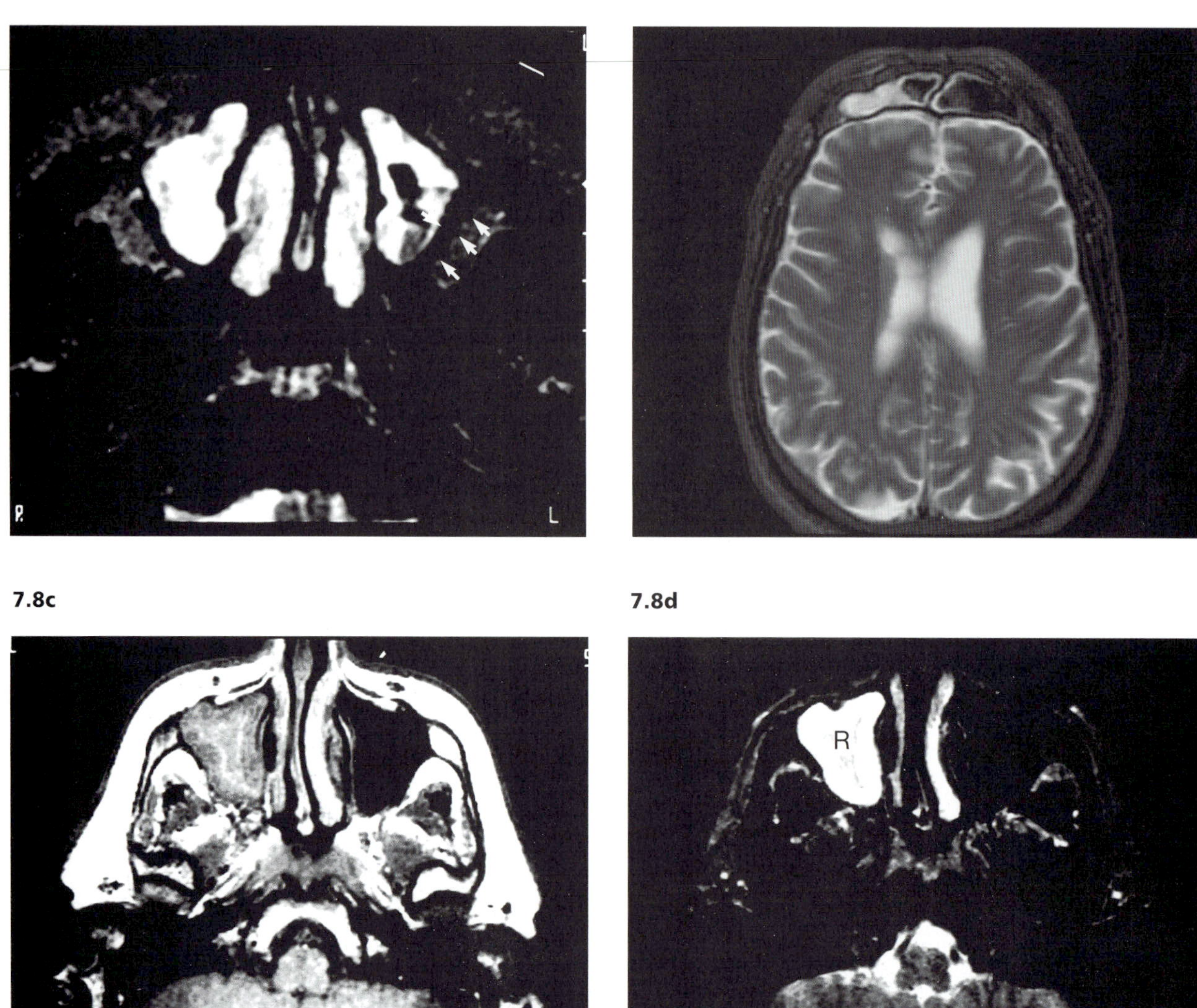

Figure 7.8 (a, b) *Chronic sinusitis*. (a) Thickened and hyperintense mucosa is seen in the maxillary sinuses. There is a small pocket of retained air in the left maxillary sinus. The chronic reactive osteitis is seen as a signal void along the lateral maxillary sinus wall (arrows). (b) T2-weighted MRI scan demonstrating hyperintense, inflamed mucosa in the frontal sinuses. (c, d) *Chronic maxillary sinusitis*. This patient presented with a history of recurrent maxillary sinus infections. (c) On this T1-weighted MRI scan, the contents of the right maxillary sinus and the apparently thickened mucosal lining are of mixed signal intensity and difficult to separate. (d) On this T2-weighted scan of the same patient, the thickened and inflamed (R) mucosal lining of the right maxillary sinus is hyperintense. The lumen of the maxillary sinus has been compromised by the mucosal edema. The purulent secretions within the lumen have a lower signal intensity due to desiccation. This is typical of maxillary sinusitis.

NASAL POLYPS (Figures 7.14–7.36)

The etiology of nasal polyps remains unclear. Chronic inflammation – allergic or infectious in origin – can result in hyperplasia and edema of the sinonasal mucosa. There is accumulation of fluid in the stroma of the polyps, possibly due to a deranged vascular mechanism. The cellularity of polyps may vary. Eosinophils are predominant in polyps derived from allergic or atopic patients.

Patients often present with a long history of nasal obstruction, rhinorrhea, recurrent sinusitis,

7.8e

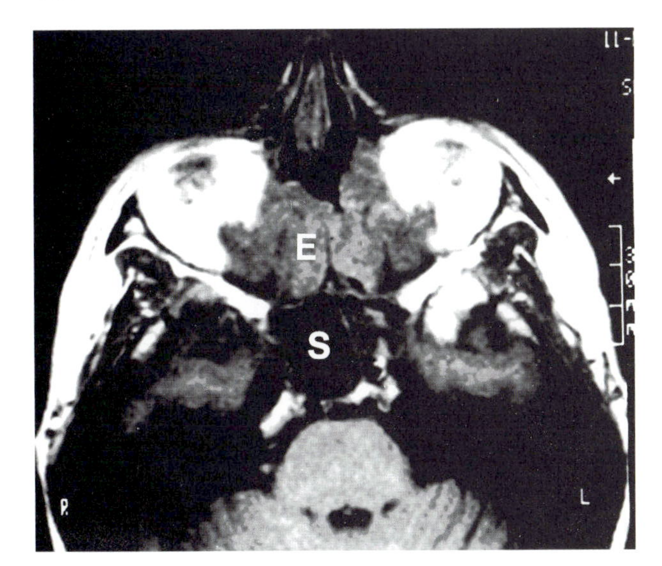

7.8f

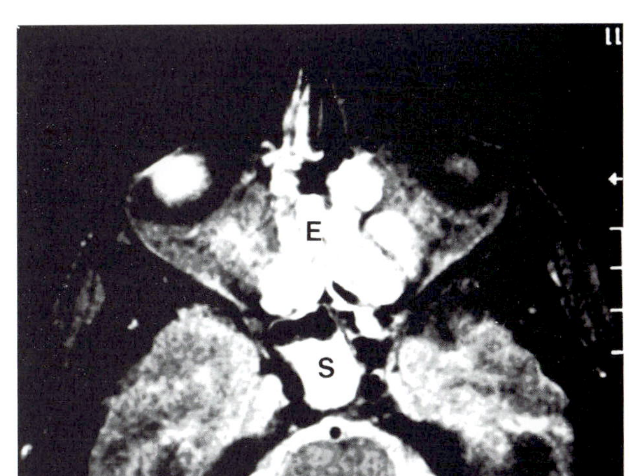

Figure 7.8 *continued* (e, f) *Ethmoid and sphenoid sinusitis*. (e) This T1-weighted MRI scan demonstrates inflammatory mucosal thickening in both posterior ethmoid sinuses (E). There is a faint suggestion of an air–fluid level within the right sphenoid sinus (S). (f) This T2-weighted scan of the same patient demonstrates hyperintensity of the inflamed mucosa in both posterior ethmoid sinuses. The hyperintense air–fluid level in the right sphenoid sinus (S) is clearly seen.

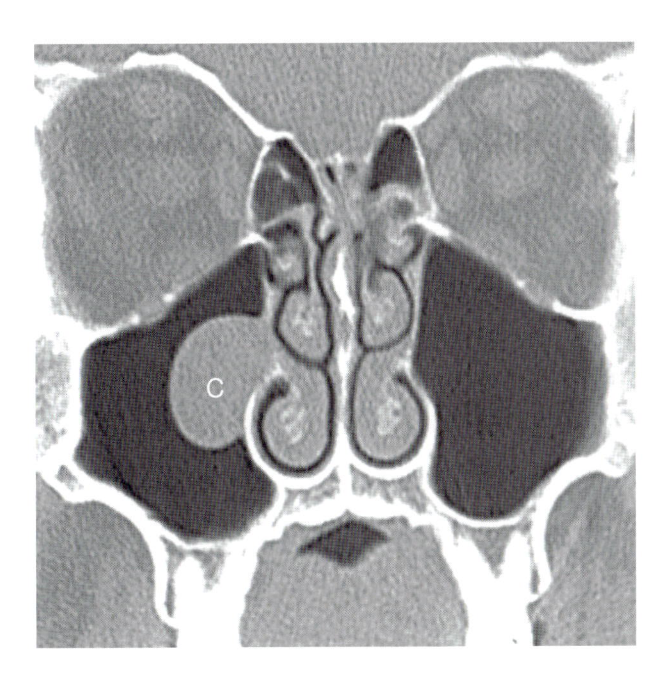

Figure 7.9 *Retention cyst*. A small retention cyst (C) is seen adherent to the medial wall of the right maxillary sinus.

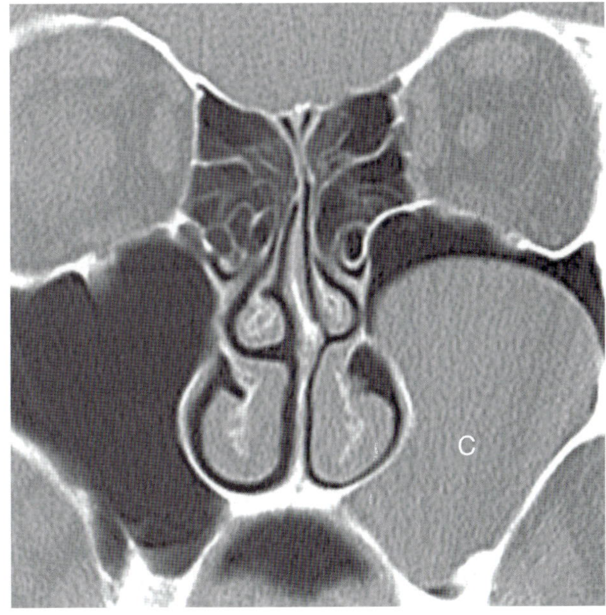

Figure 7.10 *Retention cyst*. A large retention cyst (C) is seen occupying the left maxillary sinus.

and/or headaches. Rarely, hypertelorism or proptosis may arise in those with diffuse polyposis. Both of the nasal cavities are usually filled with polyps, but the finding of unilateral polyps should raise clinical concern of more sinister pathology.

CT appearance of sinonasal polyposis

Nasal polyps are demonstrated on CT by the finding of unilateral or bilateral soft tissue masses within the nasal cavity and paranasal sinuses. Bony rarefaction

7.11a

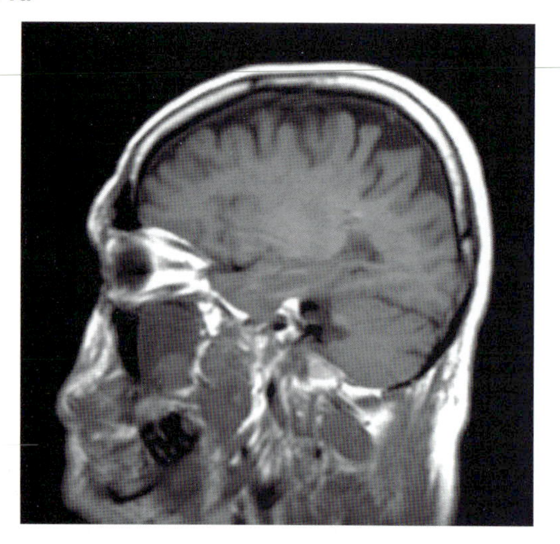

7.11b

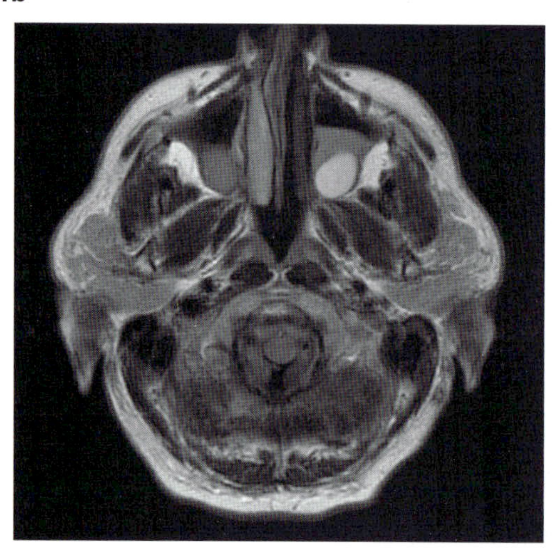

7.11c

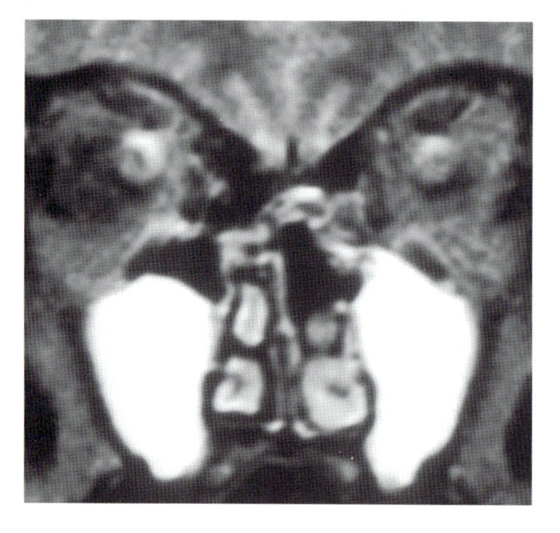

Figure 7.11 *Retention cyst.* (a) T1-weighted MRI scan demonstrating a hypointense lesion in the left maxillary sinus. (b) Gd-DTPA-enhanced MRI scan from same patient demonstrating a large retention cyst with an enhancing polyp in the left maxillary sinus. (c) T2-weighted MRI scan on a different patient demonstrating bilateral large hyperintense mucous retention cysts.

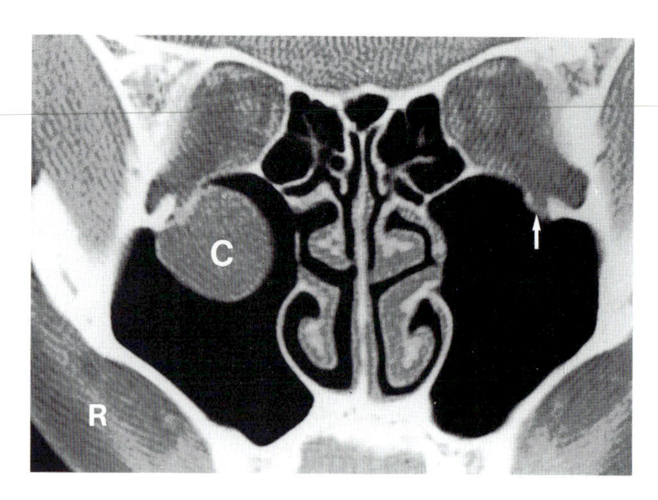

Figure 7.12 *Mucous retention cyst.* This patient presented with right facial pain. This coronal scan demonstrates a mucous retention cyst (C) adjacent to the right infraorbital canal. The left infraorbital canal is demonstrated (arrow).

of the turbinates and walls of the sinuses and ethmoid septa may occur.

The images of the polypoid tissue often demonstrate an alternating mucoid and soft tissue density. This feature can be accentuated by examination with narrow window settings.

Administration of intravenous contrast may show enhancing curvilinear looping strands within the polypoid tissue. The enhancing areas represent areas of mucous membrane surrounded by the mucoid material within the polyp.

Long-standing disease may cause hypertelorism due to expansion of the sinus walls from chronic pressure.

The finding of mixed density or alternating radiating bands of high and low density associated with polyposis may lead to suspicion of fungal sinusitis. The presence of calcification is an unusual feature in inflammatory polyps. Visualization of calcification should raise suspicion of fungal polyposis or foreign-body granulomatous sinusitis.

It has been shown endoscopically that most nasal polyps arise from the ethmoid, the most frequent sites of origin being areas of contact between the infundibulum, the middle turbinate, and the uncinate process. In many other patients, polyps arise from the anterior aspect of the bulla ethmoidalis and protrude into the middle meatus. In up to 50% of patients, polyps are found in the frontal recess. Polyps have also been identified arising in the concha bullosa and the lateral recess. The latter is most

7.13a

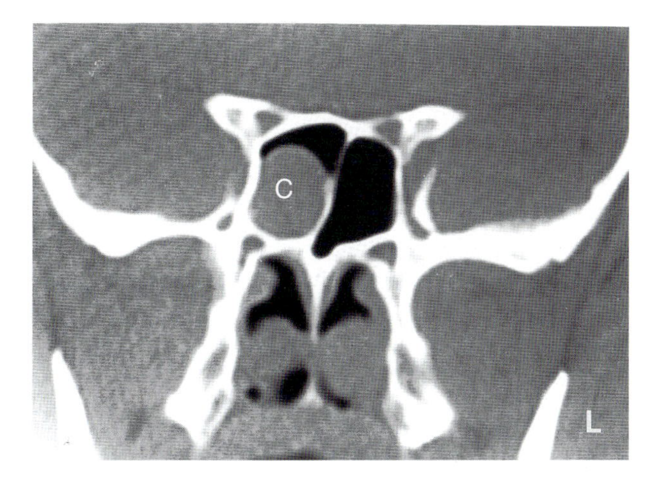

7.13b

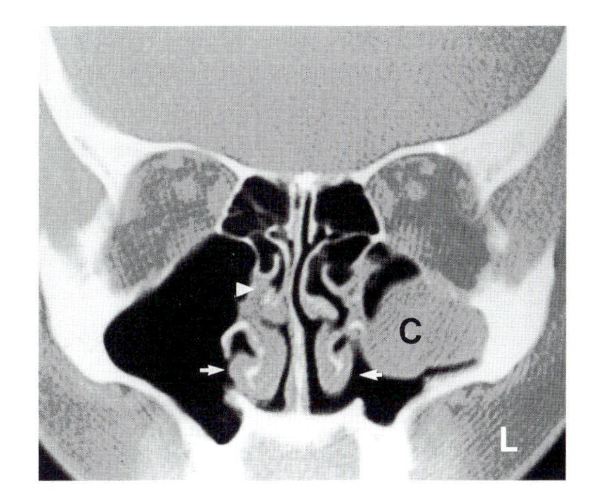

Figure 7.13 (a, b) *Mucous retention cyst*. (a) Coronal scan demonstrating a sphenoid sinus with a retention cyst (C) in the right lateral recess. (b) This patient presented with a history of previous sinus surgery for recurrent sinusitis. This coronal scan demonstrates bilateral intranasal antrostomies (arrows). There remains bilateral ostiomeatal complex disease with inflammatory disease in the right middle meatus (arrowhead). A small retention cyst or polyp is seen within the lumen of the left maxillary sinus (C). Most cysts are situated in the dependent part of the sinus cavity.

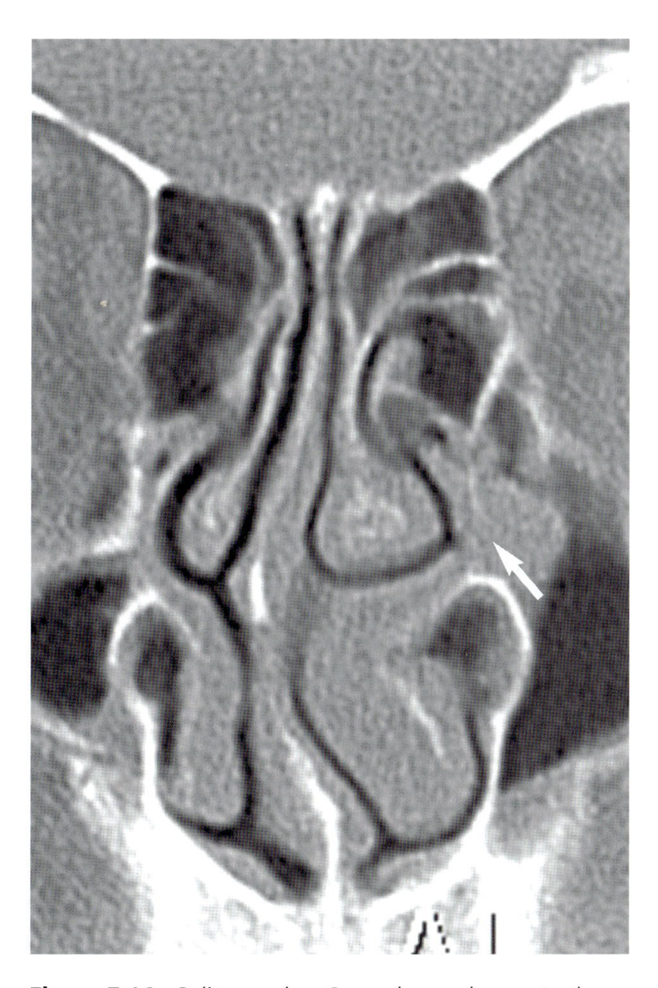

Figure 7.14 *Solitary polyp*. Coronal scan demonstrating a small polyp in the left ostiomeatal complex (arrow). Although easily demonstrated on the CT scan, this could not be identified on clinical examination.

frequently affected when there is simultaneous polypoid involvement of the posterior ethmoid sinus. In uncomplicated polyposis, the anterior ethmoid is almost always involved. Isolated polyps have not been identified arising solely from the posterior ethmoid sinus, except around tumors. Only 8% of sphenoid sinuses show any polypoid change. Relatively minor polypoid change in the ostiomeatal complex revealed by diagnostic endoscopy may be found to be extensive when the patient is examined by CT.

It may be difficult to interpret accurately CT scans of patients with massive polyposis if they have undergone previous surgery. There may be extensive resorption of bone following pressure necrosis, and all that may be seen is an amorphous mass of polypoid tissue, indicating the need for a radical procedure – which may be at variance with the decision based on diagnostic endoscopy. Surgical decisions should not be based solely on radiographic findings. However, in those who have undergone previous surgery, CT is of value in demonstrating the presence of critical bony defects as well as the precise location of disease.

There are no unique radiological features that will lead to a definite diagnosis of nasal polyposis. The presence of aggressive destructive change can raise the suspicion of neoplasm, and biopsy may be

7.15a

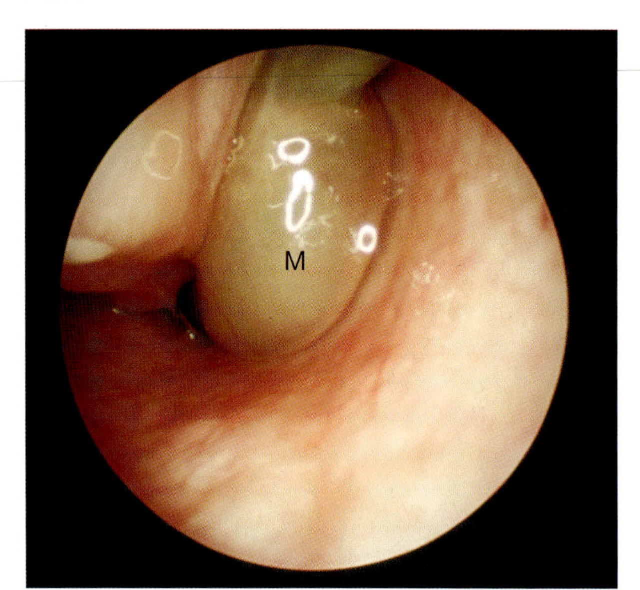

7.15b

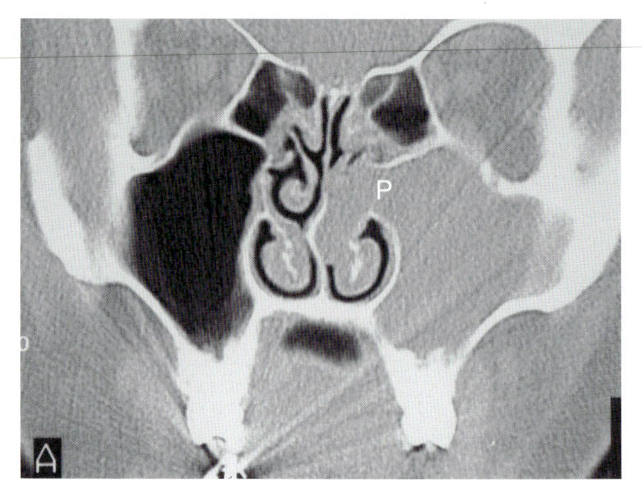

7.15c

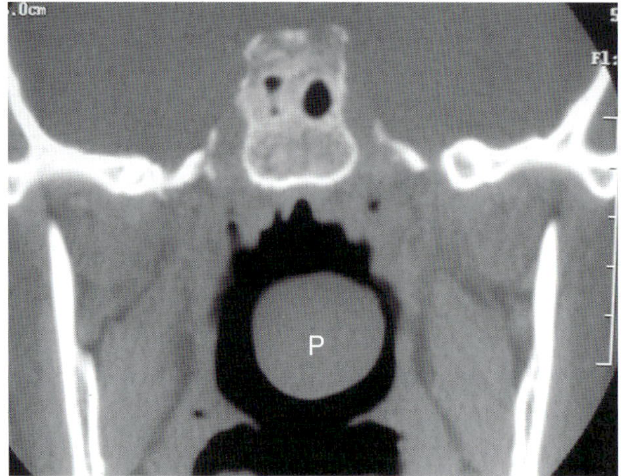

7.15d

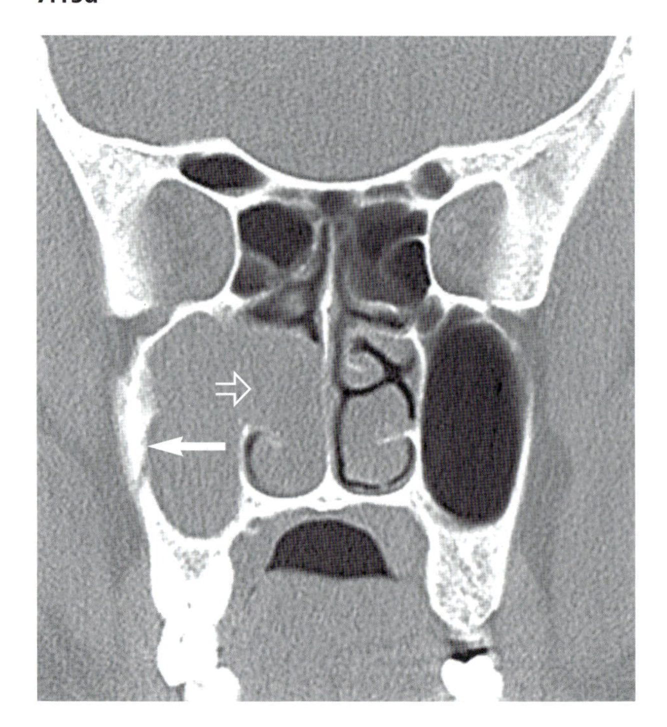

Figure 7.15 *Antrochoanal polyp.* (a) Endoscopy demonstrating a mass (M) in the middle meatus. (b, c) Coronal scans demonstrating a large inflammatory antrochoanal polyp (P) that extends from the left maxillary sinus into the middle meatus. The polyp is seen protruding into the nasopharynx. (d) Coronal scan demonstrating a large antrochoanal polyp that extends from the right maxillary sinus into the middle meatus. There is reactive osteitis of the maxillary sinus wall (arrow). Medial wall remodeling is apparent, with widening of the maxillary sinus ostium (open arrow).

warranted. Associated calcification may be suggestive of a chronic inflammatory process, but is also associated with inverting papilloma or fungal sinusitis. The CT attenuation of the polypoid mass may help to differentiate it from a mucocele, which is usually non-enhancing compared with polyps, which will show enhancement. The differential diagnosis of hyperdense masses on CT is shown in Table 7.3.

CT is the imaging modality of choice for benign sinonasal polyposis. MRI is reserved for complex cases of sinonasal polyps, where there is a question of superimposed fungal sinus infection, or intracranial or intraorbital extension of disease.

7.16a

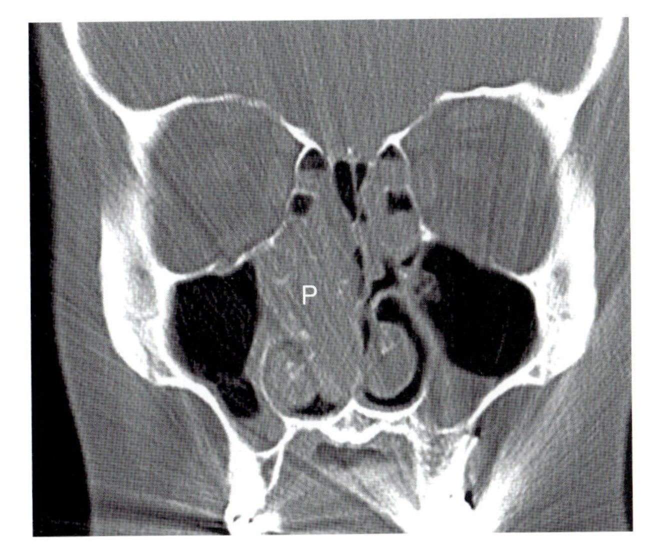

7.16b

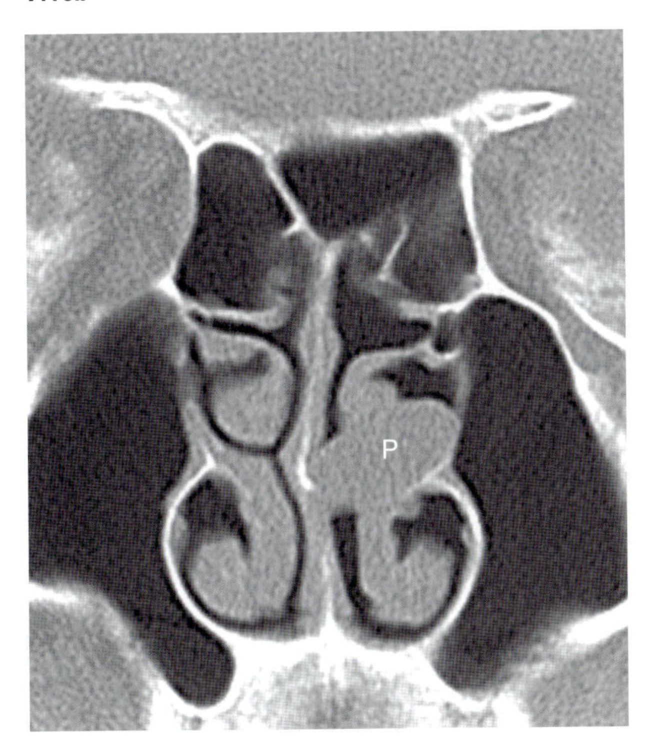

7.16c

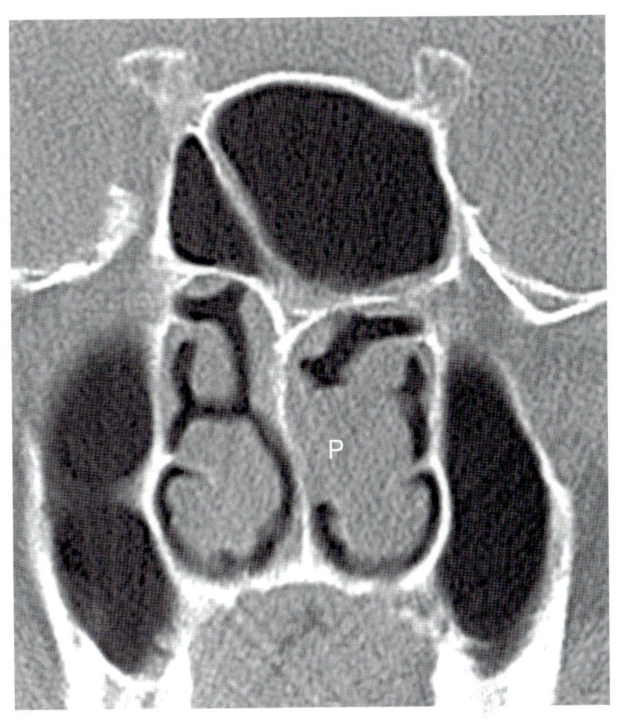

Figure 7.16 (a–c) *Middle meatal polyps*. The middle meatus is a common site for polyps. These polyps are seen protruding between the inferior and the middle turbinates (P).

MRI features of sinonasal polyposis

The characteristic MRI feature of sinonasal polyposis is a reflection of the rich proteinaceous and watery contents of these polyps. Most polyps are of the same signal intensity as water. With time, the amount of free available hydrogen protons decreases as the water content decreases. This results in variable MRI signal characteristics. A hyperintense appearance on T1-weighted MRI scans is usually due to an increase in protein content or to hemorrhage within the polyps.

The hyperintense signal on T2-weighted MRI scans is due to the high water content. Chronic inspissated mucus can give rise to low T1 and T2 signals.

ANTROCHOANAL POLYPS

(Figure 7.15)

The etiology of these unilateral polyps is unclear, although they are histologically similar to inflammatory nasal polyps. An antrochoanal polyp has two components: a cystic part filling the maxillary sinus, which originates most commonly from the posterolateral wall, and a solid part, which extends by a stalk through the maxillary ostium, or frequently via an accessory ostium into the middle meatus.

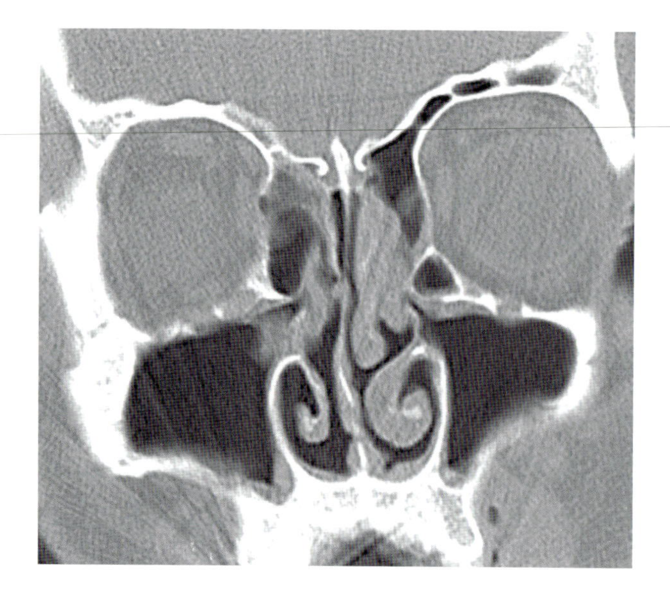

Figure 7.17 *Frontal recess polyps*. Early polyp formation can be seen in the left frontal recess.

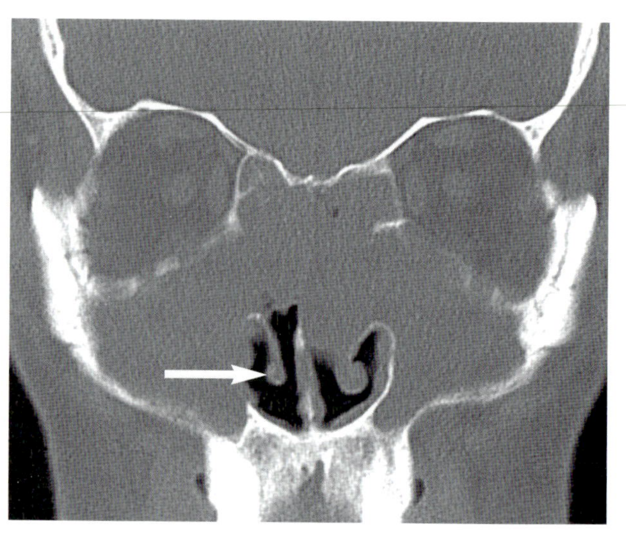

Figure 7.19 *Nasal polyposis*. Coronal CT scan demonstrating extensive polyposis occluding the entire sinonasal cavity in a patient who has undergone several prior surgical procedures. There is loss of much of the normal bony septa. The inferior turbinates are small and shrunken from chronic use of topical decongestants (arrow).

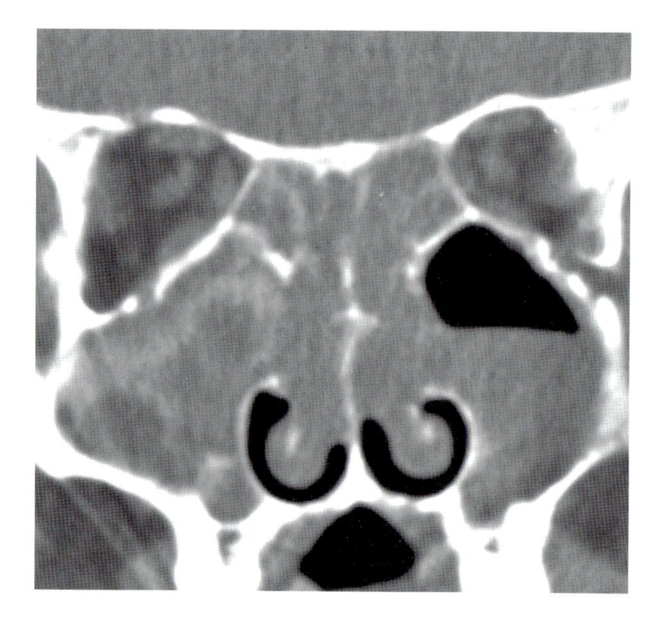

Figure 7.18 *Nasal polyposis*. Multiple high-density polyps are seen packed in the right maxillary sinus lumen and there is an air–fluid level in the left maxillary sinus. The differential diagnosis includes allergic fungal sinusitis and chronic granulomatous fungal sinusitis.

This latter component progressively expands to reach the posterior choana. Antrochoanal polyps occur more frequently in children and young adults and have a tendency to recur if inadequately excised.

Plain radiographs shows a homogeneous mass in the maxillary sinus and an opacified nasal cavity. A lateral view may demonstrate the smooth posterior margin of the polyp hanging in the nasopharynx.

CT scans show a mass within the antrum that is contiguous with a soft tissue mass of uniform density in the ipsilateral nasal cavity.

The sinus ostium and the nasal cavity may be widened due to pressure remodeling. Occasionally, the surrounding bone may exhibit a mixture of resorption and reactive osteitis.

FUNGAL INFECTION OF THE PARANASAL SINUSES

(Tables 7.1 and 7.2; Figures 7.37–7.45)

Fungal sinusitis is an unusual condition that is being recognized with increasing frequency. It can affect healthy patients, but more commonly affects immunocompromised individuals. The symptoms may include nasal obstruction, purulent rhinorrhea, and facial pain, all of which are resistant to treatment with antibiotics. There may be a long history of sinusitis refractory to conventional medical therapy. In most cases, the diagnosis is rarely made from the clinical findings alone, and these patients are usually investigated by a CT scan.

Aspergillus molds are the commonest cause of fungal infection seen in the population at large.

Table 7.1 Classification of fungal sinusitis

- Allergic fungal sinusitis
- Indolent, slowly progressive invasive disease
- Non-invasive local disease: aspergilloma
- Fulminant invasive type occurring in the immunocompromised host

Table 7.2 Predisposing factors for fungal sinusitis

- Chronic sinusitis and sinonasal polyposis
- Immunosuppression
- Diabetes mellitus
- Stagnant mucus as a result of poor ventilation, decreased mucociliary activity

Table 7.3 MRI signal characteristics of various sinus abnormalities[a]

Abnormality	*Appearance on T1-weighted MRI*	*Appearance on T2-weighted MRI*
Sinusitis	Thick mucosa, hypointense	Thick mucosa, hyperintense
Retention cysts	Hypointense	Hyperintense
Polyposis	Hypointense	Hyperintense
Long-standing polyps	Variable	Variable
Mucocele (high water content)	Hypointense	Hyperintense
Mucocele (less water and more protein)	Hyperintense	Hyperintense
Mucocele (thick, pasty content)	Hypointense	More hypointense to signal void
Mucocele (desiccated, dry, and no mobile hydrogen)	Signal void	Signal void
Hemorrhage (acute)	Hypointense	Hypointense
Hemorrhage (chronic)	Hyperintense	Hyperintense
Mycetomas ('cheesy' content)	Hypointense or isointense	More hypointense or signal void
Mycetomas (dry content)	Signal void	Signal void

[a]Signal intensity relative to brain: hypointense (dark); hyperintense (bright); isointense (same as brain); signal void (black); variable (hypo-, hyper-, isointense, or signal void).

These fungi are commonly found in the soil and in decaying fruits and vegetables. The three species of *Aspergillus* that are most commonly responsible for sinus and respiratory infections are *A. fumigatus* (the most common), *A. niger*, and *A. flavus*. The sinonasal and the pulmonary forms of aspergillosis are unrelated, with the pulmonary form primarily occurring among immunocompromised patients.

Imaging findings in patients with fungal sinusitis include the following:

- Nodular mucoperiosteal thickening. The inflamed sinus mucosa is usually hyperintense on MRI scans. The signal characteristics of various abnormalities such as hemorrhage, polyps, and tumors are summarized in Table 7.3.
- Absent air–fluid levels, opacification of the ethmoid sinuses, and bony erosion.
- Areas of increased attenuation in a diseased sinus are suggestive of fungal infection. These are thought to be due to the presence of metal metabolites such as iron, magnesium, calcium, and manganese. These metals are also responsible for the signal void that can be seen on MRI scans.
- Sclerotic thickening, or reactive osteitis, of the bony walls of the sinuses with both remodeling and erosion or destruction can be seen in some cases. When there is extensive bony destruction, it may be impossible radiologically to differentiate fungal sinusitis from malignancy and tissue sampling will be required (Table 7.4).

Table 7.4 Differential diagnosis of hyperdense masses on CT scans in the sinonasal cavity

- Thick pus
- Desiccated secretions in nasal polyps
- Fungal sinusitis
- Thrombus or intrasinus hemorrhage
- Foreign bodies and foreign-body granulomatous sinusitis
- Bony tumors surrounded by inflammation
- Sarcomas with dystrophic calcification
- Dystrophic calcifications in inverting papilloma

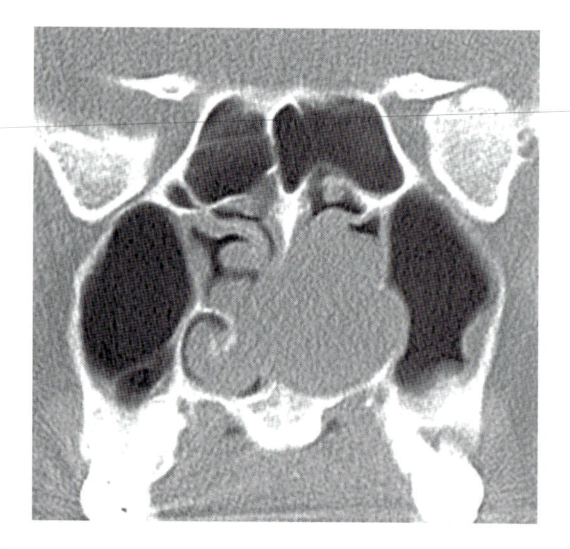

Figure 7.20 *Large nasal polyp*. There is a large smooth polypoid mass in the left nasal cavity, with remodeling of the nasal cavity. Based on the CT features, it would be impossible to differentiate between a benign tumor and an inflammatory polyp.

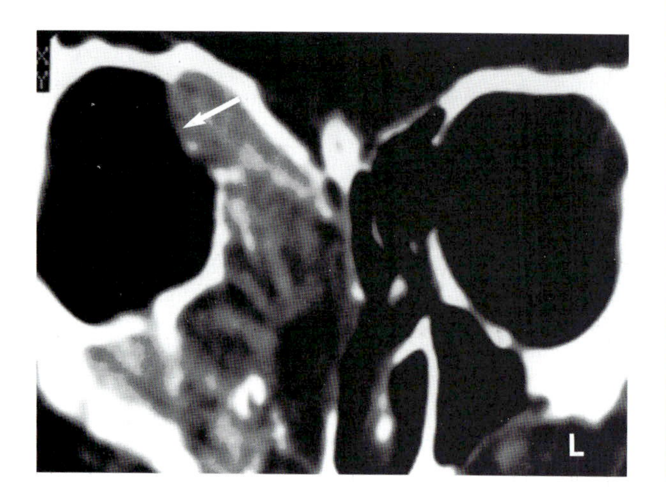

Figure 7.21 *Nasal polyposis*. Coronal scan, examined with a narrow window, demonstrating benign nasal polyps associated with a mucocele in the right ethmoid sinus following obstruction of the ostia. The alternating densities are due to the mucoid material in the polyp (low density) and the dense mucosal folds. The superomedial margin of the orbit is eroded (arrow). Image courtesy of Dr Mario Chiu, St Michael's Hospital, Toronto.

7.22a

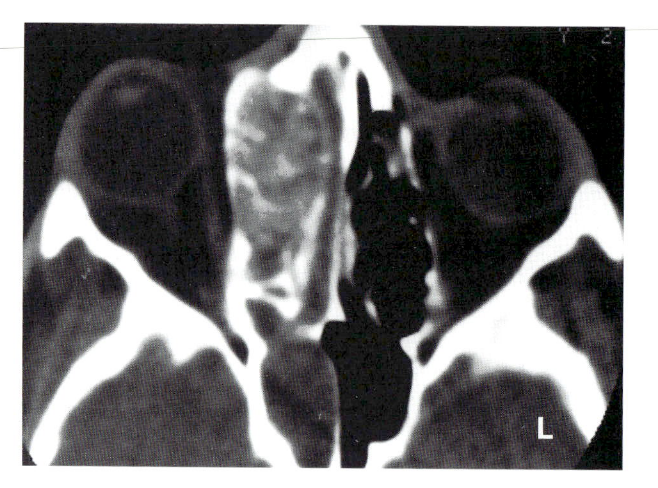

7.22b

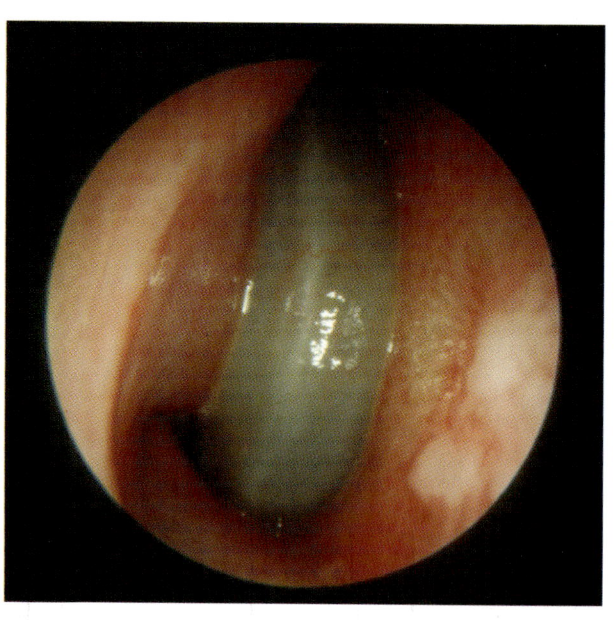

Figure 7.22 *Nasal polyposis*. (a) Narrow-window axial scan of the same patient as in Figure 7.21, demonstrating widening of the ethmoid labyrinth into the right orbit with preservation of some of the bony septa that separate the ethmoid air cells. This has some of the features of an ethmoid polypoidal mucocele. The lamina papyracea is thickened and sclerotic. (b) Endoscopic examination demonstrating a bluish-green benign polyp in the middle meatus.

- CT scans may show compromise of the ostiomeatal complex, which is a predisposing factor for recurrent infection.

In the immunocompromised patient, fungal sinusitis can be life-threatening. Significant clinical features such as fever, rhinorrhea, sinus tenderness, and facial edema may give rise to only mild mucosal thickening on cross-sectional imaging, as these patients are often unable to mount a significant inflammatory response. With time, intracranial extension of disease and cavernous sinus thrombosis

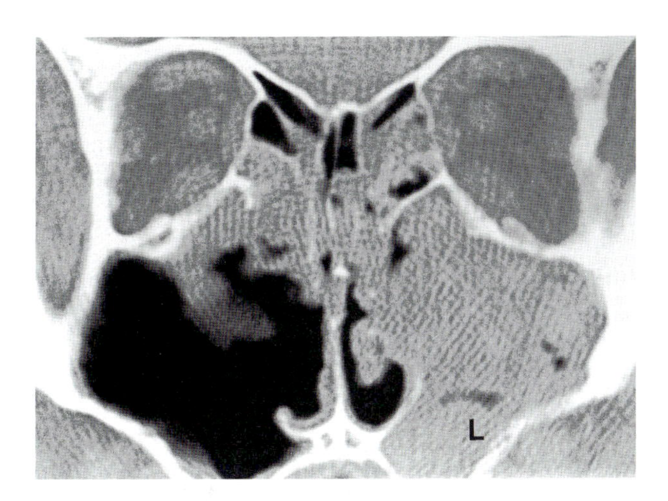

Figure 7.23 *Recurrent nasal polyps*. Coronal scan, examined with a wide window demonstrating the tissue defect from a radical drainage procedure conducted for chronic maxillary sinusitis. The medial wall of the maxillary sinus and the middle and inferior turbinates on the right side have been removed. The remainder of the sinuses are filled with apparently homogeneous soft tissue.

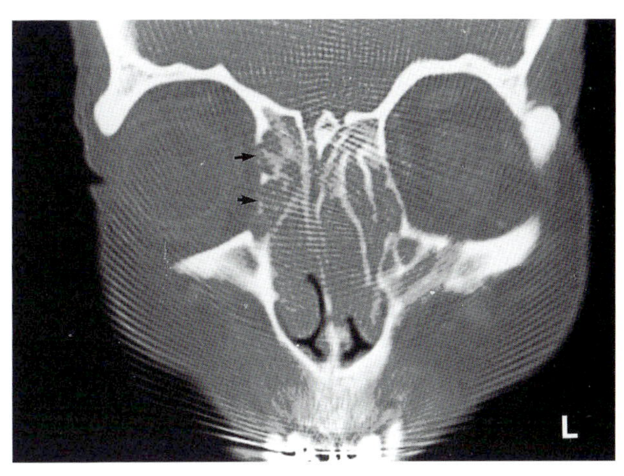

Figure 7.25 *Polypoidal mucocele*. Coronal scan demonstrating extensive soft tissue filling the ethmoid air cells. The bony erosion seen in the right lamina papyracea (arrows) raises the possibility of either polypoid disease or a mucocele. The smooth expansion characteristic of a mucocele is absent.

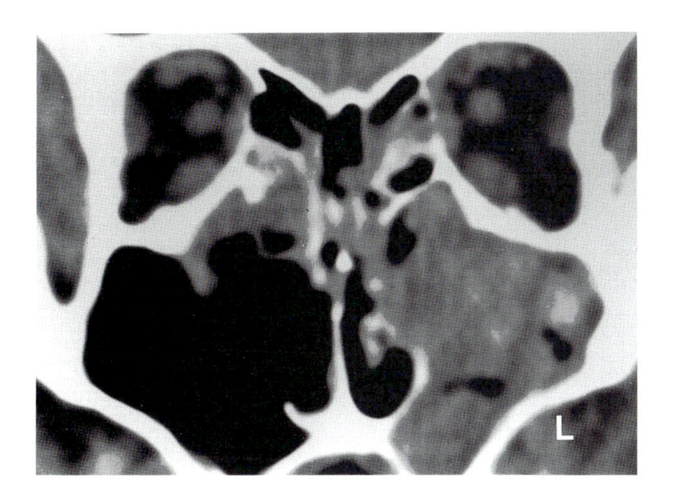

Figure 7.24 *Recurrent nasal polyps*. Narrow-window coronal scan of the same patient as in Figure 7.23 demonstrating alternating high and low densities in the left maxillary sinus consistent with recurrent polypoid tissue.

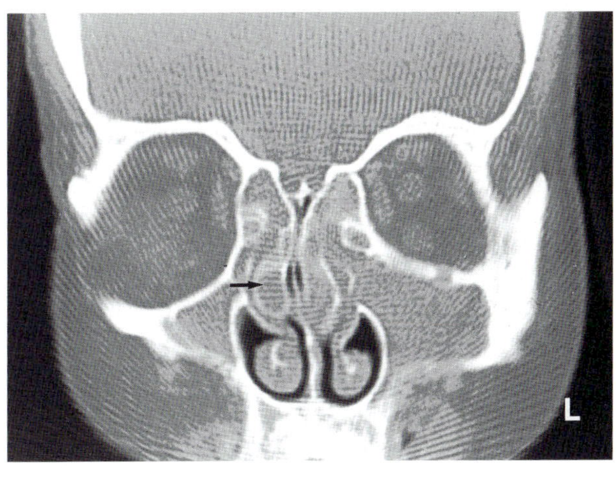

Figure 7.26 *Polypoidal mucocele*. This coronal scan is more posterior than that in Figure 7.25. The extensive soft tissue seen throughout the paranasal sinuses is due to polyposis. There is a diseased concha bullosa on the right (arrow).

can arise. Mycotic intracranial aneurysms and intracranial hemorrhage can also occur.

Diabetic patients with ketoacidosis are at increased risk of an aggressve form of invasive fugnal sinus disease secondary to mucormycosis. Necrosis of the turbinates with black crusting in the nasal cavity is suggestive of this aggressive form of invasive fungal sinusitis. Mucormycosis can develop into an aggressive rhinocerebral infection that is often fatal. The diagnosis can be confirmed by careful examination of nasal scrapings and mucosal biopsies.

Treatment of fungal sinusitis requires surgical debridement and re-establishment of ventilation to the sinus, as well as systemic antifungal therapy in those patients who have invasive fungal disease, together with steroids.

7.27a

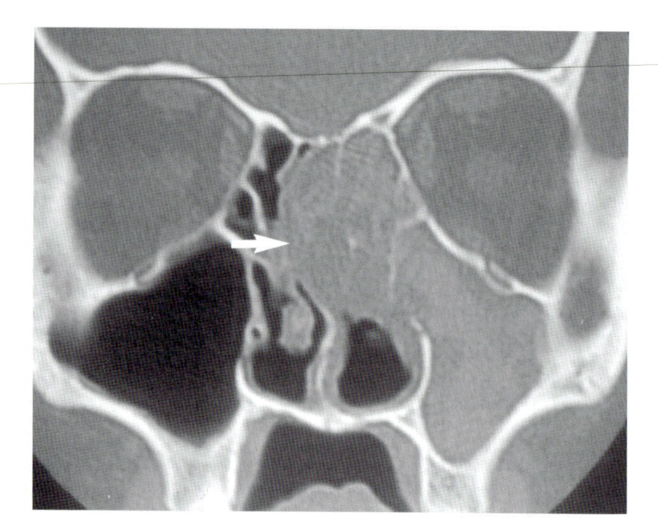

7.27b

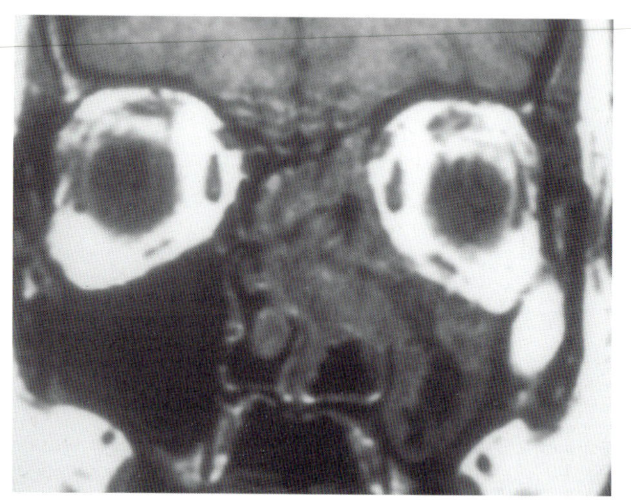

7.27c

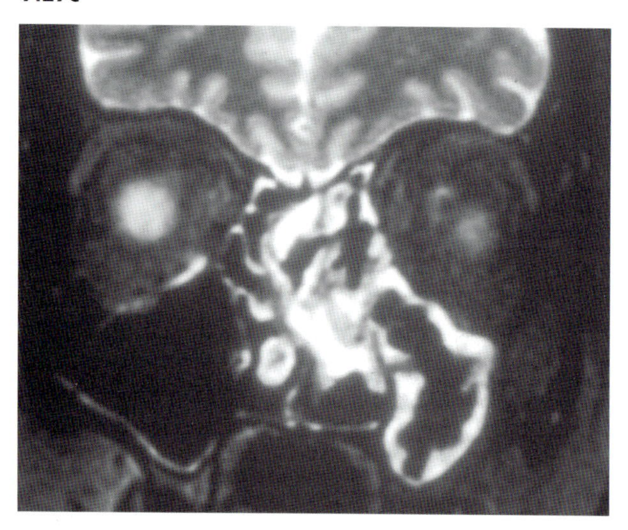

Figure 7.27 *Inspissated polyps.* (a) CT scan demonstrating the presence of high-density masses in the left maxillary and ethmoid sinuses. (b) On T1-weighted MRI, the polyp in the lumen of the sinus is hypointense and the surrounding mucosa is hypertrophic, reactive, and complex in its signal characteristics. (c) On T2-weighted MRI, the polyp is signal void and the surrounding mucosa is hyperintense in its signal characteristics. The findings are due to the lack of water in the polyp.

ATROPHIC RHINITIS

(Figures 7.46 and 7.47)

Atrophic rhinitis is a poorly understood disease, characterized by atrophy of the nasal mucosa and reabsorption of the underlying bone. Patients usually complain of nasal obstruction. Other clinical features include anosmia and an offensive purulent rhinorrhea. Atrophic rhinitis may occur as a primary disease of the nasal cavity or it may follow intranasal surgery. Imaging may show resorption of the bony walls of the nasal cavity and mucosal atrophy of the inferior and middle turbinates. Enlargement of the nasal cavity as a result of lateral bowing of the lateral nasal wall can occur. The process is usually symmetrical, but may occur unilaterally. Hypoplasia of the maxillary sinuses and mucosal thickening in the paranasal sinuses may be seen.

SINUS HEMORRHAGE (Figure 7.48)

Hemorrhage within the paranasal sinuses results in higher CT attenuation than does serous fluid. It may be difficult to differentiate fluid from blood and thickened mucosa on CT scanning. MRI is ideal for assessing an opacified sinus. The signal

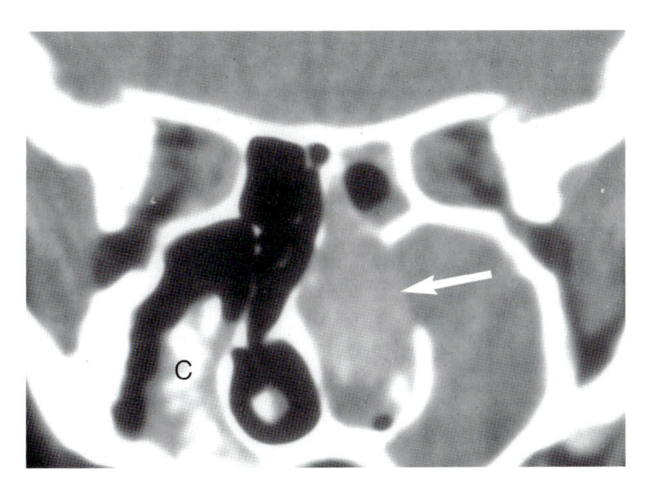

Figure 7.28 *Foreign-body polypoidal granulomatous sinusitis*. This 30-year-old female presented with chronic nasal discharge and recurrent sinusitis. The CT scan demonstrates the presence of coarse calcifications (C) in the right maxillary sinus lumen. In addition, there is a mass of varying density in the left maxillary sinus, with some destruction to the medial wall (arrow). The differential diagnosis includes fungal sinusitis, talc, cocaine, or other foreign-body reactive sinusitis.

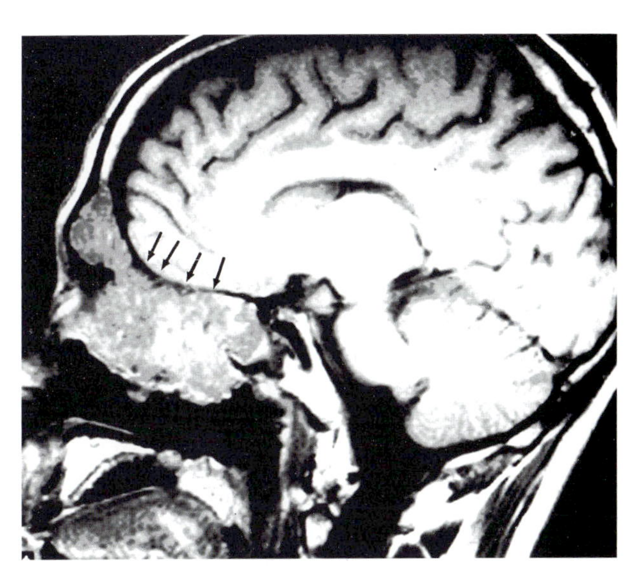

Figure 7.30 *Benign nasal polyposis*. Sagittal T1-weighted MRI scan showing the masses in the frontal, sphenoid, and ethmoid sinuses to be of mixed signal intensity. The bone (signal void) appears to be intact (arrows).

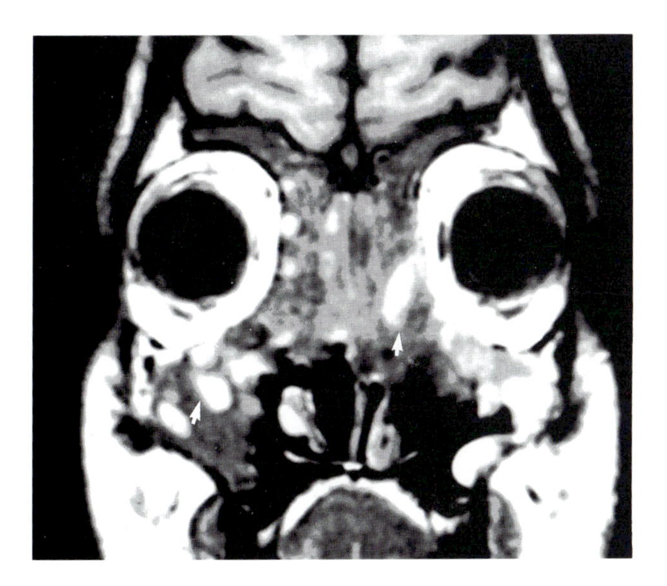

Figure 7.29 *Nasal polyposis*. This patient has undergone several operations for massive sinonasal polyposis. This T1-weighted MRI scan demonstrates the nasal polyps to be of varying signal intensities (arrows).

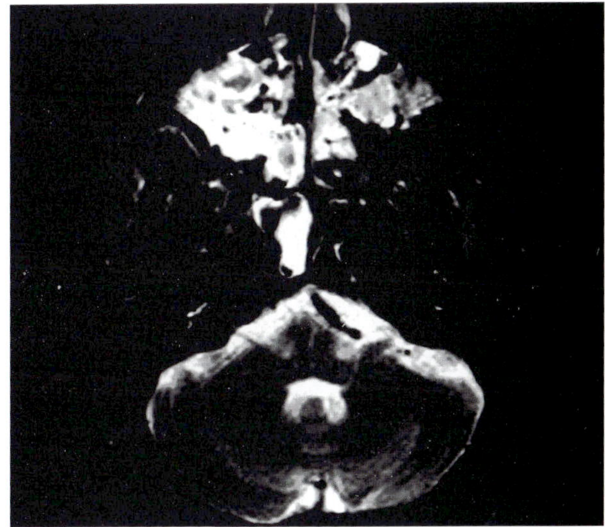

Figure 7.31 *Sinonasal polyposis*. T2-weighted MRI scan in the axial plane demonstrating the varying signal intensities ranging from signal void to hyperintensity. This MRI appearance is classic for the benign nature of these polyps – as opposed to malignant polyps, which are usually of intermediate signal intensity with all imaging sequences.

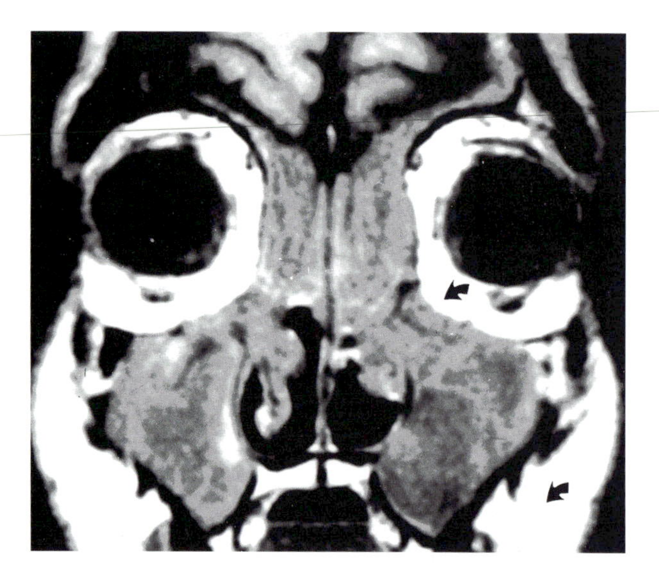

Figure 7.32 *Sinonasal polyposis*. This patient underwent multiple polypectomies and an ethmoidectomy. A T1-weighted MRI scan demonstrates masses of intermediate signal intensity in the maxillary and ethmoid sinuses bilaterally. Hypertelorism is evident. The bright signals seen in the orbits and the cheeks are due to fat (black arrows).

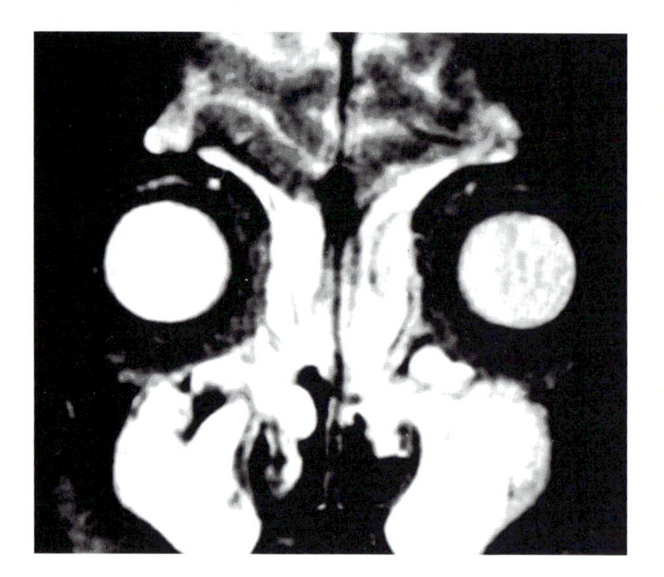

Figure 7.33 *Sinonasal polyposis*. In the same patient as in Figure 7.32, a T2-weighted MRI scan demonstrates hyperintensity of the bilateral large polyps in the maxillary sinuses and in the ethmoid complexes.

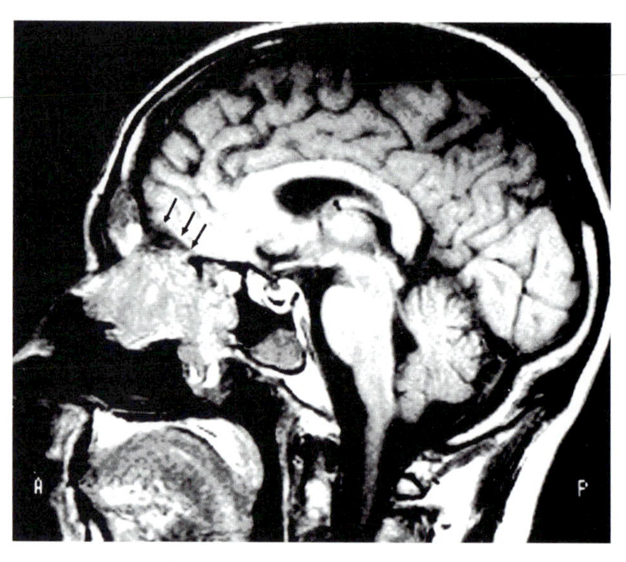

Figure 7.34 *Sinonasal polyposis with skull base erosion*. Sagittal T1-weighted MRI scan demonstrating the erosion of the skull base anteriorly (arrows) secondary to the polyps. The non-homogeneous appearance of the polyps characterizes the benign nature of this disease, despite the erosions seen on the scans.

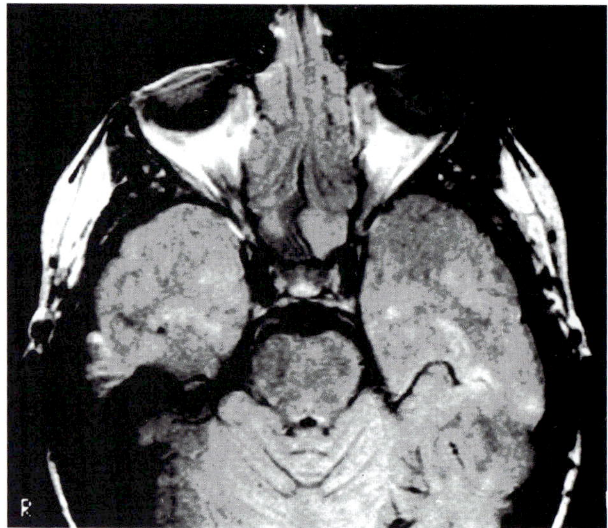

Figure 7.35 *Nasal polyposis*. Axial proton density-weighted MRI scan demonstrating the masses in the ethmoid sinuses to be of intermediate signal intensity. The bony septa in the ethmoid complex are well preserved.

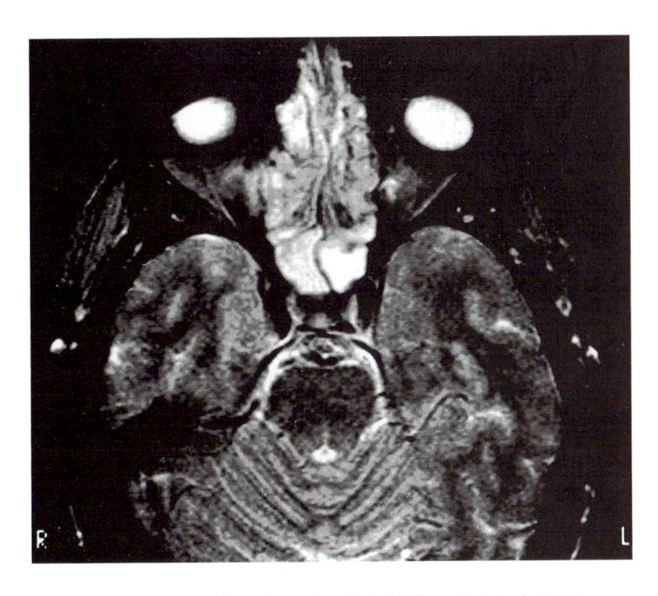

Figure 7.36 *Nasal polyposis*. Axial T2-weighted MRI scan of the same polyps as in Figure 7.32 demonstrating the masses to be hyperintense in signal intensity.

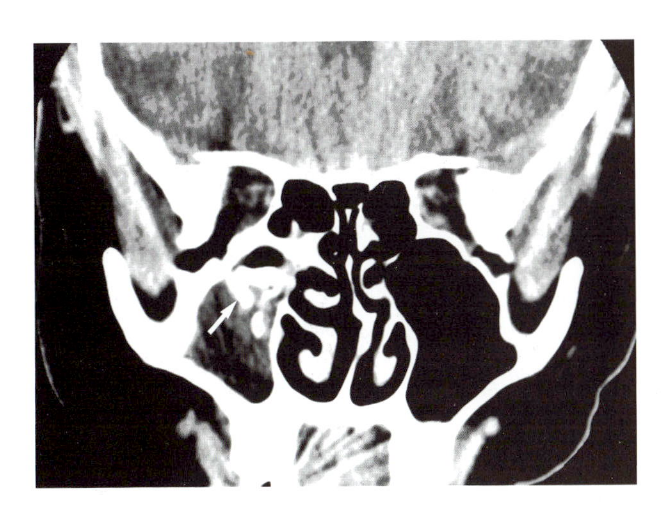

Figure 7.37 *Fungal sinusitis*. A 34-year-old female presented with a long-standing history of sinusitis unreponsive to antibiotics. This coronal CT scan demonstrates sinusitis in the left maxillary sinus with dystrophic calcifications in the fungus ball (arrow).

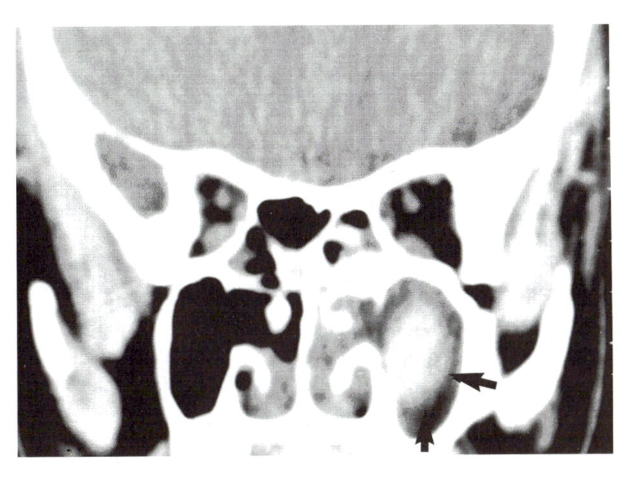

Figure 7.38 *Fungal sinusitis*. A 52-year-old female presented with recurrent sinusitis. This coronal CT scan demonstrates a high-density mass in the left maxillary sinus, with a rim of inflamed sinus mucosa, which is of low density (black arrows). The high-density mass is also seen in the ethmoid complex.

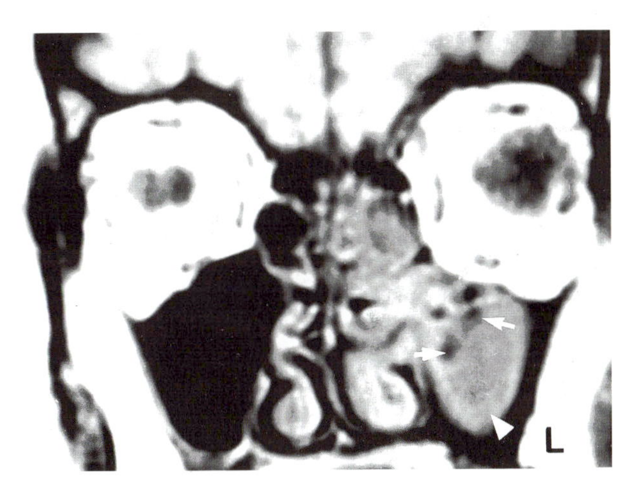

Figure 7.39 *Fungal sinusitis*. T1-weighted MRI scan of the same patient as in Figure 7.37 demonstrating an area of signal void in the isointense antral (arrows). Ferromagnetic compounds and calcium in the mycelia of the fungus give rise to the signal void. There is also an inhomogeneous increase in signal from the inflamed sinus mucosa (arrowhead).

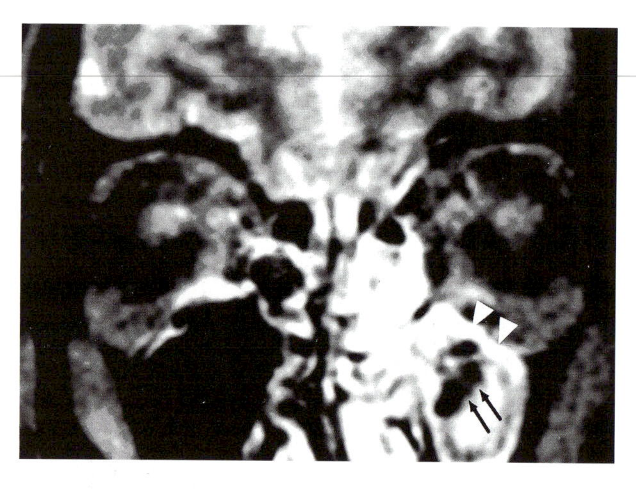

Figure 7.40 *Fungal sinusitis*. Proton density-weighted MRI scans (not shown) demonstrated a further decrease in the signal intensities of the contents of the maxillary sinus. This T2-weighted MRI scan shows the fungal concretions as an area of signal void (black arrows). This is surrounded by intensely bright high signal intensity from the inflamed maxillary sinus mucosa (arrowheads).

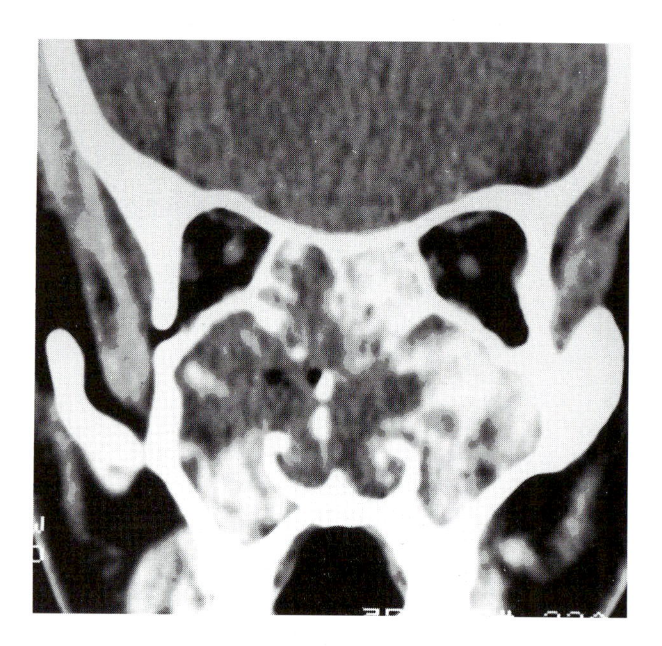

Figure 7.41 *Allergic fungal polyposis and fungal sinusitis*. A 38-year-old male presented with a history of chronic recurrent sinusitis and recurrent nasal polyposis. This CT scan shows the maxillary and posterior ethmoid sinuses to be completely filled with a material that is of greatly varying radiodensity. This appearance is characteristic of allergic fungal sinusitis. At the time of surgery, the material within the sinus was seen to consist of khaki-colored, gritty and rubbery inspissated mucus. The areas of increased radiodensity are believed to be the result of the accumulation of heavy metals.

7.42a

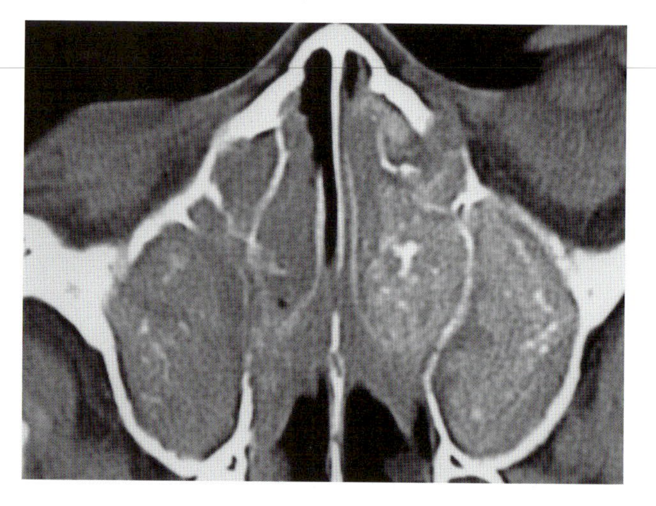

7.42b

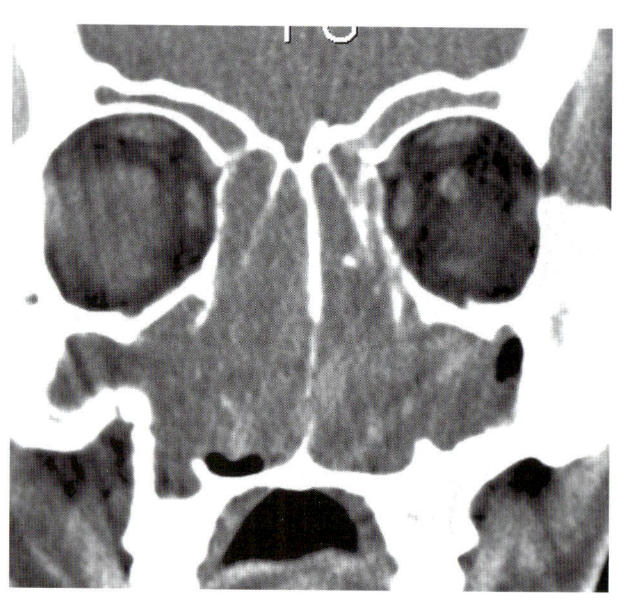

Figure 7.42 (a, b) *Allergic fungal polyposis and fungal sinusitis*. In this patient, there are polyps with amorphous calcifications tightly packed in the sinus cavities.

characteristics of blood vary according to the chemical form in which the blood products are present. The constituents of blood undergo several changes with degradation over time. Oxyhemoglobin in red blood cells will be converted into deoxyhemoglobin, which is subsequently oxidized to methemoglobin. Following red blood cell lysis, intracellular methemoglobin becomes free extracellular methemoglobin. Hemosiderin is the final degradation product. Each of these components will show different characteristic T1 and T2 signal intensities.

7.43a

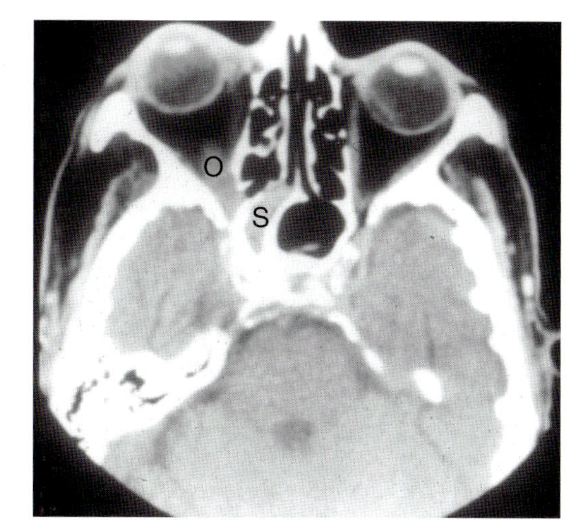

7.43b

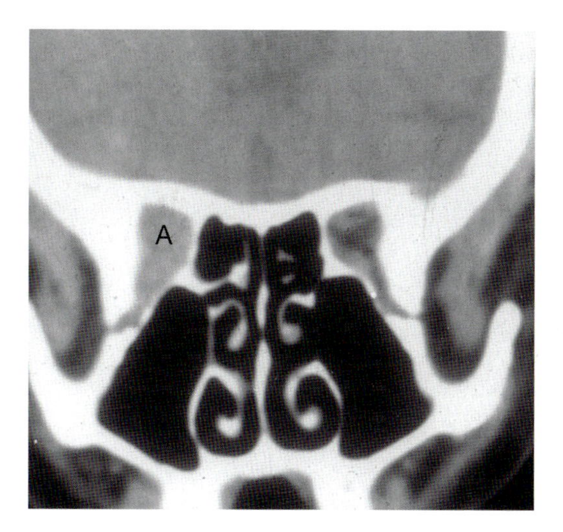

7.43c

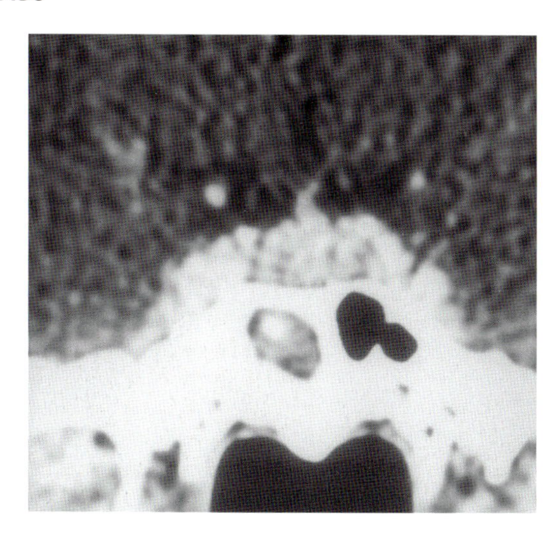

Figure 7.43 *Invasive Aspergillus fungal sinusitis.* A 60-year-old female with diabetes mellitus presented with a 3-day history of decreased vision, orbital pain, nausea, and vomiting. (a, b) CT scans demonstrating the presence of a mass in the sphenoid sinus (S) associated with loss of fat plane in the superior orbital fissure (A) on the right side. The optic nerve (O) is swollen. (c) A high-density fungus ball is present in the sphenoid sinus. This patient responded well to antifungal therapy.

Fresh bleeding releasing oxyhemoglobin will show low–intermediate T1 and high T2 signals. Deoxyhemoglobin will show low T1 and T2 signals. Intracellular methemoglobin will be hyperintense on T1-weighted and hypointense on T2-weighted scans. Extracellular methemoglobin is hyperintense on both T1- and T2-weighted scans. Hemosiderin is hypointense on both T1- and T2-weighted scans.

If the sinus is not completely filled with blood and has residual air in it, the blood oxidizes more rapidly. Following oxidation, the sinus contents are predominantly intracellular methemoglobin, which is hyperintense on T1-weighted scans and hypointense on T2-weighted scans. Once the cells break down, the intracellular methemoglobin becomes extracellular and is hyperintense on T1- and T2-weighted scans. It is not uncommon to see blood in the paranasal sinuses. Blood is often associated with trauma, bleeding dyscrasias, and hemorrhage from benign or malignant lesions. Hemorrhage following trauma can produce an inflammatory reaction of the sinus mucosa, which can be mistaken for sinonasal polyposis.

7.44a

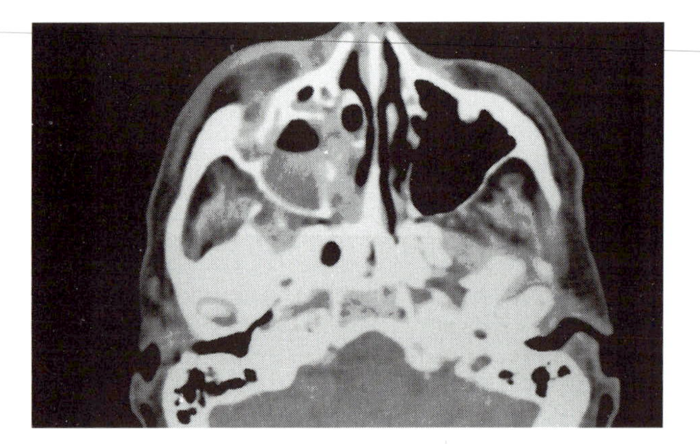

7.44b

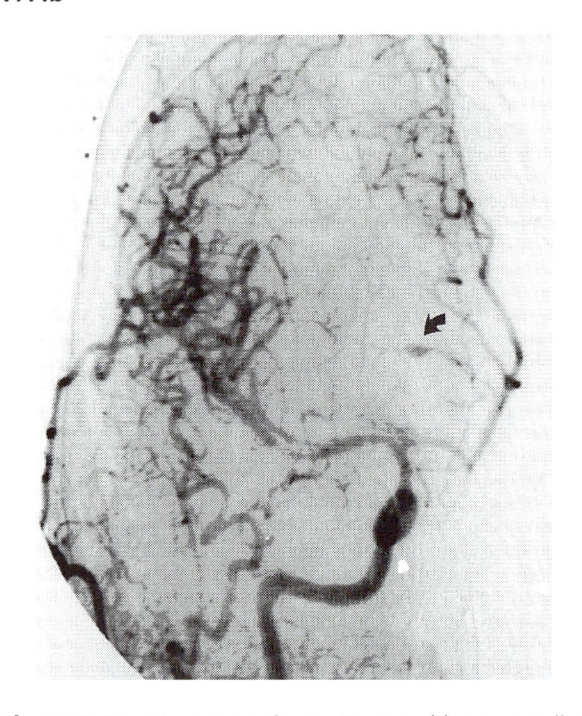

Figure 7.44 *Mucormycosis*. A 54-year-old uncontrolled diabetic had undergone root canal therapy 4 days previously. He presented in the emergency department with severe pain in the right cheek area. Endoscopic examination of the nasal cavity revealed the presence of black fungal debris and crusting. An axial CT scan (a) demonstrated an acute sinusitis with an air–fluid level involving the right maxillary and ethmoid sinuses in addition to cellulitis of the right orbit. On the day after admission, the patient had an acute cerebrovascular event. An emergency angiogram (b) identified a mycotic aneurysm (arrow) which was the most likely cause of the intracranial hemorrhage.

7.45a

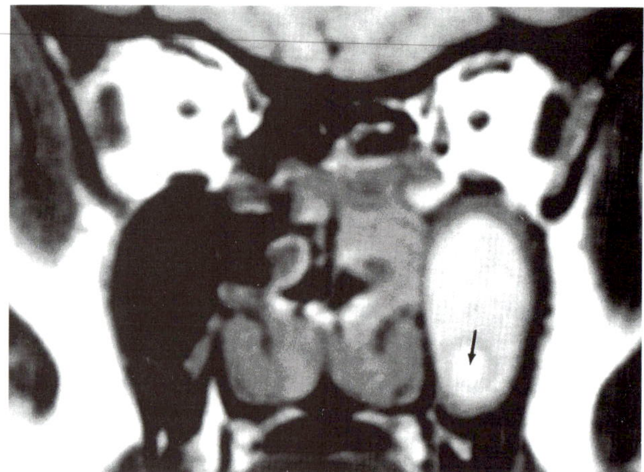

7.45b

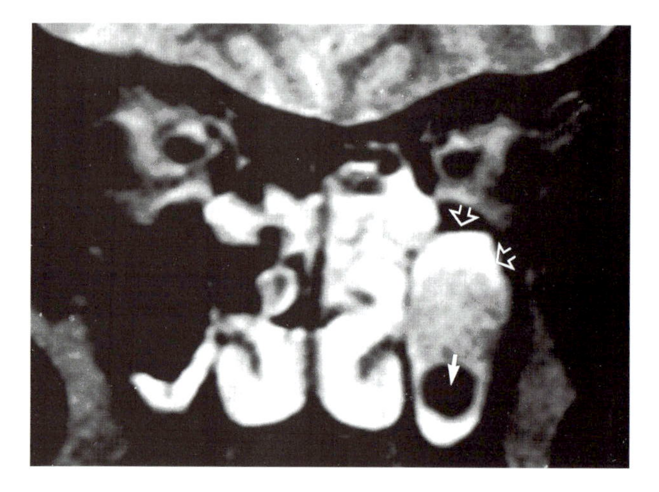

Figure 7.45 *Fungal sinusitis*. (a) T1-weighted MRI scan demonstrating a hyperintense mass in the left maxillary sinus surrounded by hypointense fluid (arrow). A second hyperintense focus is seen in the maxillary sinus. (b) T2-weighted MRI scan demonstrating the hyperintense focus in the left maxillary sinus to be signal void (arrow). The remaining contents of the sinus are decreased in signal intensity in comparison with the T1-weighted scan in (a). The inflamed sinus mucosa is hyperintense (open arrows). This progressive decrease in the signal intensity on T2-weighted scans when compared with T1-weighted scans is typical of fungal infection in the sinuses. Intrasinus hemorrhage can resemble fungal sinusitis: the difference is in the T2-weighted scan, where the hemorrhagic area is decreased in signal intensity – but not to the extent that is seen in fungal sinusitis. The inflamed sinus mucosa is hyperintense.

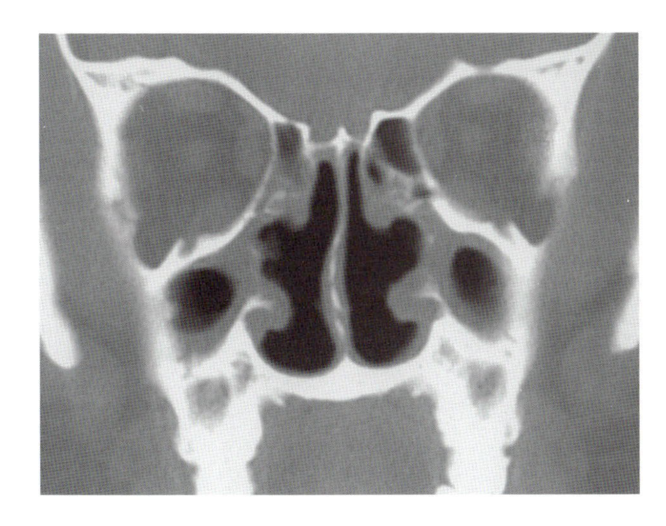

Figure 7.46 *Atrophic rhinitis*. Patients present with nasal obstruction, foul-smelling discharge, and nasal dryness. This coronal CT scan demonstrates inflammatory mucosal thickening in both maxillary sinuses. The middle and inferior turbinates have atrophied and there are few bony septa in the ethmoid labyrinth. The nasal cavities appear to be enlarged.

7.47a

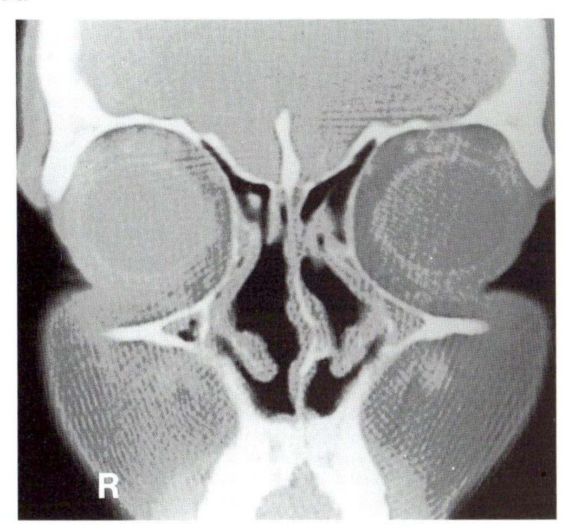

7.47b

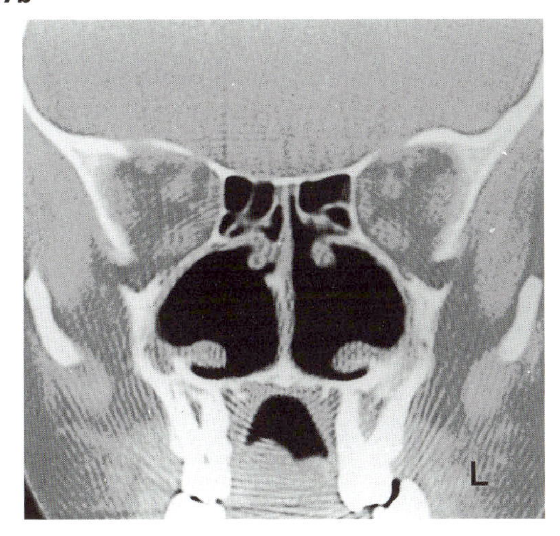

Figure 7.47 *Atrophic rhinitis*. (a, b) Coronal scans demonstrating expanded nasal cavities due to the resorption of both the turbinates and the bony walls of the nasal cavities. Despite the 'spacious' nasal cavities, patients often complain of nasal obstruction.

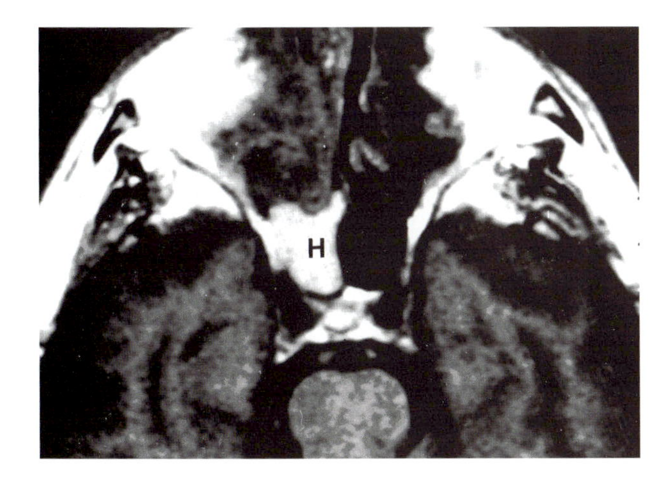

Figure 7.48 *Sinus hemorrhage*. T1-weighted MRI scan demonstrating a hyperintense hemorrhage (H) in the right sphenoid sinus.

8

Complications of sinusitis

INTRODUCTION

The complications of sinusitis are usually related to infection escaping from within the paranasal sinuses and invading the adjacent anatomical structures. The commonest complications are secondary to disease of the frontoethmoid complex and can be life-threatening. In the pre-antibiotic era, it was not uncommon to see osteomyelitis of the frontal bone or intraorbital abscesses. With the widespread use of antibiotics, there has been a significant decline in the incidence of such complications and these now more commonly occur in association with resistant bacteria or immunocompromised patients, such as those with AIDS.

The complications of sinusitis can be divided into three groups: local, orbital, and intracranial. These complications need immediate treatment with high-dose intravenous antibiotics and frequently require surgical drainage. If such treatment is instituted without delay, permanent ocular and neurological damage may be avoided.

The various complications are listed in Table 8.1. The factors that predispose to complications from sinusitis are as follows:

- Congenital deficiencies of the sinus walls such as defects in the wall of the sphenoid sinus
- Facial fractures
- Surgical defects
- Erosion of the bony walls by infection or tumor
- Retrograde phlebitis – retrograde spread of infection through various venous portals, including those along the interstitium surrounding the veins, through the emissary foramina, and through the diploic veins
- Extension along pre-existing anatomical pathways – perineural spread may occur around the branches of the olfactory nerve traversing the cribriform plate, via nerves that communicate into the pterygopalatine fossa, the Vidian nerve, or the maxillary division of the trigeminal nerve

Table 8.1 Complications of sinusitis

Local	*Orbital*	*Intracranial*
Mucocele	Periorbital cellulitis	Meningitis
Pyocele	Subperiosteal abscess	Epidural empyema or abscess
Empyema	Orbital abscess	Brain abscess
Osteitis	Optic neuritis	Superior orbital fissure syndrome[a]
Osteomyelitis	Occlusion of central retinal artery	Cavernous sinus thrombosis
Facial cellulitis		Superior sagittal sinus thrombosis[a]

[a]Detailed discussion is outside the scope of this book.

- Hematogenous spread as part of a generalized septicemia

The diagnosis of a complication of sinusitis is usually confirmed with computed tomography (CT). While magnetic resonance imaging (MRI) has some diagnostic value, these patients are usually too ill and uncooperative to undergo this lengthier examination. Multiplanar CT scans are easily obtained by the 64-slice CT scanners without any discomfort to the patient. CT ideally is conducted in both the axial and the coronal planes following the administration of intravenous contrast. The scans should be examined with both wide and narrow window settings to allow adequate assessment of the sinus cavities, the bony walls, and the adjacent soft tissue structures.

MUCOCELE (Figures 8.1–8.23)

By definition, a mucocele is the result of prolonged obstruction of the drainage pathway of a sinus. The mucosa lining the sinus cavity continues to secrete a thick white clear uninfected mucus, which cannot escape from the sinus. The increasing pressure from the accumulating mucus gradually causes resorption of the bony walls of the sinus. The net effect of smooth, gradual enlargement of the sinus cavity is the hallmark of mucoceles. A mucocele is the most common expansile lesion seen in the paranasal sinuses. The sinuses involved in decreasing order of frequency are the frontal, the ethmoid, the maxillary, and the sphenoid sinuses. Mucoceles can also occur in a concha bullosa or any other pneumatized cell.

Mucoceles commonly present as painless masses adjacent to the superomedial margin of the orbit, with or without exophthalmos and diplopia. Mucoceles of the frontal sinus present with swelling of the upper eyelid and inferior displacement of the globe. There may also be swelling over the anterior wall of the frontal sinus, with the characteristic 'eggshell crackling' on palpation.

Pathologically, a mucocele appears to be a normal sinus that is filled under pressure with mucus. It is the increasing pressure of the secreted mucus that is responsible for the slow expansion that may lead to compression of the adjacent structures. The causes are multifactorial and include obstruction of the ostium with chronic inflammation or polyps, trauma (surgical or accidental), allergy, and tumor. Mucoceles are associated with smooth expansion of the sinus walls without bony destruction. These bony changes are best demonstrated on CT scans and can be easily overlooked on MRI scans. Frontal sinus mucoceles cause erosion of the incomplete septa normally found within the frontal sinus cavity. This leads to loss of the normal scalloped appearance and a smooth outline. There may be an associated reactive sclerosis of the bone. With increased expansion, the anterior and posterior bony walls of the sinus may become dehiscent, risking intracranial extension and sepsis or escape of the mucocele into the upper eyelid. Mucoceles may occur in any sinus cavity, and occasionally multiple mucoceles may occur in the same patient.

CT features of a mucocele

- In the early stages, the changes are non-specific when compared with those of allergy or inflammatory disease.
- As the mucus accumulates within the sinus, there is gradual expansion of the sinus cavity, with thinning and loss of the peripheral bony margins.
- With continuous increase in the intrasinus pressure, bone remodeling will change to bony erosion, and malignancy will enter the differential diagnosis.
- The contents of the mucocele usually appear homogeneous and are isodense or hypodense relative to brain tissue. The contents do not usually enhance following administration of intravenous contrast.
- Should the mucocele become acutely infected, and develop into a pyocele, the administration of intravenous contrast will demonstrate rim enhancement.

MRI and mucoceles

MRI, while poorly demonstrating bony defects, has superior ability to differentiate contrast between soft tissues and may help in the differentiation of mucoceles from solid tumors. The MRI signal intensity of mucoceles varies according to the amount

8.1a

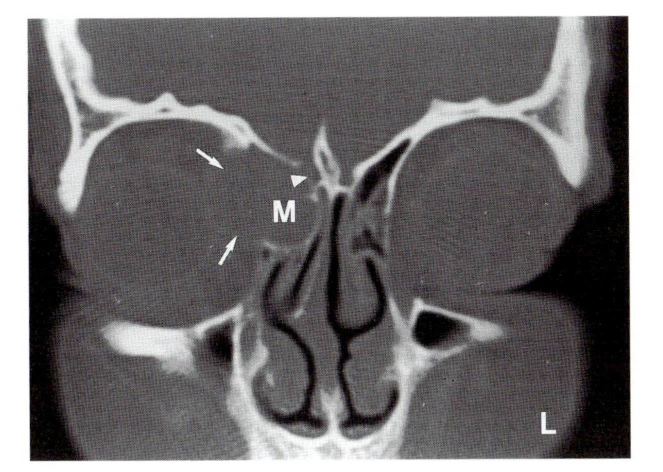

8.1b

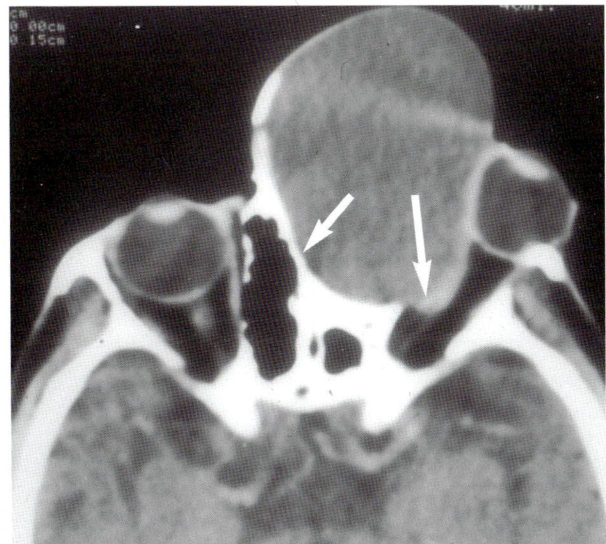

8.1c

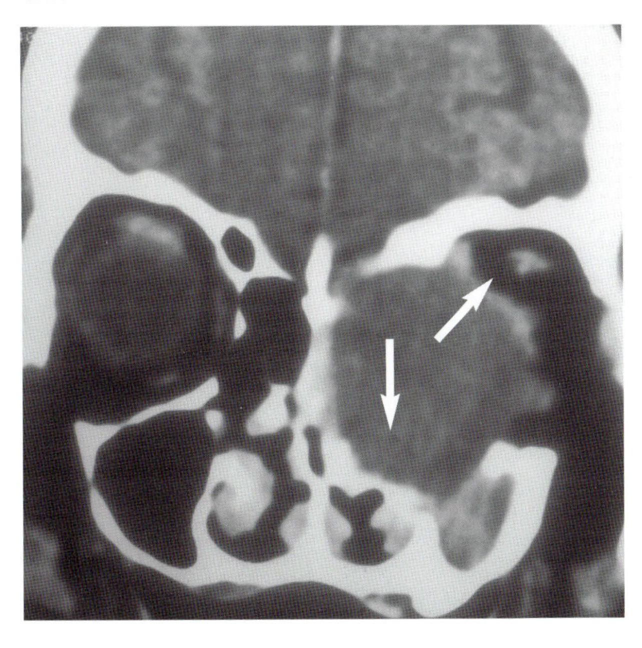

Figure 8.1 *Ethmoid mucocele*. This 55-year-old female presented with right-sided exophthalmos. (a) Coronal CT scan demonstrating an isodense soft tissue mass with expansion and erosion of the fovea ethmoidalis (arrowhead) and the superomedial margin of the orbit (arrows). This has the features of a mucocele (M). The scan also demonstrates the limited surgical access, as there is encroachment of the middle turbinate and of the deviated nasal septum onto the middle meatus. (b) Axial and (c) coronal CT scans of the ethmoid sinuses demonstrating a large expansile mass in the left ethmoid sinus that has pushed the eyeball laterally. There is smooth erosion (arrows) of the walls of the ethmoid sinus to such an extent that there is no bone in some parts of the mucocele wall.

of hydrogen protons and glycoprotein complexes present within the mucocele.

Chronic obstruction to the ventilation and drainage pathway of a sinus results in the prolonged retention and accumulation of mucus. The retained secretion within the sinuses may change its biochemical characteristics over a period of time. Water is slowly absorbed, resulting in a thicker fluid. If obstruction of the sinus continues, then the chronic reaction may stimulate the goblet cells of the lining epithelium to produce a fluid that is rich in protein. Goblet cell metaplasia will be seen on histology. As a consequence, water is slowly absorbed and the secretions become protein rich. This makes the fluid gelatinous, thick, and viscous. As protein molecules are known to shorten T1 and T2 relaxation times, a proteinaceous fluid is bright or hyperintense on T1-weighted and T2-weighted MRI. With an increase in the amount of glycoprotein production, there is an increase in the binding of hydrogen atoms. This further reduces the amount of mobile hydrogen protons. The decrease in water content further reduces the T1 relaxation time, and the reduced motion of the glycoprotein complex results in a shorter T2 relaxation time. The pasty thick material may eventually be replaced by a

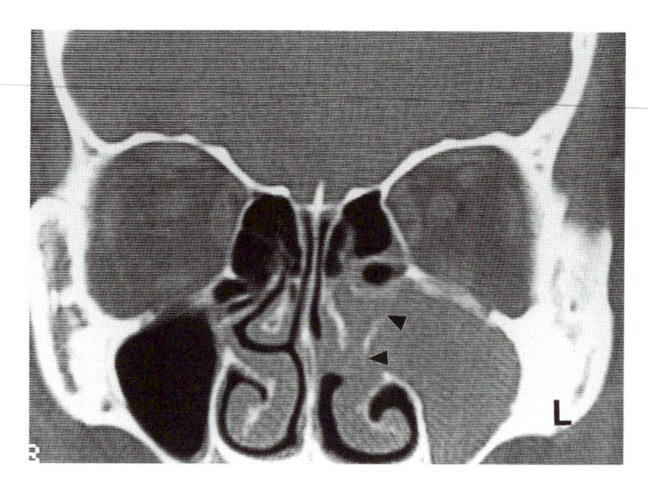

Figure 8.2 *Maxillary sinus mucocele.* Coronal CT scan demonstrating an expansile soft tissue density within the maxillary sinus, with bowing of the medial wall of the maxillary sinus (arrowheads).

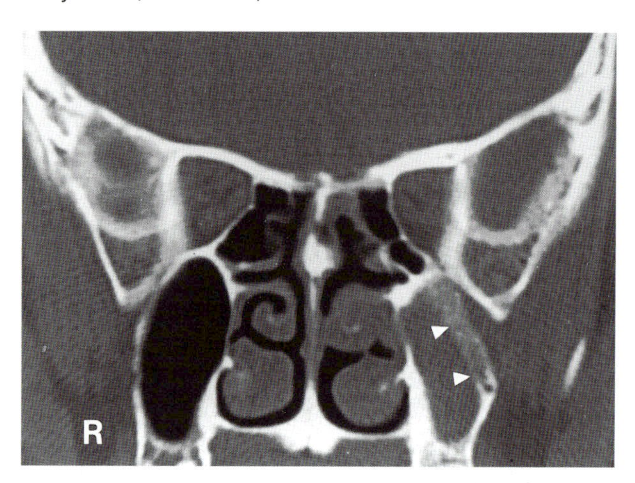

Figure 8.3 *Maxillary sinus mucocele.* Taken more posterior than that in Figure 8.2, demonstrating irregular bony resorption in the lateral wall (arrowheads) of the maxillary sinus. This was found to be a pyocele.

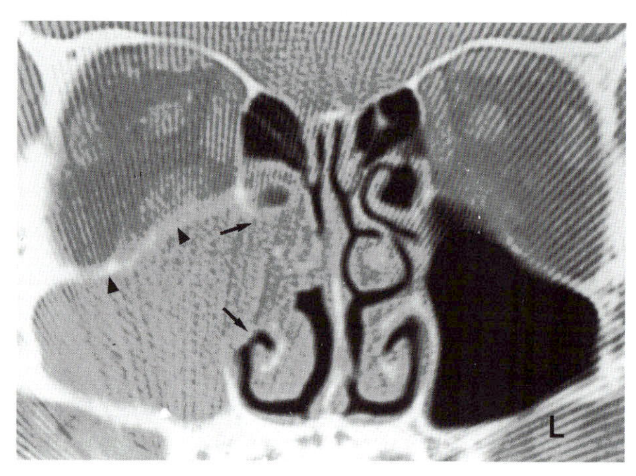

Figure 8.4 *Maxillary sinus mucocele.* Narrow-window coronal scan showing the maxillary sinus cavity to be filled with low-density matter. The secondary changes caused by mucoceles, such as medial expansion of the maxillary sinus lumen (arrows) and reactive sclerosis of the orbital floor (arrowheads), are at an early stage.

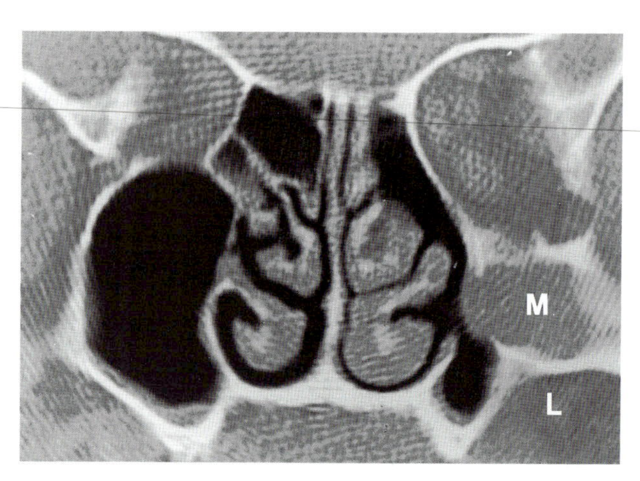

Figure 8.5 *Maxillary sinus mucocele.* If the patient has had surgery to the maxillary sinus, the mucocele may be lateralized within a small compartment and the surrounding wall may be sclerotic. This coronal scan demonstrates the bony defect from previous intranasal antrostomy. As a result of scarring, a mucocele (M), limited to the lateral compartment of the septated maxillary sinus, has developed. The difference in size between the maxillary sinuses suggests postoperative hypoplasia of the left maxillary sinus.

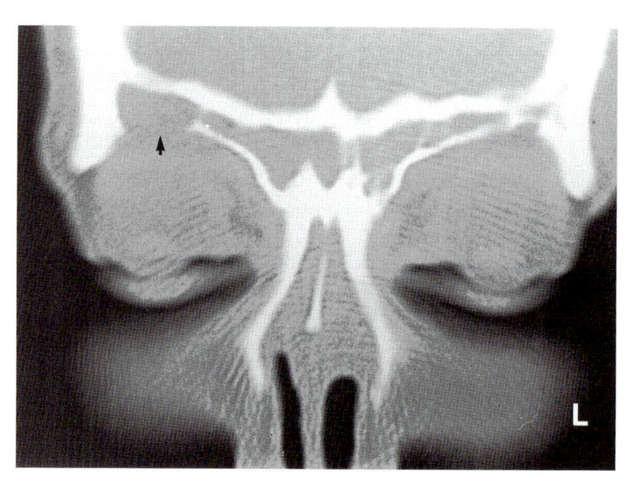

Figure 8.6 *Frontal sinus mucocele.* Coronal scan demonstrating a defect in the floor of the right frontal sinus (arrow). The patient had polypoidal disease with a small mucocele in the lateral part of the frontal sinus. This is unusual, as most frontal sinus mucoceles occur close to the superomedial margin of the orbit.

dry desiccated material in the sinus lumen. As there are no more free mobile hydrogen protons, the substance essentially has an extremely short spin echo time and is seen as signal-void (black) areas on T1-weighted and T2-weighted images. These dynamic biochemical and physiological changes in an

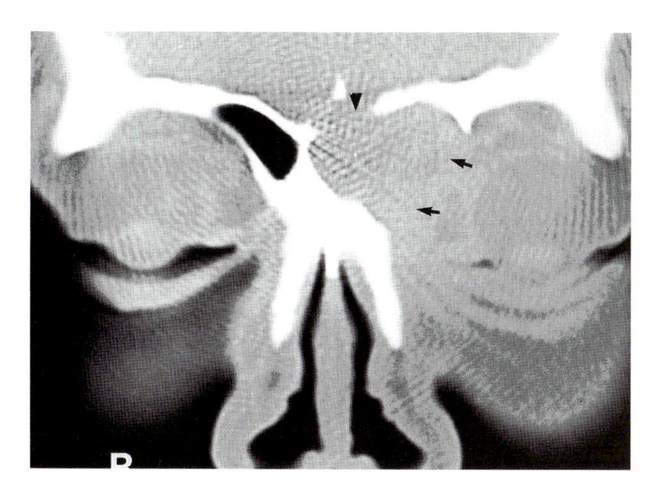

Figure 8.7 *Left frontoethmoid mucocele.* This patient, who had previously undergone sinus surgery for chronic sinusitis, presented with a mass in the superomedial aspect of the orbit. This coronal scan demonstrates a smooth, expansile, soft tissue mass with erosion of both cribriform plates (arrowhead) and the superomedial aspect of the orbit (arrows). This mucocele can be considered as a 'late' complication of the previous sinus operation in which postoperative scarring occluded drainage of the frontal recess on the left side.

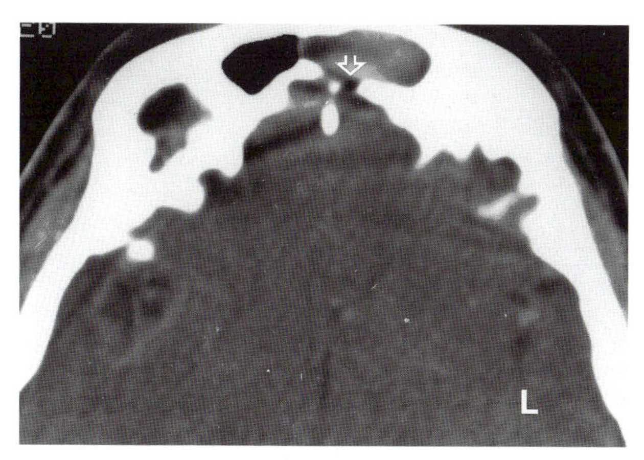

Figure 8.9 *Frontoethmoid mucopyocele.* This patient presented with a painful expansile mass in the forehead. This axial CT scan demonstrates an expansile, soft tissue mass that has eroded through the posterior wall of the frontal sinus (open arrow). There is enhancement of the mucous membrane consistent with a mucopyocele of the left frontal sinus.

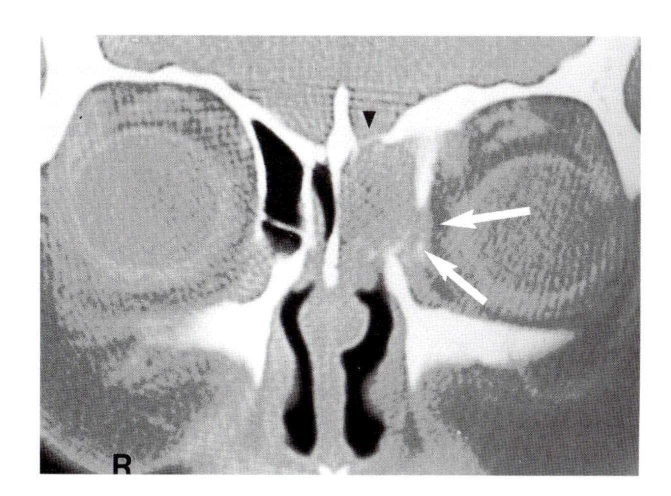

Figure 8.8 *Left frontoethmoid mucocele.* Coronal CT scan, taken posterior to that in Figure 8.7, demonstrating a smooth, expansile, soft tissue mass with erosion of the left lamina papyracea (arrows), and of the left cribriform plate (arrowhead). The soft tissue images of the orbital contents show the globe to be displaced inferolaterally on the left.

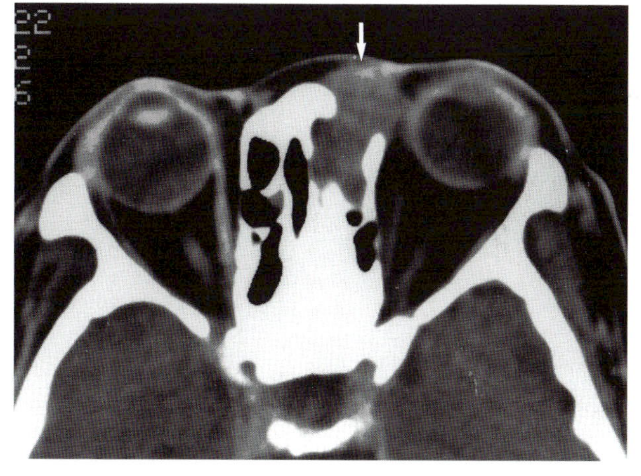

Figure 8.10 *Frontoethmoid mucopyocele.* Axial CT scan demonstrating an expansile, soft tissue mass that has eroded through the anterior margin of the ethmoid sinus (arrow). There is enhancement of the mucous membrane in keeping with a mucopyocele of the ethmoid sinuses.

obstructed sinus form the basic ingredients that will influence the MRI appearance of fluid on the various spin echo MRI sequences.

MRI features of a mucocele

- A mucocele that contains serous secretions with a high water content is hypointense on T1-weighted, intermediate signal on proton density-weighted, and hyperintense on T2-weighted MRI.
- The water within a mucocele that has been present for a few months is slowly absorbed and is replaced by protein-rich secretions from the seromucinous glands. This makes the mucocele

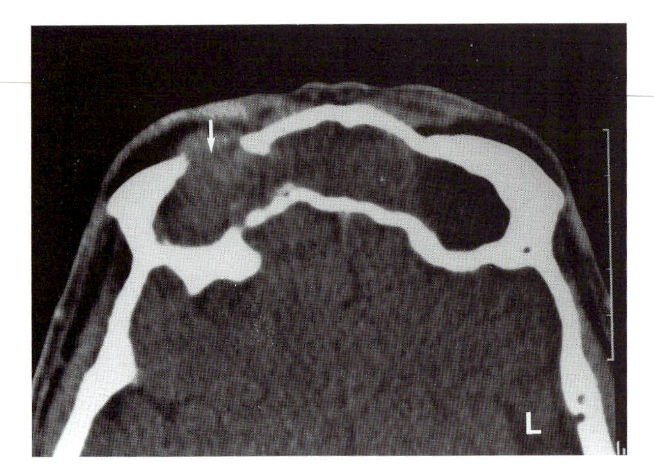

Figure 8.11 *Frontal mucocele.* Axial CT scan demonstrating an enhancing mass that has eroded the anterior wall of the frontal sinus (arrow). Reactive sclerosis of the sinus walls is noted. This was a frontal sinus mucocele. When erosion is the dominant feature, the mucocele may be difficult to differentiate radiologically from a malignant tumor.

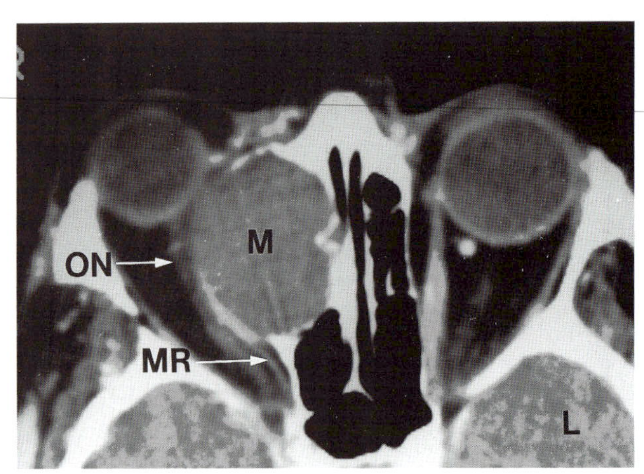

Figure 8.13 *Ethmoid mucocele.* This patient presented with right-sided exophthalmos. A smooth expansile mass with thinning of the lamina papyracea is seen in the right ethmoid sinus. The medial rectus (MR) muscle is stretched over the mucocele (M). The smooth margins and erosions suggest the presence of a mucocele. The optic nerve (ON) is displaced laterally.

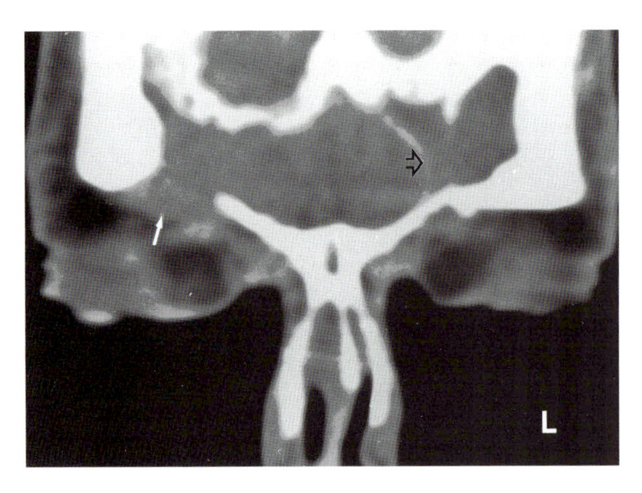

Figure 8.12 *Frontal sinus mucocele.* Coronal CT scan, of the same patient as in Figure 8.11, demonstrating the laterally placed frontal sinus mucocele with erosion of the floor of the lateral part of the sinus (arrow). The intersinus septum is bowed to the left (open arrow).

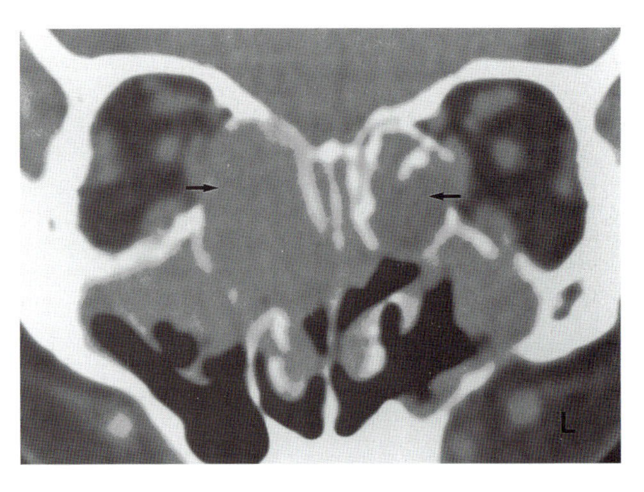

Figure 8.14 *Multiple mucoceles.* This patient had a history of multiple sinus operations. Large mucoceles erode and displace the lamina papyracea laterally. This coronal CT scan demonstrates large bilateral ethmoid sinus mucoceles (arrows) with expansion and erosion of the wall of the ethmoid and frontal sinuses and the lamina papyracea.

intermediate in signal intensity on T1-weighted and hyperintense on T2-weighted MRI.

- With a further loss of free mobile hydrogen protons and an increase in protein content, the mucocele contents become thick and pasty. This appears as hyperintense on T1-weighted and T2-weighted MRI.
- The contents of a long-standing mucocele are dry and desiccated. There are no free hydrogen protons, and the mucocele is now seen as a signal-void cavity on T1-weighted and T2-weighted MRI. These mucoceles pose a problem as they can be easily misinterpreted as a normal air-filled sinus. A CT scan will identify this by demonstrating the desiccated material in the sinus in addition to the expansion of the sinus by the mucocele.
- If the expansile nature of the mucocele is overlooked, these long-standing mucoceles can be

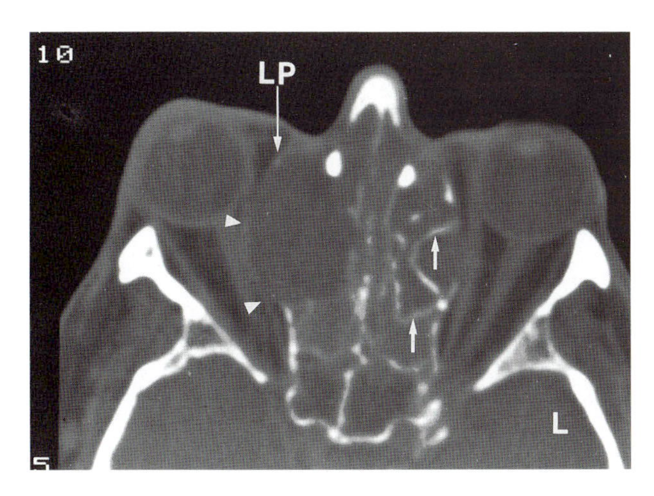

Figure 8.15 *Ethmoid sinus polypoidal mucoceles with bilateral exophthalmos.* This axial scan demonstrates a smooth expansile mass in the right ethmoid sinus, with eggshell thinning of the lamina papyracea (LP). The bony septa in the left ethmoid sinus are sclerotic (arrows) and the labyrinth is expanded, in keeping with the diagnosis of a polypoidal mucocele. The right medial rectus muscle is stretched over the mucocele (arrowheads).

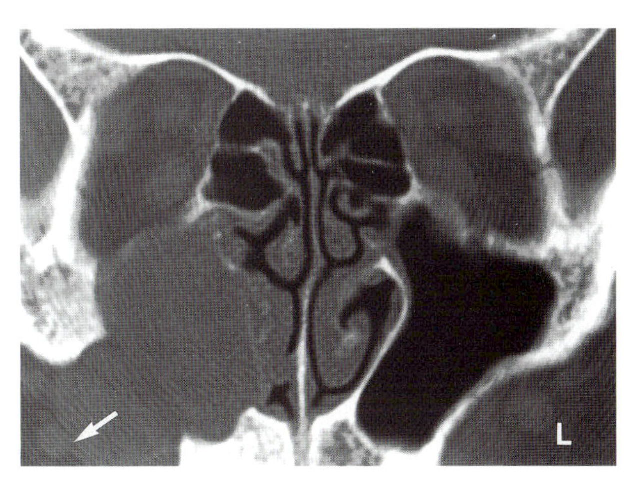

Figure 8.17 *Maxillary sinus mucocele.* This patient presented with a mass in his right cheek (arrow). This wide-window coronal scan demonstrates a large, expansile mass in the right maxillary sinus that is of similar density to water. Smooth expansion of the maxillary sinus with erosion of the inferolateral wall and the roof of the maxillary sinus has occurred.

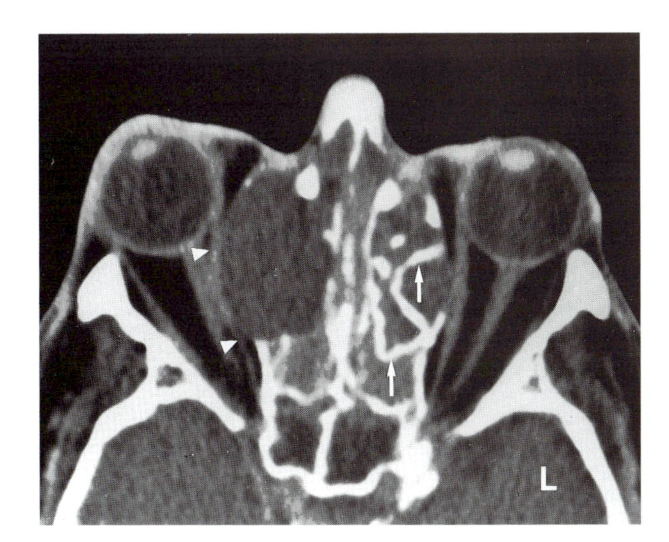

Figure 8.16 *Ethmoid sinus polypoidal mucoceles with bilateral exophthalmos.* Narrow-window axial CT scan (as in Figure 8.15) demonstrating the smooth, expansile mass in the right ethmoid sinus to be isodense. The bony septa in the left ethmoid sinus appear sclerotic (arrows) and the labyrinth is expanded, in keeping with the diagnosis of a polypoidal mucocele. The right medial rectus muscle is stretched over the mucocele (arrowheads).

misinterpreted as a normal sinus on MRI because air in a normal sinus presents as a signal void.

- In addition to expansion of the bony walls, the sinus mucosa appears hyperintense on T2-weighted MRI. Mucosa will also enhance following gadolinium-diethylenetriaminepenta-acetic acid (Gd-DTPA) administration.
- Signal-void areas may be misinterpreted as a normal sinus on MRI if a CT scan is not available for correlation. Clotted blood, fibrotic scar, mycetomas, calcium, tooth, bone, or a pocket of air can also cause a signal void in a sinus.

Specific anatomical mucoceles

Ethmoid sinus mucoceles

(Figures 8.1, 8.13, and 8.14)

Mucoceles of the ethmoid sinus tend to cause proptosis and lateral displacement of the globe. There may be an associated swelling in the superomedial quadrant of the orbit, and both of these features may cause diplopia. Encroachment on the lacrimal apparatus causes epiphora. Ethmoid mucoceles are best demonstrated by CT scans. CT will show expansion of the ethmoid sinus by a smooth mass filled with mucus, loss of the fine bony septa dividing the air cells, and erosion of the lamina papyracea. Supraorbital extension may be indicated by thinning or loss of the superomedial orbital rim and the adjacent roof of the orbit.

8.18a

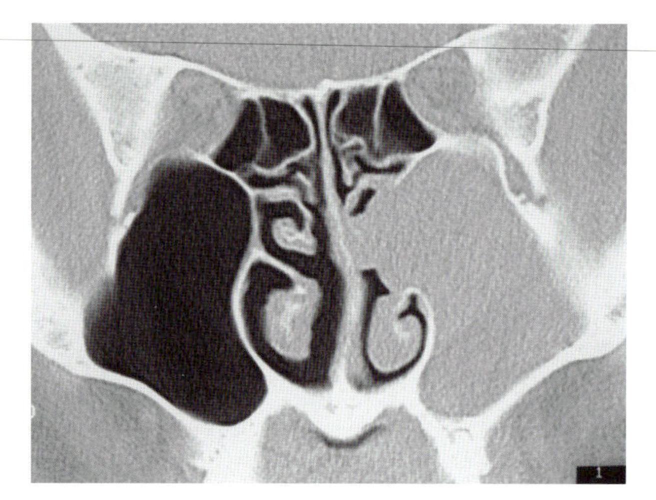

8.18b

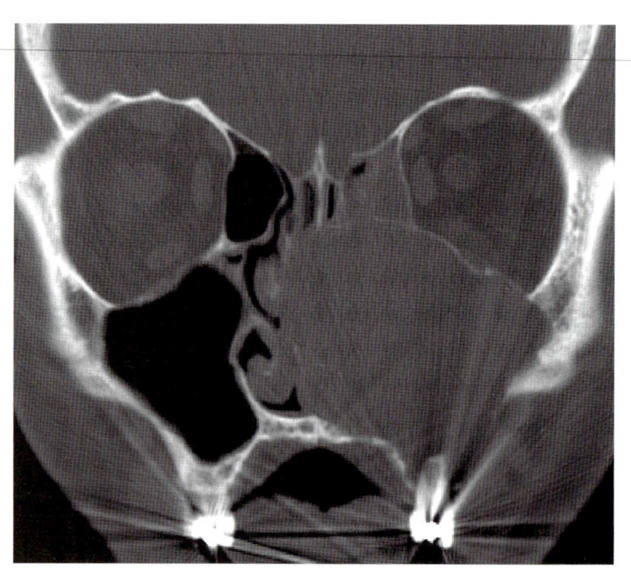

8.18c

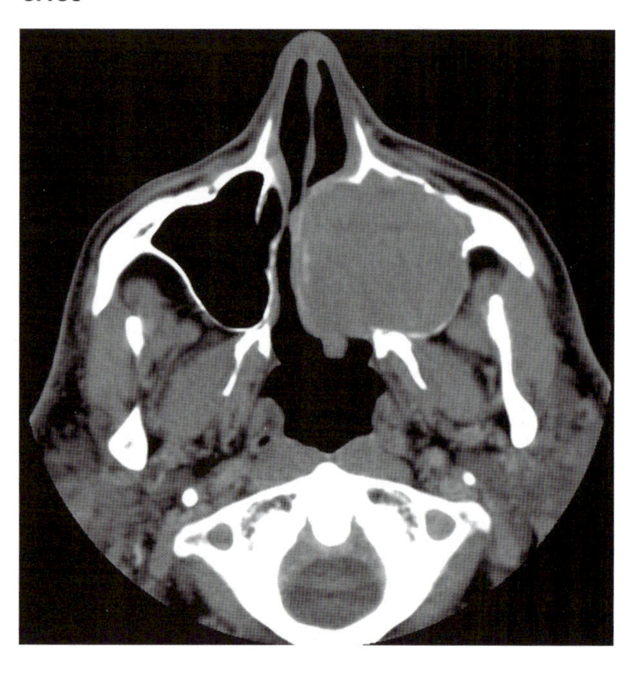

Figure 8.18 *Maxillary sinus mucocele*. (a) CT scan demonstrating the early changes due to the presence of an expansile mass in the left maxillary sinus, with smooth erosion of the medial sinus wall and extension into the nasal cavity. The lumen contents are fluid and homogeneous. (b, c) This mucocele demonstrates advanced prolonged effects of mucocele on the walls of the left maxillary sinus (expansion, thinning, and erosion). The smooth expansile erosion is the classic appearance of a benign process.

Ethmoid sinus polypoidal mucoceles with bilateral exophthalmos (Figures 8.15 and 8.16)

The polypoidal mucocele is a separate entity in which patients present with diplopia and proptosis. It exhibits involvement and expansion of the whole ethmoid labyrinth, with preservation and sclerosis of the lamina papyracea and the bony leaflets separating the ethmoid air cells. These lesions have also been noted to enhance slightly following the administration of intravenous contrast, which is at variance with the behavior of the classic mucocele. These polypoid mucoceles are usually associated with multiple sinus inflammatory disease and not infrequently with other mucoceles developing in the supraorbital ethmoid air cells.

Maxillary sinus mucoceles (Figures 8.2–8.5, 8.17, and 8.18)

Mucoceles of the maxillary sinus may present in many ways. These include presentation as a mass in the nasal cavity if there is medial extension, with diplopia if there is superior extension, with cheek swelling if there is anterior expansion, and with

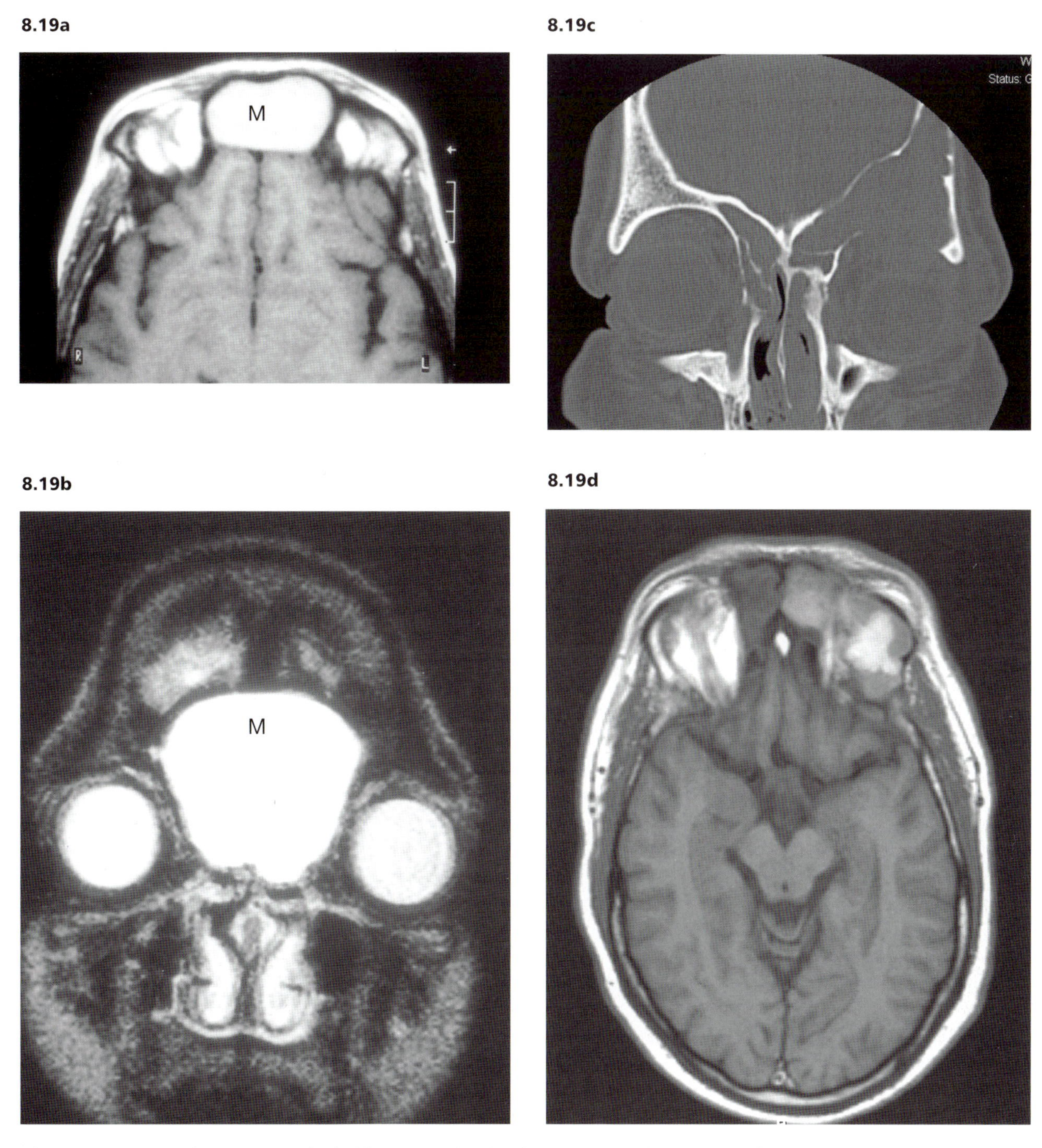

Figure 8.19 *Frontal sinus mucocele.* (a, b) MRI examination demonstrating the presence of a midline expansile mass (M) that is hyperintense on T1-weighted (a) and T2-weighted (b) images. (c, d) CT scans demonstrating an expansile mass in the left frontal sinus. The walls of the sinus are eroded.

swelling of the gums if there is extension into the alveolus. Recurrent infection suggests that the dental roots should be examined, as disease in the roots may be a predisposing factor. Maxillary sinus mucoceles in the early stage will exhibit opacification of the sinus on plain radiographs. As the mucocele expands, the bony walls become thinned and displaced medially into the nasal cavity, superiorly into the orbit, posteriorly into the pterygopalatine fossa, or laterally reversing the natural convexity of the lateral antral wall. The fluid is less dense than muscle and isodense with brain. The differential diagnosis includes malignancy, especially if bony erosion is present. A significant number of maxillary sinus

8.19e

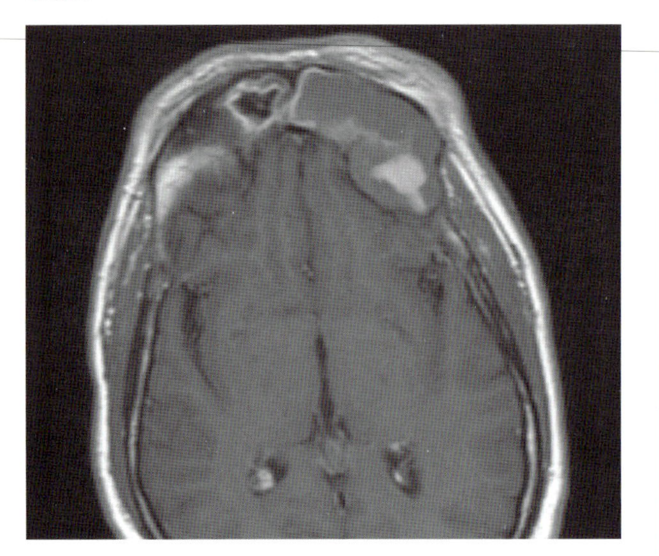

8.19f

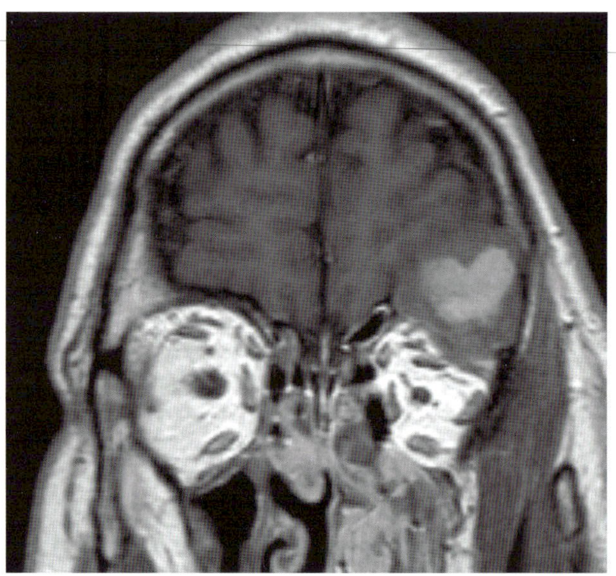

8.19g

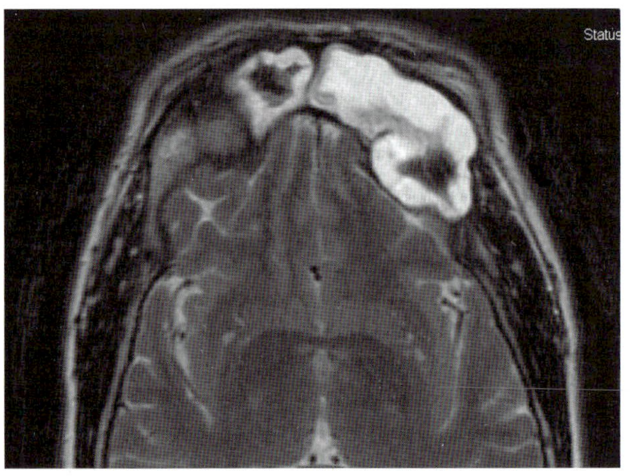

Figure 8.19 *continued* (e) T1-weighted MRI scan demonstrating the frontal sinus lumen content to be of mixed signal intensity. (f) Gd-DTPA-enhanced MRI scan demonstrating that the contents do not enhance. There is a thin rim of sinus mucosa that enhances. (g) T2-weighted MRI scan demonstrating the frontal sinus cavity contents to be hyperintense, with some signal-void areas. Image courtesy of Dr Herman Schuttevaer.

mucoceles follow surgical procedures of the maxillary sinus, and these are characteristically found to be laterally placed in the sinus as opposed to filling the entire antrum.

Frontal sinus mucoceles

(Figures 8.6–8.12 and 8.19–8.21)

Frontal sinus mucoceles cause resorption of the incomplete septa normally found within the sinus cavity. This leads to loss of the normal scalloped appearance and gives rise to a smooth outline. There may be an associated sclerosis of the bone. With increased expansion, the anterior and posterior walls of the sinus may become dehiscent, risking intracranial sepsis or infection spreading to the upper eyelid.

Mucocele of the sphenoid sinus

(Figures 8.22 and 8.23)

Sphenoid sinus mucoceles tend to present with headaches or with retro-orbital or periorbital pain. They may expand into the cavernous sinus and the orbital apex, causing ophthalmoplegia and retro-orbital pain known as 'the orbital apex syndrome'. There may be an associated gradual loss of vision, papilledema, and optic atrophy. These patients can also present with multiple cranial nerve palsies. Sphenoid sinus mucoceles may be localized unilaterally within the sinus or may expand to fill the whole sinus. Early features include a hemispherical opacity of the sinus. There may be displacement of the intersinus septum to the opposite side, and the lesion may then expand anteriorly

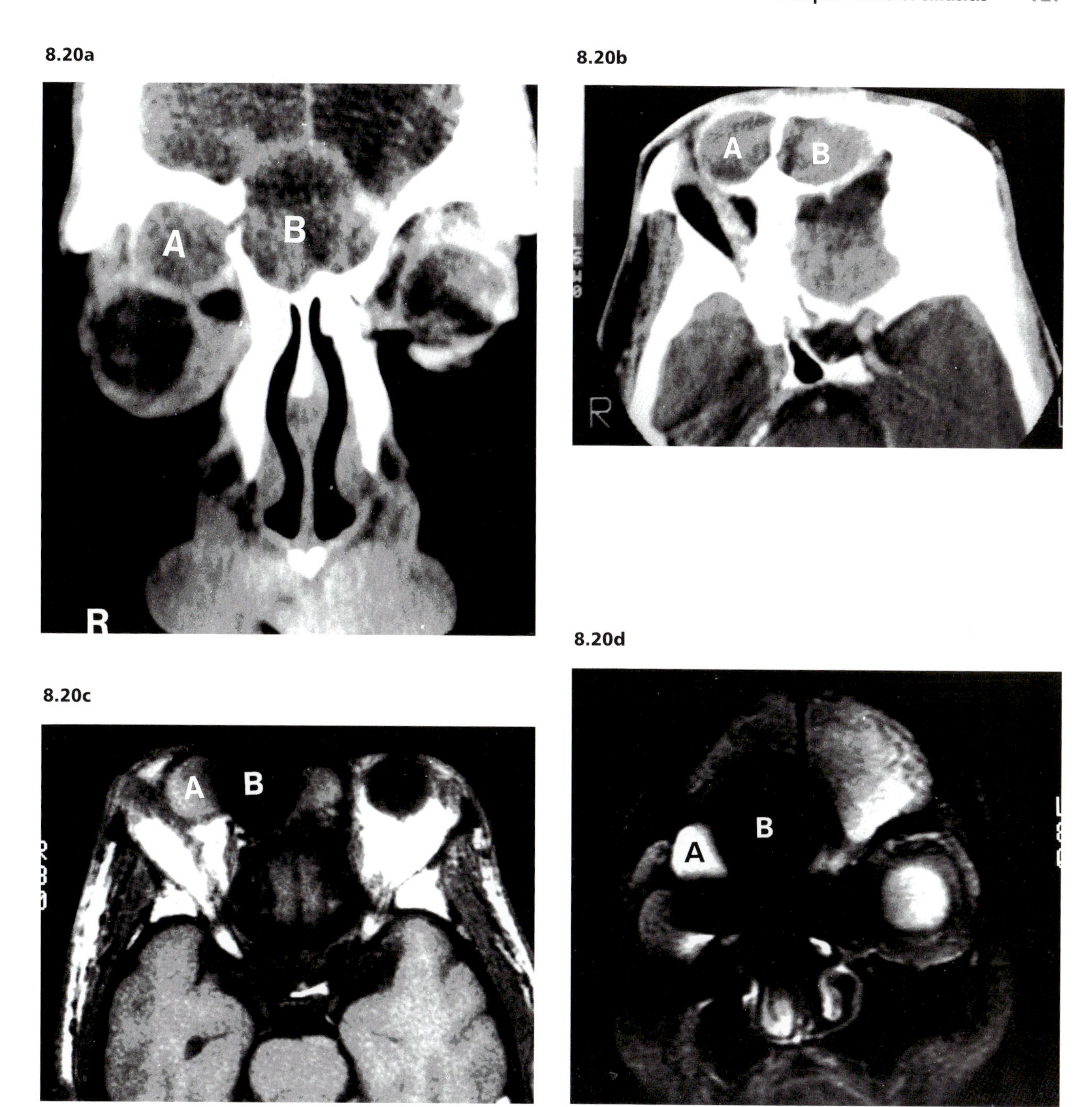

Figure 8.20 *Frontal sinus mucocele.* This patient presented with exophthalmos. (a) Coronal CT scan demonstrating a large mucocele with smooth erosion of the bony wall, extending into the right orbit. (b) Axial CT scan demonstrating two mucoceles (A and B) separated by a sclerotic and thickened bony septum in the frontal sinuses. The collections in the two mucoceles are similar in densitiy. (c) Axial T2-weighted MRI scan demonstrating the signal intensity of the contents in the two mucoceles to be markedly different. One of these mucoceles (A) is isointense with brain, while the other (B) is signal-void because its contents are inspissated. (d) T2-weighted MRI scan demonstrating the mucocele as a signal-void area (B). If the expansion of the sinus wall is subtle, then such a mucocele can be easily overlooked on MRI scans. Mucoceles have variable signal intensities, depending upon their contents. A thick viscid mucoid material that has few hydrogen protons will be signal-void (B), whereas a fluid that has abundant hydrogen protons will be hyperintense on T2-weighted images (A).

into the posterior ethmoid and the sphenoethmoid recess. If it is extensive, the mucocele will be seen expanding into any of the related anatomical regions, such as the cranial cavity, the nasopharynx, the pterygopalatine fossa, the infratemporal fossa, or the orbit. Expansion into the orbit may be associated with widening of the superior orbital fissure. This extensive appearance may be sugges-

8.21a

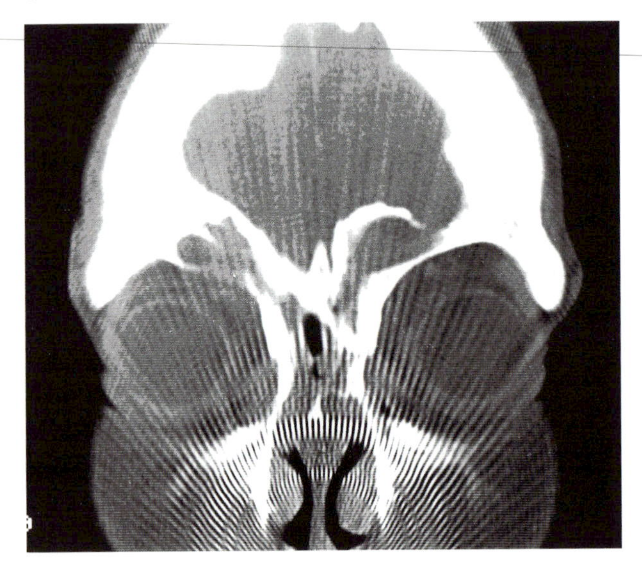

8.21b

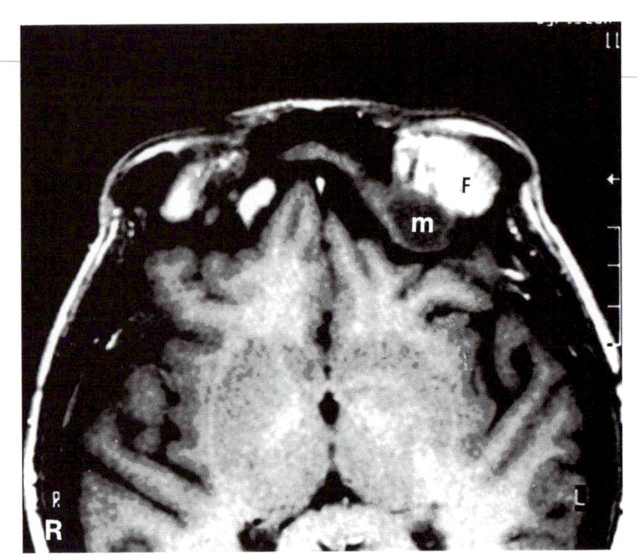

8.21c

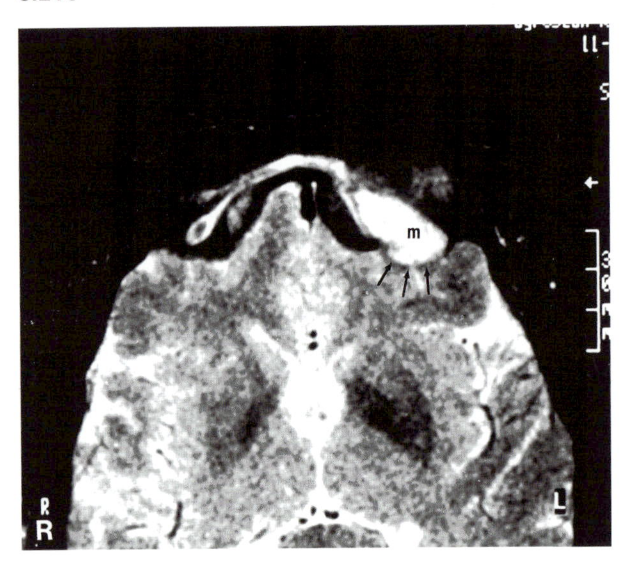

Figure 8.21 *Postoperative mucocele.* This patient presented with a history of recurrent symptoms of sinusitis following, obliterative surgery (an osteoplastic flap with obliteration of the frontal sinus by the insertion of a free fat graft into the sinus cavity). She had a history of frontal sinus mucoceles. (a) Coronal CT scan demonstrating the postoperative changes. The cause of the recurrence of the patient's symptoms could not be ascertained from the CT scan. She was referred for an MRI scan because her headaches continued and the CT scan was inconclusive. (b) T1-weighted MRI scan demonstrating high signal intensity from fat (F) and a hypointense well-circumscribed lesion (m) posteriorly in the left frontal sinus. (c) The T2-weighted MRI scan showing the mucocele (m) to be hyperintense. The posterior wall of the mucocele is eroded (arrows).

tive of malignancy. MRI scans are useful in the evaluation of mucoceles of the sphenoid sinuses, as the relationship of the internal carotid artery, optic nerve, and cavernous sinuses to the mucocele is well demonstrated.

Lacrimal sac mucoceles

Lacrimal sac mucoceles are an uncommon finding and can occur in infants. These mucoceles present with a swelling in the region of the medial canthus. These are usually related to congenital anomalies of the nasolacrimal duct. CT is an invaluable aid in confirming the diagnosis as it will demonstrate a cystic mass in the medial canthus in continuity with an expanded nasolacrimal duct and a contiguous submucosal intranasal mass.

PYOCELE (Figures 8.24–8.26; see also Figures 8.2 and 8.3)

A pyocele is a mucocele that has become secondarily infected. This usually exacerbates the symptoms. The radiological features are similar to those of mucoceles, but following the administration of intravenous contrast there is usually a ring of

8.22a

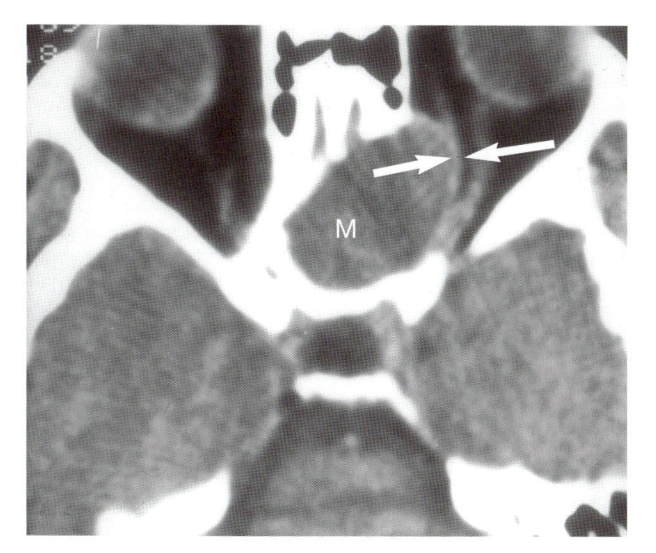

8.22b

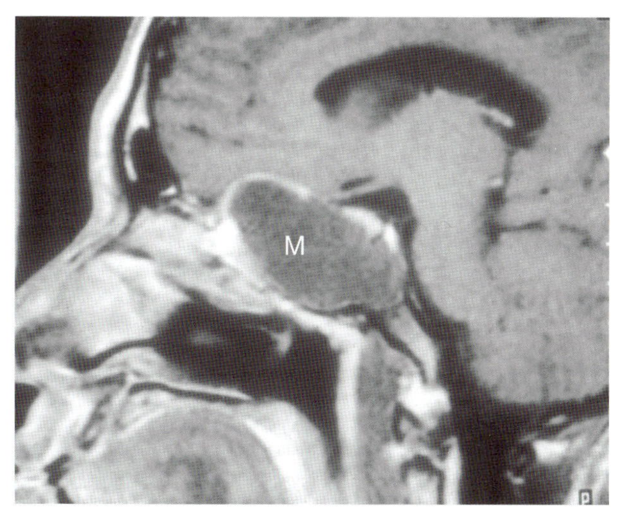

8.22c

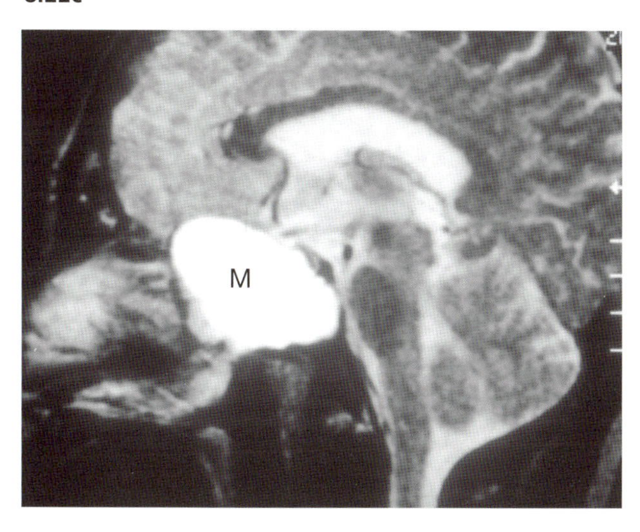

Figure 8.22 *Sphenoethmoid mucocele*. (a) CT scan demonstrating a homogeneous expansile mass (M) in the left sphenoethmoid complex. There is almost complete bony resorption, with a thin layer of mucoperiosteum separating the mucocele from the structures in the orbit (arrows). (b, c) MRI examination demonstrating the contents to be hypointense on T1-weighted (b) and hyperintense on T2-weighted (c) scans.

enhancement within the cavity of the pyocele representing the inflamed mucosa.

EMPYEMA (Figure 8.27)

An empyema is a purulent collection in a sinus. Unlike a pyocele, the affected sinus does not demonstrate any preexisting inflammatory process or bony changes. The bony walls of the sinus do not bow outwards and there is no expansion of the sinus lumen. On CT, however, rarefaction of the sinus walls may be seen in addition to the opacification of the sinus, and will indicate that a major complication is imminent if the infection is not controlled.

OSTEOMYELITIS (Figures 8.28–8.30)

Clinically, osteomyelitis of the frontal bone presents with a soft doughy swelling overlying the frontal bone. The patient is unwell, with a fever, rigors, diffuse headache, and spreading edema of the forehead. Osteomyelitis affects the frontal bone most commonly, with the maxillary sinus being the second most commonly affected. Osteomyelitis of the frontal bone either is spontaneous or occurs following trauma (accidental or operative). The sepsis spreads into the bone either by direct extension or via thrombophlebitis of the diploic veins. Osteomyelitis occurs with infection of diploic bone and is different to osteitis, which is infection of com-

8.23a

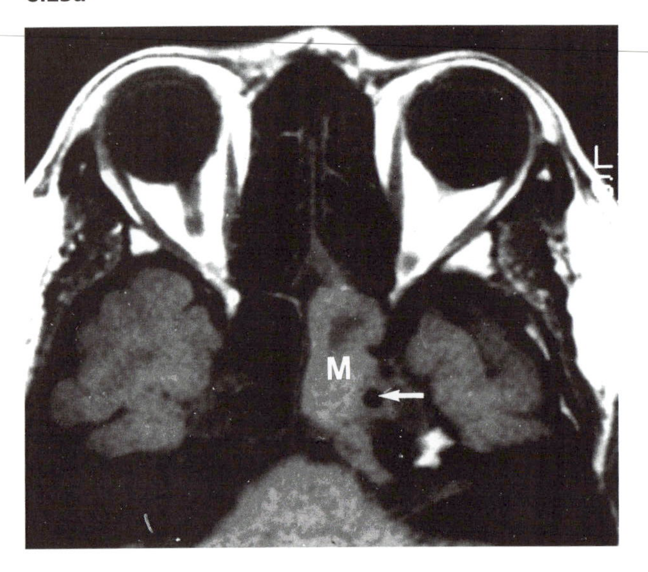

8.23b

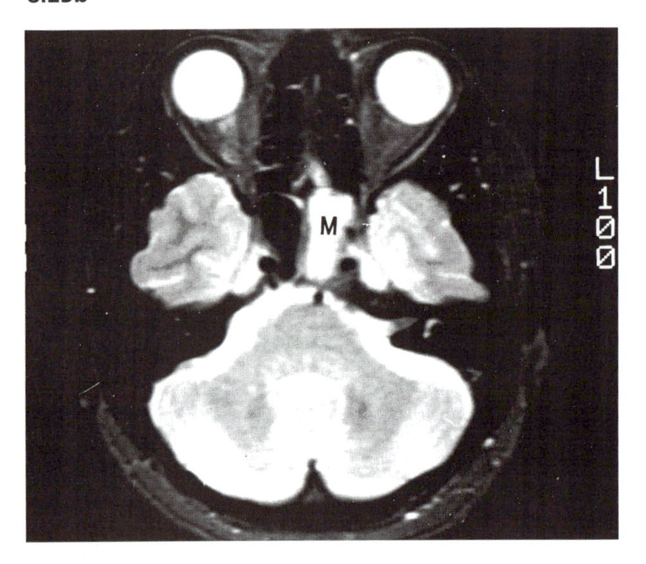

Figure 8.23 *Mucocele of the sphenoid sinus.* (a) T1-weighted MRI scan demonstrating a mucocele of the sphenoid sinus (M) as an isointense mass with a hypointense center, surrounding the left internal carotid artery (arrow) and encroaching onto the prepontine cisterns. T1-weighted imaging defines the relationship to vital neurovascular structures. (b) T2-weighted scan demonstrating the mucocele (M) to be hyperintense due to its high water content.

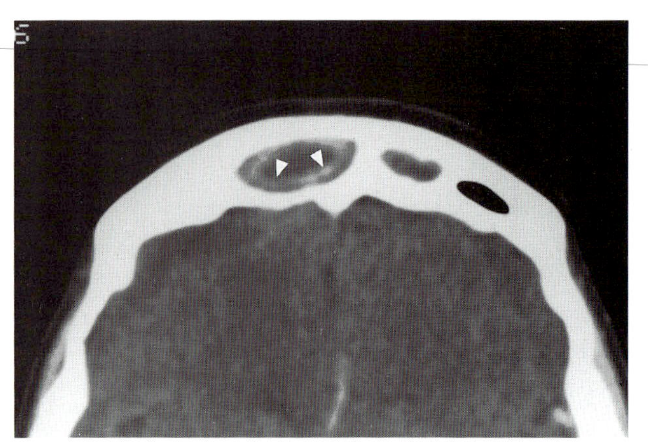

Figure 8.24 *Pyocele.* This patient presented with a furuncle on the forehead, which developed into a draining sinus. CT following the administration of intravenous contrast demonstrates mucosal enhancement (arrowheads) in the frontal sinus. The mucosal enhancement is suggestive of an acute inflammatory process. The erosion through the anterior wall of the frontal sinus is not demonstrated on this scan, but was the drainage pathway of the pyocele.

pact bone, such as is found in the floor of the frontal sinus. For this reason, surgical drainage of an acute frontal sinusitis should only be undertaken through the sinus floor.

Osteomyelitis tends to manifest itself as a subperiosteal abscess, which is limited by the attachment of the periosteum, or intracranially by the dura as an extradural abscess. This association of an extradural abscess, subperiosteal abscess, and intervening osteomyelitis is known as Pott's puffy tumor.

Radiographic appearance of osteomyelitis

- There may be little radiological evidence for 7–10 days if the osteomyelitis is untreated.
- There is poor definition of the sinus walls, with disruption of the mucoperiosteal lining.
- Uncontrolled sinusitis, despite high-dose antibiotics, progresses to rarification of skull bone, with lytic lesions appearing in the adjacent bone. The appearance on plain radiographs is similar to that on CT, with multiple lytic foci being unevenly distributed.
- Bony sequestra are less common in chronic osteomyelitis of the facial bones or skull than in chronic osteomyelitis of the long bones.
- In chronic cases, sclerotic changes are superimposed upon areas of rarefaction and the margins of the sinus become indistinct.
- Following the administration of intravenous contrast, the acutely inflamed mucosa exhibits

8.25a

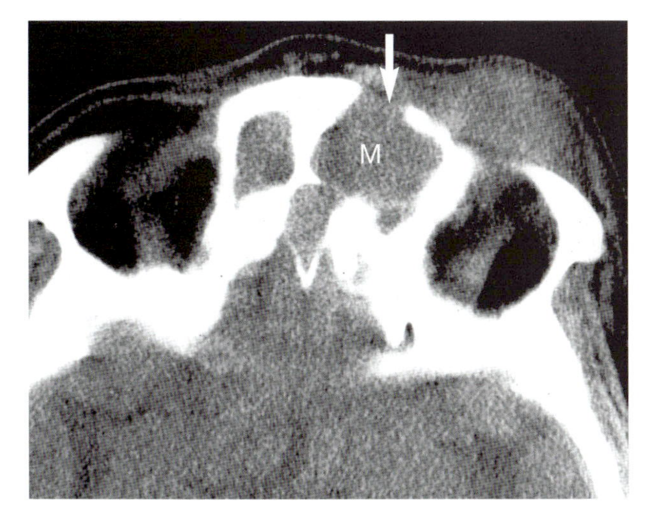

8.25b

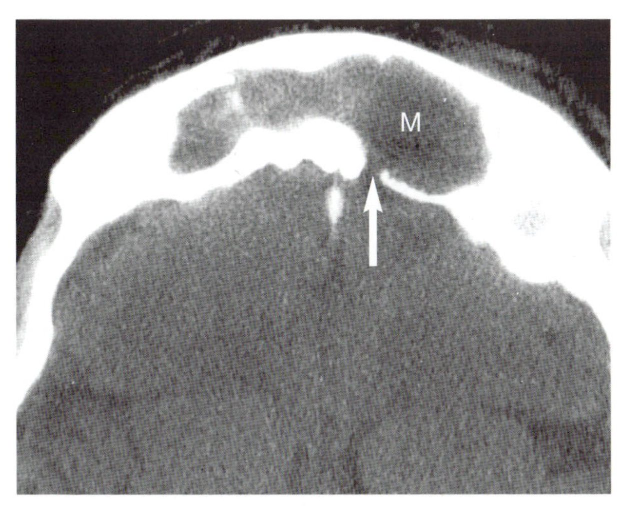

Figure 8.25 *Frontal sinus mucopyocele.* (a, b) Axial CT scans demonstrating an expansile mass (M) in the frontal sinus with erosion (arrows) of the anterior and posterior walls of the frontal sinus associated with left eyelid edema. Image courtesy of Dr Herman Schuttevaer.

8.26a

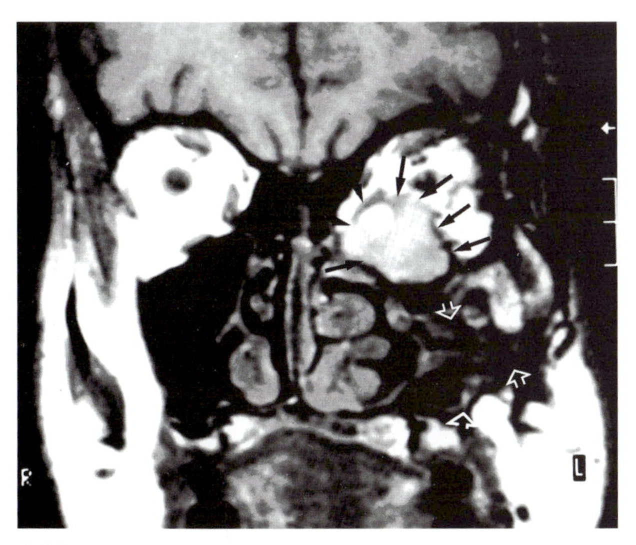

8.26b

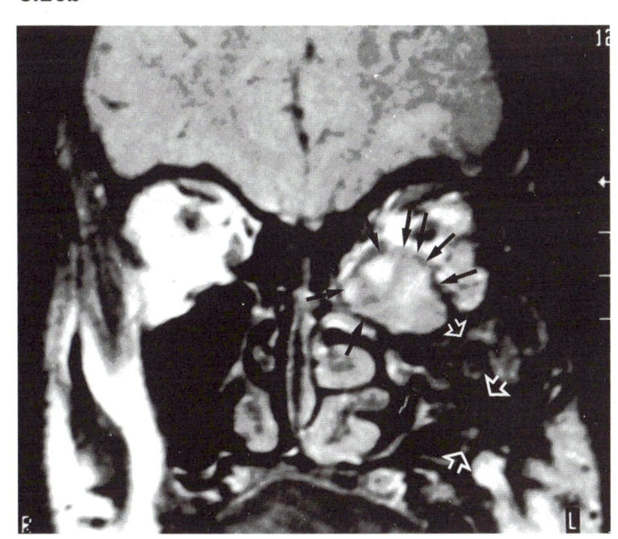

8.26c

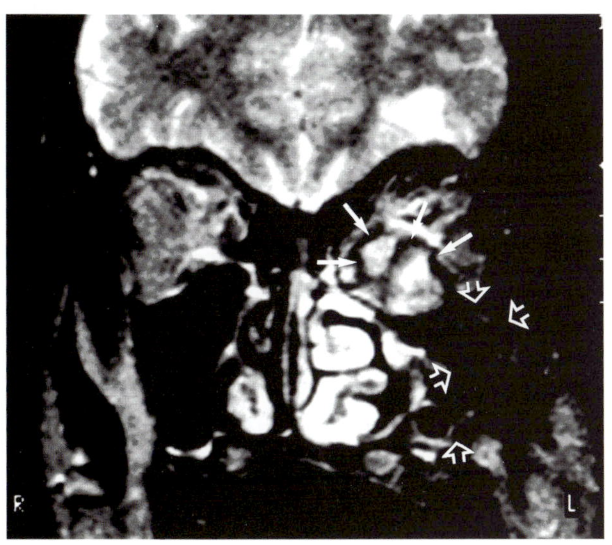

Figure 8.26 *Post-traumatic pyocele and scarring.* (a) T1-weighted MRI scan demonstrating an expansile mass in the inferomedial aspect of the orbit (arrows). This patient had previously undergone surgery for multiple fractures to the sinuses and the facial bones. The left maxillary sinus lumen is replaced by linear strands of varying signal intensities (open arrows). (b) Proton density-weighted MRI scan demonstrating unchanged signal intensity of the pyocele. The scarring in the maxillary sinus appears darker (open arrows). (c) T2-weighted MRI scan demonstrating the pyocele as an unusual multiseptated mass (arrows) with contents that are hyperintense in signal intensity. The fibrosis and scarring (open arrows) are further reduced in signal intensity. This progressive decrease in signal intensity is more in keeping with scarring. Active inflammatory reaction would be hyperintense on a T2-weighted scan.

8.27a

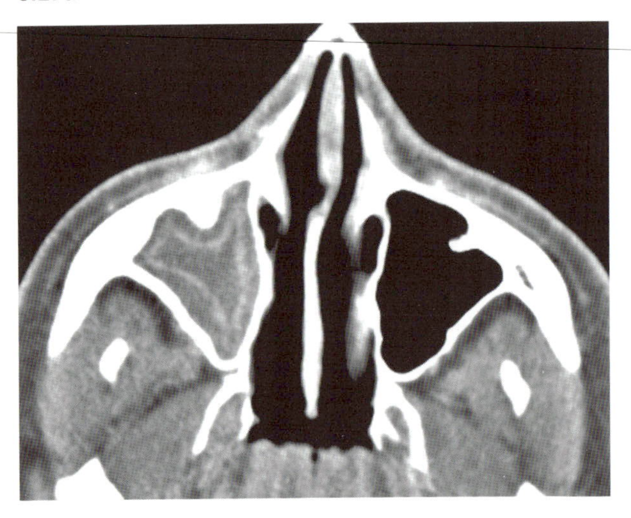

8.27b

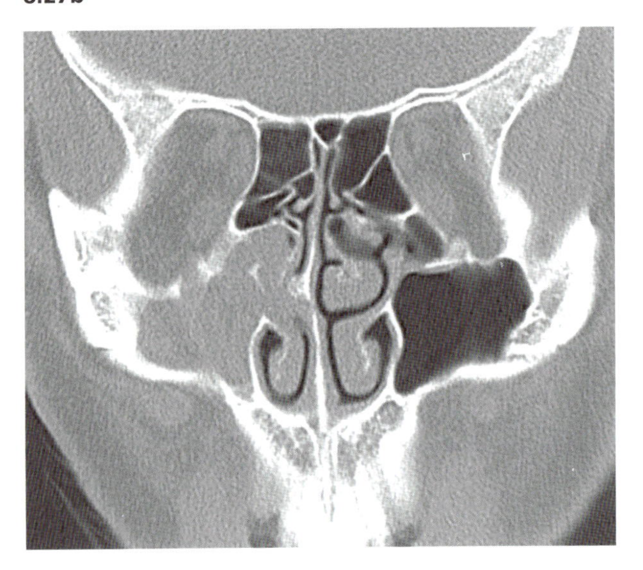

Figure 8.27 *Maxillary sinus empyema following root canal therapy*. Axial contrast-enhanced CT scan (a) and coronal CT scan (b) demonstrating fluid in the maxillary sinus lumen associated with enhancement of the mucosa.

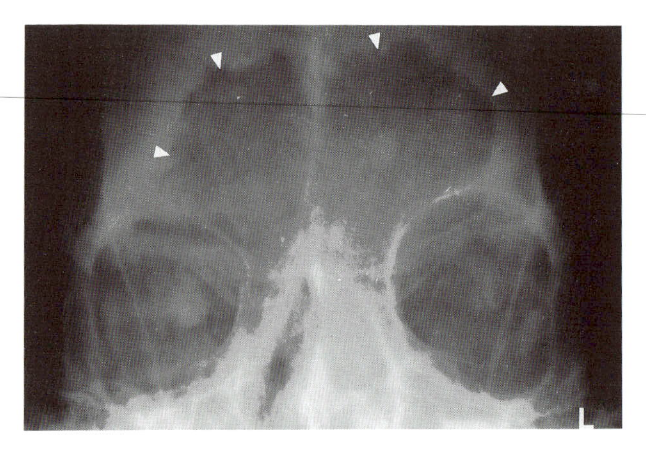

Figure 8.28 *Osteomyelitis*. This patient presented with the onset of headache following a 5-week history of sinusitis refractory to medical management. This plain radiograph demonstrates extensive destruction of the frontal bone (arrowheads) with opacification of the frontal and the ethmoid sinuses consistent with frontoethmoid sinusitis and osteomyelitis.

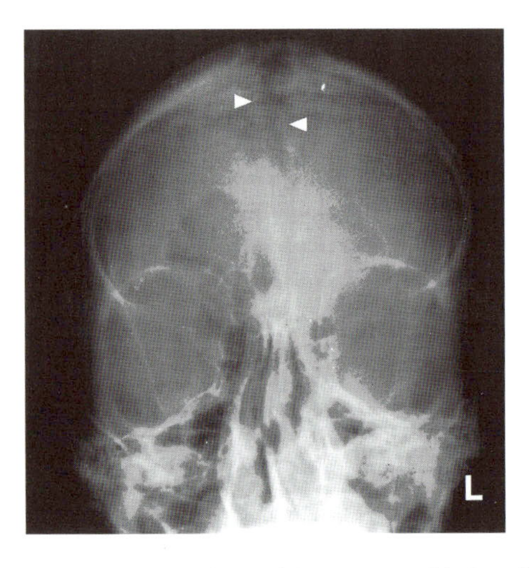

Figure 8.29 *Osteomyelitis*. This 15-year-old female presented with a history of acute frontal sinusitis, fever, and headaches. This plain radiograph demonstrates left-sided frontal sinusitis with poor definition of the sinus walls and disruption of the mucoperiosteal lining. Rarefaction is seen progressing along the sagittal suture (arrowheads).

intense enhancement. This needs to be differentiated from the enhancement of pyoceles. The smooth expansion of the sinus walls associated with pyoceles is usually absent with osteomyelitis.

Osteomyelitis of the maxilla usually affects the alveolar bone, which is cancellous between two plates of thin compact bone. It may occur both in adults and in infants. The commonest cause is dental infection, which may lead to a subperiosteal abscess spreading across the maxilla. Radiological features are minimal in some cases, with slight opacity of the maxillary sinus. In some cases, there may be marked sclerosis of the maxilla.

OSTEITIS

Condensing osteitis is a reaction of the bone to sinus infection. The reaction is in the form of bone production brought about by a good immune response

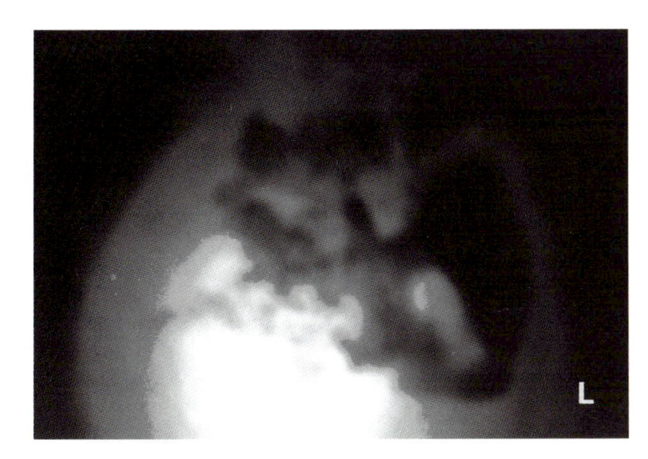

Figure 8.30 *Osteomyelitis*. CT scan of the same patient as in Figure 8.29 demonstrating progression of acute frontal sinusitis to osteomyelitis. Widespread lytic lesions are seen in the frontal bone.

from the patient, as opposed to rarefaction, which results in fragmentation and demineralization of the skull and facial bones. This is seen as a focal area of increased density and localized deformity of the sinus wall or the frontal bone, which is often the site of osteitis secondary to frontal sinus disease.

FACIAL CELLULITIS

Antiobiotic therapy has reduced the incidence of facial cellulitis. Periorbital and facial cellulitis may be manifestations of a more ominous major intraorbital complication. This is more prevalent in the pediatric age group, drug abusers, and immune-compromised individuals. CT demonstrates this as enhancing thickened cutaneous and subcutaneous structures.

ORBITAL COMPLICATIONS (Figures 8.31–8.35)

Orbital complications include orbital cellulitis, subperiosteal abscess, orbital abscess, optic neuritis, and retinal artery occlusion. These complications are usually associated with infection of the frontal and/or ethmoid sinuses or with a pansinusitis. The usual route of spread is either through bony dehiscences of the sinus wall or through the venous pathways. The patient may become blind if immediate treatment is not started. Treatment includes high-dose intravenous antibiotics, abscess drainage, and orbital decompression if indicated.

PERIORBITAL CELLULITIS

An important clinical differentiation must be made in this group regarding the site of the infection in relation to the orbital septum. The orbital septum is the fibrous band that spans from the orbital margins to the tarsal plate of the upper eyelid. Both preseptal and postseptal orbital inflammation present with swelling of the upper eyelid.

Preseptal orbital cellulitis

- The skin of the eyelid assumes a dusky, reddish-blue hue.
- CT of preseptal inflammation shows a diffuse increase in density with thickening of the eyelid.
- The conjunctiva is usually unaffected.
- Abscess formation is indicated by an area of low density, which may or may not exhibit rim enhancement following the administration of intravenous contrast.
- The eye is in its normal position, and normal movements of the eye can be observed if the lids are separated.
- The globe does not exhibit proptosis and occasionally is displaced slightly posteriorly.

Postseptal orbital cellulitis

Postseptal inflammation requires a different management and is divided into three groups:

- Extraconal – subperiosteal
- Intraconal – within the periosteum/orbital cavity
- Combined – both intraconal and extraconal

Features of extraconal orbital cellulitis

- The commonest cause of medial extraconal inflammation is ethmoiditis. Anterolateral displacement of the globe with inflammatory exudate in the subperiosteal space is seen.

8.31a

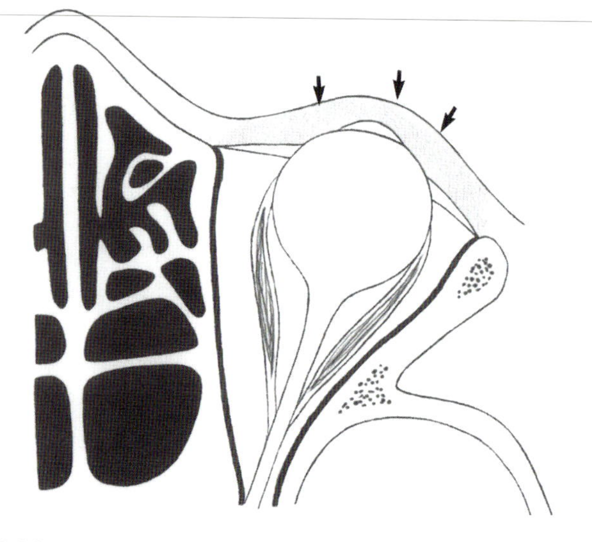

8.31b

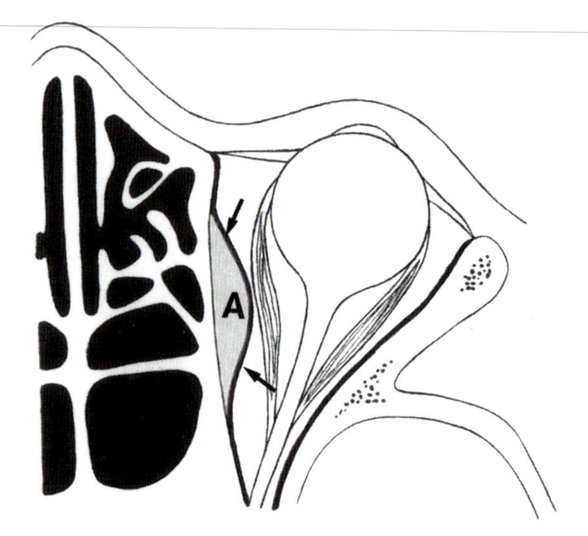

8.31c

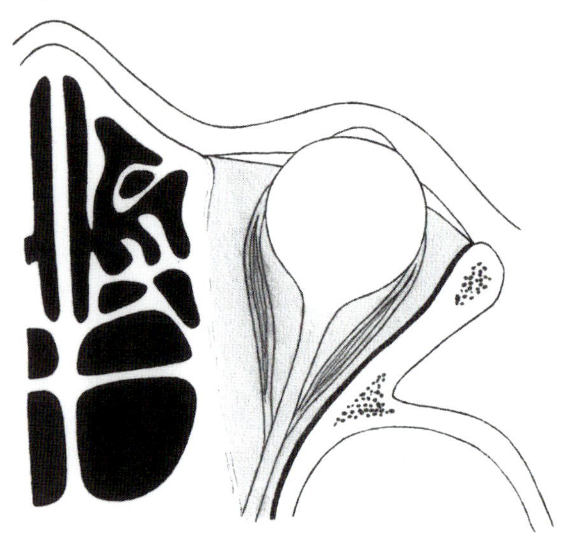

Figure 8.31 *Orbital cellulitis.* (a) Preseptal stage of orbital cellulitis, where there is swelling of the eyelids (arrows). (b) Postseptal orbital cellulitis inflammatory process restricted to the subperiosteal space, with infection spreading from the ethmoid sinus into the orbit. The protective periosteum (arrows) is stripped from the medial wall of the orbit by the abscess (A). (c) Postseptal orbital cellulitis spread of infection into the entire orbital cavity, including the retro-orbital fat.

- The clinical signs include proptosis of the globe, restricted eye movements, chemosis of the conjunctiva, and loss of vision, color vision first.
- With subperiosteal inflammation, the exudate accumulates between the lamina papyracea and the loose periosteum. Initially, this may only be a phlegmonous reaction, but if inadequately treated, it will progress to abscess formation. The infection is limited by the periosteum and rarely spreads into the intraconal space.
- The CT characteristics are similar for both subperiosteal phlegmon and subperiosteal abscess. The medial rectus muscle is displaced laterally, is broadened from inflammatory edema, and may enhance slightly. The elevated periosteum is displaced laterally and is demonstrated as an enhancing line running alongside the medial rectus muscle. The thickened periosteum may be indistinguishable from the medial rectus muscle. An abscess becomes apparent by the development of an area of low density, which may be localized or may spread along the entire medial wall of the orbit. The inflammation may cause demineralization of the lamina papyracea or even osteitis, which becomes evident with bony loss or thinning.
- This condition requires aggressive treatment with intravenous antibiotics and surgical drainage of any abscess collection using the same approach as for an external ethmoidectomy. Orbital decompression may also be indicated.

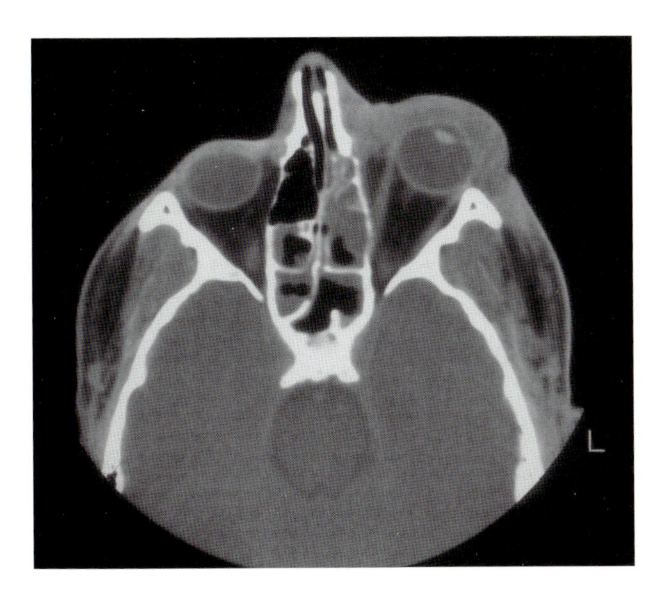

Figure 8.32 *Preseptal periorbital cellulitis.* Axial CT scan demonstrating diffuse swelling of the left eyelid associated with ethmoid sinusitis.

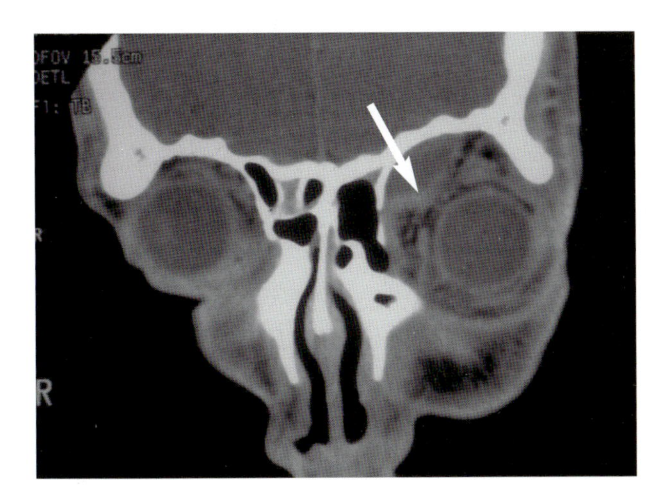

Figure 8.33 Subperiosteal abscess. Coronal CT scan demonstrating the presence of a subperiosteal abscess (arrow) adjacent to the roof of the orbit.

Features of intraconal orbital cellulitis

- The clinical features include proptosis, restricted eye movements, and chemosis. If intraorbital abscess formation occurs, there is usually marked proptosis and a rapid decrease in visual acuity. There is a grave risk of retrograde infection causing cavernous sinus thrombosis which may lead to papilledema.

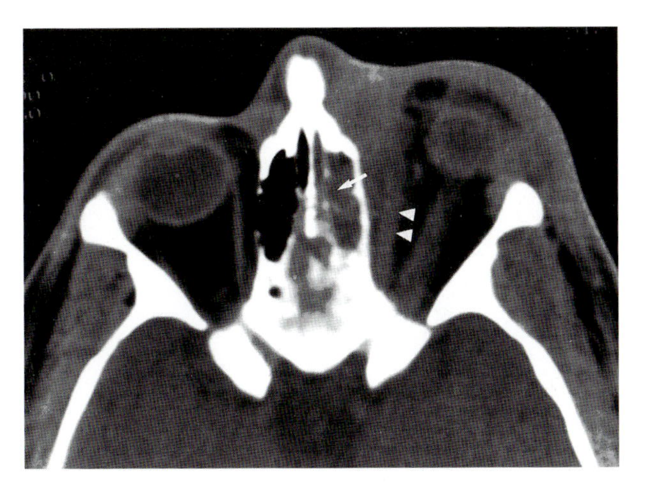

Figure 8.34 *Subperiosteal abscess.* This patient presented with fever, sinusitis, and orbital cellulitis. On this CT scan, the non-enhancing mass along the medial aspect of the left ethmoid complex (arrow) is a subperiosteal abscess. The medial rectus muscle and the elevated periosteum (arrowheads) are seen as an enhancing linear density lateral to the abscess. This abscess is the result of spread of infection into the orbit from the ethmoid sinus through the lamina papyracea. Image courtesy of Dr J Cairnes and Dr D Kirkpatrick, Dalhousie University, Halifax, Nova Scotia, Canada.

- CT will demonstrate intraconal inflammation as loss of definition of the extraocular muscles and the optic nerve. The fat in the intraconal space is infiltrated with linear strands of inflammatory reaction, making it difficult to distinguish either the extraocular muscles or the optic nerve. Abscess formation is indicated by the characteristic development of an area of low density with an enhancing rim or air in the orbital fat. Again, treatment consists of aggressive antibiotic therapy and orbital decompression.

Features of diffuse intraconal and extraconal orbital cellulitis

- This is the least common type.
- The infection initiates in the intraconal or extraconal compartments.
- There is severe proptosis, with the possibility of spread of infection to the infratemporal fossa and cavernous sinus if left untreated.
- The CT findings usually demonstrate obliteration of the muscles and of the optic nerve by inflammatory exudate.

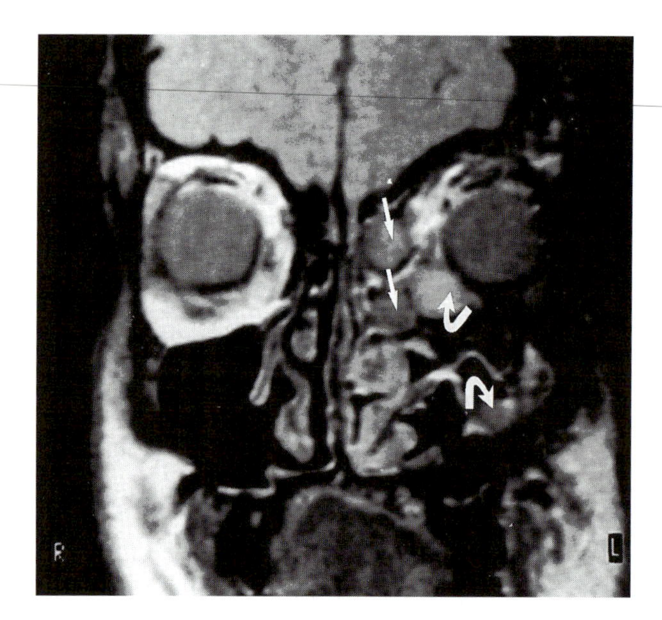

Figure 8.35 *Pyocele and orbital cellulitis*. This patient had a history of a previous facial injury, with multiple fractures of the sinuses and orbit on the left side. This T2-weighted MRI scan demonstrates large signal-void masses (arrows), which are mucoceles of the left ethmoid complex compressing the orbital contents. The hyperintense masses are the infected pyocoeles (curved arrows). The irregular hyperintense area of inflammation represents the inflammatory reaction in the orbit.

ORBITAL ABSCESS

While orbital abscess and cellulitis are more common complications from ethmoid sinusitis, intracranial complications are more frequent with frontal sinusitis. The abscess may occur intraconally or extraconally. On CT imaging, the inflammatory process in the orbital fat leads to streaky areas of increased density, resulting in obliteration of the optic nerve outline.

OPTIC NEURITIS

Optic neuritis may result from compression and ischemia of the optic nerve by the inflammatory process in the orbit or from a direct insult to the optic nerve where the nerve is the site of inflammatory neuropathy. Infection can spread to the optic nerve through the venous plexus of the orbital apex, which surrounds the optic nerve sheath. The compromised vision shows rapid improvement with successful treatment of the sinusitis, and this may be a reflection of the immune reaction to the inflammatory process in the sinuses, which causes vasomotor changes and decreased blood flow with stagnation and engorgement around the optic nerve.

OCCLUSION OF THE CENTRAL RETINAL ARTERY

Compression of the central retinal artery or the ophthalmic artery branches occurs as a direct effect of the inflammatory process in the orbit. In some rare cases, the central retinal artery flow may decrease or cease. This should be suspected when the optic disk becomes edematous and the retinal veins engorged. Profound visual loss is inevitable if the arterial circulation is not reestablished immediately.

INTRACRANIAL COMPLICATIONS

(Figures 8.36 and 8.37)

Intracranial sepsis is a rare but life-threatening complication of uncontrolled sinus disease. Complications include meningitis, extradural abscess, subdural abscess, intracerebral abscess, and cavernous sinus thrombosis. These complications usually occur as a consequence of inadequate antibiotic treatment or of the presence of resistant bacteria, or in patients who are immunosupressed.

The clinical features of intracranial sepsis include the following:

- There is generalized malaise and progressively severe headache.
- The clinical picture depends on the site of intracranial infection. A high index of suspicion is needed to make the appropriate diagnosis and arrest the infection before serious neurological sequelae occur.
- Focal signs and convulsions may occur, as well as changes in personality and conscious level. Vomiting and papilledema occur at a late stage.
- Examination of the cerebrospinal fluid may be of value by identifying elevated protein and leukocyte levels and reduced glucose levels, as well as sampling for bacteriological culture.

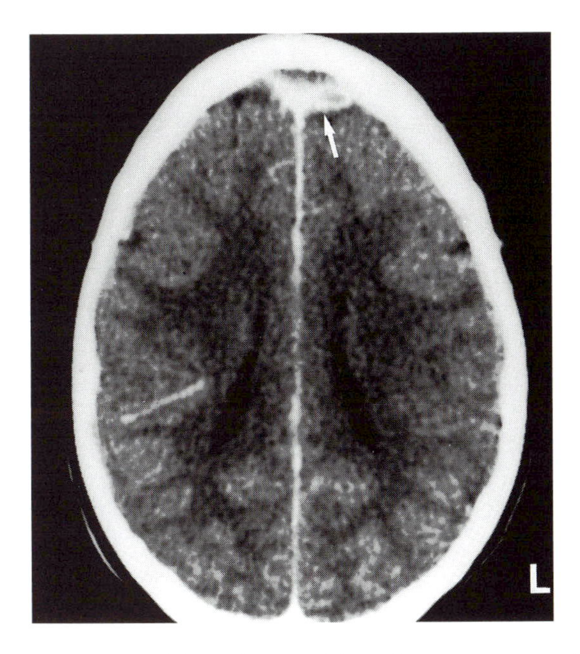

Figure 8.36 *Epidural abscess*. This patient (the same as in Figures 8.29 and 8.30) presented with acute frontal sinusitis and fever, which rapidly progressed to osteomyelitis. A small epidural abscess (arrow) developed adjacent to the infected sinus.

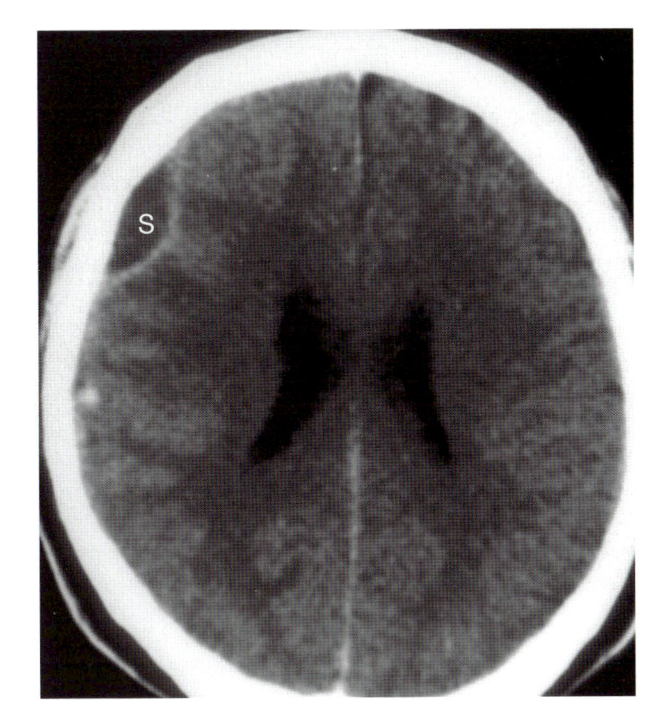

Figure 8.37 *Subdural empyema*. This patient presented as an emergency with a 1-week history of sinusitis refractory to oral antibiotics and increasing headache. This CT scan demonstrates a right subdural empyema (S).

CT appearance of intracranial infection

Meningitis

If meningitis is localized to the base of the skull, multiple cranial nerve palsies may present. Obstruction to the flow of cerebrospinal fluid leads to dilatation of the ventricles and hydrocephalus. Cortical and gyral enhancement may be seen following the administration of intravenous contrast.

Epidural empyema or abscess

An extradural abscess occurs between the bone of the calvarium and the dura mater. CT will usually demonstrate a collection that is lentiform in shape and will be limited by the dural attachment to the suture lines between the individual skull bones. The adjacent brain is usually hypodense because the surrounding tissue is edematous.

Subdural abscess

If an abscess forms in the subdural space lying between the dura and the arachnoid, it tends to have a semilunar shape. It may extend into the interhemispheric fissures or along the margins of the tentorium. Both the periosteum and the meninges will enhance following the administration of intravenous contrast. The collection of pus will vary in density, depending on the contents and the length of time for which the abscess has been present. Air may be seen in the fluid collection.

Brain abscess

A brain abscess may result from direct spread of infection from the sinus into the cerebral tissue, or following septic embolization. In the former situation, the abscess is usually in close proximity to the infected sinus responsible, whereas in the latter, the abscess may be distant to the infected sinus. Infection of the frontal sinus is frequently responsible for intracerebral abscesses, which may reach some size before the diagnosis becomes clinically evident. CT findings will vary, depending on the stage of development that the abscess has reached at the time of the scan. Early in the process of abscess formation, there may be only a poorly defined hypodense area exhibiting little enhancement. If left untreated, this will progress, to exhibit a well-demarcated, encapsulated lesion surrounding an area of pus. The capsule enhances brightly following the administration of intravenous contrast. The surrounding brain appears hypodense, demonstrating the edema in the tissue.

Cavernous sinus thrombosis

Cavernous sinus thrombosis is a further rare intracranial complication of sinusitis. It is predisposed to by acute thrombophlebitis secondary to infection in an area with venous drainage into the cavernous sinus, such as acute sphenoiditis or the mid-third of the face. The clinical features include fever, headache, and rigors. There is edema of the eyelids, exophthalmos, chemosis, ophthalmoplegia, and low-grade papilledema. The white cell count is elevated and blood cultures are often positive. On CT, a normal cavernous sinus is seen as a brightly enhancing structure surrounding the pituitary fossa, with a sharply defined lateral border. Usually, the intracavernous part of the internal carotid artery is indistinguishable from the surrounding venous structure. In contrast, in cavernous sinus thrombosis, the venous structure fails to enhance and the internal carotid arteries become very prominent as enhanced tubular structures.

CHOLESTEROL GRANULOMA OF THE SINUSES (Figure 8.38)

This is a rare complication of sinusitis. The expansile lesion has all the radiological features of a mucocele. These lesions are unlike petrous apex cholesterol cysts and are acquired as a result of a chronic inflammatory process in the sinus cavity. The congenital type, petrous apex cholesterol granulomas, arise from epithelial rests. On MRI, they appear as hyperintense masses on all sequences due to the fluid content being hemorrhagic. Histopathologically, these masses are characterized by the presence of cholesterol crystals. Their treatment is surgical. The congenital type needs complete resection, while the acquired type often needs drainage into the adjacent sinus

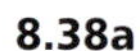

8.38a

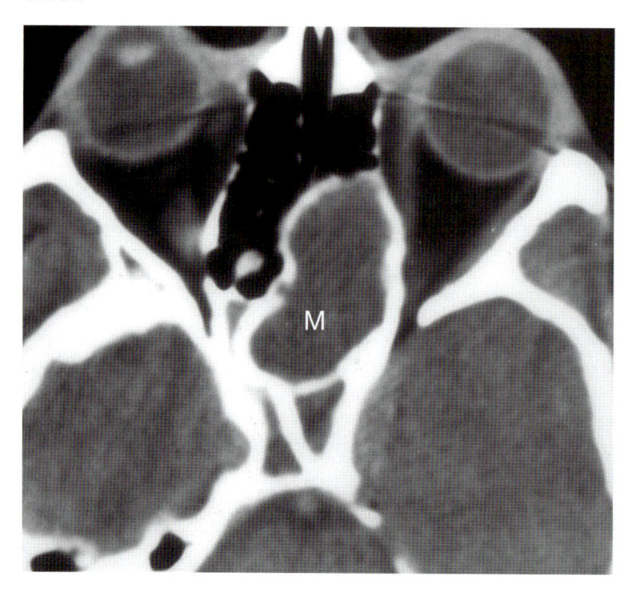

8.38b

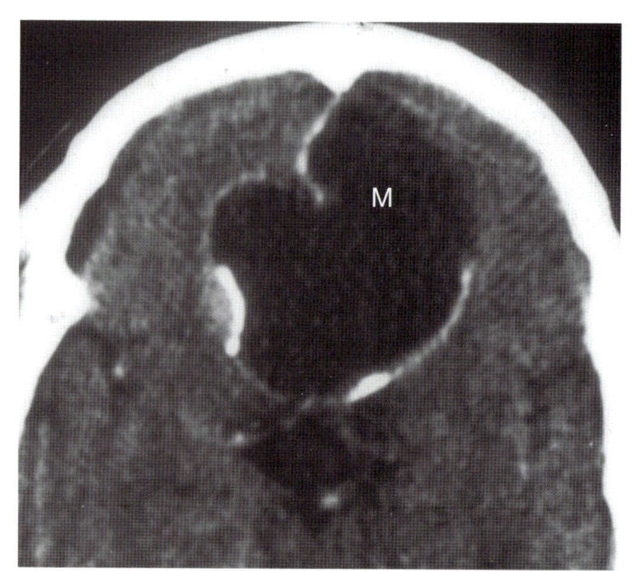

Figure 8.38 (a, b) *Cholesterol granuloma of the posterior ethmoid sinus.* A large expansile well-defined hypodense mass (M) is seen on the axial CT scan, with reactive osteitis and thinning of the sinus wall. This mass has expanded intracranially. The granuloma is seen to push the frontal lobe superiorly without any invasion or edema. The lumen contents contained cholesterol crystals and chronic inspissated mucus.

8.38c

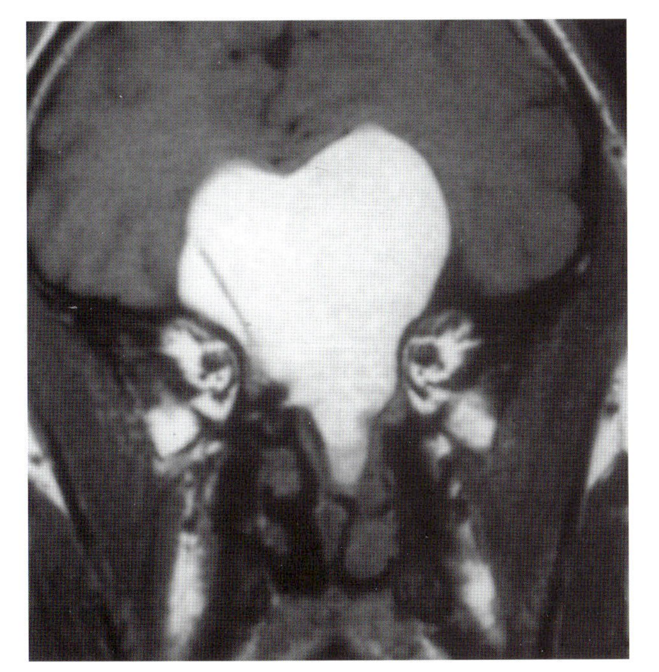

8.38d

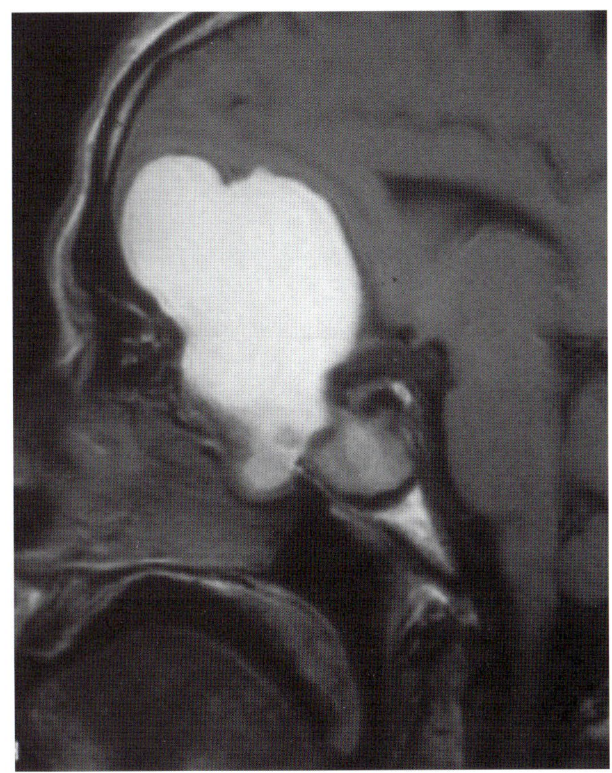

8.38e

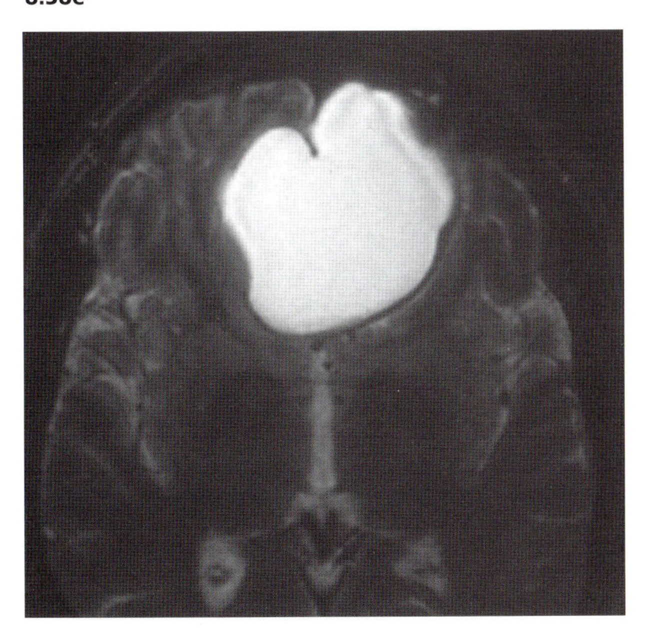

Figure 8.38 *continued* (c, d, e) MRI T1 and T2 weighted *Cholesterol granuloma of the ethmoid sinus.*

9

Tumors and tumor-like conditions of the sinonasal cavity

A comprehensive overview of all tumor and tumor-like conditions of the sinonasal cavity is beyond the scope of this book. This chapter will examine some of the more common disease entities likely to be encountered. A comprehensive classification is shown in Table 9.1. The differential diagnosis of the signal-void appearance of some sinonasal lesions on magnetic resonance imaging (MRI) is shown in Table 9.2.

BENIGN TUMORS

Osteoma (Figures 9.1 and 9.2)

Osteomas are benign slowly growing tumors containing mature compact or cancellous bone. These occur most frequently in the frontal sinus, but can also be found in the ethmoid and maxillary sinuses. Osteomas are usually asymptomatic and are an incidental finding in up to 1% of radiographs conducted for an unrelated reason. They can present with headache. Osteomas may block the drainage pathway of a sinus and lead to recurrent sinus infections or the development of mucoceles. Large frontal sinus osteomas can erode the inner table and either produce pneumocephalus or allow a sinus infection to spread intracranially. Rarely, osteomas arising in a sinus can enlarge, leading to proptosis, secondary to expansion into the orbit. Visual deterioration may occur if the osteoma extends backwards into the sphenoid sinus, thus compromising the optic nerve.

The radiological features consist of a uniformly calcified dense mass on computed tomography (CT). There is no enhancement with intravenous contrast. The bony margins are sharply defined and the mass may appear either pedunculated or broadly based. Both bone and air are seen as an area of signal void on MRI scans and therefore osteomas are poorly visualized on MRI.

The development of multiple osteomas precedes the development of multiple colonic polyposis in patients with Gardner's syndrome. This is an autosomal dominant condition consisting of the triad of colonic polyposis, osteomas, and soft tissue tumors, including sebaceous cysts and desmoid tumors.

Odontogenic cysts and tumors

These lesions originate from the dental apparatus or the alveolar ridge. Primordial cysts arise from supernumerary teeth. These masses expand into the maxillary sinuses, similarly to dentigerous cysts, which are more common and arise from unerupted teeth.

Dentigerous cysts (Figures 9.3–9.6)

These represent 25–30% of odontogenic cysts. They are predominant in Black males in the 2nd–4th decades of life. The most common location is in the region of the 3rd mandibular molar. The maxillary teeth can also be involved. The cysts form as a result of fluid accumulation around the crown of an unerupted tooth. Dentigerous cysts can present as expanding masses and may lead to facial asymmetry. Imaging reveals a radiolucent area in the upper or lower jaw that incorporates the crown of an unerupted tooth. The lesion is usually unilocular

Table 9.1 Tumors

Benign tumors
Epithelial
• Squamous papilloma
• Inverting papilloma
Glandular
• Mixed tumor/pleomorphic adenoma
Mesenchymal
• Myomatous leiomyoma, rhabdomyoma
• Neurogenic neurofibroma, ectopic meningioma
• Fibroma
• Lipoma
• Hemangioma/lymphangioma
• Juvenile angiofibroma
Bony/cartilaginous/odontogenic
• Osteoma
• Osteochondroma
• Osteoblastoma
• Keratocyst/odontogenic cysts
• Ameloblastoma
Tumor-like conditions
• Fibrous dysplasia
• Giant cell granuloma
• Ossifying fibroma
Malignant tumors
Epithelial
• Squamous cell carcinoma
• Adenocarcinoma
• Undifferentiated carcinoma
Glandular
• Adenocystic carcinoma
• Mucoepidermoid carcinoma
Mesenchymal
• Rhabdomyosarcoma
• Malignant fibrohistiocytoma
• Esthesioneuroblastoma
Bony/cartilaginous/odontogenic
• Osteosarcoma
• Chondrosarcoma
• Ewing's sarcoma
• Ameloblastoma
Miscellaneous
• Plasmacytoma
• Melanoma
• Lymphoma
Metastasis
• Direct extension from: Nasopharynx, oral cavity, orbits, pituitary, and infratemporal fossa
• Hematogeneous spread from primary sites: Lungs, breast, kidneys, prostate

Table 9.2 Sinonasal lesions – signal void on MRI

Inflammatory
• Inspissated secretions in mucocele
• Inspissated polyps
• Fungus ball
Tumors
• Chondroid tumors
• Osteomas
Miscellaneous
• Proteinaceous material
• Hemorrhage
• Foreign body
• Teeth
• Fibrosis
• Amyloidomas

and surrounded by sclerotic bone. As the cyst grows, it may extend into the maxillary sinus. A thin characteristic rim of calcification, representing the elevated sinus periosteum, and the associated tooth will be visible.

Periapical cysts (Figure 9.7)

This is the most common type of odontogenic cyst and is the result of dental caries. It can affect any age and has no sexual predilection. It appears as a lucent zone in the region of the tooth apex or along the lateral root. Lesions in the maxilla can extend into the adjacent maxillary sinus and elevate the periosteum. Secondary odontogenic sinusitis can develop.

Ameloblastoma (Figure 9.8)

Ameloblastoma arises from the epithelial components of the embryonic tooth. The most common site is the premolar–molar area, where it presents as an expansile painless mass in the 3rd–4th decades of life. As the tumor enlarges, symptoms from obstruction, bleeding, and pressure occur.

The unilocular cystic variety presents as an expansile mass with smooth erosion of the underlying bone. These tumors cannot easily be differentiated from dentigerous cysts and may have an unerupted tooth within them. They respond to removal and curettage.

The multilocular variety tends to recur, and to extend into the adjacent infratemporal fossa, orbit, and intracranial structures. On CT, the multilocular

9.1a

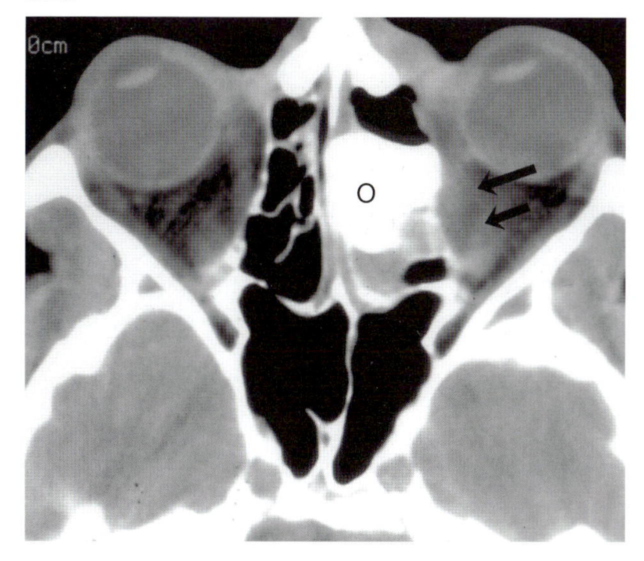

9.1b

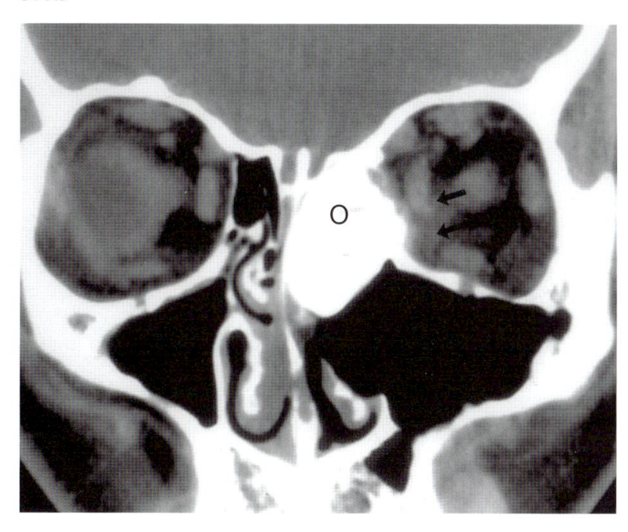

Figure 9.1 *Osteoma*. Axial (a) and coronal (b) CT scans demonstrating a large osteoma (O) with inflammatory reaction in the orbit surrounding the medial rectus muscle (arrows) in a patient who presented with orbital cellulitis.

variety presents as an inhomogeneous mass in the maxillary sinus, with erosion of the bony walls. These tumors are of intermediate signal intensity on T1-weighted, and intermediate to high intensity on T2-weighted scans. Occasionally, papillary and nodular types of mucosal enhancement within the tumor may be seen on MRI scans. The multilocular type is treated by resection of the involved bone. Recurrences are treated with repeated attempts to remove the tumor surgically and by irradiation. Histologically, these tumors can be benign or malig-

9.2a

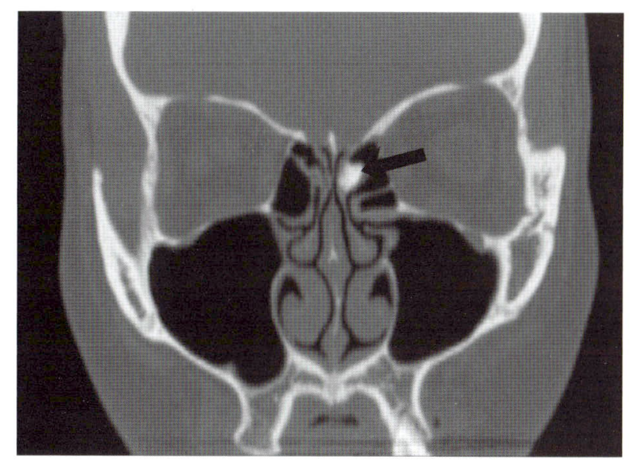

9.2b

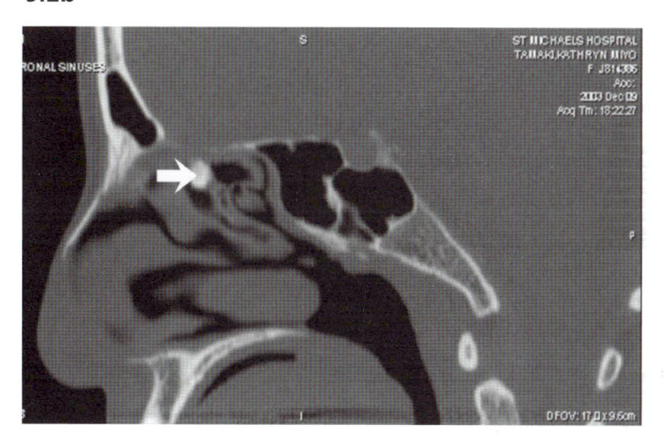

Figure 9.2 *Osteoma*. A bony mass (arrow) is identified in the ethmoid sinus on the coronal CT scan (a) and the sagittal reconstruction (b) of the sinuses.

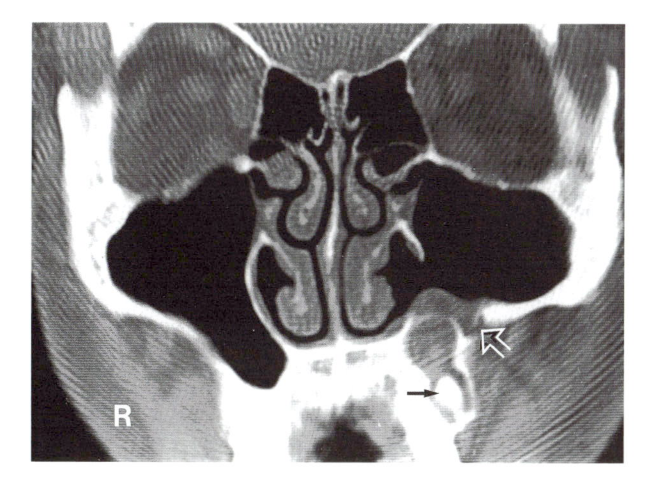

Figure 9.3 *Odontogenic keratocyst*. Coronal CT scan demonstrating a cystic lesion in the left alveolar ridge; it has a smooth scalloped margin. The uneruped tooth can be seen in the base of the cyst (arrow). The defect in the anterior bony wall of the maxilla (open arrow) is evidence of a previous Caldwell–Luc procedure. Incomplete resection results in recurrence. These cysts can be multioculated.

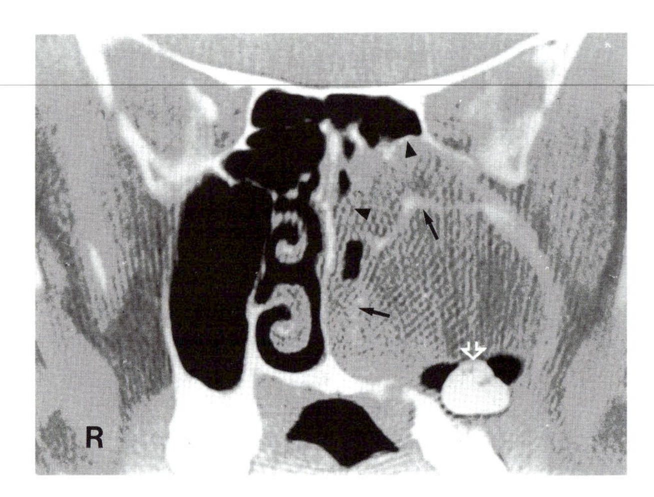

Figure 9.4 *Dentigerous cyst.* CT scan demonstrating a large expansile cyst (arrow) containing an unerupted tooth (open arrow). The maxillary sinus walls are remodeled and the inferolateral wall of the maxillary sinus is eroded. The sinus extends medially into the nasal cavity (arrowheads).

nant. The benign variety can be as life-threatening as the malignant type because of its size and extension through the skull base. The malignant type may recur locally, despite repeated resections and irradiation. These tumors can metastasize to the local lymph nodes and lungs. The differential diagnosis includes aneurysmal bone cysts, odontogenic tumors, and giant cell tumors.

Hemangioma (Figure 9.9)

Hemangiomas are benign vascular lesions composed of vascular channels of varying size. They are subtyped into capillary, cavernous, and mixed types. They occur rarely in the sinonasal cavity, with the most common location being the nasal septum, where they can remodel and displace the nasal septum and lateral wall of the nose. Affected patients present with nasal obstruction and epistaxis. Hemangionas tend to arise in females between the ages of 20 and 50 years. They may complicate the second trimester of pregnancy and may regress spontaneously following delivery (granuloma gravidorum). Hemangiomas enhance following the administration of intravenous contrast. These tumors are intermediate to mildly high in signal intensity on T1-weighted MRI sequences and are hyperintense on T2-weighted scans. CT scans demonstrate an intensely enhancing soft tissue mass.

Angiofibroma (Figure 9.10)

Angiofibromas are histologically benign vascular, but highly aggressive, lesions of the nasal cavity consisting of fibrous tissue with intermixed thin-walled vessels. They arise almost exclusively in adolescent males. Due to their vascular nature, these tumors bleed profusely and outpatient biopsy is contraindicated. They are thought to originate in the region of the sphenopalatine foramen in the nasal cavity. From here, they can either spread into the nasal cavity, or extend into the pterygopalatine fossa and then through the superior orbital fissure into the orbit. Spread via the foramen rotundum and Vidian canals allows entry into the cavernous sinus. These extremely vascular, non-encapsulated lesions derive their blood supply from the external carotid system via the internal maxillary and ascending pharyngeal arteries. Those lesions with intracranial extension can also receive a supply from the internal carotid circulation.

Imaging demonstrates an enhancing soft tissue mass within the posterior nasal cavity. There can be widening of the pterygopalatine fossa, with erosion of the pterygoid plates and extension into the infratemporal fossa. MRI can show vascular flow voids. Conventional angiography and embolization is used to help reduce intraoperative blood loss during surgical excision. The benefits of radiation treatment are not clear. The tumor usually undergoes fibrosis and involutes with treatment.

Inverting papilloma (Figures 9.11–9.20)

Inverting papillomas are benign lesions composed of hyperplastic squamous epithelium with an endophytic growth pattern. They commonly arise from the lateral nasal wall in the vicinity of the middle turbinate. They occur more commonly in men than in women, with the greatest incidence being seen in the 6th and 7th decades. Inverting papillomas are slowly growing lesions that have a propensity to recur, especially if the initial excision is incomplete. This is partly related to the fact that the adjacent mucosa often shows evidence of squamous metaplasia and hyperplasia. There is also a risk for developing metachronous and/or synchronous squamous cell carcinoma. The clinical features include nasal obstruction, anosmia, rhinorrhea, and epistaxis. Pain and facial paresthesia are not characteristic fea-

9.5a

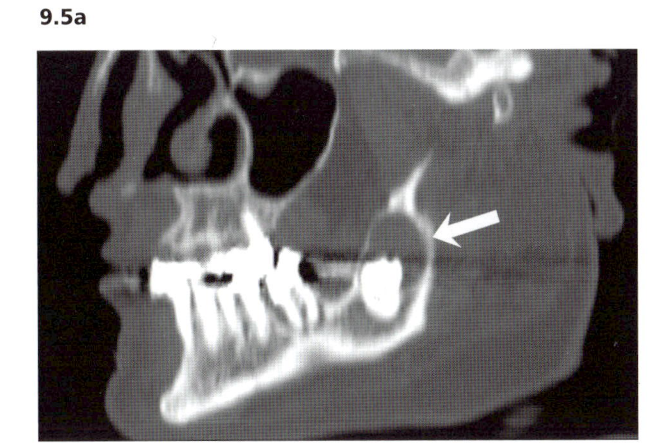

9.5b

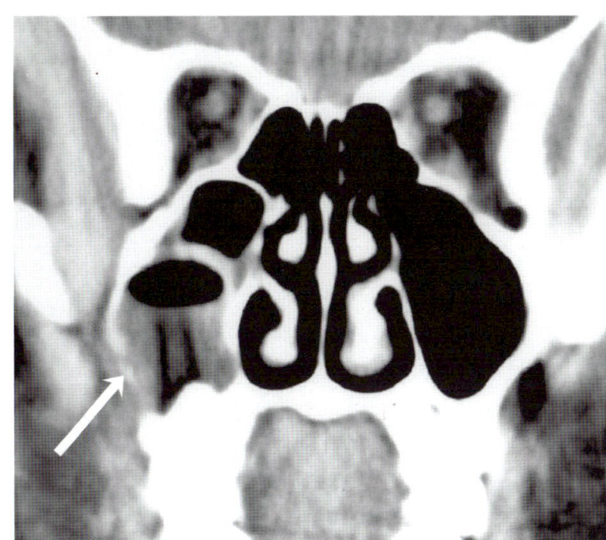

9.5c

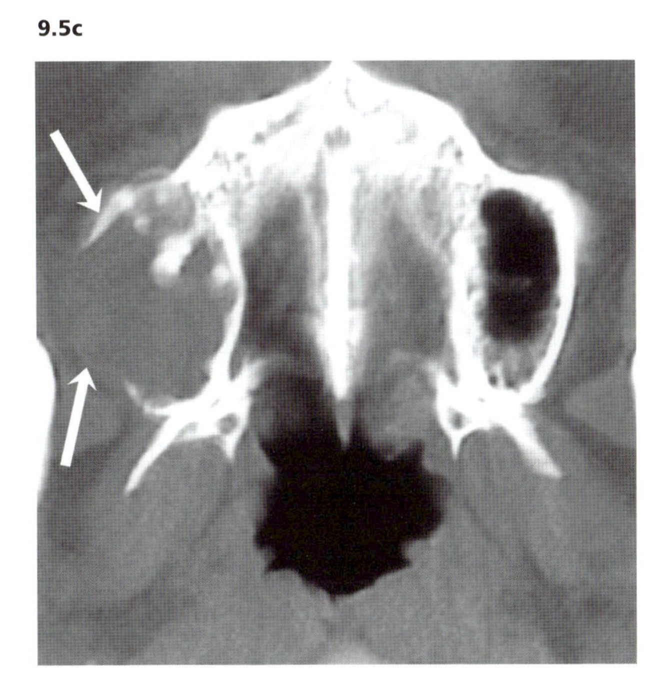

9.5d

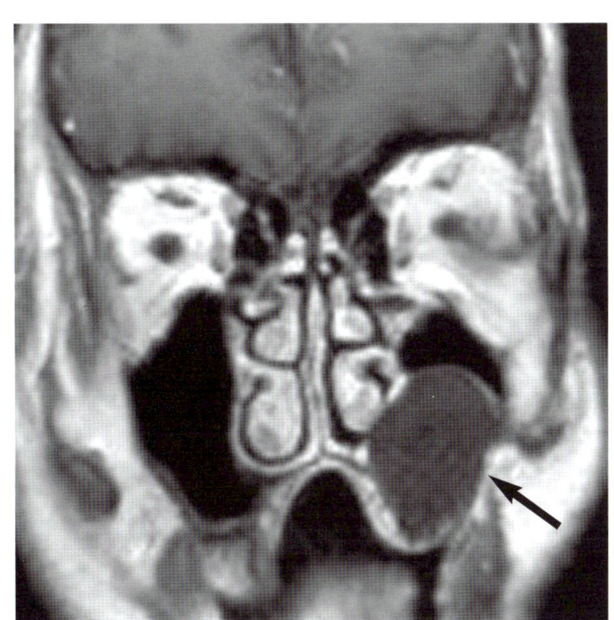

Figure 9.5 *Dentigerous cyst*. (a) Sagittal reconstruction of a CT scan of the facial bones demonstrating a cyst (arrow) surrounding the apical region of the molar tooth. (b, c) This patient presented with sinusitis refractory to antibiotic therapy. CT examination demonstrates the presence of an infected dentigerous cyst (arrows). The lateral wall of the cyst is eroded and there is an air–fluid level in the infected cyst. (d) Coronal MRI scan of the sinus demonstrating the presence of a cyst (arrow) close to the floor of the maxillary sinus.

tures of inverting papillomas, but may be indicative of concurrent malignancy. As mentioned above, the most common site of origin is within the middle meatus, but extension into the adjacent sinus occurs frequently. The maxillary antrum is involved in 69% of cases, followed by the ethmoid, sphenoid, and frontal sinuses in decreasing order of frequency. Inverting papillomas arising from the nasal septum are uncommon and bilateral disease is rare. Obstruction of the sinus ostia in the middle meatus may lead to the accumulation of secretions in the obstructed sinus and a secondary sinusitis. Rarely,

9.6a

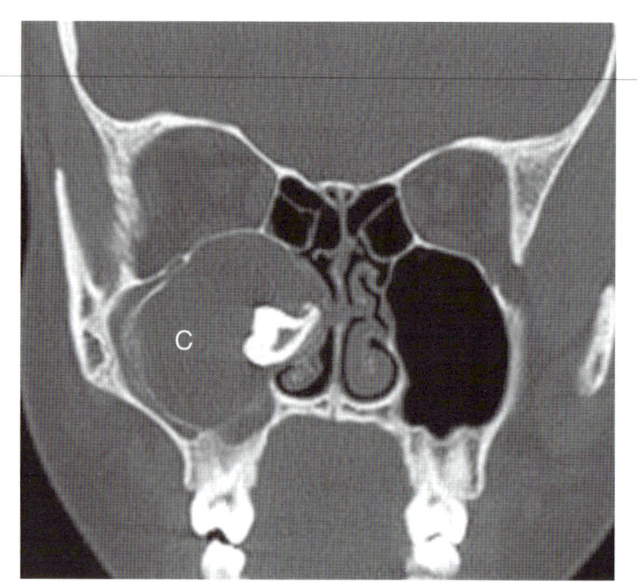

9.6b

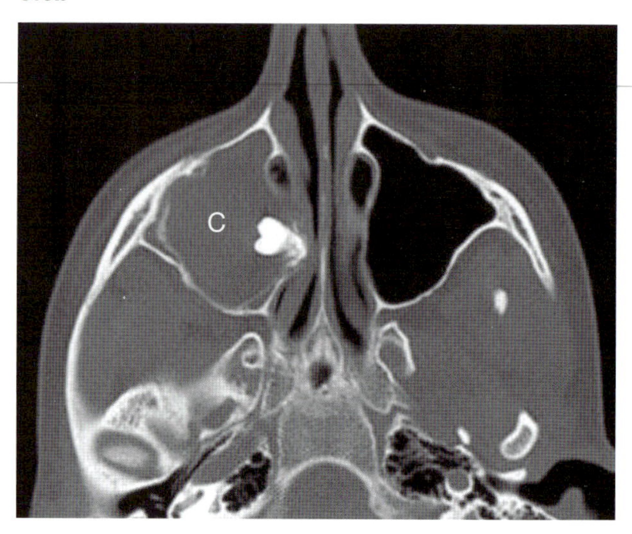

9.6c

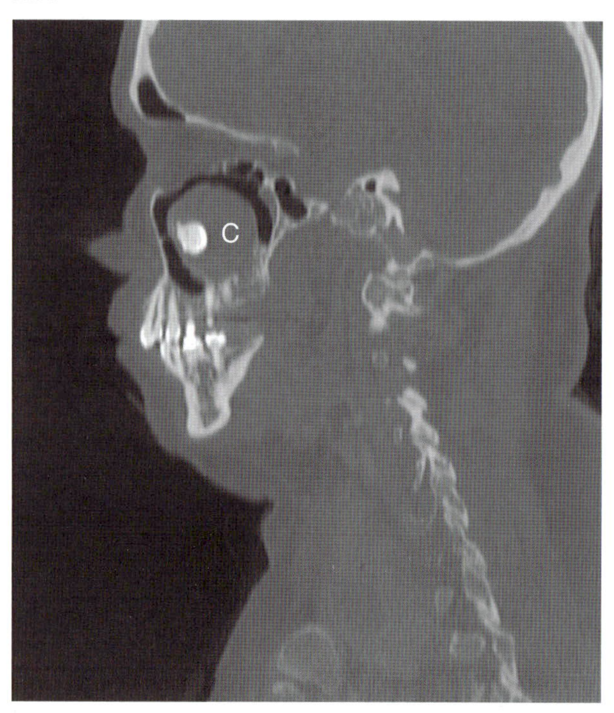

Figure 9.6 *Dentigerous cyst*. Coronal (a), axial (b), and sagittal reformatted (c) CT scans showing an expansile cystic lesion (C) within the right maxillary sinus. The presence of a thin calcific rim and a tooth embedded within the wall is highly characteristic of a dentigerous cyst. The sagittal scan (c) demonstrates a rim of air in the maxillary sinus around the dentigerous cyst (C).

one of the paranasal sinuses may be involved primarily, with no evidence of tumor extension into the nasal cavity.

Imaging demonstrates the presence of a soft tissue mass within the nasal cavity. CT can delineate bony erosion, and both CT and MRI can show extension of the lesion beyond the confines of the nasal cavity and the paranasal sinuses. It is not uncommon to find tumor extending into the nasopharynx. The tumor may extend into the retrobulbar space, causing exophthalmos, and through the cribriform plate into the anterior cranial fossa or through the greater wing of the sphenoid into the middle cranial fossa. The frequent finding of mucosal disease from concurrent allergic rhinitis or sinusitis may be misinterpreted as further extension of disease. This is especially true if CT scanning is used in isolation. MRI may be helpful

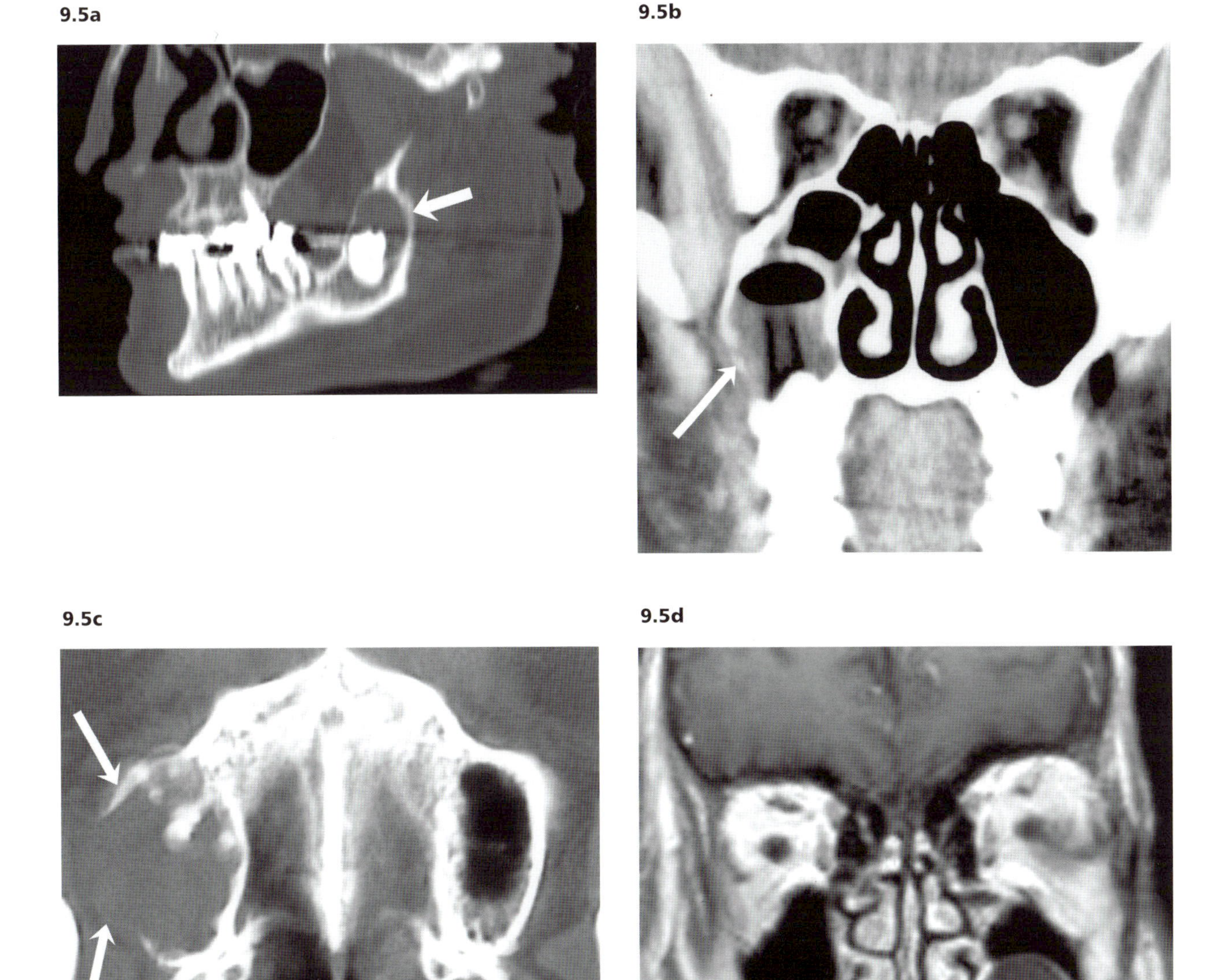

Figure 9.5 *Dentigerous cyst*. (a) Sagittal reconstruction of a CT scan of the facial bones demonstrating a cyst (arrow) surrounding the apical region of the molar tooth. (b, c) This patient presented with sinusitis refractory to antibiotic therapy. CT examination demonstrates the presence of an infected dentigerous cyst (arrows). The lateral wall of the cyst is eroded and there is an air–fluid level in the infected cyst. (d) Coronal MRI scan of the sinus demonstrating the presence of a cyst (arrow) close to the floor of the maxillary sinus.

tures of inverting papillomas, but may be indicative of concurrent malignancy. As mentioned above, the most common site of origin is within the middle meatus, but extension into the adjacent sinus occurs frequently. The maxillary antrum is involved in 69% of cases, followed by the ethmoid, sphenoid, and frontal sinuses in decreasing order of frequency. Inverting papillomas arising from the nasal septum are uncommon and bilateral disease is rare. Obstruction of the sinus ostia in the middle meatus may lead to the accumulation of secretions in the obstructed sinus and a secondary sinusitis. Rarely,

9.6a

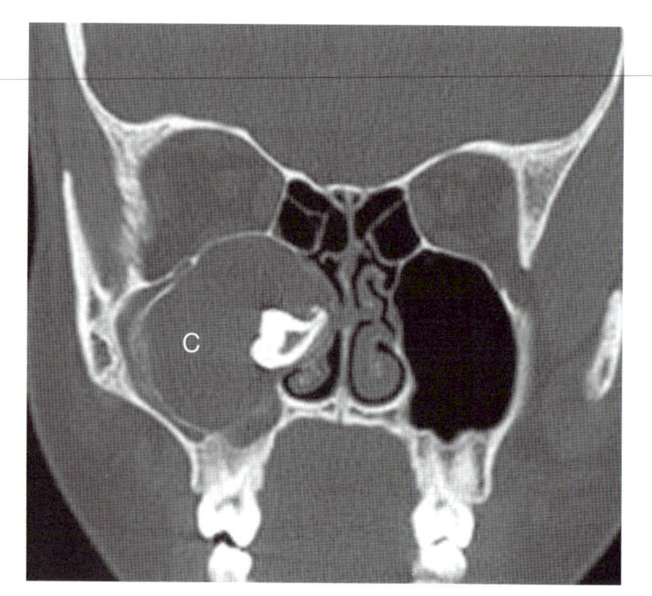

9.6b

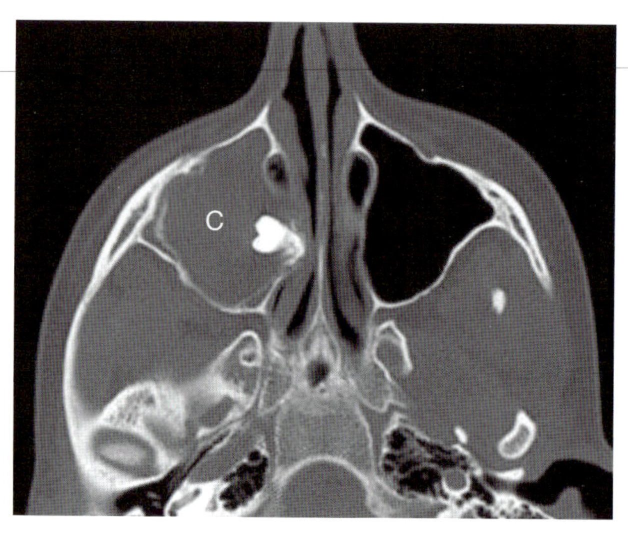

9.6c

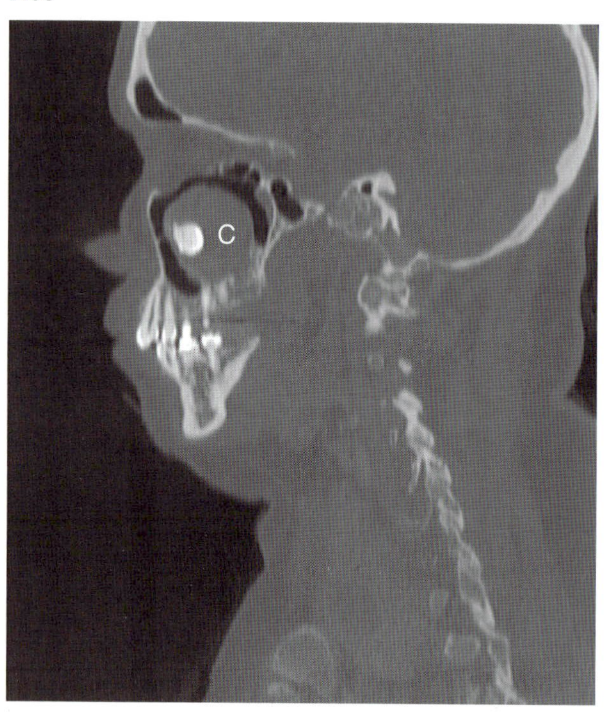

Figure 9.6 *Dentigerous cyst*. Coronal (a), axial (b), and sagittal reformatted (c) CT scans showing an expansile cystic lesion (C) within the right maxillary sinus. The presence of a thin calcific rim and a tooth embedded within the wall is highly characteristic of a dentigerous cyst. The sagittal scan (c) demonstrates a rim of air in the maxillary sinus around the dentigerous cyst (C).

one of the paranasal sinuses may be involved primarily, with no evidence of tumor extension into the nasal cavity.

Imaging demonstrates the presence of a soft tissue mass within the nasal cavity. CT can delineate bony erosion, and both CT and MRI can show extension of the lesion beyond the confines of the nasal cavity and the paranasal sinuses. It is not uncommon to find tumor extending into the nasopharynx. The tumor may extend into the retrobulbar space, causing exophthalmos, and through the cribriform plate into the anterior cranial fossa or through the greater wing of the sphenoid into the middle cranial fossa. The frequent finding of mucosal disease from concurrent allergic rhinitis or sinusitis may be misinterpreted as further extension of disease. This is especially true if CT scanning is used in isolation. MRI may be helpful

9.7a

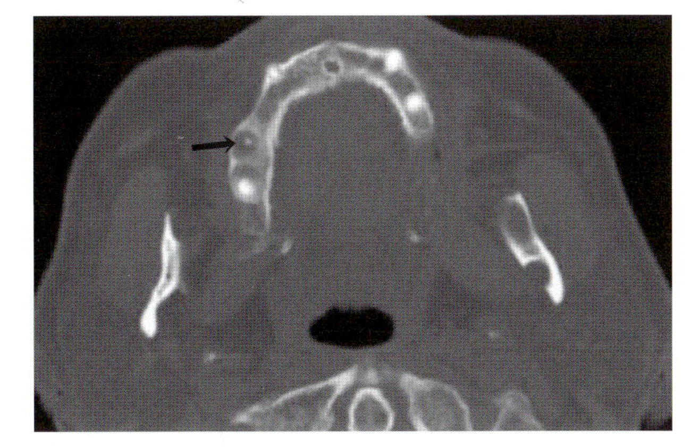

9.7b

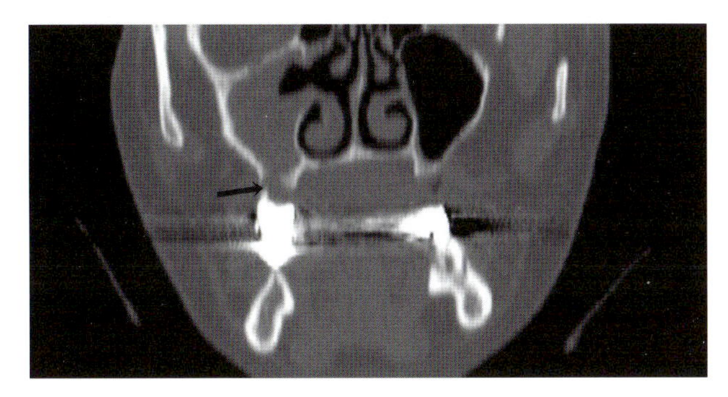

9.7c

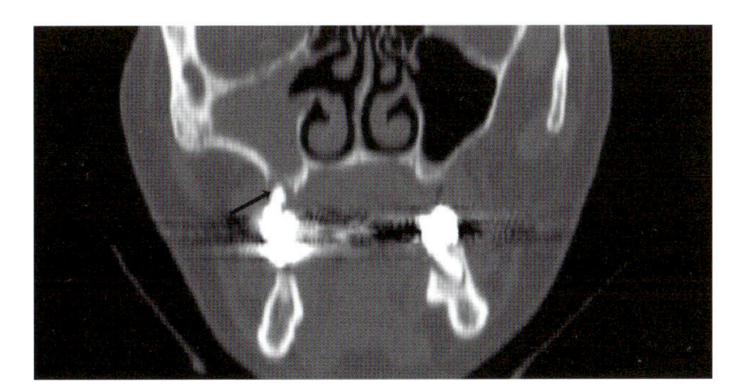

Figure 9.7 *Periapical cyst with sinusitis*. Axial (a) and reconstructed coronal (b, c) CT scans showing periapical lucency (arrow) surrounding teeth in the right maxillary alveolus. There is dehiscence of the floor of the maxillary antrum and secondary inflammatory sinusitis.

for further clarification, as these tumors exhibit low to intermediate signal intensity. Gadolinium contrast may also be of help. Both CT and MRI may demonstrate a heterogeneous texture to the lesion.

Sclerosis of the bony sinus walls has been noted in association with inverting papilloma, although this may well be related to long-standing sinusitis associated with the tumor. The radiological

9.8a

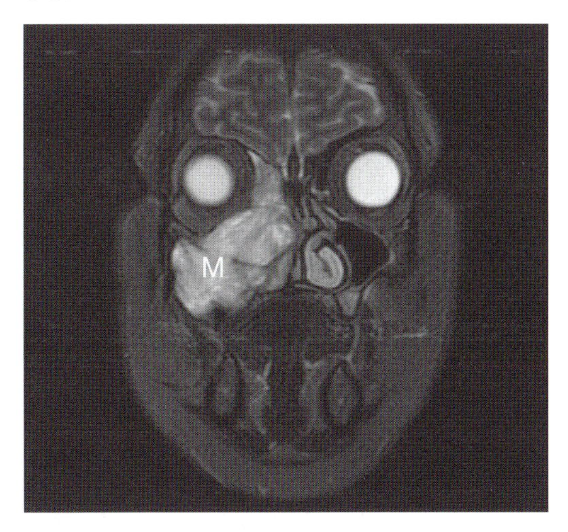

9.8b

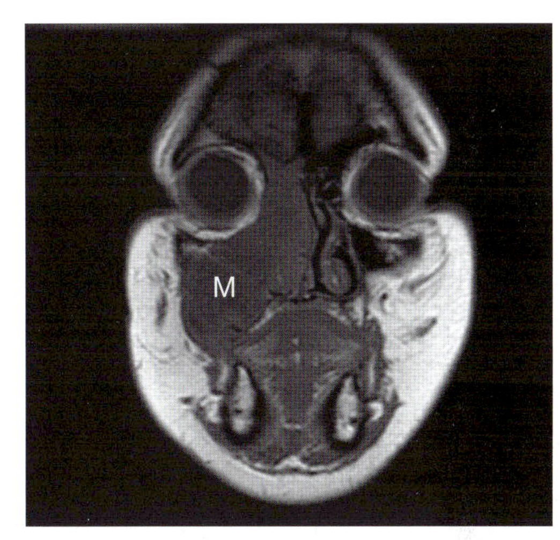

9.8c

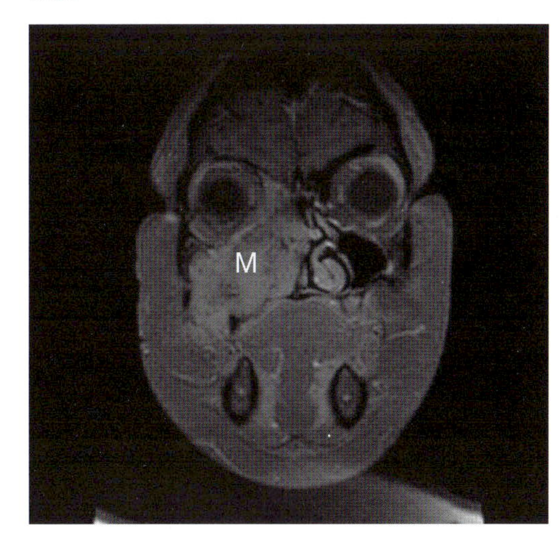

Figure 9.8 *Ameloblastoma*. (a–c) A multiloculated mass (M) in the sinus cavity is seen extending into the nasal cavity. This mass is hyperintense on T2-weighted MRI and demonstrates inhomogeneous enhancement following Gd-DTPA administration.

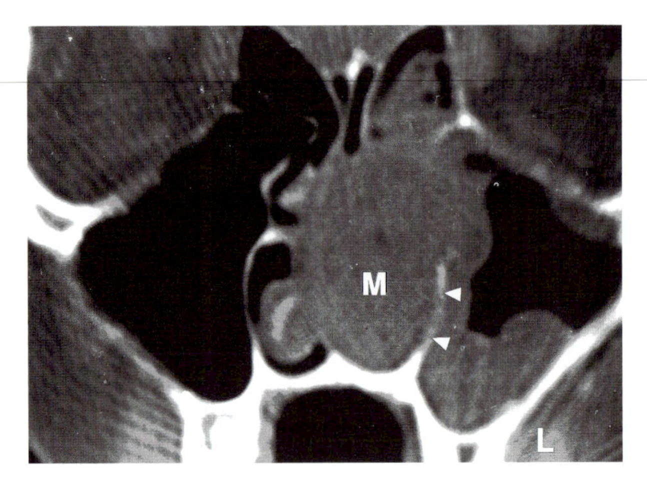

Figure 9.9 *Hemangioma*. CT scan demonstrating a soft tissue mass (M) in the left nasal cavity. As a result of chronic pressure, there is smooth expansion of the nasal cavity with marked lateral bowing of the lateral nasal wall of the nose (arrowheads). The ostiomeatal complex is occluded by the large mass and as a result there is mucosal thickening in the maxillary sinus. This proved to be a benign hemangioma, but there are no specific radiological characteristics that can point to the diagnosis on CT scans.

appearance of the bony walls of the paranasal sinuses can be variable in the presence of an inverting papilloma. If the tumor is slowly growing, the bony wall may be thinned or eroded. Opacity of the sinus will depend on the position and extent of the papilloma in relation to the ostia. Occasionally, areas of calcification will be demonstrated within the mass of the papilloma.

TUMOR-LIKE CONDITIONS

Fibrous dysplasia (Figures 9.21–9.23)

Fibrous dysplasia is a developmental disease of bone related to a defect in osteoblast maturation. On CT, these lesions may appear sclerotic, lytic, or mixed. Histology reveals myxofibrous tissue intermixed with haphazard woven bone. This condition typically presents in childhood and adolescents and in most cases arises before the age of 20 years. In the

9.10a

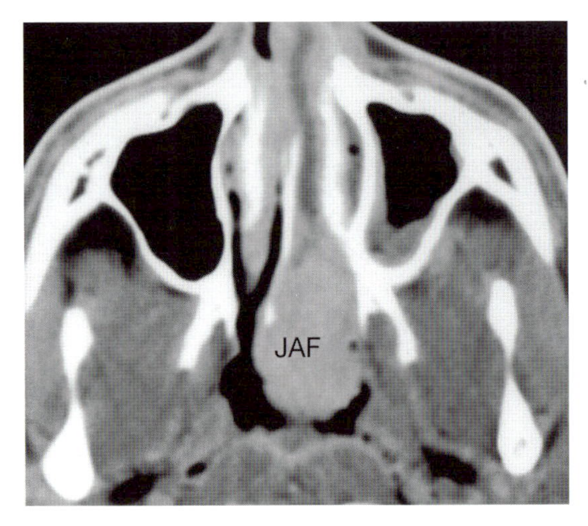

9.10b

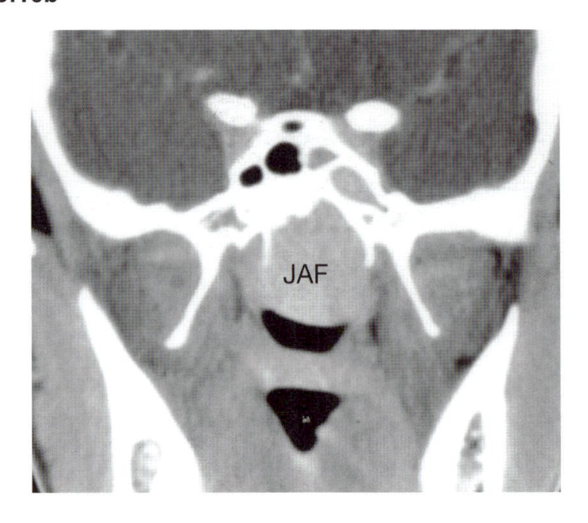

9.10c

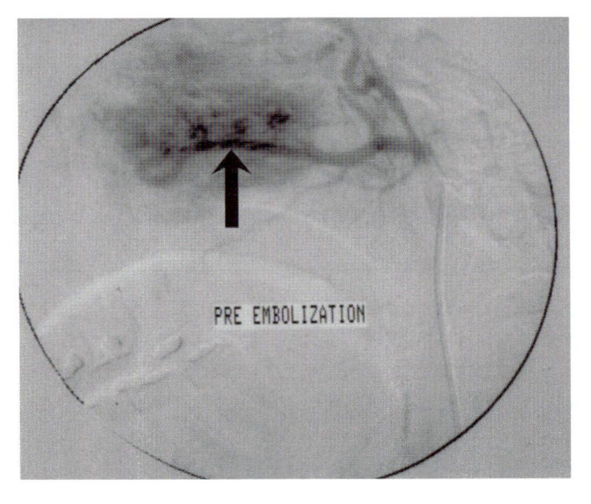

Figure 9.10 *Juvenile angiofibroma*. This 15-year-old patient presented with epistaxis. (a, b) Axial and coronal contrast-enhanced CT scans demonstrating an enhancing mass (JAF) in the nasopharynx and nasal cavity. (c) Pre-embolization angiogram demonstrating a tumor blush (arrow) in the nasopharynx.

9.11a

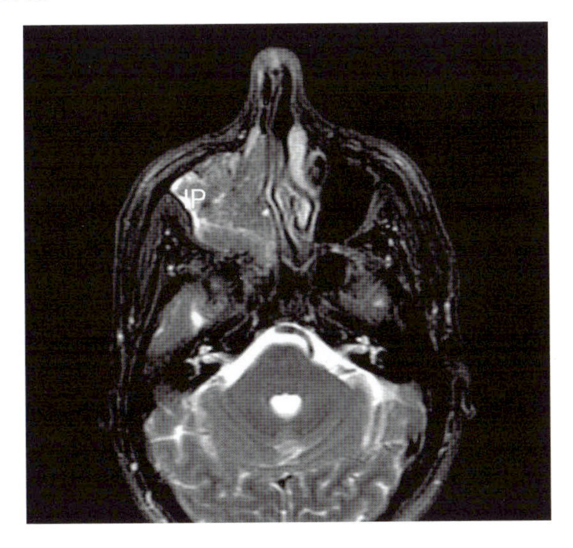

9.11b

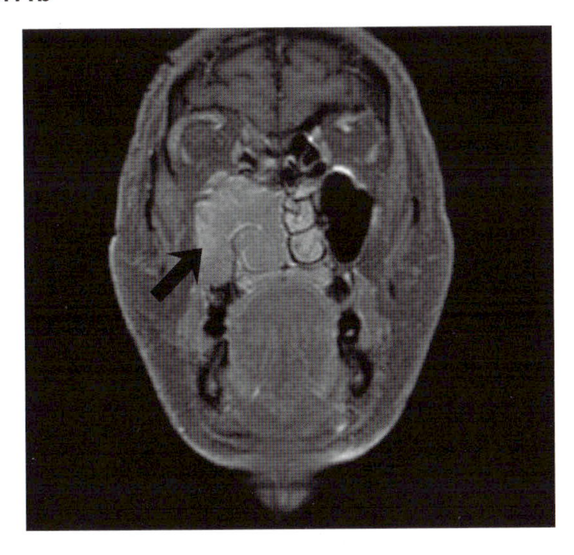

Figure 9.11 *Inverting papilloma*. Axial T2-weighted (a) and coronal contrast-enhanced T1-weighted (b) MRI scans of an inverting papilloma (IP in (a) and arrow in (b)) involving the right maxillary sinus and the ipsilateral nasal cavity. The lesion shows heterogeneous low T2 signal and mild contrast enhancement.

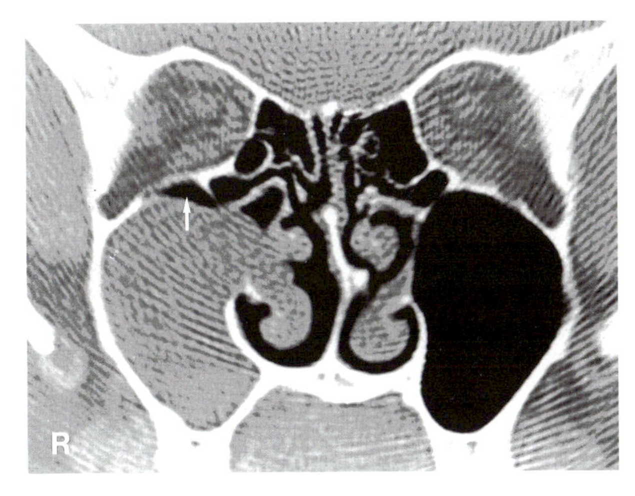

Figure 9.12 *Inverting papilloma*. CT scan demonstrating a well-defined soft tissue mass with a meniscus of air in the maxillary sinus. The mass is seen protruding into the posterior part of the middle meatus. There is no calcification in the mass and there are areas of reactive new bone formation. There are no radiological features of this mass to distinguish it from an antrochoanal polyp. A meniscus of air above the mass (arrow) is more a feature of polypoid disease rather than a mucocele.

head and neck region, the maxilla is affected more frequently than the mandible, and such cases usually present with bony swelling. Fibrous dysplasia may also affect the zygoma, the frontal bone, and the sphenoid bone, resulting in considerable deformity. Fibrous dysplasia is usually monostotic (70–80%). The remaining cases of fibrous dysplasia are polyostotic (20–30%). Polyostotic disease more frequently involves the facial bones, has a younger age of onset, and is associated with a worse prognosis. Extensive fibrous dysplasia can narrow the cranial nerve foramina, producing compression neuropathy. Cosmetic deformity can also result, including hypertelorism and exophthalmos.

Malignant change is rare (1%), although the development of various types of sarcomas has been documented. Malignant change is higher in polyostotic disease and in those with a history of prior radiation.

McCune–Albright syndrome is a rare disease consisting of a triad of polyostotic fibrous dysplasia, pigmented skin lesions, and precocious puberty.

The radiological features vary depending on the quantity of fibrous tissue that is present. The bone appears expanded and has areas of increased density that reflect the calcified cartilage and osteoid. There is often a characteristic 'ground glass' texture that is well demonstrated by CT. Adjacent sinuses can be encroached upon and narrowed, and the process may involve neighboring structures such as the orbit, cranial cavity, and adjacent soft tissue spaces. MRI often demonstrates a bizarre area of predominantly low and mixed signal attenuation. There can be areas of gadolinium enhancement. Cystic change can also be present.

9.13a

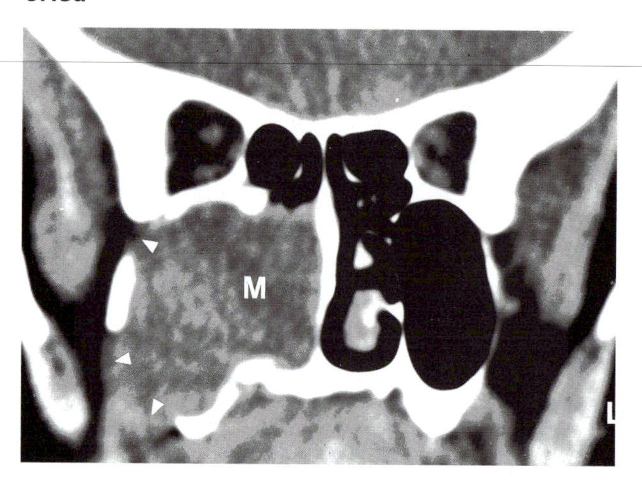

9.13b

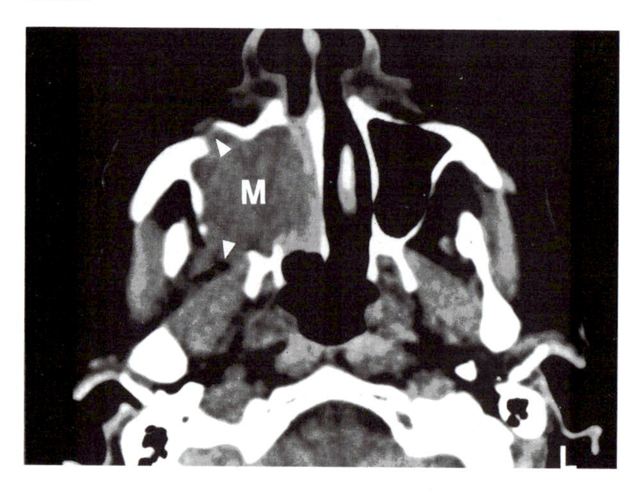

Figure 9.13 *Inverting papilloma*. Coronal (a) and axial (b) CT scans demonstrating a smooth expansile mass (M) in the right maxillary sinus. There is erosion of the anterior, posterior, medial, and inferolateral walls of the sinus (arrowheads). In benign disease of the paranasal sinuses, bony erosion occurs in close proximity to the natural ostia, i.e. near the infraorbital foramen and the medial sinus wall. In this case, the erosion has occurred in atypical sites and the radiologist should be suspicious that this is not a benign polyp.

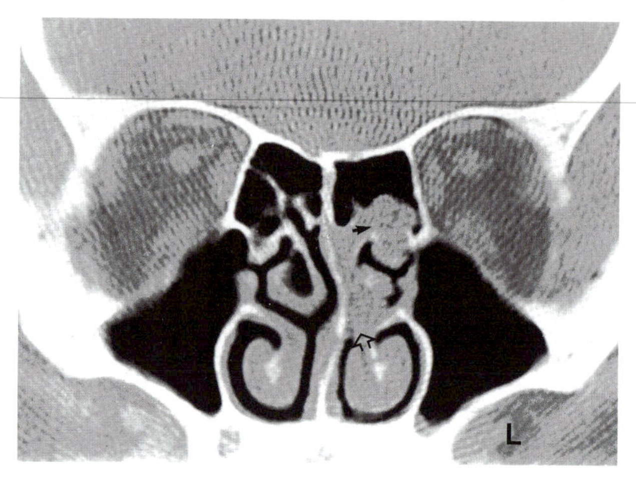

Figure 9.14 *Inverting papilloma*. Coronal CT scan of the paranasal sinuses demonstrating a unilateral soft tissue mass (arrow) arising from the superior meatus, extending from above the horizontal plate of the middle turbinate medially into the nasal cavity just alongside the free margin of the middle turbinate. The mass is in close proximity to the inferior turbinate on the left side (open arrow). The middle meatus appears normal. There is no evidence of erosion of the underlying bones. Clinically, this proved to be an inverting papilloma arising from the posterior ethmoid air cells and the superior meatus.

Ossifying fibroma (Figure 9.24)

This lesion consists of a vascular fibrous stroma with intermixed trabeculae surrounded by a rim of ossified lamellar bone. As with fibrous dysplasia, this entity can also cause deformity, sinonasal obstruction, and neural compression. Most cases involve the mandible, and there is a noted female predominance. Ossifying fibroma can be challenging to distinguish from fibrous dysplasia, both histologically and radiographically. The former has been reported to have a central area of relative lucency, corresponding to the fibrovascular matrix, with a surrounding peripheral rim of ossification. Thus, it may have a more well-circumscribed appearance. Both lesions can demonstrate bony expansion.

Wegener's granulomatosis (Figure 9.25)

Wenger's granulomatosis can result in destruction and erosion of the tissues of the midface including the sinuses and nasal cavity. This necrotizing granulomatous process typically involves the upper and lower respiratory tracts. There are often associated systemic symptoms, such as fever, malaise, and weight loss. Systemic progression may occur through the involvement of the pulmonary, renal, and musculoskeletal systems. Disease may arise in the sinuses and nasal cavity. There may be orbital involvement, such as conjunctivitis, corneal–scleral ulceration, uveitis, or optic neuritis. This may be the result of primary disease of the orbit or may be related to spread of the disease from the adjacent paranasal sinuses. Treatment for Wegener's granulomatosis includes high-dose steroids and immunosuppressants.

9.15a

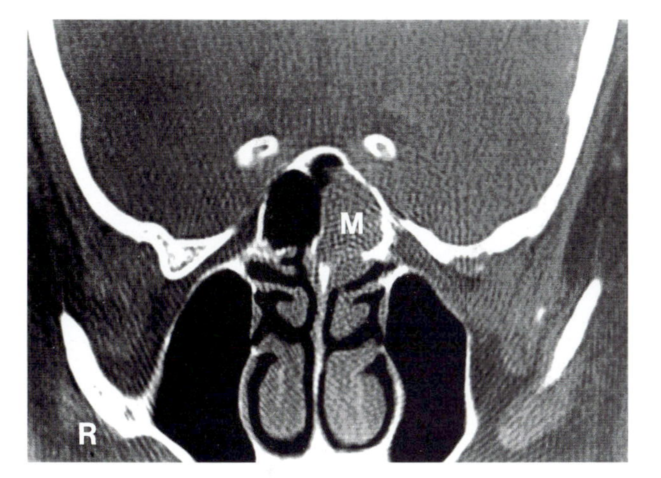

9.15b

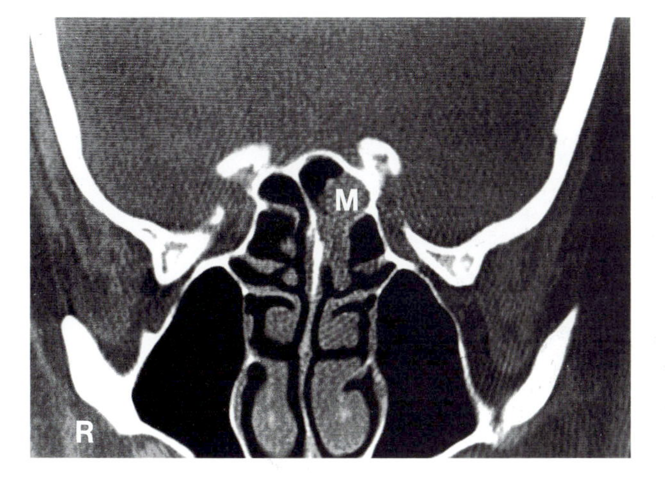

Figure 9.15 *Inverting papilloma*. (a, b) One of the unusual presenting sites for an inverting papilloma is the sphenoid sinus. The mass (M) that arose in the left sphenoid sinus has caused erosion of the floor of that sphenoid sinus and can be seen on these CT scans protruding into the sphenoethmoid recess. There is reactive bony sclerosis of the lateral wall of the left sphenoid sinus. Note in (b) how the tumor has extended into the superior meatus.

9.16a

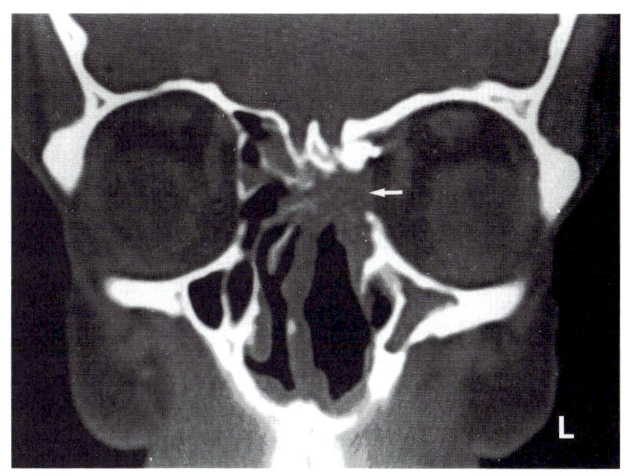

9.16b

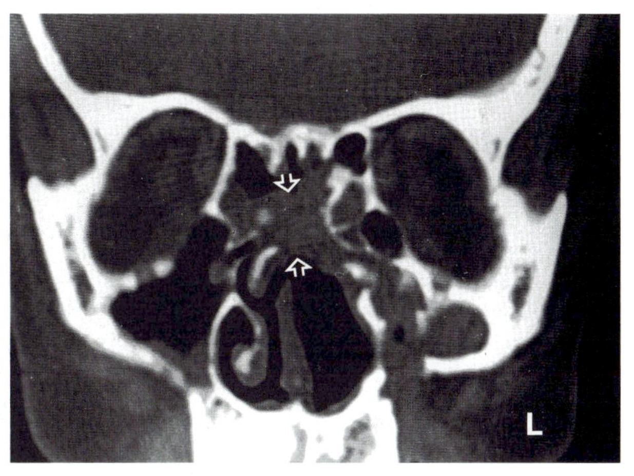

Figure 9.16 *Inverting papilloma*. (a, b) Postoperative CT scans of the sinuses demonstrating a defect in the lamina papyracea from a previous external ethmoidectomy (arrow) with removal of the ethmomaxillary plate. There is soft tissue proliferation, extending to involve the nasal septum and the opposite ethmoid sinuses (open arrows). This patient had a recurrent inverting papilloma. It is unusual for the papilloma to involve both nasal cavities. The bony septa in the ethmoid air cells indicate that the previous ethmoidectomy was incomplete.

The radiological features of Wegener's granulomatosis initially appear similar to those of chronic inflammatory disease, with mucosal thickening in the sinonasal cavity. Subsequently, the nasal septum or turbinates may be thickened and focal soft tissue lesions may develop. If the disease progresses to a destructive stage, erosion of the nasal septum and turbinates may occur. The sinuses may become sclerotic, with the sinus lumen compromised by fibro-osseous proliferation. In some cases, a secondary bacterial infection within the nose and paranasal sinuses can account for the bony sclerosis that is often demonstrated on CT scans. Non-specific irregular densities may be seen within the orbit, associated with scleral–uveal thickening and muscle swelling. MRI may show the granulomatous lesions to be of low signal on both T1-weighted and T2-weighted sequences. High T2 signal can also be seen.

Rhinoliths (Figure 9.26)

A variety of objects – both animate and inanimate – have been recovered from the nasal cavity. If a

9.17a

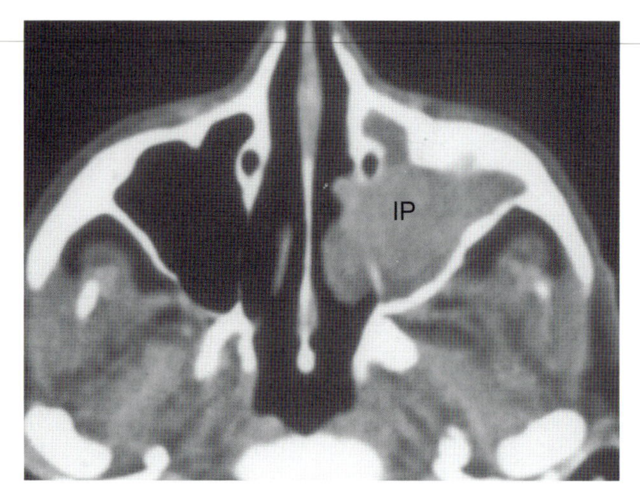

9.17b

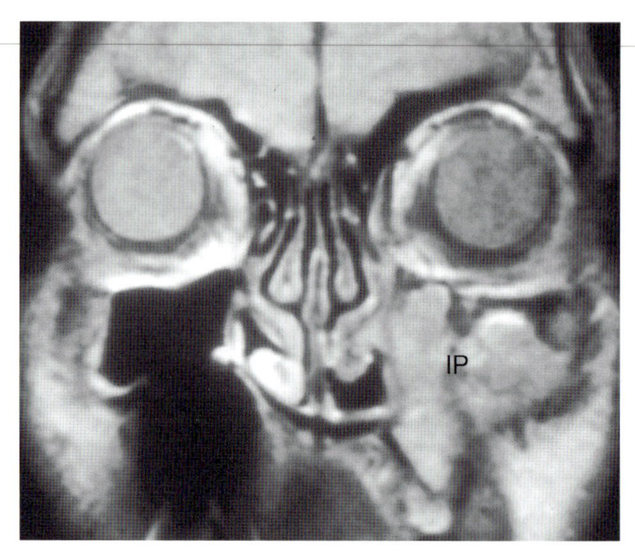

9.17c

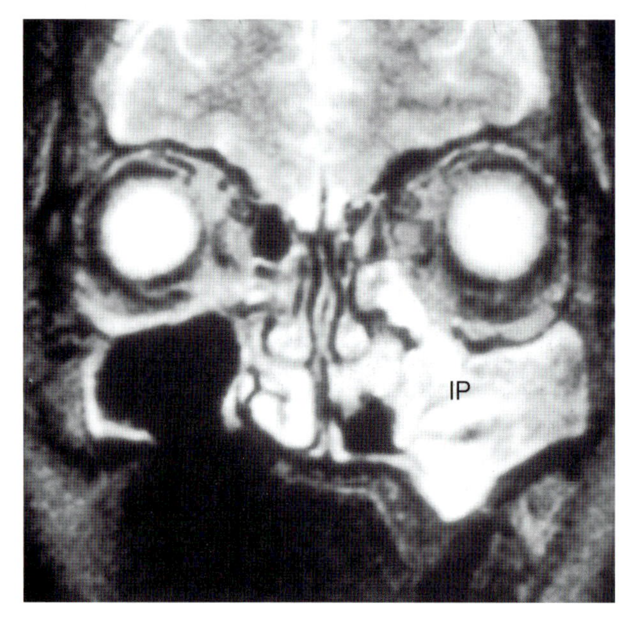

9.17d

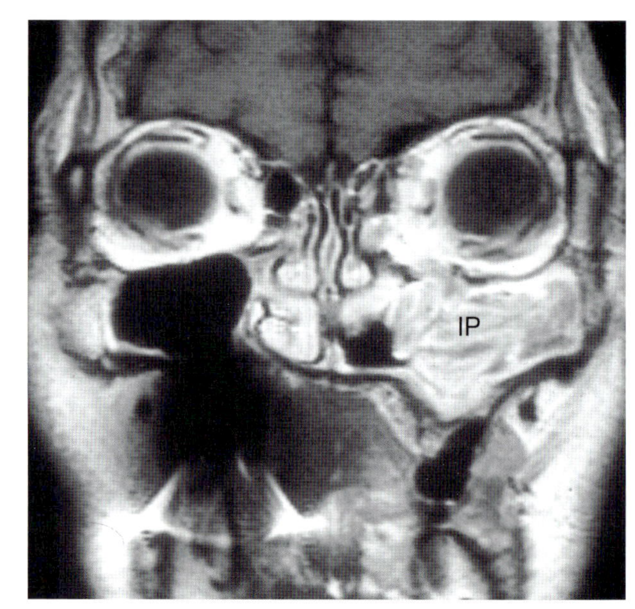

9.17e

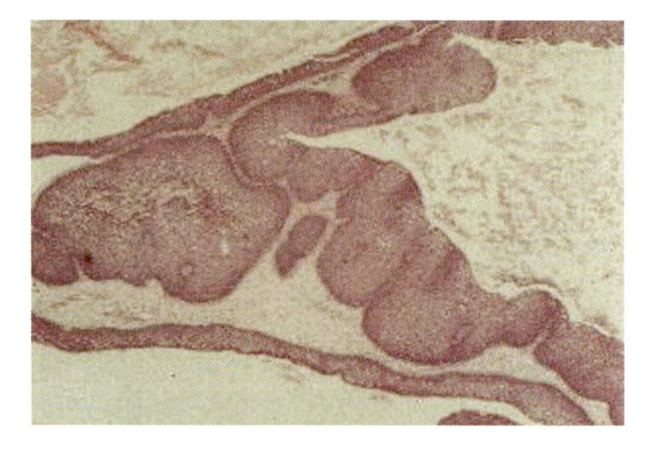

Figure 9.17 *Inverting papilloma*. (a) Axial CT scan demonstrating a mass (IP) in the maxillary sinus. (b, c) Coronal T1-weighted (b) and T2-weighted (c) MRI scans demonstrating the mass (IP) to be of intermediate signal intensity. (d) Gd-DTPA-enhanced MRI scan demonstrating striated and convoluted enhancement of the tumor mass. This correlates with the unique classical histopathological appearance of an inverting papilloma, shown in (e), where the lesion has a thickened epithelial covering with extensive endophytic growth of the hyperplastic epithelium into the underlying stroma.

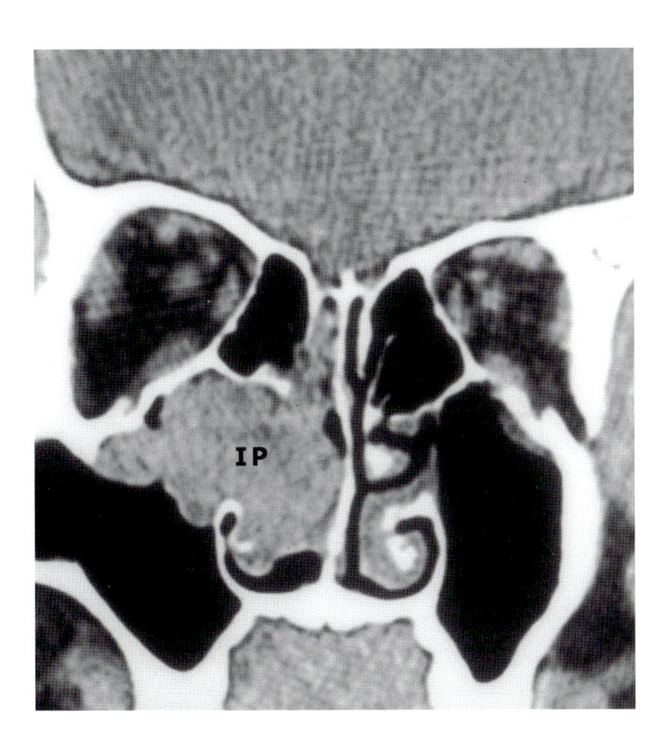

Figure 9.18 *Inverting papilloma*. There is a lobulated mass (IP) in the right ostiomeatal complex. This has eroded the lateral nasal wall, and the mass is protruding into the maxillary sinus. There is no associated sinusitis. No dystrophic calcification is seen in the mass.

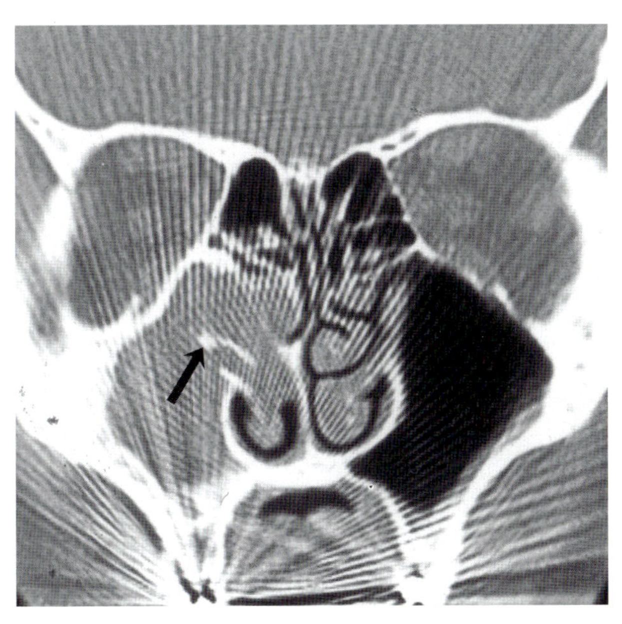

Figure 9.19 *Inverting papilloma with dystrophic calcifications*. Nodular or curvilinear calcifications (arrow) when seen can be mistaken for fungal sinusitis.

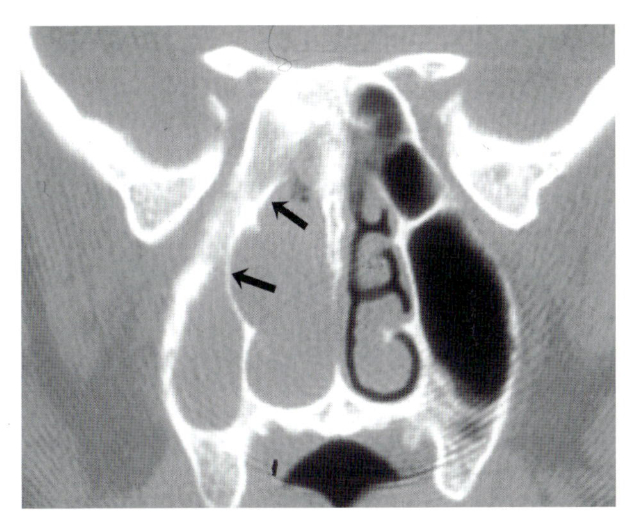

Figure 9.20 *Inverting papilloma*. There is a lobulated mass in the nasal cavity associated with bowing (arrows) of the nasal wall. There is opacification of the maxillary sinus.

foreign body remains undisturbed for some time, it will become covered in salts of calcium and magnesium. These are usually phosphates, oxalates, and carbonates. Over a period of years, the rhinolith can enlarge and become molded to the shape of the cavity in which it is situated. A rhinolith may present with nasal obstruction and a foul-smelling unilateral rhinorrhea. If sufficiently large, it may require disimpaction under general anesthesia. The rhinolith is readily demonstrated on CT as a radio-opaque lesion with sharply demarcated borders.

MALIGNANT TUMORS

(Figures 9.27–9.36)

Malignant tumors of the nose and paranasal sinuses are rare, accounting for 0.2–0.8% of all malignancies. Because of the concealed nature of the anatomy and the relatively innocuous nature of the early symptoms, these tumors often reach an advanced stage prior to diagnosis.

Initial symptoms may be similar to those of chronic sinusitis, with persistent rhinorrhea and facial pain. Progression of the symptoms to a more persistent pain or paresthesia should warrant further investigation. Evidence of bone erosion or asymmetrical sclerosis may be suggestive of an underlying malignancy.

The symptoms associated with malignancy in the paranasal sinuses will also depend upon the site of origin of the tumor. These may include facial

9.21a

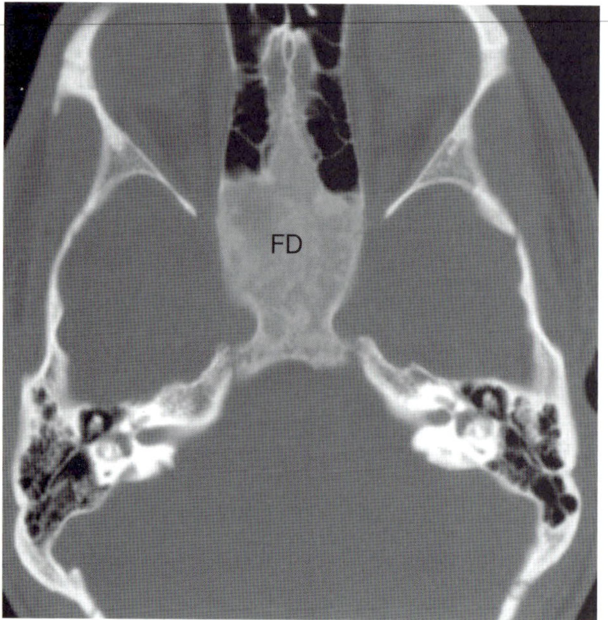

9.21b

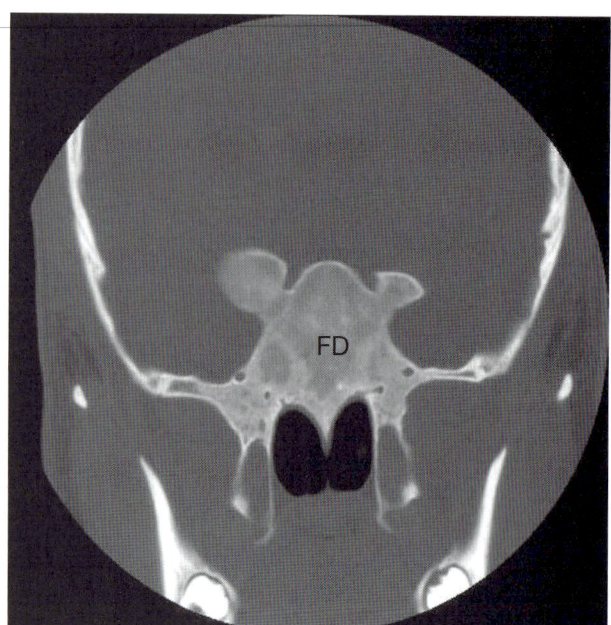

9.21c

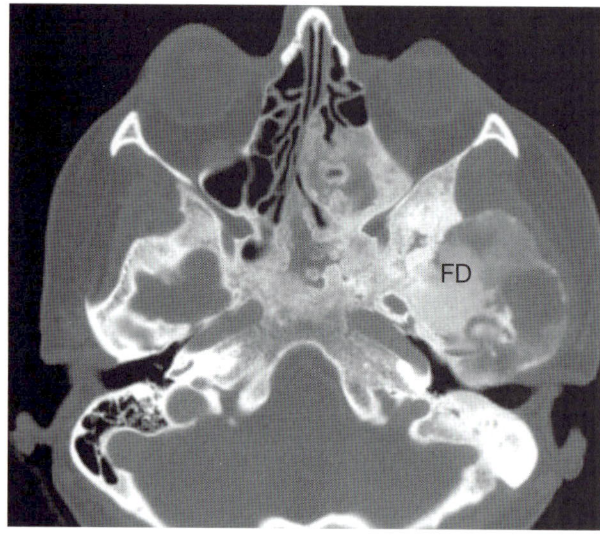

9.21d

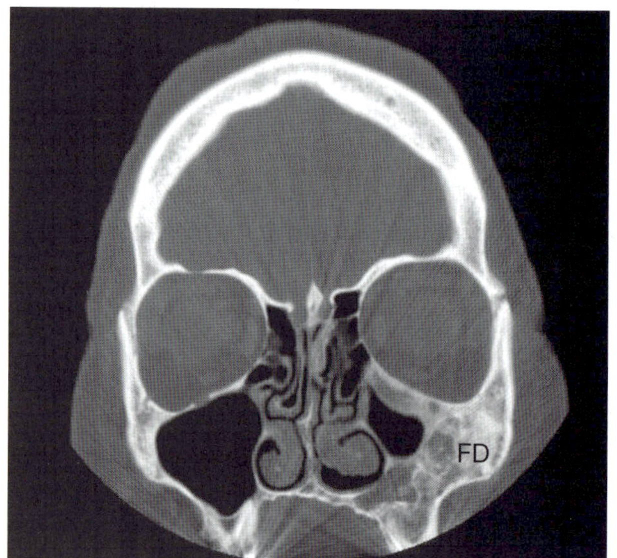

Figure 9.21 *Fibrous dysplasia*. (a, b) Axial (a) and coronal (b) CT scans depicting fibrous dysplasia (FD) involving and obliterating the sphenoid sinus. There is extension of disease to involve the sphenoid bone and anterior clinoid processes. The ground-glass-like attenuation is characteristic. (c, d) Axial (c) and coronal (d) CT scans of fibrous dysplasia (FD) involving the left maxillary sinus wall, sphenoid sinus, ethmoid sinus, and the greater wing of the sphenoid. This example demonstrates the marked degree of expansion and deformity that can arise. Areas of ground-glass opacity are interspersed with areas of cystic degeneration.

pain and paresthesia, loosening of the teeth, change in the fit of a dental plate, exophthalmos, epiphora, nasal obstruction, and a persistent discharge that may be blood-stained. In the more advanced stages of the disease, the tumor often involves more than one sinus.

The commonest site of malignancy in the paranasal sinuses is the maxillary antrum. The

9.22a

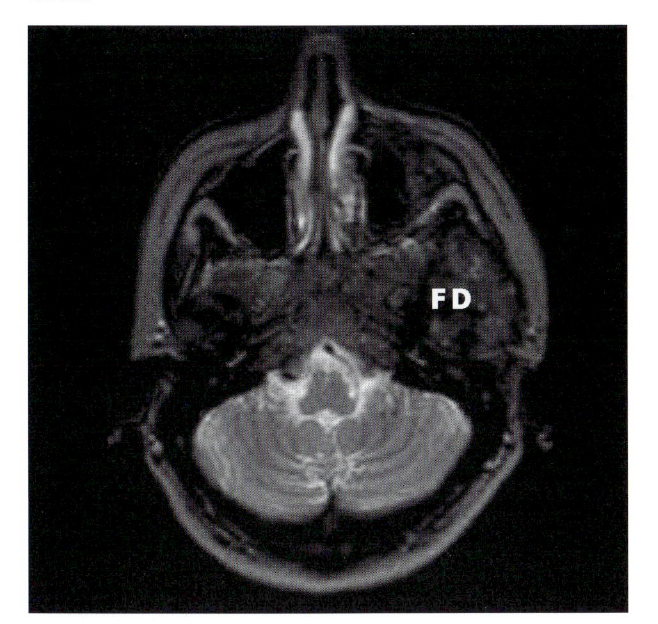

9.22b

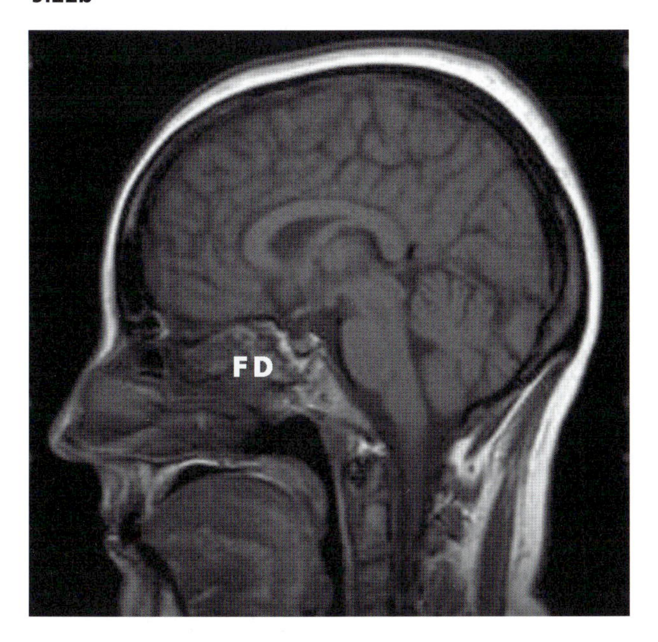

Figure 9.22 Axial T2-weighted (a) and sagittal T1-weighted (b) MRI scans of the same patient as in Figure 9.21. MRI of fibrous dysplasia shows a very heterogeneous expansile lesion within the sphenoid sinus (FD). Involvement of the left maxillary–zygomatic junction and the greater wing of the sphenoid is again seen.

9.23a

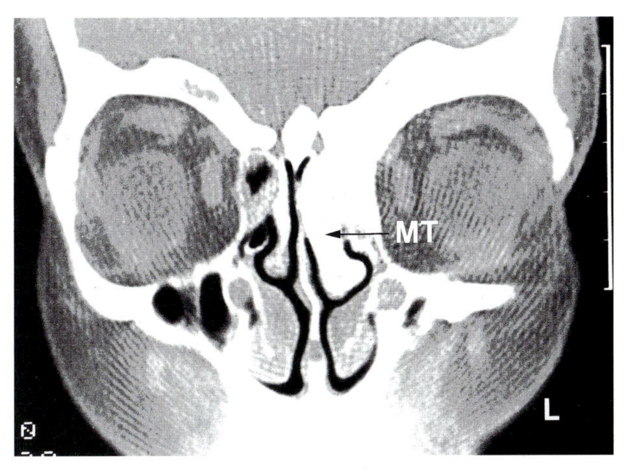

9.23b

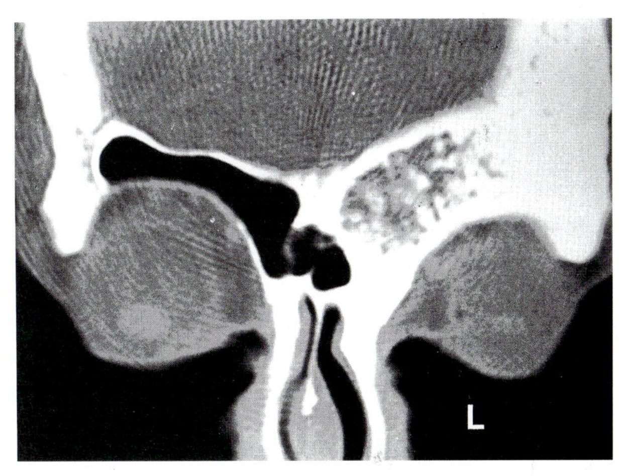

Figure 9.23 *Fibrous dysplasia*. (a) CT scan demonstrating thickening of the roof and superomedial aspect of the orbit. The entire left middle turbinate (MT) is thickened and replaced by abnormal bone. (b) Wide-window CT scan demonstrating the characteristic ground-glass appearance of fibrous hyperplasia affecting the left frontal bone. If the sinuses are viewed with a narrow window, this abnormality can be mistaken for inflammatory disease in the left frontal sinus.

second most common site is the ethmoid sinus. It is rare for tumors to arise in either the frontal or sphenoid sinuses.

The commonest cell type of sinonasal malignancy is squamous cell carcinoma, followed by undifferentiated carcinoma, adenoid cystic carcinoma, and adenocarcinoma. Other less common malignancies occur, including lymphoma, malignant melanoma, esthesioneuroblastoma, plasmacytoma, sarcoma, and metastases, as well as the malignant variety of ameloblastoma (discussed earlier in this chapter).

The diagnosis of paranasal sinus malignancies requires an accurate history and a thorough clinical examination that includes endoscopy and tissue biopsy.

Tumors arising in the maxillary sinus are staged according to the TNM ('tumor, node, metastasis')

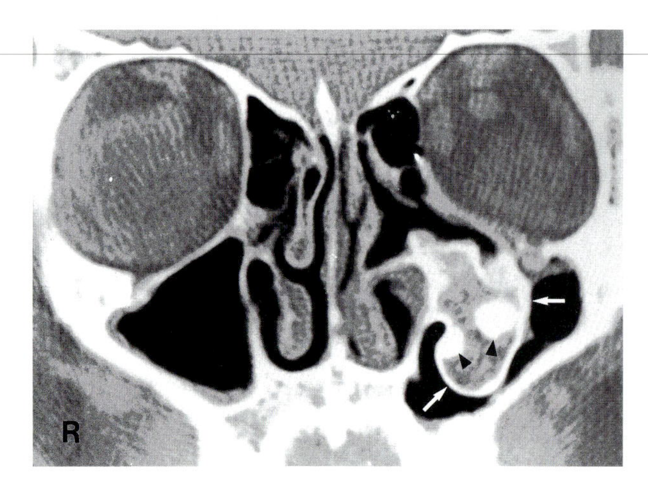

Figure 9.24 *Ossifying fibroma.* CT scan demonstrating an unusual mass in the left maxillary sinus. This has the radiology features of an ossifying fibroma. Note the sclerotic margins of the mass (arrows) and the ovoid areas of calcification (arrowheads) within the mass.

classification (Table 9.3), but as yet there are no adequate staging protocols for malignancies of the frontal, ethmoid, or sphenoid sinuses. The TNM staging classification is used by radiotherapists, oncologists, and surgeons to help determine the most appropriate form of treatment. Historically, maxillary sinus tumors were staged depending upon their position relative to Ohngren's line. This is a plane extending from the medial canthus of the eye to the angle of the mandible, which divides the maxillary antrum into an anteroinferior and a posterosuperior portion.

Accurate imaging plays an important role in the management of patients with malignancies in the sinuses or nasopharynx. Both MRI and CT are used to define the margins and extent of the tumor, and for the assessment of any involvement of vital structures such as the cranial nerves, orbit, and intracranial structures. Postoperative and postirradiation follow-up is best undertaken with both of these modalities. Neither modality can distinguish between the various histological types of malignancy.

CT and MRI of sinonasal malignancy

The symptoms of sinonasal malignancy and benign inflammatory disease have many similarities. Imaging is indicated if:

- Symptoms of rhinosinusitis persist for more than 2 months despite aggressive antibiotic treatment
- Suspicious clinical features arise, such as facial paresthesia, the presence of a palpable mass, epiphora, or blood-stained rhinorrhea

9.25a

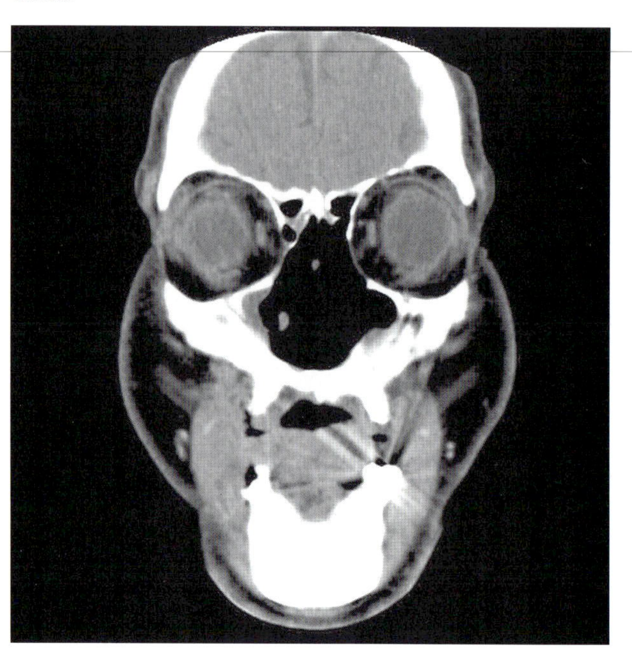

9.25b

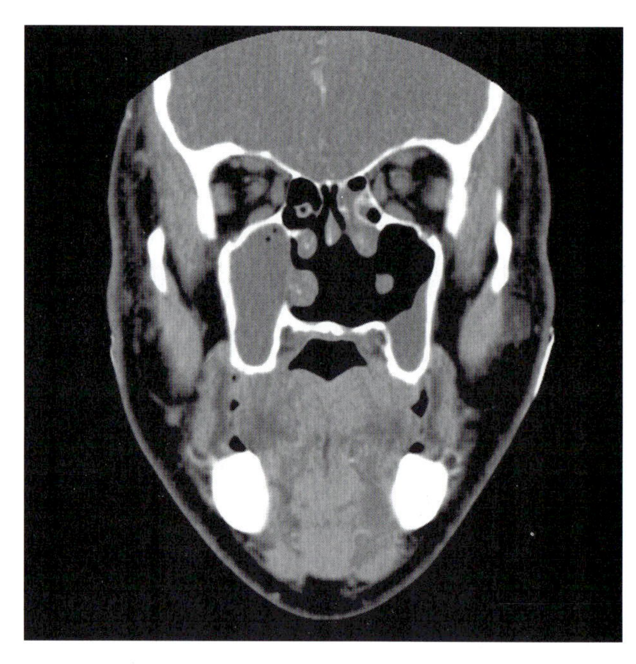

Figure 9.25 *Wegener's granulomatosis.* (a, b) Coronal CT scans showing absence of the nasal septum. Polypoid areas of mucosal opacity are seen in both maxillary antra. There is also reactive bony wall thickening.

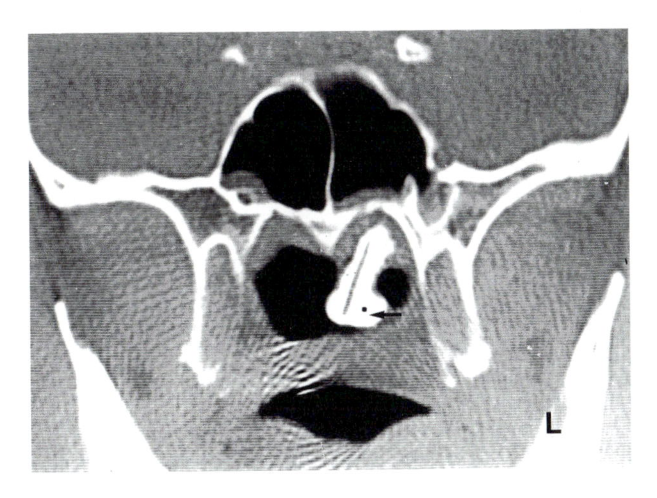

Figure 9.26 *Rhinolith*. This patient presented with a long history of halitosis and a mass was was seen in the nasopharynx on clinical examination. This CT scan shows a rhinolith in the nose that has formed around a tiddlywink. This has caused extensive inflammatory reaction, and the rhinolith (arrow) was seen molding around the inferior turbinate and into the nasopharynx.

Table 9.3 TNM classification of maxillary sinus tumors

T1	Tumor is confined to the antral mucosa of the anteroinferior portion, without bone erosion or destruction
T2	Tumor is confined to the posterosuperior portion without bone erosion or to the anteroinferior portion with erosion of the medial or inferior bony walls
T3	Tumor invades the skin, orbits, anterior ethmoid sinuses, or pterygoid muscles
T4	Tumor invades the cribriform plate, posterior ethmoid sinuses, sphenoid sinuses, pterygoid plates, nasopharynx, or skull base
N0	No clinically positive lymph nodes
N1	A single clinically positive, ipsilateral lymph node < 3 cm in diameter
N2	A single clinically positive, ipsilateral lymph node 3–6 cm in diameter, or multiple ipsilateral nodes < 6 cm in diameter
N3	Massive ipsilateral nodes, bilateral nodes, or a contralateral node
M0	No distant metastases
M1	Distant metastases present

CT is often the first imaging modality utilized in such instances. Scans are conducted in both the axial and coronal planes following the administration of a bolus of intravenous contrast. It is important to scan the whole sinus as well as the surrounding soft tissue areas to identify any tumor that has extended beyond the confines of the sinus cavity.

The benefit of CT is its ability to detect bone destruction, which suggests an aggressive process. Bone destruction of the sinus walls is usually suggestive of a squamous cell carcinoma. New bone formation is occasionally seen with tumors of the paranasal sinuses such as osteosarcoma and chondrosarcoma. The type of bony change seen in such lesions will differ from the chronic bony reactive changes seen in long-standing sinus inflammatory disease. However, the absence of bone destruction does not exclude the possibility of an early malignant lesion, and biopsy should be performed if clinically indicated.

Intravenous contrast demonstrates a variety of enhancement patterns, depending on the tumor histology and vascularity. Necrotic areas enhance less and have lower CT attenuation. The contrast also helps define the surrounding blood vessels and their relationship to the tumor mass. Despite the sensitivity of CT in identifying abnormal soft tissue within the sinonasal cavities, it is rarely possible to differentiate benign inflammatory disease from neoplastic disease in the absence of destruction of bony walls. In many instances, tumors may show homogeneous enhancement and have well-defined margins. MRI can play a more significant role in differentiating between inflammatory mucosa and tumor. Hyperintense tissue within the sinus on T2-weighted scans is almost always due to inflammatory change. Following radiotherapy, vascularized scar tissue may appear identical in both recurrent and residual tumor on both CT and MRI, even following the administration of contrast. In these cases, the radiologist has an important role to play in identifying abnormal tissue and thereby helping to direct biopsy.

Both axial CT and MRI are useful for demonstrating the extension of tumors of the maxilla into the pterygopalatine fossa, infratemporal fossa, orbital apex, and soft tissue of the cheek. Images in the coronal plane are superior at demonstrating intraorbital and frontal sinus involvement, as well as spread through the cribriform plate or planum sphenoidale into the anterior cranial fossa. Tumors can extend intracranially through the many bony foramina in the skull base, as well as along the internal carotid artery to involve the cavernous sinus.

Accurate documentation of tumor extension is vital to guiding appropriate treatment. In sinonasal malignancies, it is important to trace the branches of the trigeminal nerve, which can be a vehicle for perineural spread. The tumor that is visible on clinical examination may only represent a small portion of the whole mass. This occurs when lesions are centered in the sphenoid sinus or with aggressive lesions centered outside of the sinonasal cavity, such as nasopharyngeal carcinoma. The latter are notorious for invasion and extension into the nasal cavity (T2) or sinuses (T3).

Radioisotope bone scans are sensitive for bony metastases and are useful in staging disease. If a sinonasal lesion is suspected to be of metastatic origin, then a bone scan may be helpful if multiple bony foci are revealed.

CT can demonstrate enlarged lymph nodes in the submandibular space and lateral retropharyngeal space and among the upper deep cervical lymph nodes. These nodes are usually the first to become involved by metastases from malignancy in the paranasal sinuses.

A baseline scan is performed about 6 weeks following surgery, radiotherapy, or chemotherapy. This scan is important to document the boundaries of the surgical defect. By this time, most of the soft tissue irregularities resulting from surgery will have settled and the margins of any cavity should be smooth. Both radiotherapy and chemotherapy cause an acute inflammatory response that is seen on images. This usually subsides within 6–8 weeks following completion of treatment. It is unlikely that soft tissue recurrence will be visible at this stage, and thus future follow-up scans can be compared with this baseline examination. Any newly documented soft tissue changes – especially those of a polypoid or focal nature – should be considered to be recurrent disease until proven otherwise.

Other features that are suggestive of recurrence include new or continued destruction of the remaining bones of the sinus. Care should be taken to differentiate bone dehiscence secondary to the surgical defect from that which may be secondary to tumor recurrence.

Both CT and MRI are sensitive to detect and stage the extent of any tumor, but neither is able to make a histological diagnosis. There are, however, certain imaging features that may be suggestive of certain tumor types. Aggressive bone erosion and the presence of calcified fragments are suggestive of squamous cell carcinoma and lymphoma. The presence of peripheral cysts in a mass that has crossed the cribriform plate and spans the nasal cavity and the anterior cranial fossa is suggestive of esthesioneuroblastoma.

Chondrosarcomas and chordomas may show areas of stippled calcification. The former are commonly centered in a parasagittal plane involving the region of the petrous apex and petroclival synchondrosis. Chordomas are usually centered in the clivus. Both lesions usually show a hyperintense signal on T2-weighted MRI scans.

Rhabdomyosarcoma (Figure 9.27)

These tumors are more common in children and are rarely seen in adults. They are primitive muscle cell tumors and are classified as among the small, round, blue cell tumors. They can occur anywhere in the body except in bone. There are three histological groups of tumor: embryonal, alveolar, and pleomorphic. The embryonal type is seen in children between the ages of 4 and 10 years. The alveolar variety of rhabdomyosarcoma occurs in the 2nd and 3rd decades and is more common in the extremities. The pleomorphic type occurs between the ages of 40 and 60 years. These are striated muscle tumors and present as masses with nasal obstruction, bleeding, local pain, headaches, and proptosis. Cranial nerve involvement is common. On CT, these tumors demonstrate destruction of the sinus wall with invasion into adjacent spaces and exhibit little or no enhancement. On MRI, they are of intermediate signal intensity in each of the imaging sequences.

Esthesioneuroblastoma (Figure 9.28)

These tumors are characteristically located close to the roof of the nasal cavity. They originate from neural crest cells in the olfactory mucosa. These tumors present in the 2nd or the 6th decade. They are slowly growing tumors that spread into the orbit, intracranial structures, and the sellar region. These tumors are currently resected via a craniofacial approach to facilitate complete removal. On MRI, they are of intermediate signal intensity, and they enhance, with both CT and MRI, following administration of contrast.

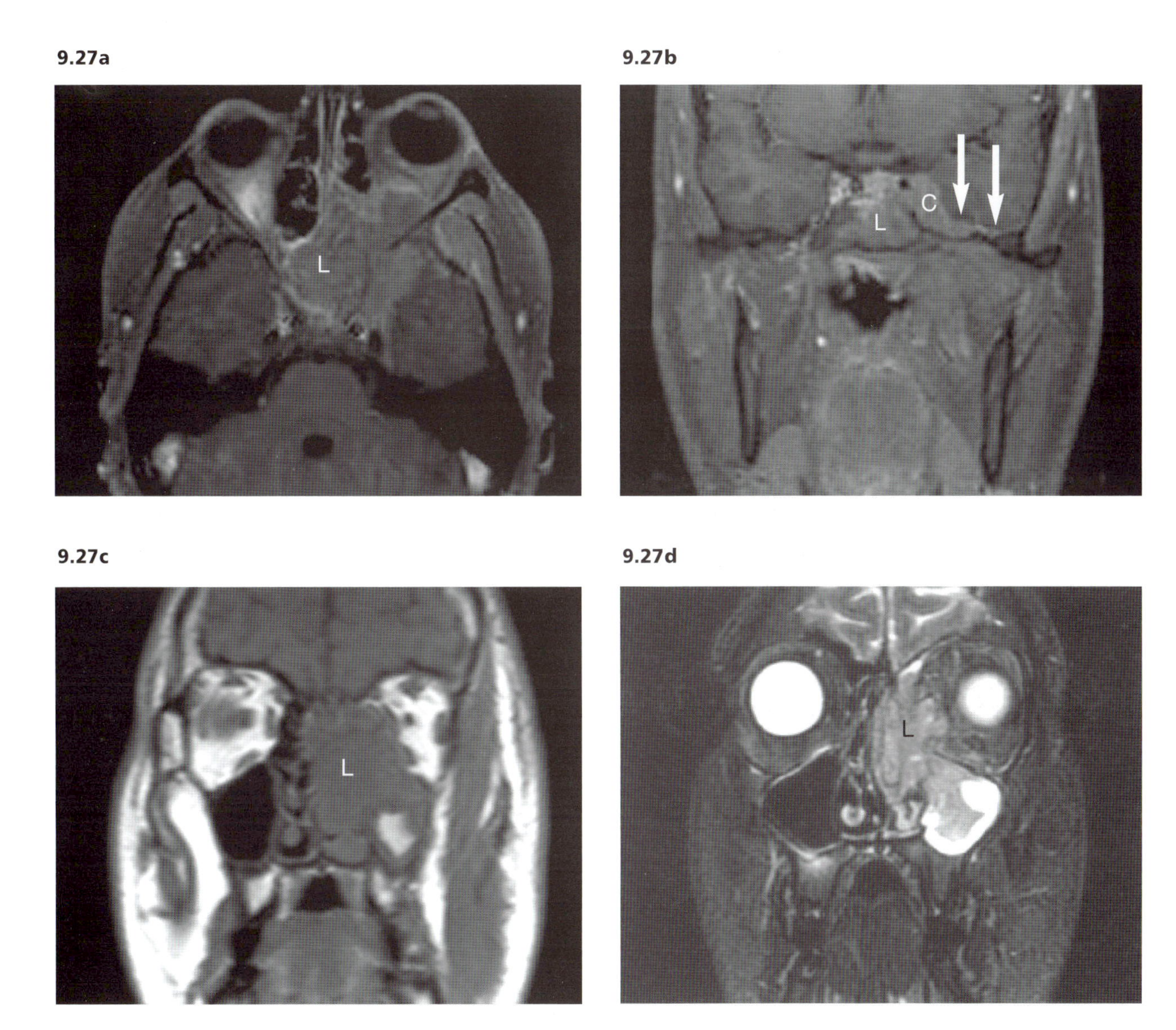

Figure 9.27 *Rhabdomyosarcoma*. Gadolinium-enhanced axial (a) and coronal (b–d) T1-weigted MRI scans showing an enhancing lesion (L) involving the sphenoid sinus with contiguous extension into the left posterior nasal cavity and left orbit. The coronal image (b) clearly show that there is involvement of the left cavernous sinus (C), with mild narrowing of the cavernous carotid artery. There is also abnormal thickening and enhancement along the floor of the left middle cranial fossa (arrows).

Melanoma (Figure 9.29)

Sinonasal melanoma has a higher propensity for both the nasal cavity and septum. Due to the paramagnetic properties of melanin and the presence of hemorrhage, the tumor can have a higher signal on T1-weighted MRI, while T2-weighted sequences may show a low to intermediate signal. This unusual MRI signal may suggest the histology of the tumor.

Plasmacytoma (Figure 9.30)

Plasmacytoma is a rare soft tissue tumor composed of plasma cells. The common presenting symptoms include a soft tissue mass, nasal obstruction, epistaxis, pain, and proptosis. It affects individuals in the 4th and 5th decades of life, with a male preponderance. On CT, these tumors are homogeneous enhancing polypoidal masses with some remodeling of the sinus walls. On MRI, they tend to have signal-

9.28a

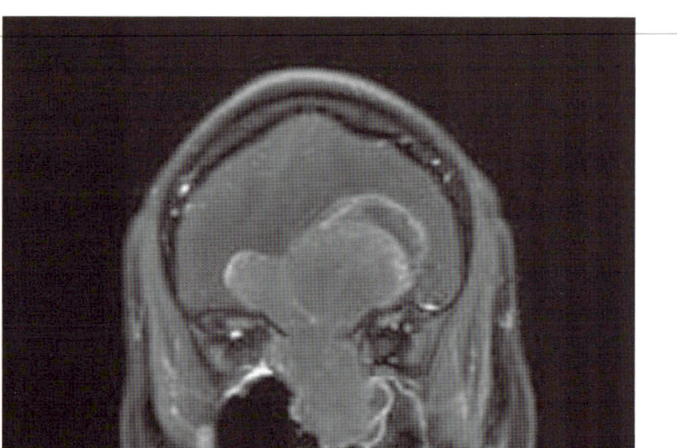

9.28b

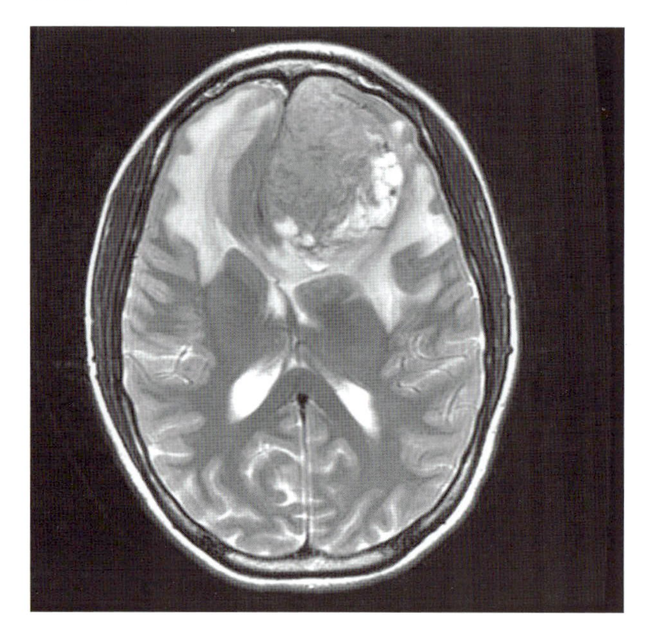

Figure 9.28 *Esthesioneuroblastoma*. (a) CT scans demonstrating a large inhomogeneously enhancing mass destroying the roof of the nasal cavity. This mass has extended into the anterior cranial fossa. Axial image (b) shows marked mass effect and edema within the displaced frontal lobes. The presence of peripheral cysts within the intracranial component is suggestive of the diagnosis of esthesioneuroblastoma.

9.29a

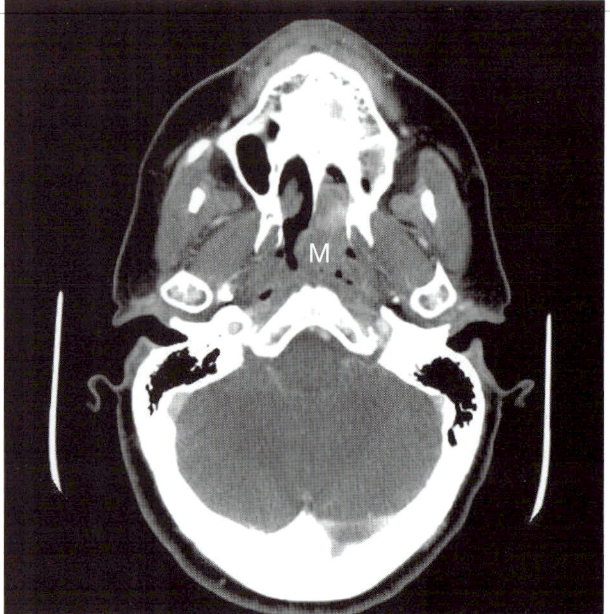

9.29b

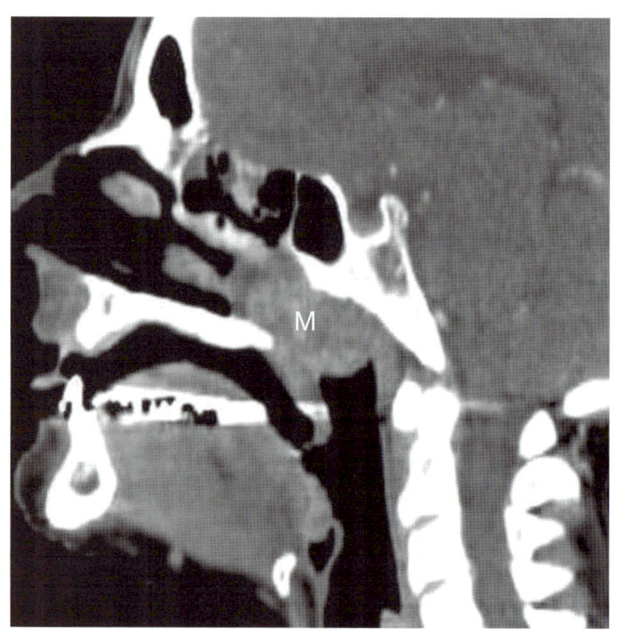

Figure 9.29 *Malignant melanoma*. Axial (a) and reconstructed sagittal (b) contrast-enhanced CT scans of the nasal cavity showing a heterogeneously enhancing mass (M) that spans the posterior nasal cavity and extends past the plane of the nasal choana into the nasopharynx. Histology revealed malignant melanoma.

9.30a

9.30b

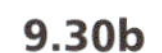

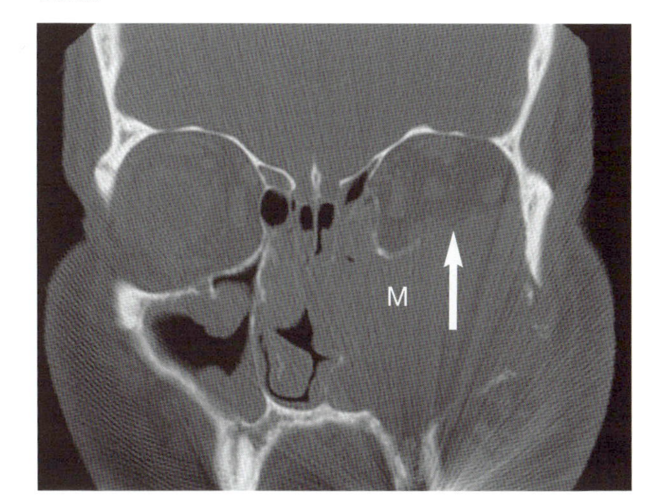

9.30c

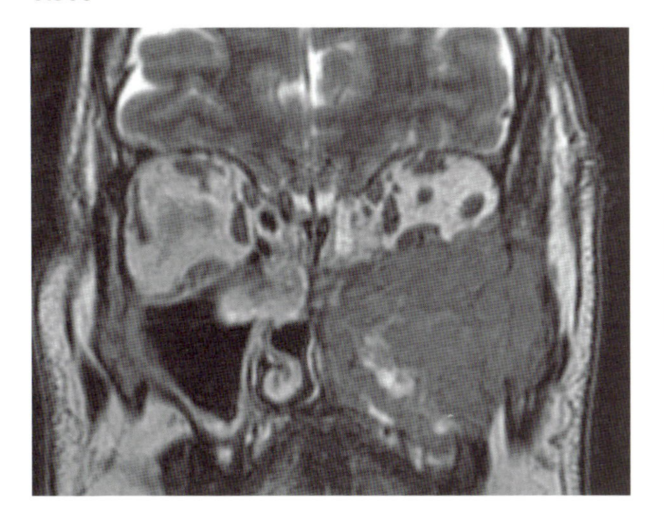

9.30d

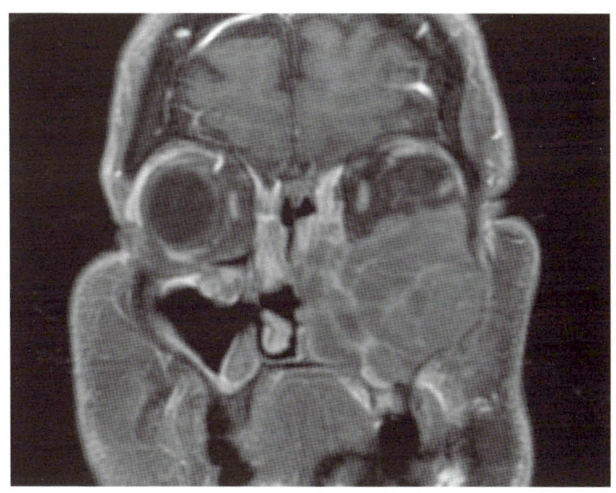

Figure 9.30 *Plasmacytoma*. (a, b) Axial (a) and coronal (b) CT scans demonstrating a large inhomogeneous mass (M) destroying the walls of the maxillary sinus. This mass has invaded the orbit and the infratemporal fossa (arrows) and the pterygoid muscles. (c, d) T2-weighted (c) and Gd-DTPA (d) MRI scans demonstrating a mass of intermediate signal characteristics, with hyperintense areas of inflammatory mucosa, and a few signal-void linear vascular areas.

void vascular channels in the tumor matrix, which is of intermediate signal intensity on all sequences.

Lymphoma (Figures 9.31 and 9.32)

Non-Hodgkin's lymphoma (NHL) is the second most common malignancy involving the sinonasal cavities. The nasal cavity and the maxillary sinuses are the most common sites of involvement. These tumors are radiosensitive and tend to be bulky neoplasms that remodel the bony walls with slight erosions. They enhance on Gd-DTPA MRI.

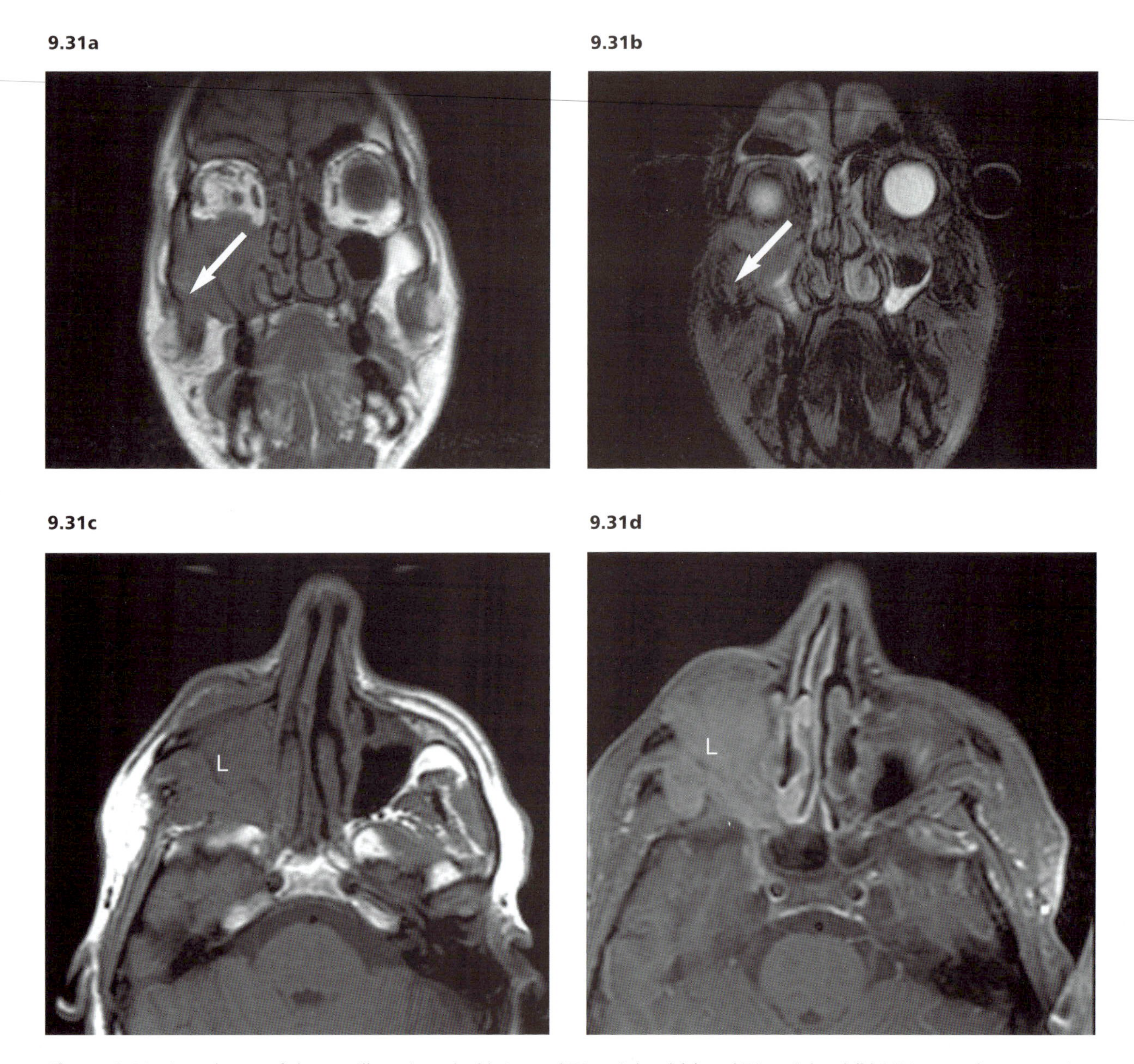

Figure 9.31 *Lymphoma of the maxillary sinus*. (a, b) Coronal T1-weighted (a) and T2-weighted (b) MRI scans demonstrating a mass invading the lateral wall of the maxillary sinus (arrows). (c, d) Axial T1-weighted (c) and T2-weighted (d) Gd-DTPA-enhanced MRI scans demonstrating the presence of a hypointense mass (L) invading the orbit and infratemporal fossa. The mass enhances following contrast administration.

9.32a

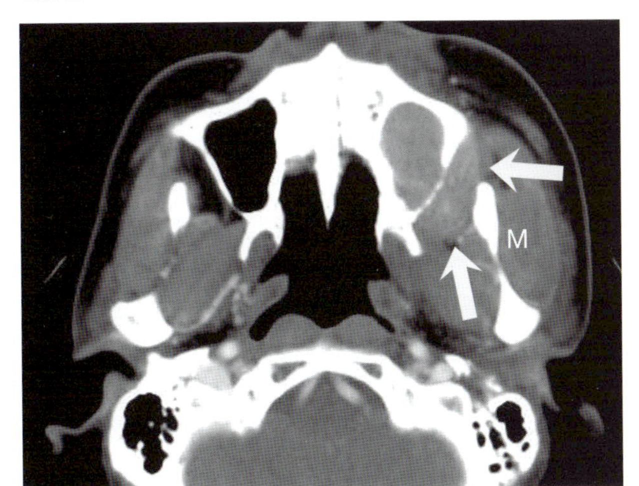

9.32b

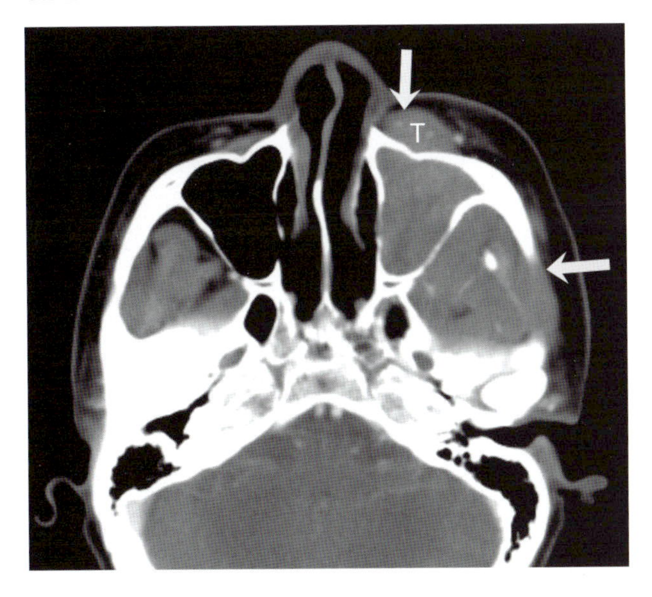

Figure 9.32 *Lymphoma of the maxillary sinus*. (a, b) Axial contrast-enhanced CT scans demonstrating a mildly enhancing mass (arrows) filling the left antrum. There is thinning of the posterolateral wall of the sinus, with tumor extension into the left masticator space (M). Loss of retroantral fat on the left is seen. Tumor invasion of the soft tissues of the face is seen anteriorly (T).

9.33a

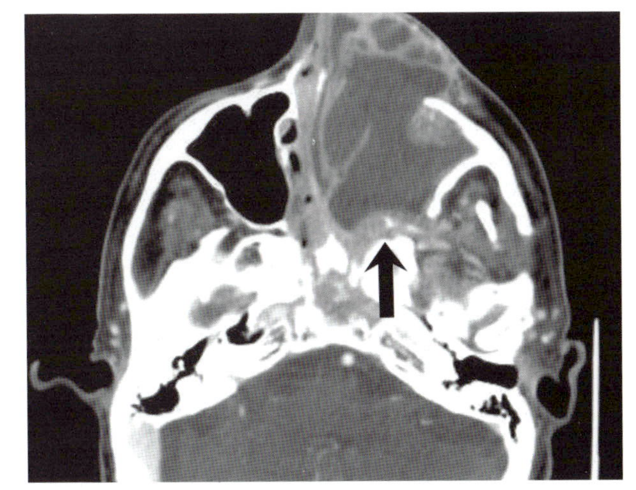

9.33b

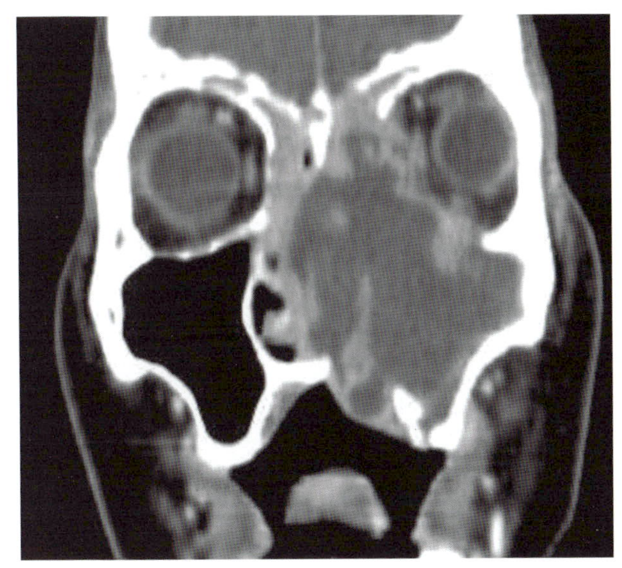

Figure 9.33 *Squamous cell carcinoma*. Contrast-enhanced axial (a) and coronal (b) CT scans showing a large necrotic squamous cell carcinoma of the sinonasal cavity. There is extension into the left orbit, and tumor is also destroying portions of the hard palate. There is strong suspicion of dehiscence of the roof of the ethmoid. The presence of soft tissue in the left pterygopalatine fossa (arrow) is consistent with involvement of the maxillary segment of the left trigeminal nerve. There is anterior tumor extension through the anterior maxillary wall to involve the overlying skin.

9.34a

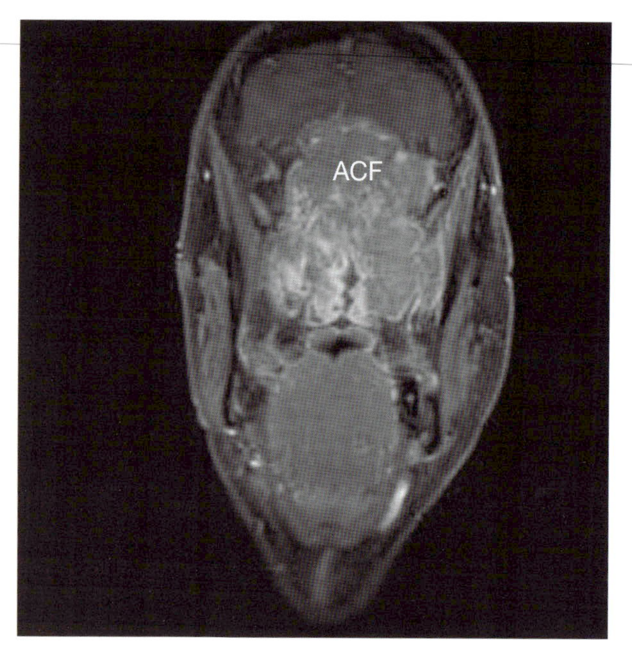

9.34b

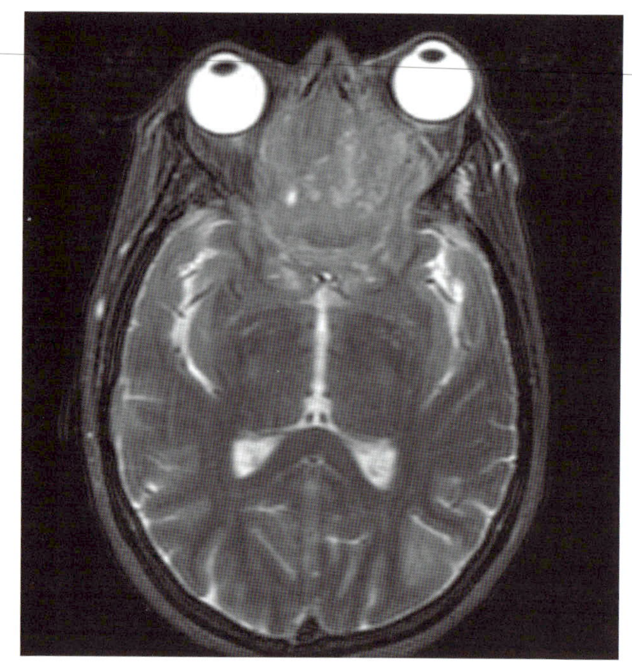

9.34c

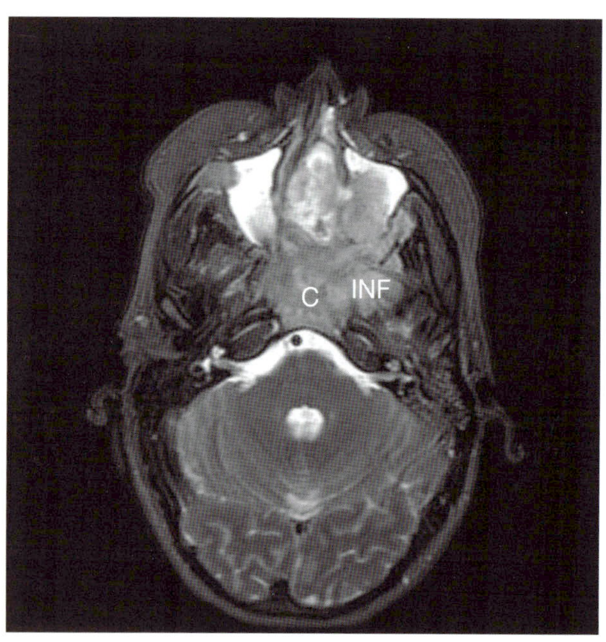

9.34d

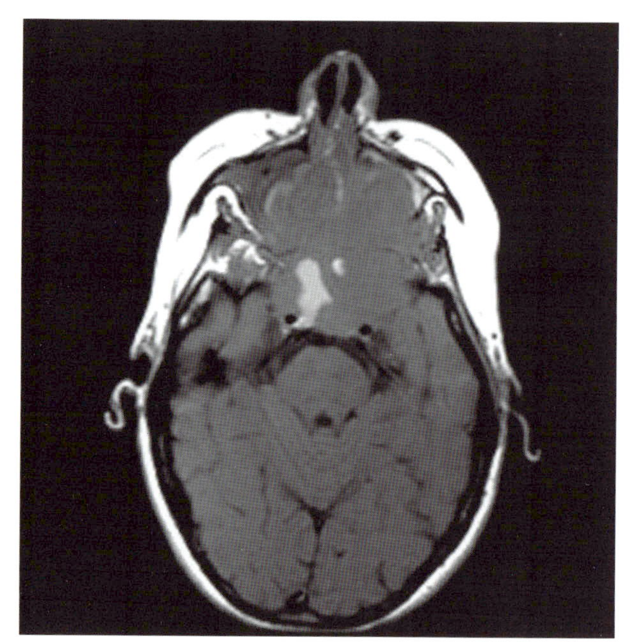

Figure 9.34 *Squamous cell carcinoma*. (a–d) Multisequence MRI of a massive squamous cell carcinoma involving the sphenoid sinus and nasal cavities. There is tumor extension into the clivus (C), left infratemporal fossa (INF), anterior cranial fossa (ACF), and orbits. Axial T2-weighted images through the level of the maxillary sinuses show that there is definite tumor extension into the maxillary sinuses, as well as a significant post-obstructive secretory component present, which is seen as hyperintense reactive fluid in the sinus cavity.

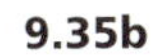

9.35a

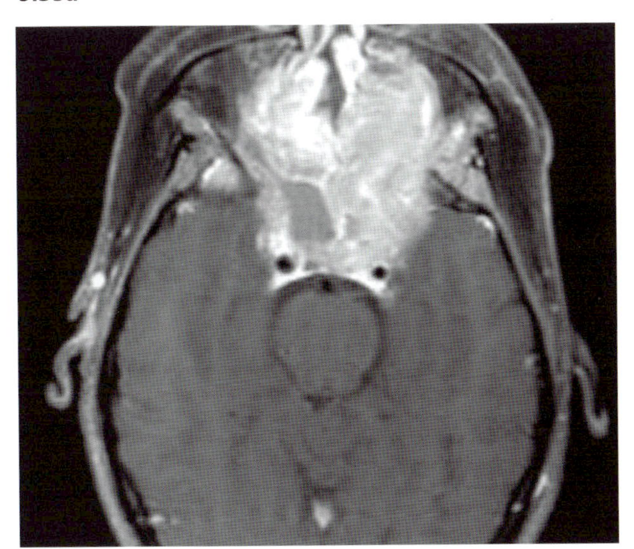

9.35b

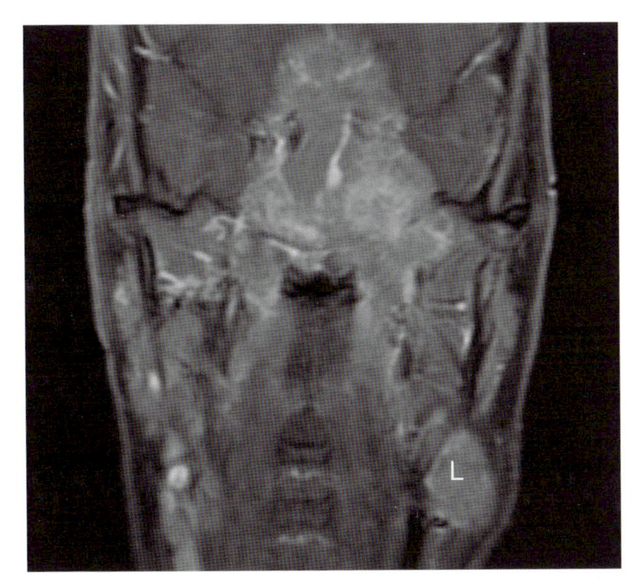

Figure 9.35 *Squamous cell carcinoma*. Axial (a) and coronal (b) Gd-DTPA-enhanced MRI scans demonstrating a large heterogeneous enhancing mass in the sinonasal cavity that has extended to involve the intracranial structures and the infratemporal fossa. Enhancing lymphadenopathy (L) is also noted in the left side of the neck.

9.36a

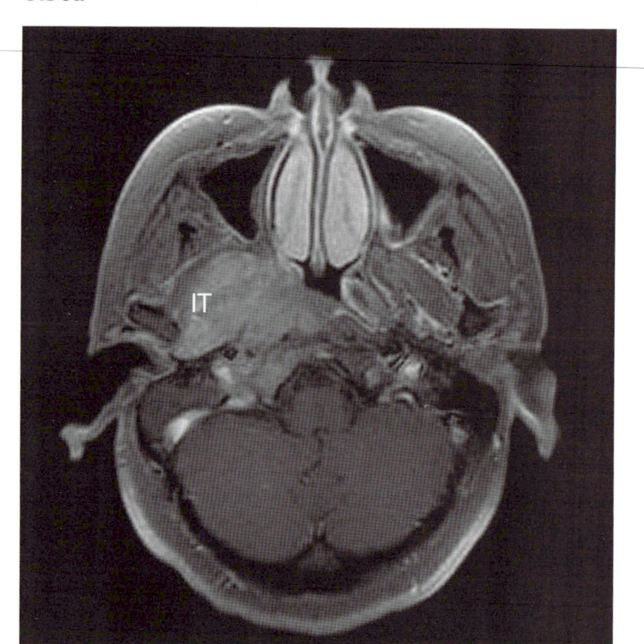

9.36b

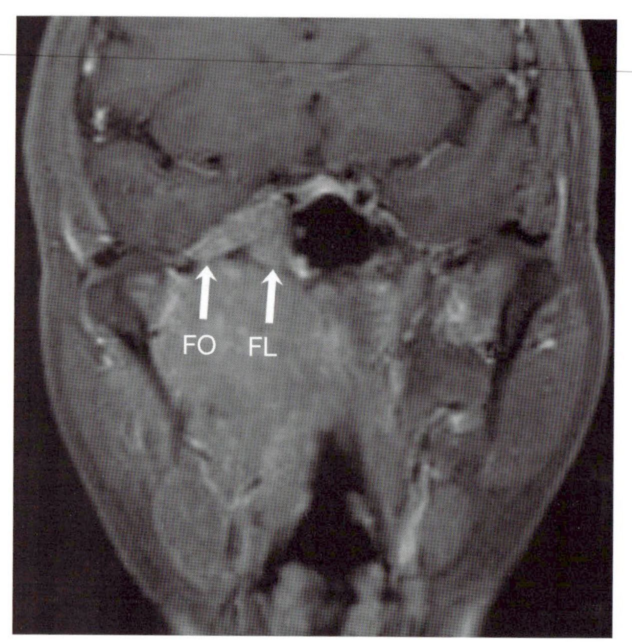

9.36c

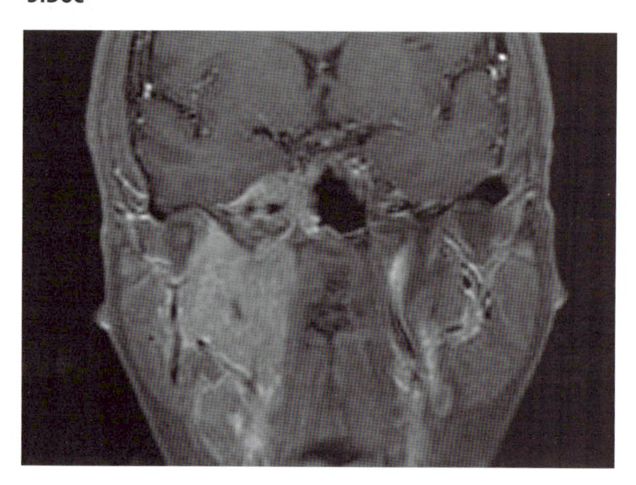

Figure 9.36 *Nasopharyngeal carcinoma*. Fat-saturated axial (a) and coronal (b, c) contrast-enhanced MRI scans of a large nasopharyngeal carcinoma demonstrating extension into the infratemporal fossa (IT). MRI is the modality of choice to show perineural disease spread. In this case, there is extension via the right V3/foramen ovale (arrow FO) into the cavernous sinus. There is also a small slip of tumor extending via the right foramen lacerum directly into the cavernous sinus (arrow FL).

10

Postoperative appearances of the paranasal sinuses

INTRODUCTION

It is important for the radiologist to have a working knowledge of the indications for sinus surgery, the variety of surgical approaches undertaken, and the surgical complications that may result from these procedures. Correct interpretation of the images requires an understanding of the expected bony defects and soft tissue changes created by the different surgical approaches. Accurate preoperative imaging will help provide a road map for the surgeon and help eliminate potential error. It is important for the radiologist to understand the reasons why the surgeon will on occasion request a postoperative computed tomography (CT) scan. A postoperative CT scan is undertaken if there is persistence of symptoms. Imaging may identify residual or recurrent disease as well as scarring reducing ventilation of the drainage channels. In addition, it is important for the surgeon to be aware of potential danger areas, such as a previous unrecognized breach of the lamina papyracea or of the cribriform plate.

CT has two important roles in the management of patients who have previously undergone sinus surgery. The first is to identify any residual or recurrent disease in symptomatic patients. Clinical evaluation alone is inadequate to assess the site of failure. Secondly, accurate radiological assessment will improve the outcome of revision surgery for treating residual disease. Magnetic resonance imaging (MRI) is superior to CT when recurrence of malignancy is suspected, and helps to direct biopsy.

Surgery conducted for the excision of an inverting papilloma or a malignant tumor requires accurate follow-up. These patients should have follow-up CT or MRI scans at 3- to 6-monthly intervals. These scans are compared with the initial baseline postoperative scan. This process identifies changes that may represent recurrent disease. The administration of intravenous contrast helps to differentiate inflammatory tissue from scar tissue or mucocele. It is important that adequate clinical information be provided to aid in the accurate interpretation of the postoperative CT and MRI scans.

POSTOPERATIVE CHANGES ON CT/MRI (Figures 10.1 and 10.2b)

CT is invaluable in the preoperative assessment of patients requiring revision sinus surgery. It identifies the extent of previous surgery, any anatomical changes that may have occurred as a consequence of the procedure, and the site of residual disease. Postoperative changes, including scarring, fibrosis, synechia, and bony sclerosis, will be demonstrated. The sclerotic changes are usually present on the interior of the sinus, resulting in a small sinus cavity with dense, thickened walls.

CAUSES OF FAILED SINUS SURGERY (Figures 10.3 and 10.4)

Surgery may fail to eradicate benign inflammatory disease of the paranasal sinuses for a variety of

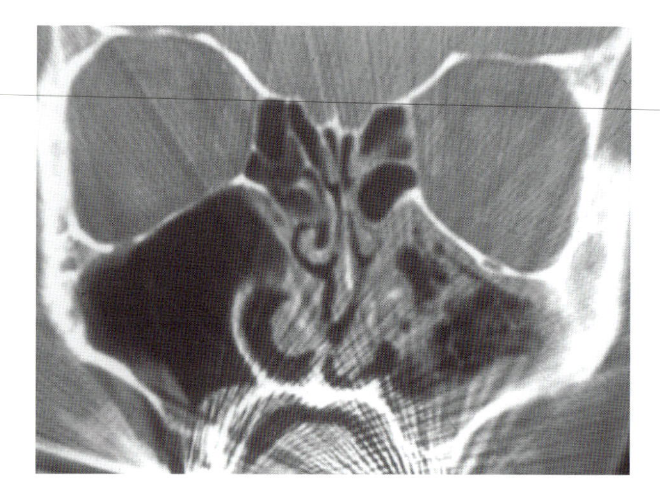

Figure 10.1 *Synechia.* Coronal CT scan demonstrating synechia and scarring with linear strands in the maxillary sinus.

reasons. The commonest cause of failure is incomplete marsupialization of the ethmoid air cells, especially those of the anterior ethmoid or agger nasi. This is common following intranasal ethmoidectomy, and the residual bony septa are seen with associated soft tissue abnormalities. Recurrent maxillary sinus infection can occur despite the absence of disease in the ostiomeatal

10.2a

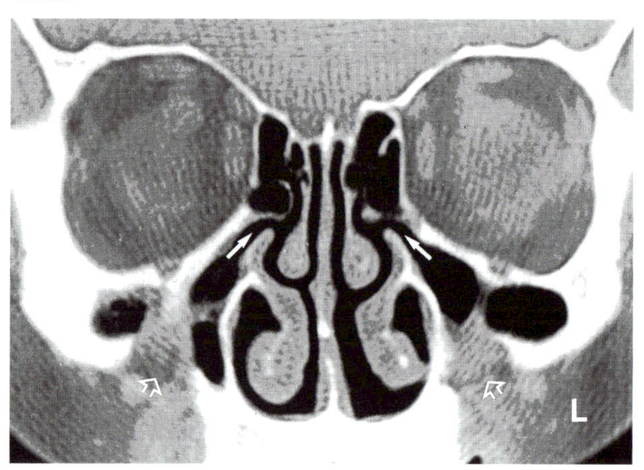

10.2b

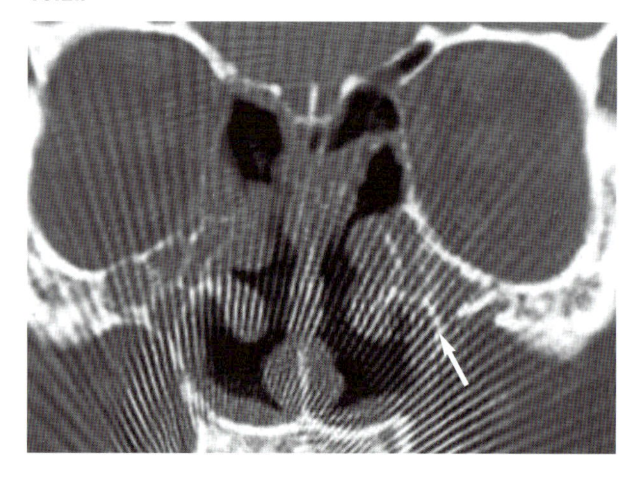

Figure 10.2 (a) *Bilateral Caldwell–Luc procedures* (open arrows). Although this patient has patent ostiomeatal complex bilaterally (arrows), scarring and compartmentalization has resulted in persistent symptoms of pain and sinus infection. (b) *Postoperative hypoplasia of the maxillary sinus.* There is thickening of the bony walls and the mucous membranes at the expense of the sinus lumen (arrow). This patient had had a Caldwell–Luc procedure several years previously.

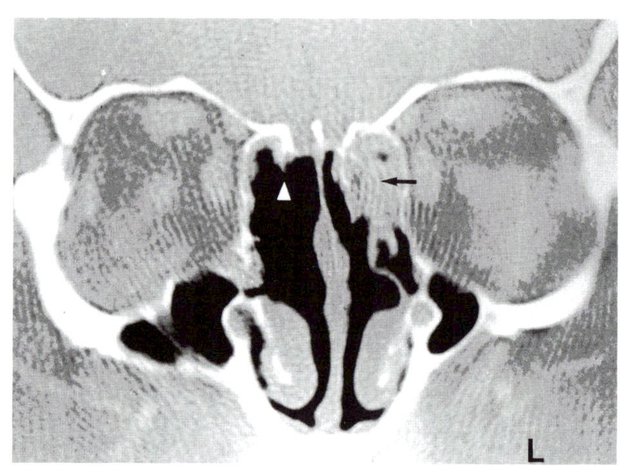

Figure 10.3 *Incomplete ethmoidectomy with residual polyps.* This patient has undergone a complete right intranasal ethmoidectomy with excision of the right middle turbinate (arrowhead). The left ethmoidectomy is incomplete and there is residual polypoid disease in the anterior ethmoid (black arrow).

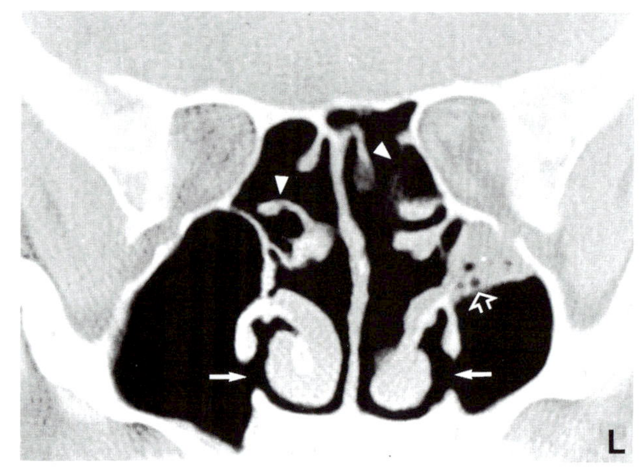

Figure 10.4 *Bilateral incomplete ethmoidectomy with recurrent polyps.* The posterior ethmoidectomies are incomplete (arrowheads). Bilateral patent inferior meatal antrostomies are present (arrows). The air bubbles within the 'soft tissue' mass in the roof of the left maxillary sinus identify this mass as thick mucus (open arrow).

complex or nasal cavity. This may be related to dental disease affecting the sinus or to disordered ciliary motility.

The aim of this chapter is to provide brief descriptions of the indications, surgical technique, and related radiographic features of the more frequently performed sinus procedures.

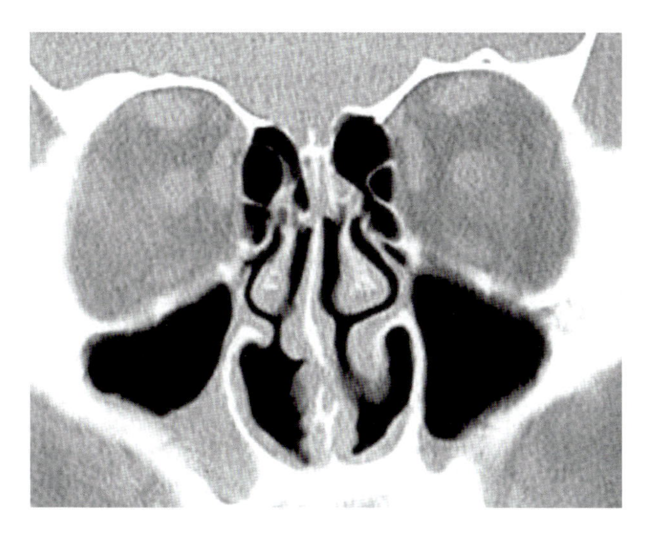

Figure 10.5 *Inferior turbinectomy*. This patient has had a right inferior turbinectomy.

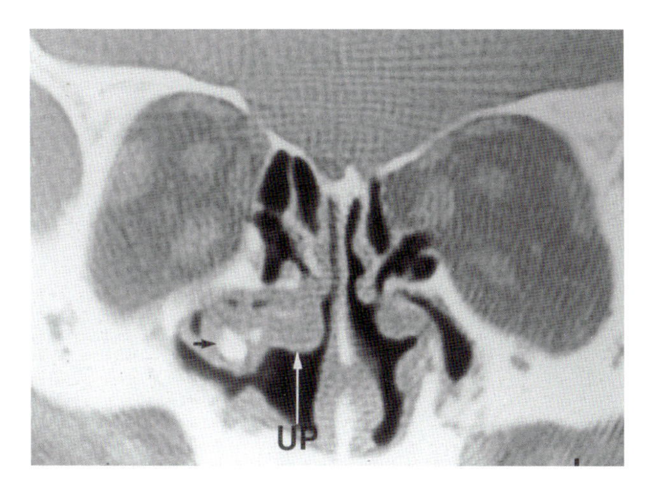

Figure 10.6 *Inferior turbinectomy*. This patient has had a right inferior turbinectomy, following which there was a fracture of the medial wall (arrow) of the maxillary sinus, resulting in scarring and synechiae of the ostiomeatal complex. UP, uncinate process.

INFERIOR TURBINECTOMY
(Figures 10.5 and 10.6)

Indication

To improve airflow through the nasal cavity.

Technique

Inferior turbinectomy can involve partial or complete removal of the inferior turbinate. More radical removal is associated with troublesome bleeding from the posterior vessels entering through the sphenopalatine foramen. The inferior turbinate is fractured medially to allow scissors to be placed around the tissue prior to removal. Any remnant is often outfractured at the end of the procedure. This procedure is frequently undertaken with septal surgery.

Radiological features

The postoperative radiological appearance will depend upon the extent of resection. Inferior turbinectomy undertaken with septal surgery may predispose to adhesions or synechiae if there is apposition of the two raw surfaces. These appear as soft tissue on CT scans.

INFERIOR MEATAL ANTROSTOMY
(Figures 10.7, 10.8, and 10.9a)

The inferior meatal antrostomy or inferior antral window procedure is conducted infrequently today. However, many patients will have had this procedure in the past. The aim was to improve drainage through an opening in the dependent part of the maxillary sinus. This procedure has fallen out of favor, as the mucociliary mechanism is known to carry mucus towards the more superiorly placed natural ostium of the maxillary sinus despite the presence of the antrostomy.

Indications

Chronic maxillary sinusitis; biopsy of soft tissue masses within the maxillary antrum; facilitation of drainage following radiotherapy.

Technique

The inferior turbinate is retracted medially. The lateral wall of the inferior meatus is perforated and the surrounding bone is excised. The antrostomy is extended inferiorly to the floor of the nasal cavity

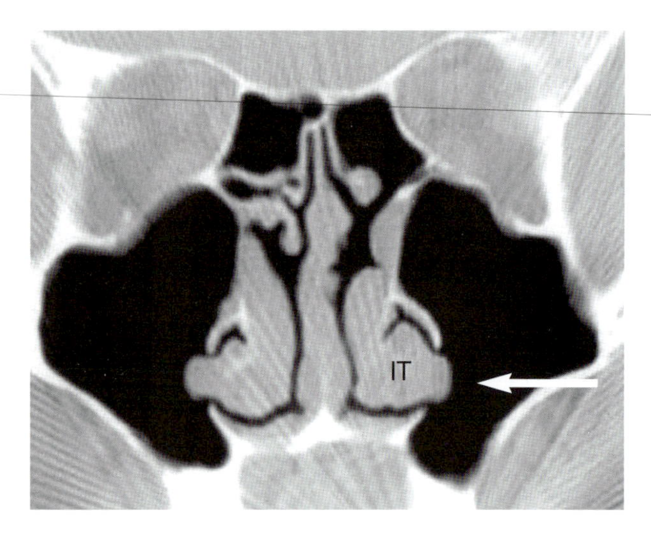

Figure 10.7 *Bilateral intranasal antrostomies*. Coronal CT scan demonstrating bilateral intranasal antrostomies with large hypertrophied inferior turbinates (IT), occluding the antrostomy sites (arrow).

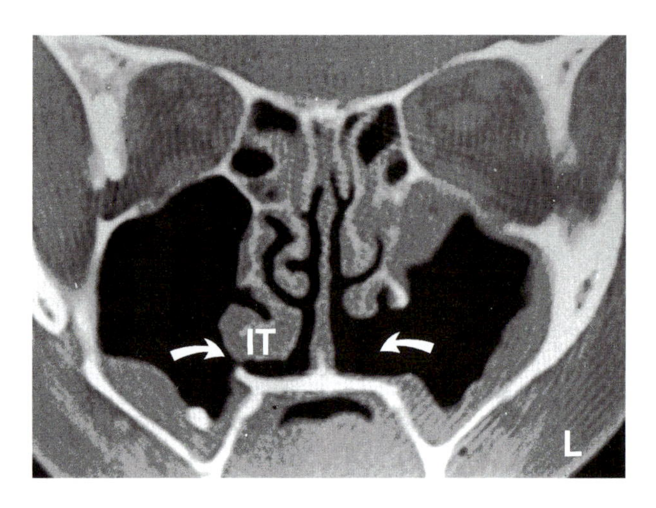

Figure 10.8 *Bilateral intranasal antrostomies*. Coronal CT scan demonstrating wide bilateral intranasal antrostomies (curved arrows). The antrostomy on the left is widely patent, whereas that on the right is blocked by an enlarged inferior turbinate (IT). There is mucosal disease in both maxillary sinuses. Failure of this procedure is due to the inflammatory disease obstructing the left ostiomeatal complex.

and both anteriorly and posteriorly to achieve a diameter of 1.5–2 cm. Some surgeons resect all or part of the inferior turbinate to facilitate antroscopy at a later date.

Radiological features

The bony defect is evident in the lateral wall of the inferior meatus. With time, this may stenose secondary to either bony or mucosal regeneration.

CALDWELL–LUC PROCEDURE

(Figures 10.2, 10.9, and 10.10)

This is one of the oldest surgical procedures described to treat chronic maxillary sinusitis. It is less commonly performed today, but older patients may exhibit bony defects.

Indications

Chronic maxillary sinusitis; removal of dental roots or foreign bodies; excision of antrochoanal polyps, mucoceles, or odontogenic or dentigerous cysts; repair of oroantral fistulae. Access with this approach is gained to the orbital floor to facilitate decompression or for elevation of the orbital floor following orbital fractures. It also facilitates access to the pterygopalatine fossa either for ligation of the internal maxillary artery for uncontrolled epistaxis or for a pterygoid (Vidian) neurectomy in patients with intractable vasomotor rhinitis.

Technique

A sublabial approach is made through the anterior wall of the maxillary sinus via the canine fossa. This is situated superolateral to the root of the upper canine tooth and inferior to the infraorbital nerve, and provides both wide exposure and access to the maxillary sinus. The sublabial antrostomy is sometimes referred to as a radical antrostomy. When this technique was used in the management of chronic sinusitis, the mucosa was then stripped from the entire antrum. If this procedure is indicated to provide access to the pterygopalatine fossa, the mucosa is left intact. An inferior meatal antrostomy is fashioned to facilitate drainage and to allow inspection of the antrum.

Radiological features

CT is valuable prior to a Caldwell–Luc procedure in order to identify any surgical hazards, such as a hypoplastic maxillary sinus. Attempting a Caldwell–Luc procedure into a hypoplastic maxillary sinus could result in perforation of the floor of the orbit and intraorbital soft tissue injury. The maxillary sinus may be divided by incomplete septa. Identification preoperatively helps to facilitate adequate drainage of the separate compartments.

10.9a

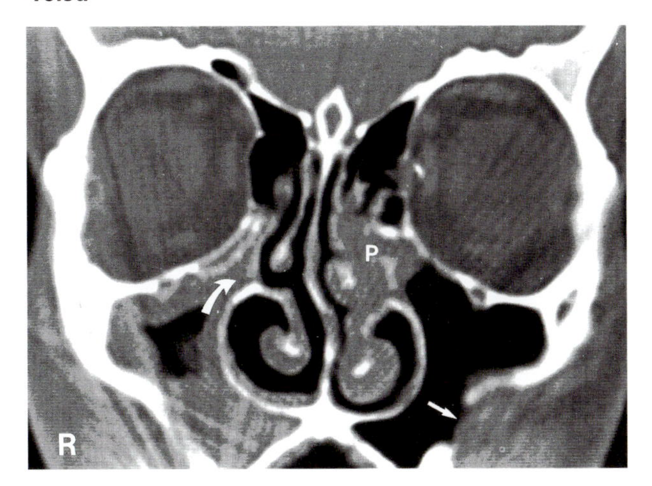

10.9b

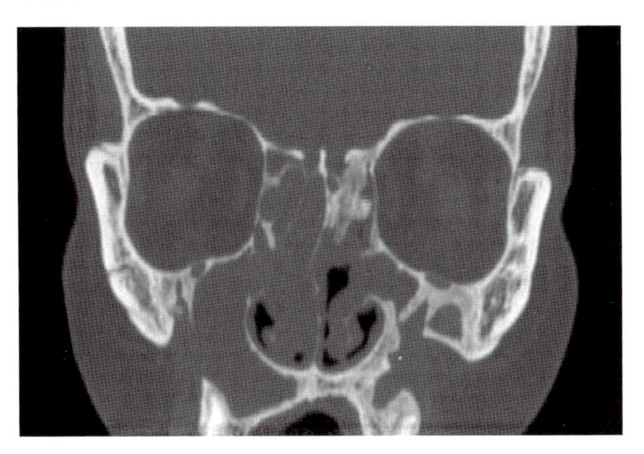

Figure 10.9 (a) *Caldwell–Luc procedures with residual disease*. Coronal scan demonstrating a large polyp in the left middle meatus (P) blocking the ostiomeatal complex in a patient who presented with persistent left malar pain and nasal obstruction despite bilateral Caldwell–Luc procedures. Excision of the polyp and reopening of the natural ostium of the maxillary sinus led to resolution of the patient's symptoms. Note the dehiscent bone in the area of the sublabial antrostomy on the left (arrow). The mucosal thickening in the right maxillary sinus is consistent with chronic sinusitis. Note the blocked infundibulum on this side (curved arrow). (b) *Scarring from Caldwell–Luc procedure*. There is soft tissue scarring in the maxillary sinuses with sclerosis of the sinus walls.

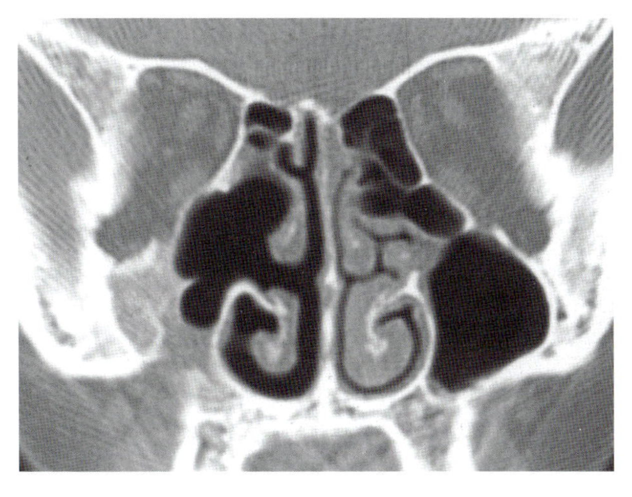

Figure 10.10 *Caldwell–Luc procedure*. A defect in the inferolateral wall of the right maxillary sinus with postoperative scarring is noted. Wide transantral middle meatal antrostomy has been performed.

Clinical and radiographic improvement occurs in about 68% of patients undergoing this form of sinus surgery. Postoperative radiographic examinations should be avoided in the first 6–8 weeks, as the presence of blood and edematous tissue may appear radiologically similar to disease. It is common to find an air–fluid level in the first few weeks following surgery, and this should not be misinterpreted as acute maxillary sinusitis. The radiologist needs to differentiate between those changes that have occurred as a consequence of the surgical procedure and those abnormalities that may reflect continuing or recurrent disease. The clinical history is of great importance, as some patients will still exhibit radiological evidence of disease, but may in fact be asymptomatic. Excessive soft tissue proliferation in the sinonasal cavity may represent polyps, loculated fluid, or scarring. Clinical information is important, as these findings can be misinterpreted as tumor, especially if bony septa have been surgically removed.

Normal aeration of the maxillary sinuses occurs in approximately 20% of maxillary antra following a Caldwell–Luc procedure and they may be partially aerated in a much greater proportion. Certain chronic changes have been noted to occur following surgery. These include fibro-osseous proliferation, antral contraction, and compartmentalization.

Fibro-osseous proliferation is thought to be secondary to the resorption of both blood and epithelium as well as to the degree of re-epithelialization. CT shows opaque thickening of the bony walls of the maxillary sinus.

Antral contraction may be associated with depression of the orbital floor and with lateralization of the lateral nasal wall with consequent enlargement of the ipsilateral nasal cavity. Fibro-osseous proliferation may also occur. Postoperative compartmentalization is an uncommon occurrence and is considered to be due to an altered tissue response during the healing process.

Both the inferior meatal antrostomy and the sublabial antrostomy may present evidence of bony irregularity. The sublabial antrostomy usually closes with fibrous tissue or new bone, although it may persist in rare cases as an oroantral fistula.

Recurrent disease in the maxillary antrum following a Caldwell–Luc procedure may be difficult to identify radiologically, because it has a similar appearance to fibrosis of the antrum. Air–fluid levels or total opacification of a previously aerated antrum are suggestive of recurrent disease. Complications following a Caldwell–Luc procedure are uncommon, although osteomyelitis and osteomas have been reported. Early complications include injury to the infraorbital nerve, dental root damage, injury to the floor of the orbit, and injury to the optic nerve or globe.

Late complications include mucocele formation, which may occur many years following surgery. CT reveals homogeneous, smooth expansion and opacification of the maxillary sinus, with thinning and occasional dehiscence of the bony margins of the antrum.

ETHMOIDECTOMY

The surgical approaches to the ethmoid sinuses are many and varied. A brief description of the more commonly performed procedures follows. The radiological features are similar in each case, with variations in the bony defects dependent on the approach used. The radiographic features are summarized together.

TRANSNASAL ETHMOIDECTOMY (Figure 10.11)

Indication

Multiple ethmoid polyps.

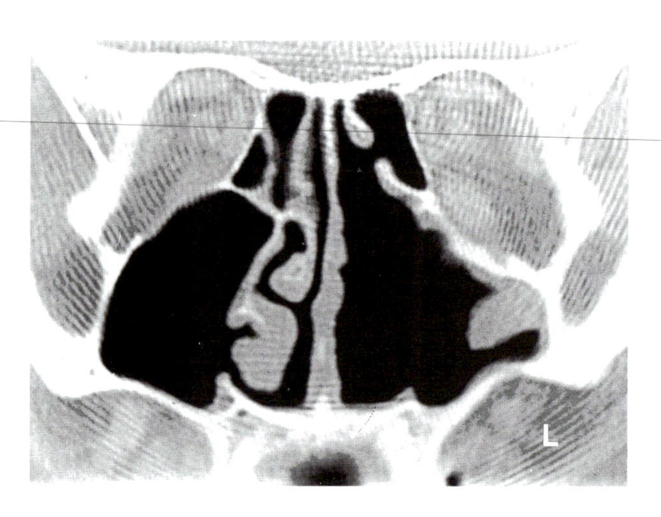

Figure 10.11 *Intranasal ethmoidectomy with exenteration of the lateral nasal wall.* Coronal CT scan demonstrating the defect following resection of the lateral nasal wall and intranasal ethmoidectomy. The resulting surgical defect allows the entire maxillary sinus to open into the empty and capacious nasal cavity.

Technique

This was the standard approach to the ethmoid sinuses before the advent of endoscopic sinus surgery. The procedure is carried out with the operative field being viewed directly through a nasal speculum and illumination being derived from a headlight. The middle turbinate is retracted medially, thereby exposing the uncinate process and the bulla ethmoidalis. The bulla is opened and removed, allowing further dissection of the ethmoid labyrinth and excision of diseased mucosa. The posterior ethmoid air cells and the sphenoid may be exposed by this approach. It is more difficult to open the agger nasi cells with this approach.

TRANSANTRAL ETHMOIDECTOMY (Figure 10.12)

Indications

Chronic maxillary and ethmoid sinusitis; orbital decompression.

Technique

This procedure was described by Jansen and Horgan and combines a Caldwell–Luc procedure

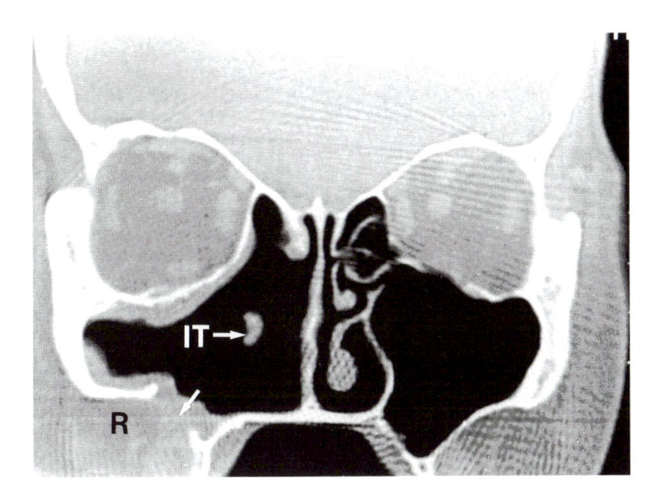

Figure 10.12 *Transantral ethmoidectomy*. Coronal CT scan demonstrating a clean ethmoid cavity following a right transantral ethmoidectomy. There is minimal residual mucosal thickening within the maxillary sinus, which is probably of no clinical significance. The defect in the anterior wall (arrow) represents the sublabial antrostomy. The middle turbinate has been removed. A remnant of the inferior turbinate (IT) appears to be 'floating' in an otherwise large and empty aerated cavity.

with partial clearance of the ethmoid labyrinth. A sublabial or radical antrostomy is performed. Forceps are then directed upwards and medially through the ethmomaxillary plate, which is located in the superomedial angle of the maxillary sinus, being directed towards the contralateral parietal eminence of the patient. This opening into the posterior ethmoid air cells is then enlarged and the accessible cells are cleared. It is not possible to clear the anterior ethmoid air cells with this procedure.

EXTERNAL ETHMOIDECTOMY

Indications

Chronic ethmoid sinusitis; recurrent inflammatory nasal polyps; approach to the pituitary fossa.

Technique

This operation was first described by Ferris Smith in 1933. A temporary tarsorrhaphy is performed to protect the cornea. A curved incision is then made in the nasofacial fold onto the nasal bones. The periosteum and lacrimal sac are elevated. The periosteum is then elevated from the superomedial wall of the orbit, the contents of the orbit are retracted laterally, and the anterior ethmoid artery is exposed. The artery is then divided and the lamina papyracea is perforated, creating an opening into the ethmoid air cells. The bony leaflets dividing the air cells are excised and the middle turbinate is then visualized. It is possible to gain access as far posteriorly as the sphenoid sinus.

TRANSORBITAL ETHMOIDECTOMY

Indications

Orbital decompression; orbital trauma.

Technique

This technique was described by Patterson. The incision is placed 1 cm below the infraorbital margin. The orbicularis oculi muscle is divided with the periosteum. The periosteum is then elevated off the floor of the orbit and the lacrimal fossa. Care is taken not to damage the origin of the inferior oblique muscle or the nasolacrimal duct. The lamina papyracea is removed superiorly to the level of the frontoethmoid suture, and the floor of the orbit is removed as far laterally as the infraorbital canal. The frontal and sphenoid sinuses may be entered with this approach.

ENDOSCOPIC SINUS SURGERY

(Figures 10.13 and 10.14)

Current thinking has focused surgery on the ventilation and drainage channels that serve the larger paranasal sinuses, especially the frontal and maxillary sinuses. The removal of disease from the fine clefts of the anterior ethmoid complex to which these channels connect promotes normal ventilation of the paranasal sinuses.

The detail with which the middle meatus can be assessed has increased dramatically with the continued development of CT and endoscopy. It is possible to identify accurately the sites of mucosal disease and anatomical variations that may influence the ventilation and drainage channels, and

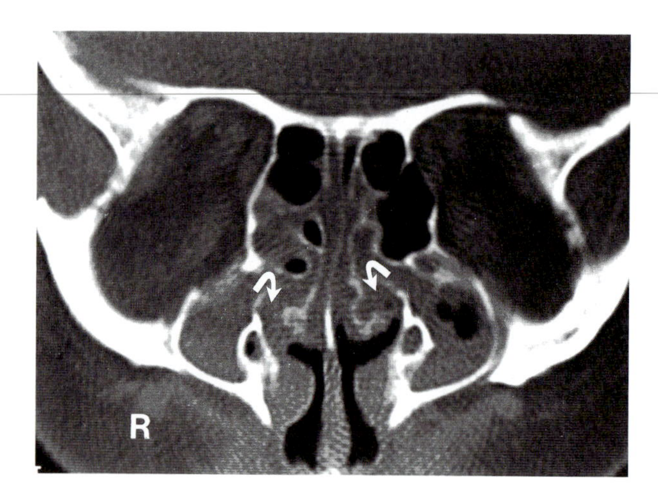

Figure 10.13 *Endoscopic ethmoidectomy: preoperative scan*. Coronal CT scan demonstrating bilateral pansinusitis. Both ostiomeatal complexes are blocked (curved arrows), and secondary infection has occurred in the maxillary sinuses.

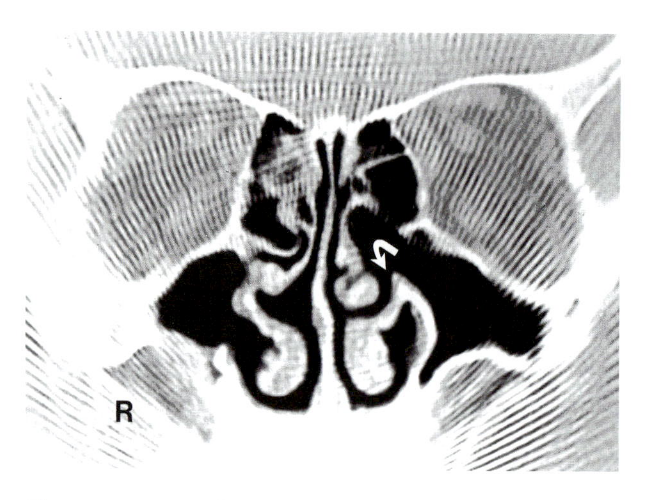

Figure 10.14 *Endoscopic ethmoidectomy: postoperative scan*. Coronal CT scan showing the surgical defect following a left endoscopic ethmoidectomy. The uncinate process has been resected and the natural ostium of the maxillary sinus has been enlarged (curved arrow). Note how the secondary infection within the maxillary sinus has resolved following the restoration of ventilation and drainage.

resect these areas using a precisely targeted, minimally invasive surgical approach.

Indications

Chronic sinusitis; recurrent inflammatory nasal polyposis; frontal, ethmoid, and maxillary sinus mucoceles; biopsy; decompression of subperiostial orbital abscesses.

Technique

Following adequate vasoconstriction, the uncinate process is resected following an incision in the lateral wall of the nasal cavity. The incision is made parallel to the free margin of the uncinate process and the lamina papyracea. This bony leaflet is then elevated and removed, exposing the ethmoid bulla and the depths of the ethmoid infundibulum. It should now be possible to visualize the natural ostium of the maxillary sinus and often that of the frontal recess. Diseased mucosa is then removed under direct vision to ensure that both passages are of adequate caliber. If indicated, the posterior ethmoid air cells may be opened by penetrating the ground lamella of the middle turbinate. Dissection through these air cells leads to the sphenoid sinus, where disease can be removed under direct vision.

RADIOGRAPHIC FINDINGS AFTER ETHMOIDECTOMY

(Figures 10.3, 10.4 and 10.15–10.21)

The ethmoid sinus is best visualized postoperatively using CT with a wide window setting, to allow adequate visualization of any remaining bony septa as well as the interface between soft tissue, bone, and air. The bony leaflets separating the ethmoid air cells are usually absent posterior to the ethmoid infundibulum. The middle turbinate may have been partially or completely resected. Ideally, a remnant of the vertical plate of the middle turbinate remains and acts as an important landmark to indicate the site of the cribriform plate, should revision surgery be needed. In some instances, partial resection of the middle turbinate may cause synechia or collapse against the lateral nasal wall, producing obstruction of the ostiomeatal unit. The posterior horizontal portion of the middle turbinate lies below the posterior ethmoid cells. It may be resected to allow greater access to the sphenoid sinus.

The ideal outcome is a single well-aerated cavity. In the first 6 weeks following surgery, there will be some opacification of the aerated cavity as a consequence of residual blood clot and edema of the remaining soft tissue. At a later stage, persistent opacification may represent scarring. This is usually

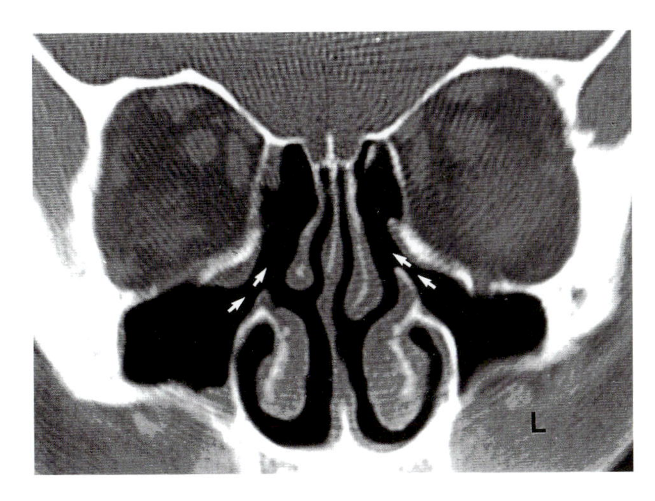

Figure 10.15 *Postoperative scan following intranasal ethmoidectomy.* Coronal CT scan following functional endoscopic sinus surgery showing that a complete bilateral anterior ethmoidectomy has been performed. The ostiomeatal complexes are patent (arrows). The uncinate process has been removed.

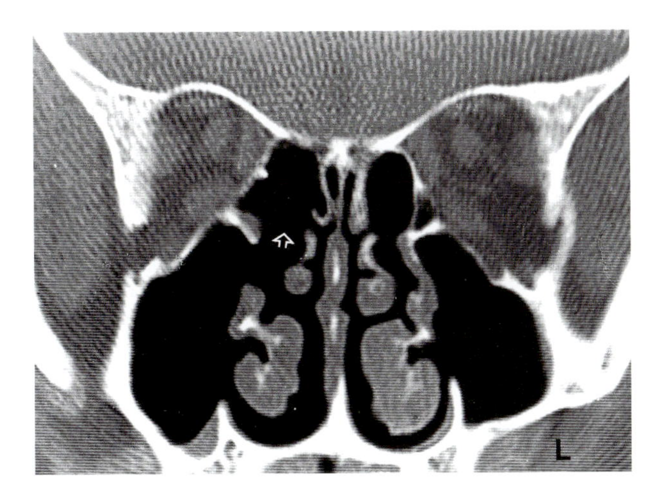

Figure 10.16 *Postoperative scan following intranasal ethmoidectomy.* Coronal CT scan (more posterior scan than Figure 10.15) showing that the right basal lamella has been perforated (open arrow), ventilating the posterior ethmoid air cells with a good result. There is no evidence of recurrent disease. Note the bilateral inferior meatal antrostomies.

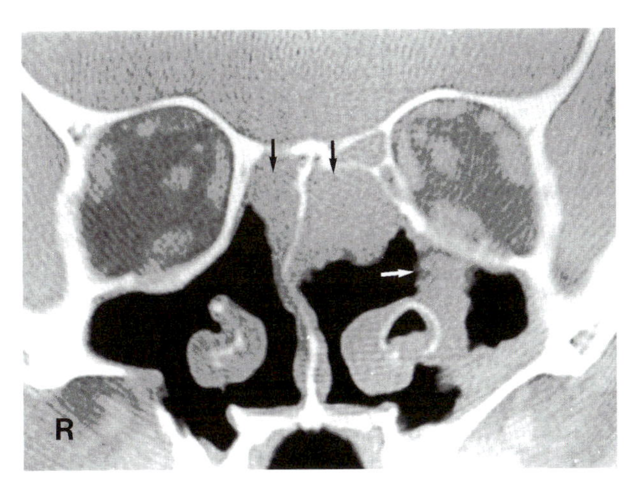

Figure 10.17 *Complete intranasal ethmoidectomy with residual disease.* This patient, with recurrent nasal polyps, had bilateral intranasal ethmoidectomies, bilateral intranasal antrostomies, a right Caldwell–Luc procedure, and resection of both middle turbinates. There is recurrent inflammatory disease in the anterior ethmoid along the roof of the nasal cavity (black arrows). Note the inflammatory tissue blocking the natural ostium of the left maxillary sinus (white arrow) and the mucosal disease within the same sinus.

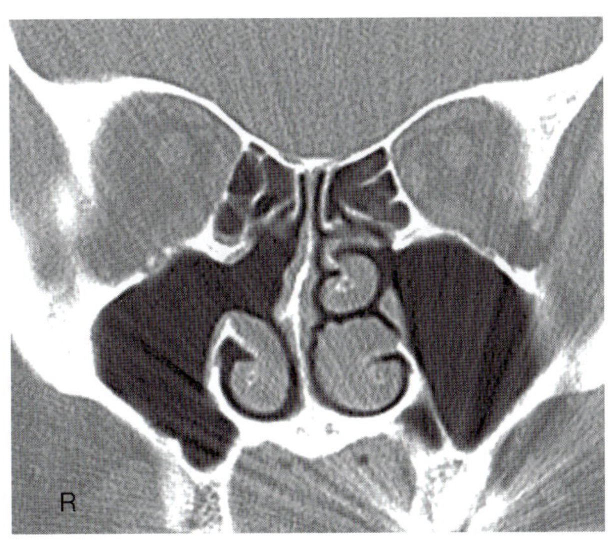

Figure 10.18 *Resection of the middle turbinate.* This patient had a right middle meatal antrostomy with resection of the middle turbinate.

of the same density as muscle and fails to enhance, unlike inflamed mucosa. Scar tissue can appear either as thin strands of tissue filling the sinus lumen or as a solid mass, which may have a nodular appearance.

The lamina papyracea is usually intact following surgery, but it may be breached during the surgical procedure. If the periosteum is incised, orbital fat will prolapse into the ethmoid cavity. There is a risk of this fat being inadvertently removed if revision surgery becomes indicated. The medial wall of the orbit may collapse medially as a late change following surgery. It then reduces the lumen of the surgical defect and reverses the usual convexity of the intact lamina papyracea. This postoperative appearance may be mimicked by an orbital blowout

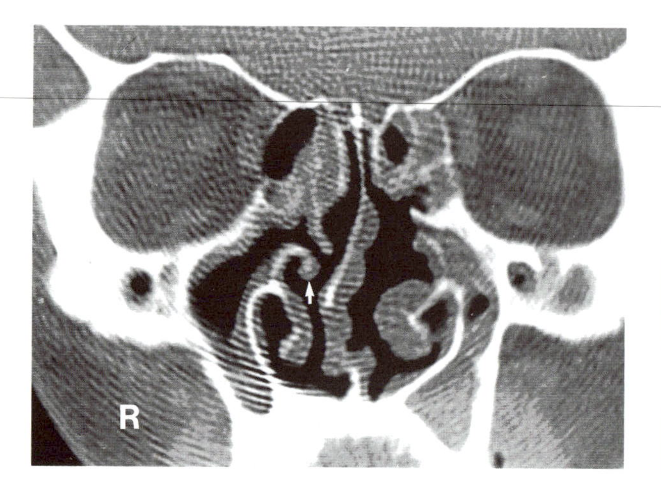

Figure 10.19 *Bilateral incomplete ethmoidectomy with residual disease*. Coronal CT scan demonstrating that the left middle turbinate has been resected and the right middle turbinate has been partially resected. An incomplete ethmoidectomy has been performed. Note the inverted uncinate process (arrow) and the fibrous and osseous proliferation in the left maxillary sinus.

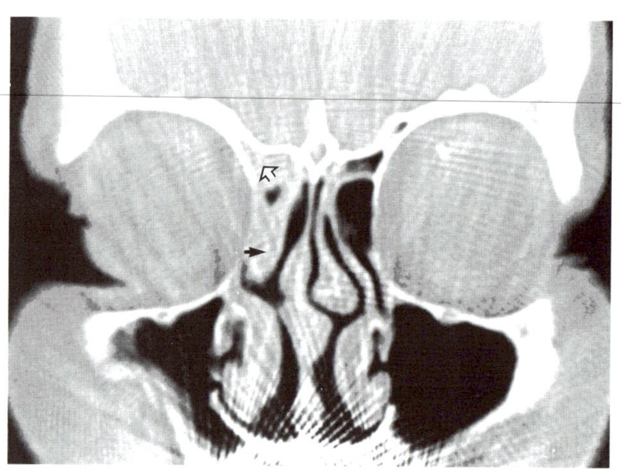

Figure 10.21 *Lateralized middle turbinate*. Coronal CT scan demonstrating lateralization of the right middle turbinate (arrow), which occurred following surgery. Fracture of the vertical insertion of the middle turbinate has resulted in its collapse, with obstruction and disease of the frontal recess (open arrow).

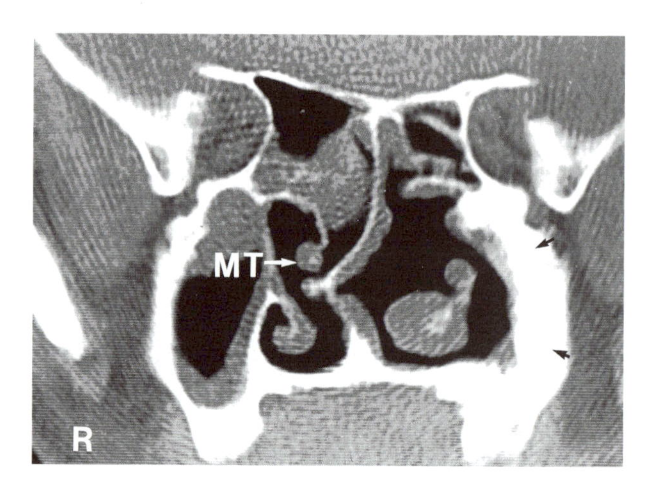

Figure 10.20 *Bilateral incomplete ethmoidectomy with residual disease*. Coronal CT scan (posterior to Figure 10.19), demonstrating that the middle turbinate on the left has been resected. Note the bilateral posterior ethmoid disease and the intact posterior portion of the middle turbinate (MT) on the right. There is marked sclerosis of the lateral wall of the left maxillary sinus (arrows).

fracture or by hypertrophy of the extraocular muscles associated with hyperthyroidism. In the latter situation, the patient may have undergone orbital decompression; if so, the medial portion of the orbital floor will be absent.

Following surgery, the lamina papyracea, the roof of the ethmoid, and any remaining bony septa may become sclerotic. This is usually secondary to reactive osteitis, which on occasion may be extensive enough to obliterate the surgical defect.

The posterior ethmoid air cells are renowned for being a difficult and hazardous area for the surgeon to operate. It is possible for untouched air cells to contain residual disease despite the surgeon's report that all of the posterior cells have been exenterated. Overzealous surgery in this area may cause injury to the surrounding vital anatomical structures, the optic nerve, the eyeball, or even the internal carotid artery.

Following transantral intranasal ethmoidectomy, the postoperative radiological features will include deficits of both the anterior and medial antral walls as well as loss of the fine bony leaflets separating the ethmoid air cells. The lamina papyracea should be intact unless the indication for surgery was to perform an orbital decompression.

Following external ethmoidectomy, a portion of the lamina papyracea will be noted to be absent below the frontoethmoid suture. The surgical defect is usually sharply demarcated, thereby differentiating it from the more gradual reduction of bone thickness caused by an erosive process.

Following transorbital ethmoidectomy for orbital decompression, the bony defect of the lamina papyracea, below the frontoethmoid suture line and the medial half of the orbital floor, will be evident on the images. Orbital fat should prolapse into the defect.

Following endoscopic sinus surgery, bony defects are usually confined to those sinus pre-chambers that were noted to be obstructed during the initial investigations. The entire ethmoid sinus is replaced by a single large space after removal of the intervening septa. This often involves resection of the uncinate process and the ethmoid bulla and the creation of a wide middle meatal antrostomy. Some patients may have undergone more radical surgery previously, and bony defects related to these procedures will remain evident.

FRONTAL SINUS TREPHINATION

(Figure 10.22)

Indication

Acute frontal sinusitis.

Technique

A short incision (1 cm) is made below the medial end of the eyebrow. The floor of the frontal sinus is perforated either with a drill or with a hammer and gouge. The opening is enlarged sufficiently to allow drainage of the purulent secretions and to allow the insertion of an indwelling catheter for frequent irrigation of the sinus. The latter remains in place until the fluid used for irrigation passes through the frontal recess into the nose.

Radiographic findings

The radiographic features should reflect a resolving sinusitis with a small bony defect in the medial part of the floor of the frontal sinus.

10.22a

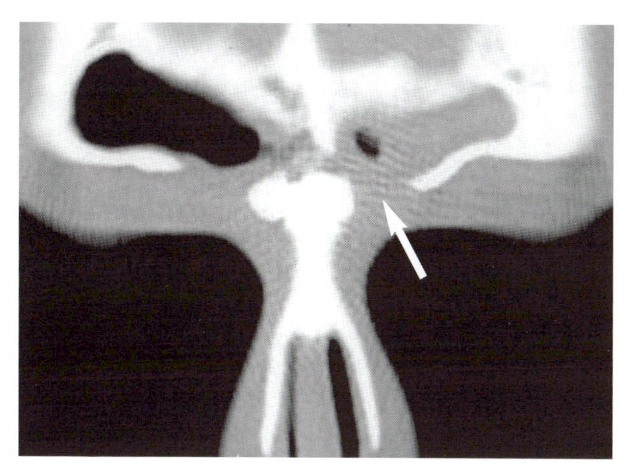

10.22b

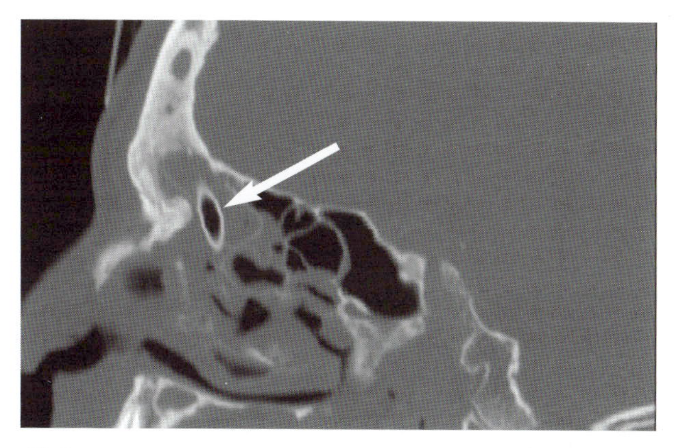

10.22c

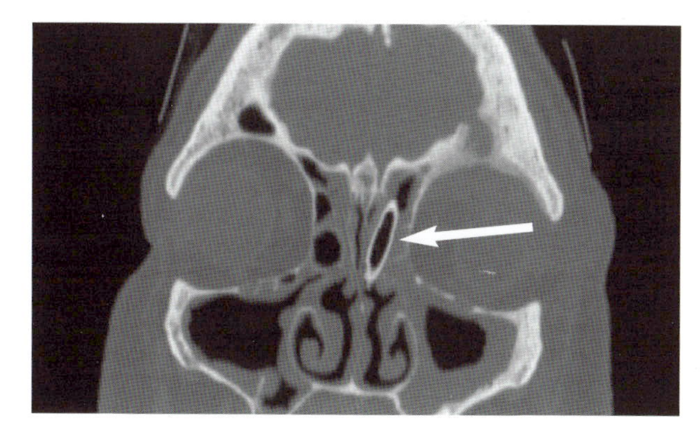

Figure 10.22 *Frontal sinus trephination*. (a) Anterior coronal CT scan demonstrating a defect in the floor of the left frontal sinus following a recent trephination (arrow). The left frontal sinus is opacified as a result of sinusitis. (b, c) A drainage tube is seen in the frontal recess (arrow).

EXTERNAL FRONTOETHMOIDECTOMY

Indications

Chronic frontoethmoid sinusitis; recurrent nasal polyposis; frontoethmoid mucoceles; complicated acute sinusitis; to provide access for transethmoid hypophysectomy, dacrocystorhinostomy, and orbital decompression.

Technique

This procedure was described by both Lynch and Howarth. A temporary tarsorrhaphy is performed to protect the cornea. An incision is placed curving from below the medial margin of the eyebrow to the pass midway between the medial canthus and the bridge of the nose. The procedure is similar to that of an external ethmoidectomy, except that it is extended to include resection of the floor of the frontal sinus and the middle turbinate. A silastic tube is often placed in the widened frontonasal duct to prevent stenosis and can remain in place for up to 3 months.

Radiographic findings

The radiological features are similar to those of an external ethmoidectomy, with additional widening of the frontal recess and excision of the floor of the frontal sinus.

OSTEOPLASTIC FLAP WITH OBLITERATION OF FRONTAL SINUS (Figure 10.23)

Indications

Chronic frontal sinusitis; excision of osteomata; excision of mucoceles; repair of frontal sinus fractures.

Technique

A template of the frontal sinus is cut from a plain radiograph. A bicoronal flap is then elevated and the outline of the frontal sinus is marked onto the frontal bone. The bone of the anterior wall of the frontal sinus is then divided obliquely with a fissure burr and the intersinus septum is divided. The bony flap is then hinged forward on an intact inferiorly based pedicle of periosteum. Meticulous excision of all diseased tissue is essential, and the sinus is obliterated with a free fat graft harvested from the anterior abdominal wall. The osteoplastic flap is then replaced.

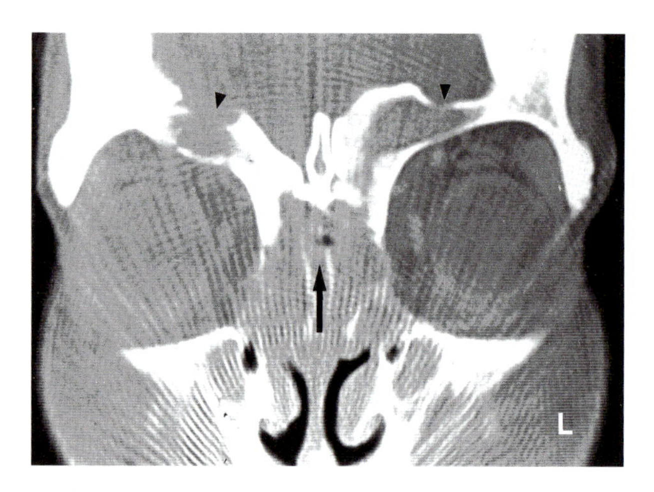

Figure 10.23 *Osteoplastic flap*. Coronal CT scan demonstrating the surgical defect of the osteoplastic flap used for the excision of a frontal sinus mucocele. There are large surgical defects in the roof of the frontal sinus (arrowheads). A small silastic tube is seen displaced medially between the frontal recess and the nasal septum (arrow).

Radiographic findings

Images of the frontal sinus following surgery will appear opaque. The outline of the sinus is often visible where the bone has been divided. In these patients, because of the opacity, it can often be extremely difficult to distinguish changes that may occur as a consequence of recurrent disease. There are a variety of different normal appearances on CT that represent different stages of fibrosis of the obliterating fat graft. The bone flap should be examined with wide window settings. This will also demonstrate the air-free frontal sinus. The sinus may appear to be air-filled if it is only examined with narrow window settings. Ideally, the bone flap should have smooth edges and be aligned with the surrounding bone. With narrow-window examinations, the fat should demonstrate a streaky appearance. This represents fibrosis in the graft. Complications include osteomyelitis of the bone flap, infection of the fat graft, and mucocele formation. If the patient presents with recurrent symptoms, care must be taken to exclude inflammatory disease in the other paranasal sinuses. If a bony complication has developed, CT is of greater value in demonstrating the lesion than MRI. The bone flap may be seen to be elevated or rotated, and there may be bone erosion or sequestrum formation. If the fat graft becomes infected, it appears of a similar density to soft tissue rather than fat and the changes may become localized. If intracranial or intraorbital complications occur, they may be better visualized by MRI.

LATERAL RHINOTOMY (Figure 10.11)

Indications

Excision of inverted papilloma and other localized tumors.

Technique

This procedure was first described in 1902 by Moure. The incision extends from the midpoint between the medial canthus and the bridge of the nose, along the natural skin crease of the nasojugal fold, around the ala of the nostrils, and into the philtrum of the upper lip. The anterior bony wall is exposed from the infraorbital canal of the maxilla to the frontoethmoid suture line. The lateral wall of the nose is excised en bloc as follows. Incisions are made: (1) along the floor of the nose into the maxillary antrum; (2) through the anterior wall of the maxillary antrum below the inferomedial angle; (3) through the nasal bone up to the level of the frontonasal suture line that demarcates the level of the cribriform plate. (4) The ethmoidal arteries are ligated and the frontoethmoid suture line is divided to the posterior ethmoid artery (the limit of safety to avoid damage to the optic nerve). (5) The orbital rim is divided with the lamina papyracea, and the lateral wall is removed in one piece. The amount of maxilla resected can be tailored depending on the pathology being treated and the extent of the disease.

Radiographic findings

The radiographic deficit includes the absence of the medial wall of the orbit extending from the infraorbital canal to the frontoethmoid suture line. A large nasoantral cavity is formed following the removal of the entire lateral wall of the nose, including the middle and inferior turbinates.

MAXILLECTOMY

Indication

Malignancy involving the maxillary antrum.

Technique

The incision used is similar to that used for a lateral rhinotomy, but it is extended along the margin of the lower lid, if the globe is being preserved, or along the margin of both eyelids if the orbit is to be exenterated. The hard palate is divided in the midline; the orbital floor is then dissected free, depending on the extent of disease; the zygoma is divided; the lateral wall of the nose is divided below the frontoethmoid suture line; and finally the pterygoid plates of the sphenoid are separated from the posterior aspect of the maxilla.

Radiographic findings

The postoperative appearance will depend on whether a partial or total maxillectomy has been undertaken. If the maxilla is removed in its entirety, the pterygoid plates usually remain and may be identified on the images. Usually, there is a clearly defined cavity that is sharply demarcated. Recurrent disease is indicated by the development of a soft tissue mass or further bony erosion.

SPHENOIDOTOMY (Figure 10.24)

Indication

Treatment of chronic sphenoid sinusitis or mucocele; to gain access to the pituitary fossa for hypophysectomy.

Technique

Traditionally, the sphenoid sinus has be entered following external ethmoidectomy or via a transseptal approach. Current approaches include via endoscopic ethmoidectomy or directly through the anterior wall of the sphenoid sinus. The sphenoid sinus, if entered from the posterior ethmoid sinuses, is found inferior and medial to the posterior wall of the latter. If directly approached from the nasal cavity, the sphenoid sinus ostium is identified in the sphenoethmoid recess in close proximity to the nasal

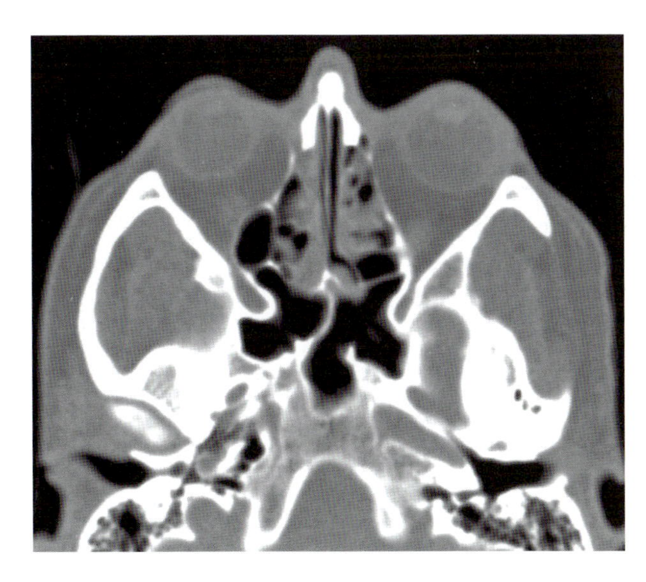

Figure 10.24 *Sphenoidotomy*. There is a defect in the anterior wall of the sphenoid sinus, which was entered via a transnasal approach.

septum, above the level of the posterior end of the middle turbinate. The ostium can be entered and bone adjacent to the ostium can be removed with a mushroom punch or bone nibbler. Care must be taken not to put traction on the intersinus septum, which is frequently attached in the vicinity of the internal carotid artery.

Radiological features

The radiological features will represent deficient bone at the anterior face of the sphenoid sinus. As with other surgical sites, healing can be accompanied by bony and soft tissue occlusion.

COMPLICATIONS FOLLOWING PARANASAL SINUS SURGERY

There are numerous neurovascular structures bordering the paranasal sinuses that are at potential risk of injury during surgery. The task of the surgeon is also complicated by variations in anatomy and pneumatization that may be misleading, or by anatomical landmarks that may be disguised by disease. Serious complications are rare, but may occur at the hands of the most experienced and well-trained surgeons. Prompt recognition of a complication and its appropriate management should allow the optimum conditions for recovery.

The complications of sinus surgery are classified into minor and major complications. (Table 10.1). Complications most commonly occur following intranasal polypectomy, intranasal ethmoidectomy, and sphenoidotomy. The risks are greater if there has been prior surgery and some of the usual landmarks may have been removed. Complications will be discussed here in relation to the nasal cavity, the orbit and optic nerve, the anterior cranial fossa, and the sphenoid sinus relations (the internal carotid artery and the cavernous sinus).

Intranasal hemorrhage
(Figures 10.25 and 10.26)

Intranasal hemorrhage is a common problem following intranasal procedures. This is usually controlled with an intranasal pack, which may be left in place for up to 48 hours. Plain gauze packs have a characteristic appearance if left in place during a postoperative CT scan. Some surgeons

Table 10.1 Complications following paranasal sinus surgery

Minor complications

Early complications
- Postoperative bleeding
- Hematoma
- Orbital emphysema

Late local complications
- Scarring and synechiae
- Mucocele
- Scarring, with obstruction of ventilation and drainage pathways

Major complications

Orbital complications
- Blindness from retrobulbar hematoma causing proptosis and stretching of optic nerve
- Injury to the lacrimal apparatus
- Ocular trauma
- Diplopia following injury to the extraocular muscles or orbital fat
- Optic nerve injury

Intracranial complications
- Cerebrospinal fluid rhinorrhea
- Intracranial hemorrhage
- Internal carotid artery injury
- Anosmia
- Brain injury
- Intracranial infection, brain abscess, and meningitis

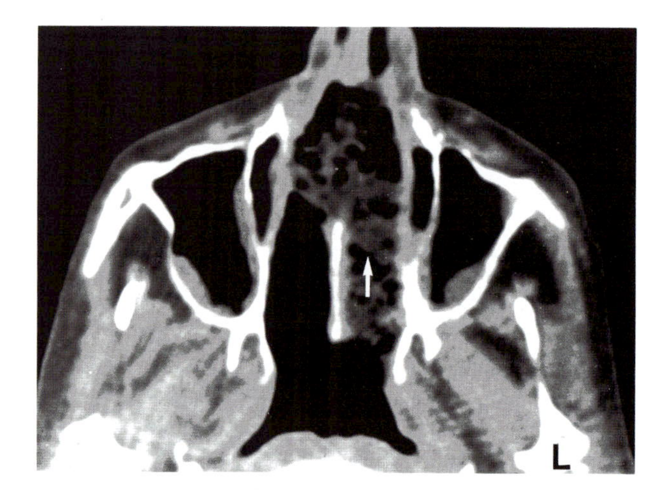

Figure 10.25 *Gauze nasal pack*. CT scan demonstrating an area filled irregularly with air and soft tissue (arrow). A gauze pack, used to control epistaxis, is present. It should not be mistaken for inflammatory disease. This patient had had a radical ethmoidectomy in the past.

prefer to use ribbon gauze that has been impregnated with bismuth–iodoform–paraffin paste (BIPP). The heavy metal bismuth will cause widespread artifact if left in place during a postoperative scan. Even following removal of the pack, small deposits of the bismuth paste will remain as small dense areas.

Late local complications

(Figures 10.1, 10.21, and 10.27–10.29)

Some late local complications include synechiae (adhesions), collapse of the lateral wall of the nose, and lateralization of the middle turbinate causing obstruction of the frontal recess. Other late

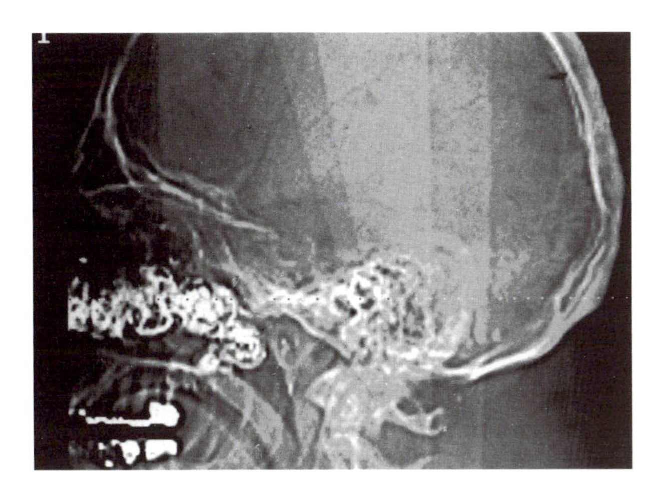

Figure 10.26 *BIPP pack*. Lateral CT view of the skull showing the radio-opaque mass of a bismuth–iodoform–paraffin paste (BIPP) intranasal pack, placed *in situ* postoperatively to control hemorrhage.

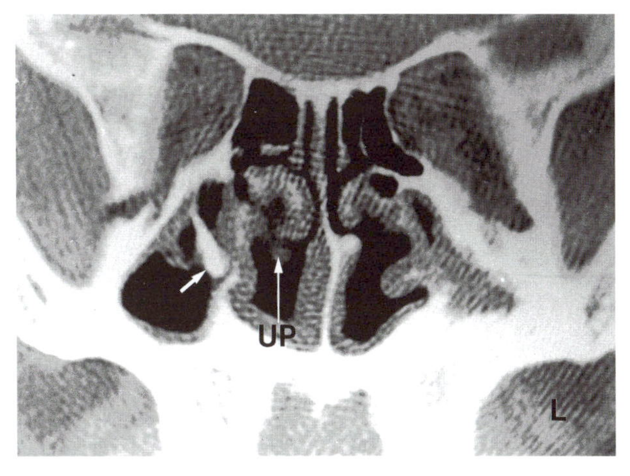

Figure 10.28 *Fracture of the lateral nasal wall*. Coronal CT scan demonstrating that the inferior turbinates have been resected too close to the lateral nasal wall (arrow). The lateral nasal wall has fractured and been displaced laterally, causing occlusion of the ostiomeatal complex and associated scarring and deformity of the partially resected inferior turbinate and uncinate process (UP).

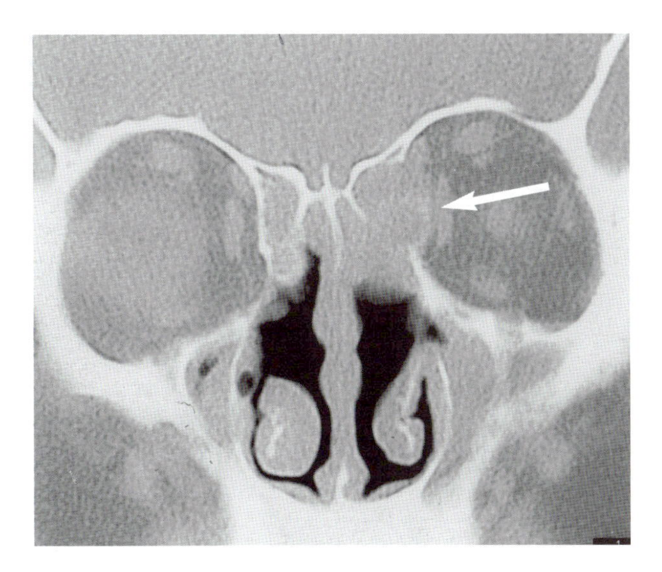

Figure 10.27 *Recurrent nasal polyp and mucocele*. This patient had undergone multiple intranasal polypectomies. The soft tissue mass filling the upper half of each nasal cavity represents recurrent polyps and a mucocele in the left side (arrow). In these patients, the scan is primarily of use to the surgeon in identifying any remaining bony structures, and in demonstrating any potential danger areas such as dehiscences of the orbital wall.

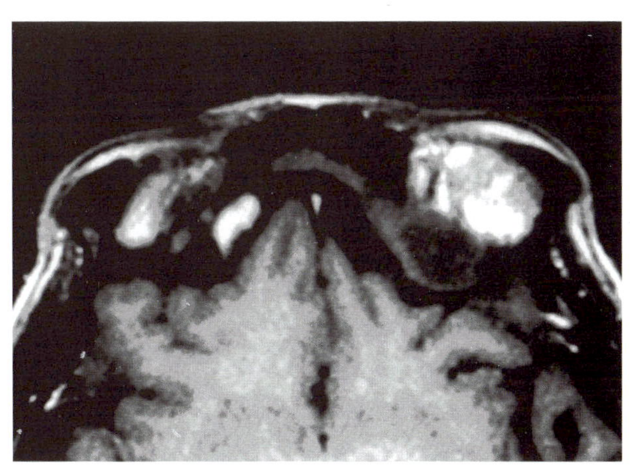

Figure 10.29 *Frontal sinus mucocele*. Axial T1-weighted MRI scan demonstrating a hypointense mass in the left orbit. This was a frontal sinus mucocele, which developed as the result of an unsuccessful obliterative procedure on the left frontal sinus.

10.30a

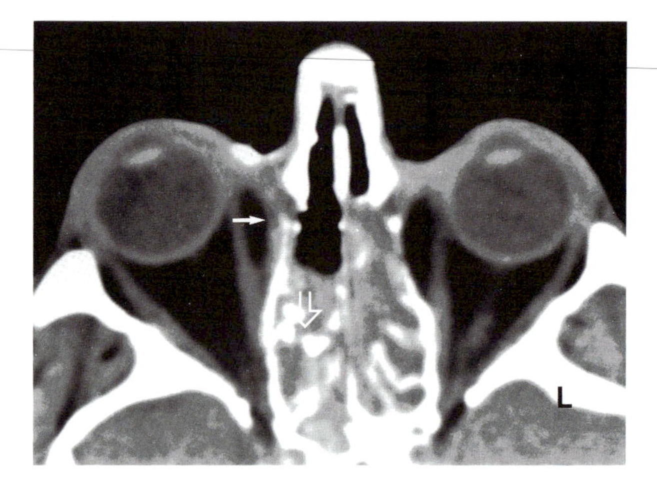

10.30b

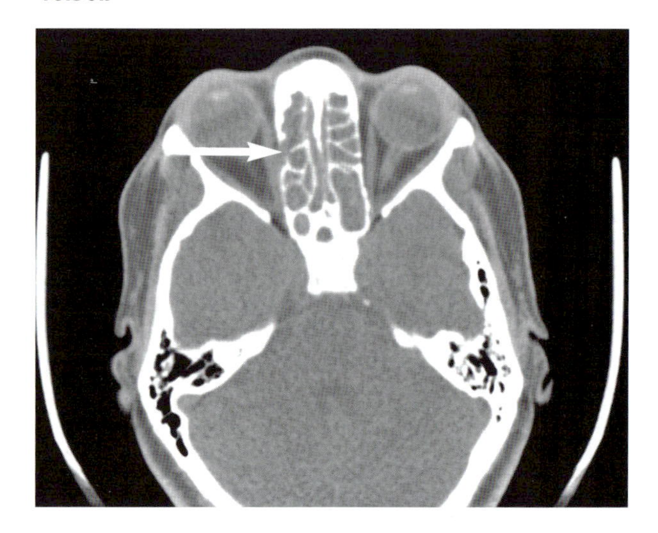

Figure 10.30 (a) *Breach of the lamina papyracea and subperiosteal intraorbital hemorrhage*. Axial CT scan demonstrating a small subperiosteal hematoma that followed breach of the lamina papyracea during intranasal ethmoidectomy (arrow). The radio-opaque material in the nasal cavity is BIPP remaining from an intranasal pack that was placed postoperatively (open arrow). (b) *Breach of the lamina papyracea and tethering of medial rectus muscle*. There is a small defect in the lamina papyracea and increased density in the medial orbital fat as a result of bleeding with tethering of the medial rectus muscle (arrow).

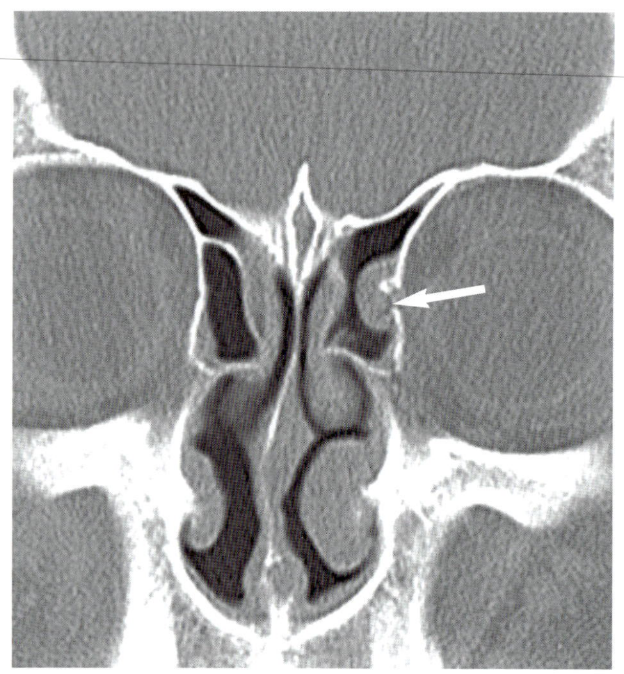

Figure 10.31 *Defect of the lamina papyracea*. Coronal CT scan demonstrating orbital fat prolapsing through a defect in the left lamina papyracea (arrow), following ethmoidectomy.

complications include mucocele formation as a result of compartmentalization and obstruction to drainage.

Orbital complications

(Figures 10.30–10.39)

Orbital complications include blindness and diplopia following injury to the optic nerve, extraocular muscles, or orbital fat. The commonest cause of blindness is a retrobulbar hematoma causing proptosis and stretching of the optic nerve. Rapid decompression of the hematoma, either endonasally or externally, may preserve optic function. Bilateral blindness has been reported following bilateral retro-orbital hematoma and also following bilateral optic nerve section. The optic nerve is particularly at risk if there is a large Onodi cell extending laterally around the nerve from the posterior ethmoid air cells. Hematoma will become evident on CT following administration of intravenous contrast. Optic nerve section becomes apparent on visualizing the injured segment of the nerve.

The lamina papyracea may be injured during intranasal ethmoidectomy. This more commonly occurs when the uncinate process is resected to facilitate middle meatal antrostomy. Portions of the lamina papyracea may be inadvertently avulsed with nasal polyps. If the orbital periosteum is breached, orbital fat will prolapse into the nasal cavity. Subperiosteal hematoma presents with periorbital ecchymosis and proptosis. CT will demonstrate an enhancing lesion running alongside the medial orbital wall. The orbit may also be accidentally injured during a transantral ethmoidectomy, when the orbital floor may be breached if it is mistaken for the ethmomaxillary plate.

10.32a

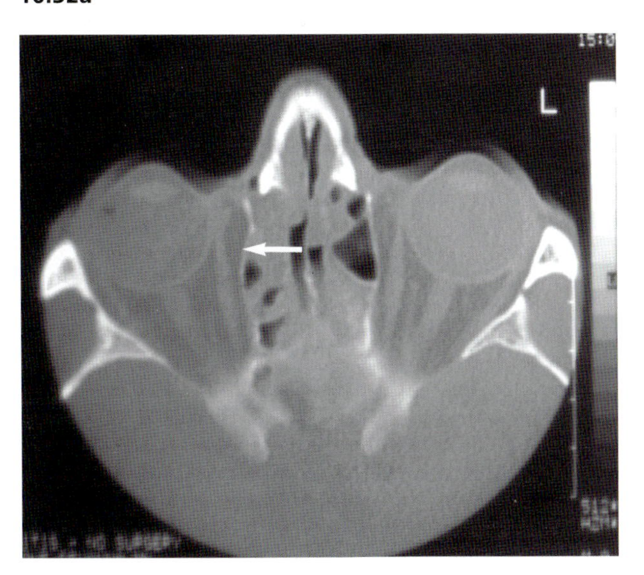

10.32b

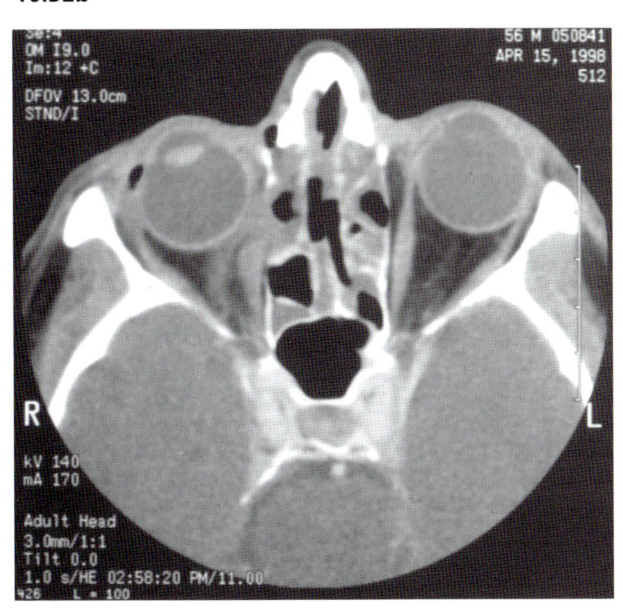

Figure 10.32 *Bisection of medial rectus muscle.* (a) Preoperative CT scan of the sinus demonstrating ethmoid disease. The lamina papyracea is intact (arrow). (b) Postoperative CT scan demonstrating that the medial rectus muscle has been bisected. There is tethering of the muscle to the medial wall of the orbit.

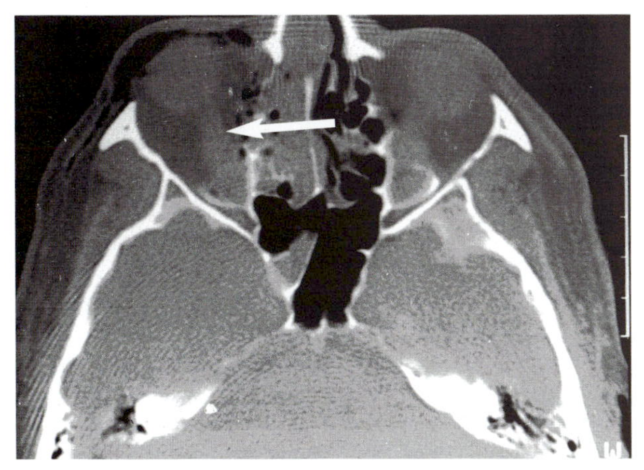

Figure 10.33 *Orbital emphysema.* Axial CT scan demonstrating air in the orbit of a patient who developed proptosis immediately following endoscopic sinus surgery (arrow).

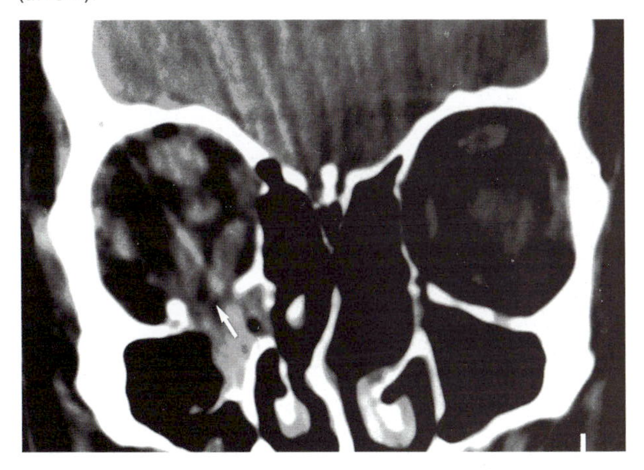

Figure 10.34 *Intraoperative orbital injury.* Coronal CT scan showing the site at which the surgeon fractured through the floor of the orbit (arrow). The higher density of the right orbital contents results from intraorbital bleeding. Note the small bubble of air in the superior aspect of the orbit.

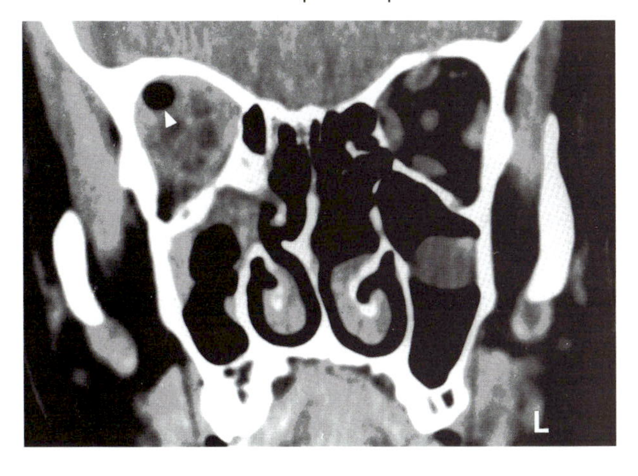

Figure 10.35 *Intraoperative orbital injury.* Coronal CT scan (more posterior than Figure 10.34), demonstrating the orbital emphysema more clearly in the superior aspect of the orbit (arrowhead). The effect of hemorrhage causes higher density and streakiness of the right orbital fat contents.

10.36a

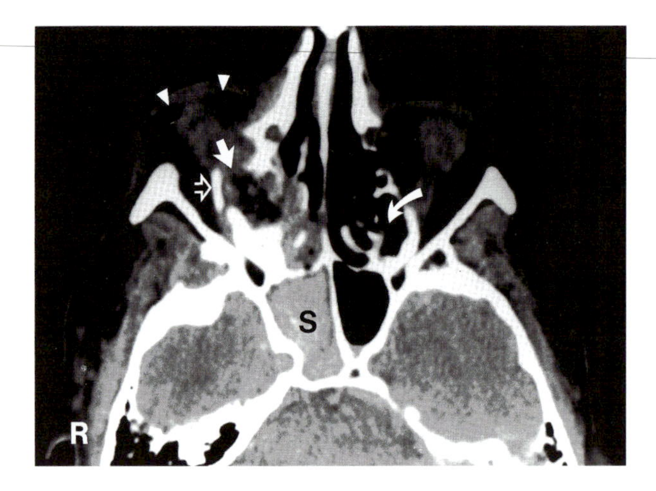

10.36b

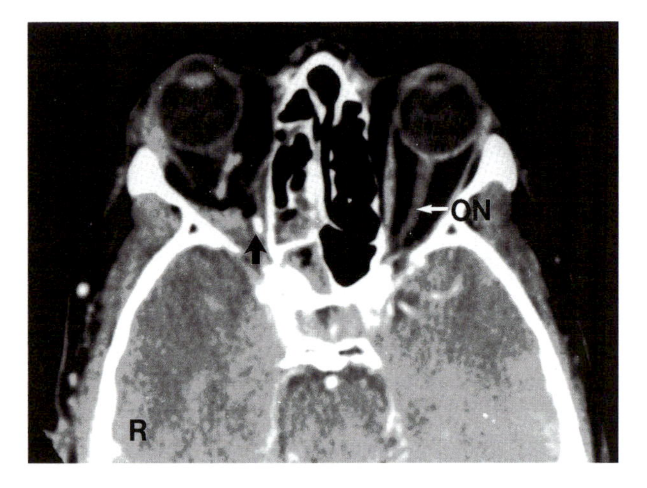

Figure 10.36 *Intraoperative orbital injury.* (a) Axial CT scan of the same patient as in Figures 10.34 and 10.35 again demonstrating orbital emphysema (arrowheads). The optic nerve has been transected (white arrow) by a large displaced portion of the lateral wall of the superior recess of the maxillary sinus (open arrow) through which the orbit was entered. The normal left superior recess of the maxillary sinus is shown (curved arrow). Note the hemorrhage in the sphenoid sinus (S). (b) Axial CT scan clearly showing the difference between the intact optic nerve on the left (ON) and the transected nerve on the right. There is retro-orbital hemorrhage adjacent to a displaced bone fragment (arrow).

Anterior cranial fossa injury (Figures 10.40–10.42)

To avoid injury to the anterior cranial fossa, particular care is needed in dissecting medially to the vertical plate of the middle turbinate. The anterior third of the middle turbinate is attached to the lateral border of the cribriform plate. Accidental avulsion of the middle turbinate may lead to a cerebrospinal fluid (CSF) leak and meningitis. If such an accident occurs and is recognized intraoperatively, then the defect should be repaired immediately. The fovea ethmoidalis, which roofs the ethmoid air cells, is part of the frontal bone. It is thicker than the cribriform plate, but still remains vulnerable to injury. Rocking of the perpendicular plate of the ethmoid should be avoided when excising it during septoplasty.

The site of CSF rhinorrhea can be identified prior to surgical closure by administering 0.2–0.5 ml of 5% sodium fluorescein solution into the spinal canal and positioning the patient with the head down for over 6 hours. This allows the dye to redistribute into the intracranial CSF. The typical yellow–green color of the dye leaking from the defect in the roof of the nasal cavity is easily located. Some centers advocate the administration of intrathecal metrizamide, which is seen on CT images and may identify the site of a leak. Bony defects are well visualized on CT, allowing for accurate targeting of repair.

Sphenoid sinus, cavernous sinus, and carotid artery injury (Figure 10.43)

Careful assessment of the anatomy of the sphenoid sinus and its vascular relations should help to prevent massive intraoperative hemorrhage from internal carotid and cavernous sinus injury. The position of the internal carotid artery can be identified and any bony dehiscences noted prior to commencing surgery. When the surgeon plans to enter the sphenoid sinus, both coronal and axial CT scans should be obtained. Axial CT scans are superior for showing the relationship of the optic nerve to the posterior ethmoid and sphenoid sinuses as well as the relationship of the internal carotid artery to the sphenoid sinus. CT has a greater role to play in the prevention of such catastrophes rather than in their immediate diagnosis and management. Interventional neuroradiologists can successfully use balloon angioplasty to occlude pseudoaneurysms that may developed following endoscopic sinus surgery.

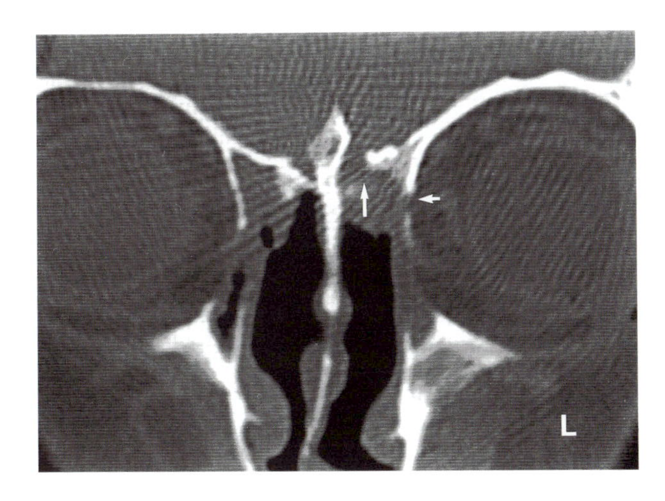

Figure 10.37 *Fracture of the cribriform plate*. Coronal CT scan obtained following bilateral complete intranasal ethmoidectomies. The cribriform plate has been avulsed at the insertion of the left middle turbinate, which was removed during the procedure (arrow). There is also a small defect in the right lamina papyracea (small arrow).

10.38a

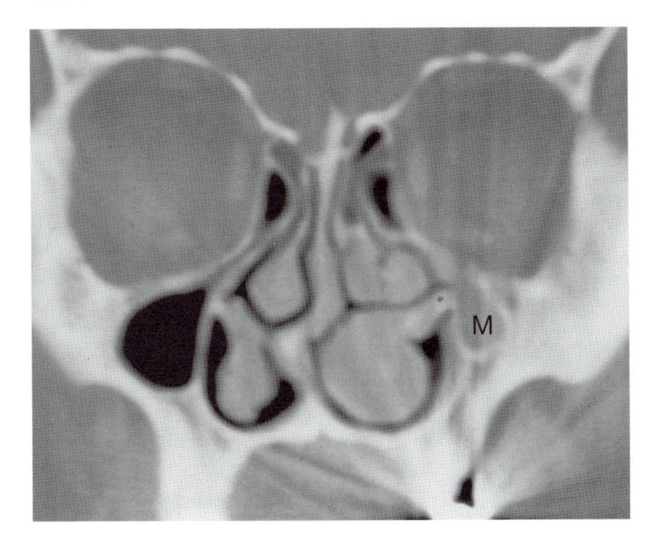

10.38b

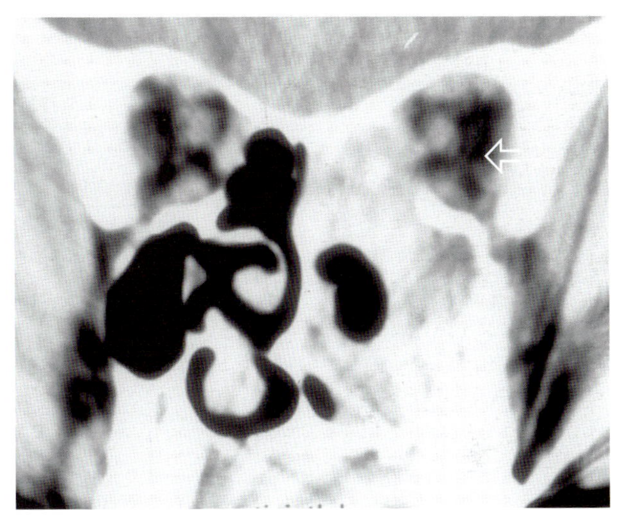

10.38c

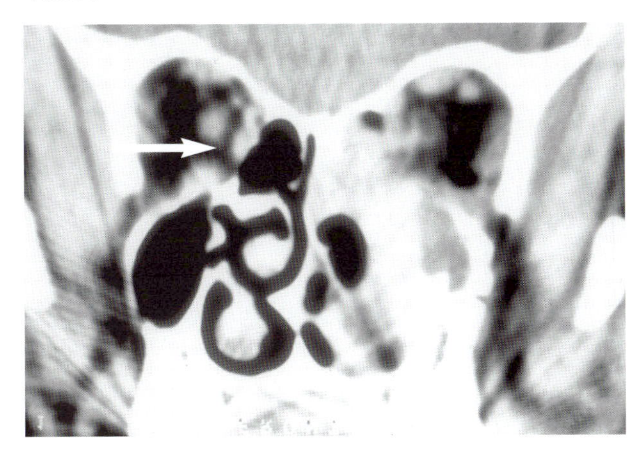

10.38d

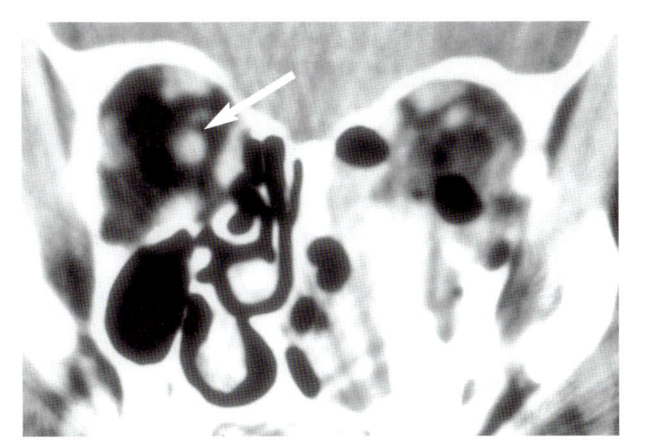

Figure 10.38 *Optic nerve injury*. (a) Preoperative CT scan of the sinus demonstrating left maxillary sinus hypoplasia (M), which is a relative contraindication for sinus surgery. (b) Postoperative CT scan showing orbital emphysema (open arrow) as a result of trauma to the floor of the orbit. (c) CT scan at a different level demonstrating the normal high-density optic nerve on the right side (arrow), while the optic nerve is absent within its covering membrane on the left side. (d) CT scan demonstrating complete severance of the left optic nerve, as it is not visualized in its normal location. The right is noted to be normal.

10.39a

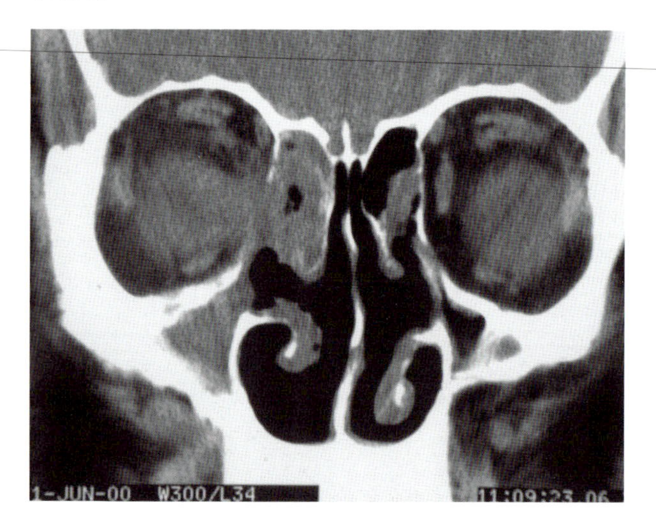

10.39b

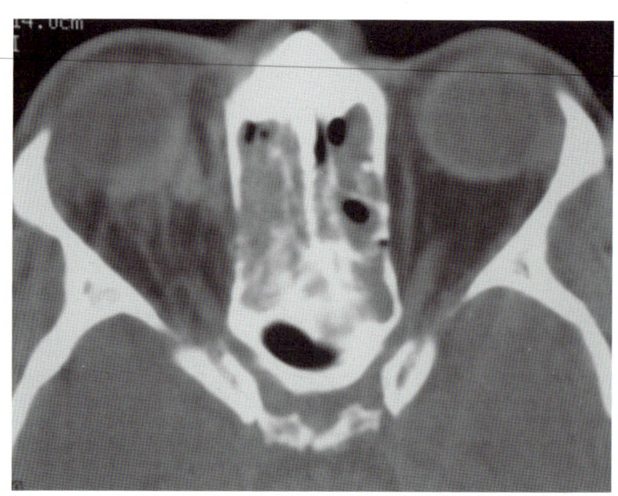

10.39c

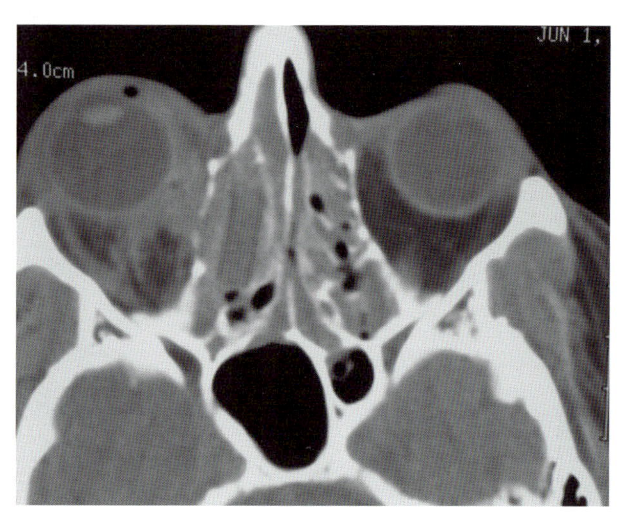

Figure 10.39 *Right ocular injury*. (a) Coronal CT following endoscopic sinus surgery which caused a fracture of the right lamina papyracea and a bleed along the medial wall of the right orbit. (b) Axial CT scan demonstrating injury to the eyeball and medial rectus muscle. (c) Axial CT scan demonstrating the breach in the lamina papyracea and the injury to the medial orbital structure.

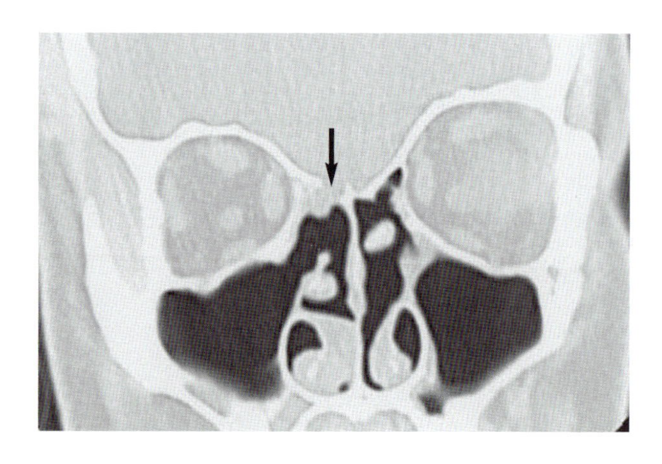

Figure 10.40 *CSF rhinorrhea*. This patient has a history of sinus surgery, following which she presented with a watery secretion from her nose. Her coronal CT scan demonstrates a defect in the right cribriform plate (arrow). This was successfully repaired with a temporalis fascia graft.

10.41a

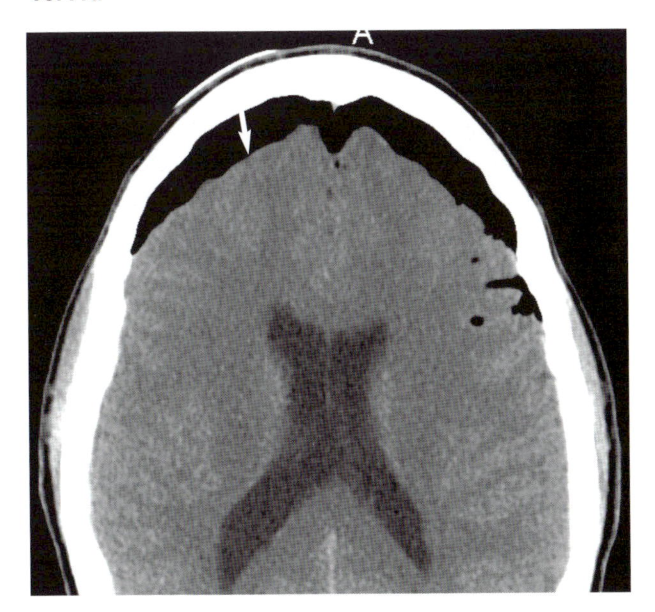

10.41b

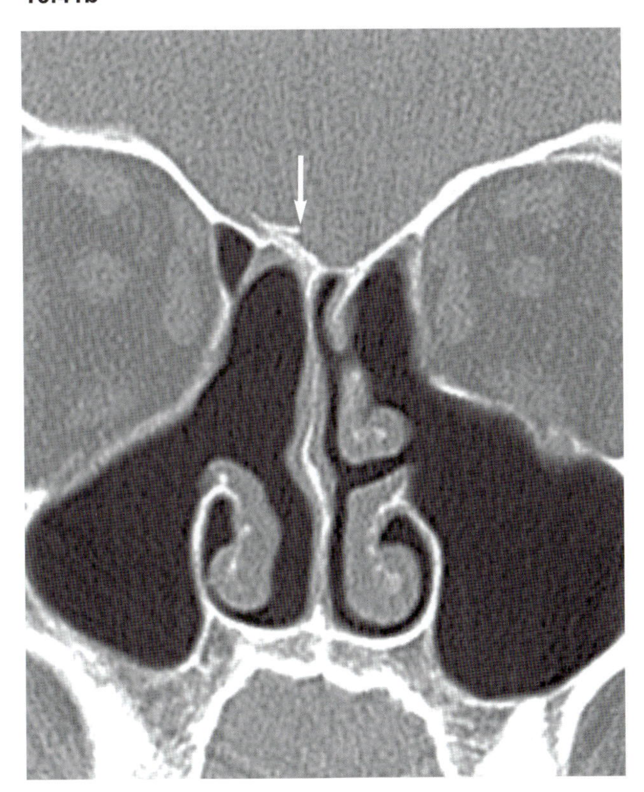

Figure 10.41 *Anterior cranial fossa injury*. (a) Axial CT demonstrating pneumocephalus, a complication of endoscopic sinus surgery, following injury to the floor of the anterior cranial fossa. (b) Coronal CT scan following repair of the defect demonstrates the breach of the floor of the anterior cranial fossa caused by removal of the middle turbinate (arrow).

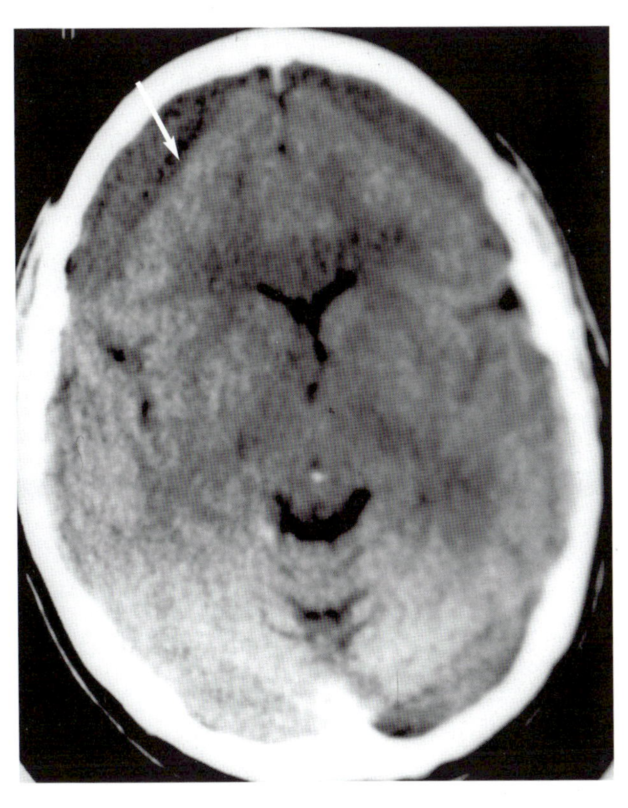

Figure 10.42 *Subdural abscess*. This patient presented with a history of recent sinus surgery and a subdural abscess as a complication of the surgery (arrow).

10.43a

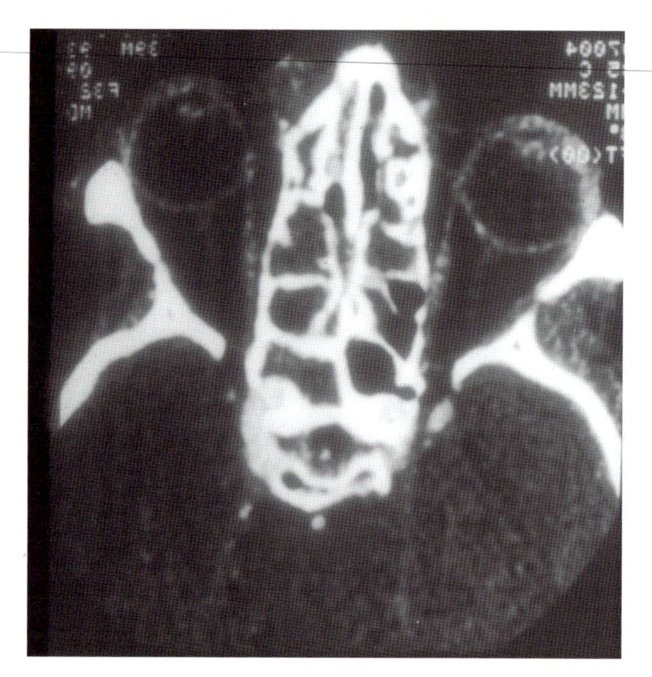

10.43b

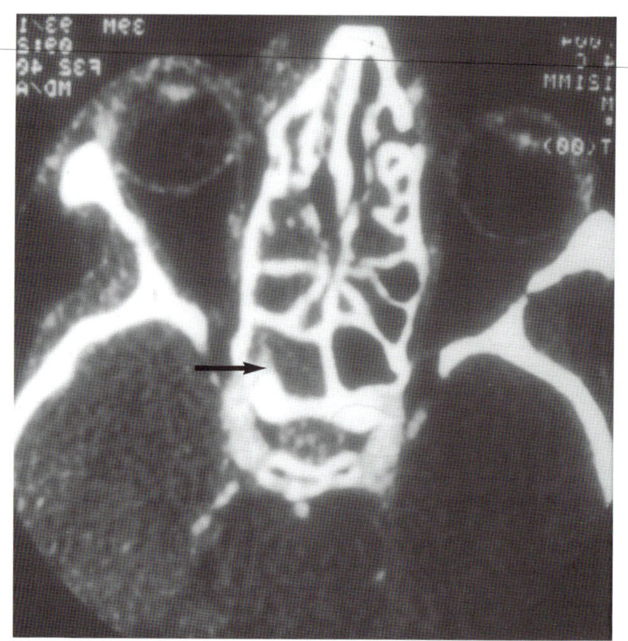

10.43c

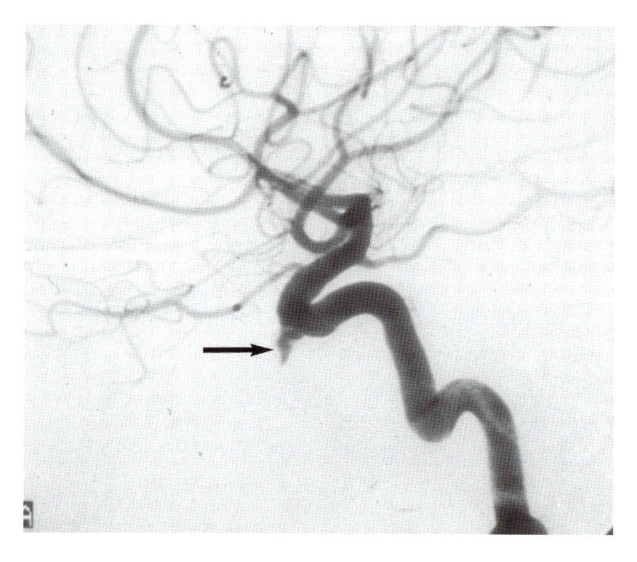

10.43d

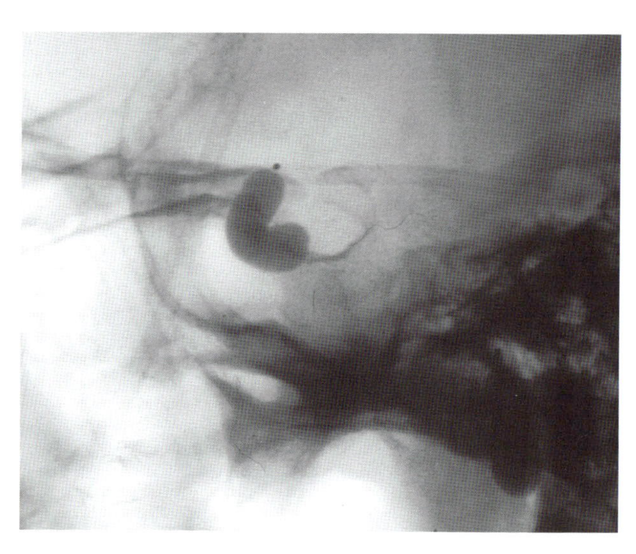

10.43e

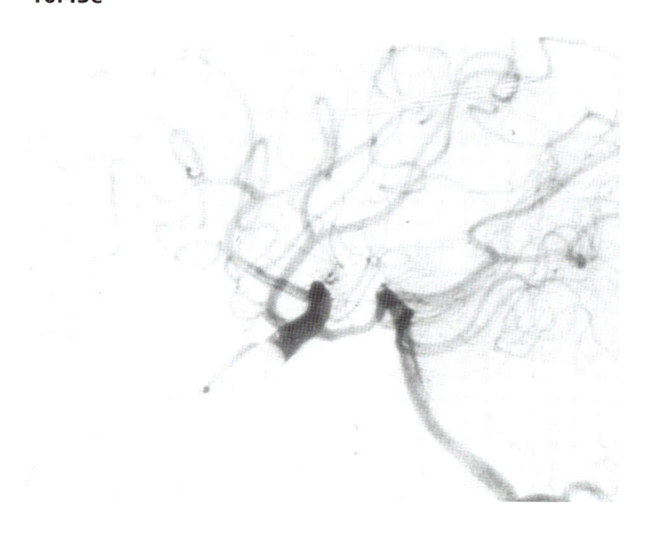

Figure 10.43 *Internal carotid artery aneurysm*. (a–e) The internal carotid artery aneurysm demonstrated is at risk during sphenoid sinus surgery. This patient continued to have fresh arterial bleeding following FESS. The post-operative CT (a,b) demonstrates a strong suggestion of a linear high density in the right ethmoid sinus indicative of aneurysm (arrow). The angiogram (c) confirms a post-traumatic pseudoaneurysm of the ICA (arrow). (d) A balloon has been introduced to occlude the aneurysm. (e) Showing successful occlusion of the ICA pseudoaneurysm (Courtesy of R. Willinsky, UHN, Toronto).

11

Congenital midface and paranasal sinus abnormalities

INTRODUCTION

This chapter discusses congenital midface anomalies, particularly relating to the nasal cavity, nasolacrimal apparatus, and craniofacial syndromes. Most congenital abnormalities of the midface require multiplanar computed tomography (CT). Targeted, small-field-of-view, high-resolution images are obtained. For detailed bony anatomy, direct coronal images are obtained. Sagittal images can be reconstructed from axial scans obtained with submillimeter multislice scanners. Three-dimensional (3D) reconstructions are useful for surgical planning. Magnetic resonance imaging (MRI) is useful to evaluate the extent of soft tissue and potential intracranial extension.

The use of gadolinium contrast with fat suppression is valuable for evaluating soft tissues with MRI. These anomalies are frequently associated with airway narrowing or anomaly, and meticulous care is needed in planning sedation and anesthesia for the necessary imaging studies.

BASIC EMBRYOLOGY OF THE MIDFACE

Craniofacial development follows closure of the anterior neuropore approximately 25 days after conception. Neural crest cells are important in the understanding of the embryology of the face. In most of the body, neural crest cells are involved in forming ectodermal components; however, in the face, neural crest cells primarily form mesenchymal cells, providing bone, cartilage, and the muscles of the face. Neural crest cells from the neural folds migrate from their dorsal position to induce formation of the branchial arch formations along with the pharyngeal endoderm. Neural crest elements along with the first branchial arch give rise to the five prominences that surround the future mouth (stomodeum). The five prominences are: a single midline frontal prominence, paired maxillary prominences, and paired mandibular prominences (Figures 11.1 and 11.2). These prominences are lined by epithelial surfaces. The epithelial surfaces disintegrate by apoptosis, eventually leading to fusion of the prominences. Grooves between the prominences are filled up by migration and proliferation of the subjacent mesenchyme. Failure of disintegration or trapping of epithelium will lead to formation of palatal and facial clefts or cyst formation, along predictable sites (i.e. the nasolabial folds, midline mandible, or globulomaxillary lines).

The frontal prominence forms the median structures of the face, including the forehead, glabella, and nasal bridge. Additionally, the olfactory nerves induce the formation of ectodermal thickenings or nasal placodes at the inferolateral border of the frontal processes at about 3 weeks of age. The lateral and medial limbs of these ectodermal thickenings are called the median and lateral nasal prominences. The inferior tip of the median nasal prominence is called the globular process.

As the maxillary prominences grow, they push the nasal processes superiorly and towards each

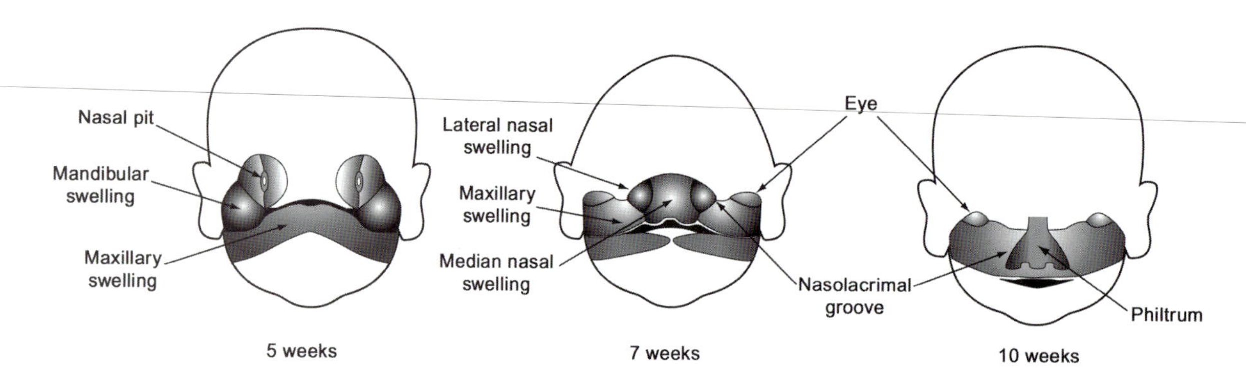

Figure 11.1 *Embryology of facial development.* The facial prominences are fused by 10 weeks of development. The lines of fusion are potential lines of clefting.

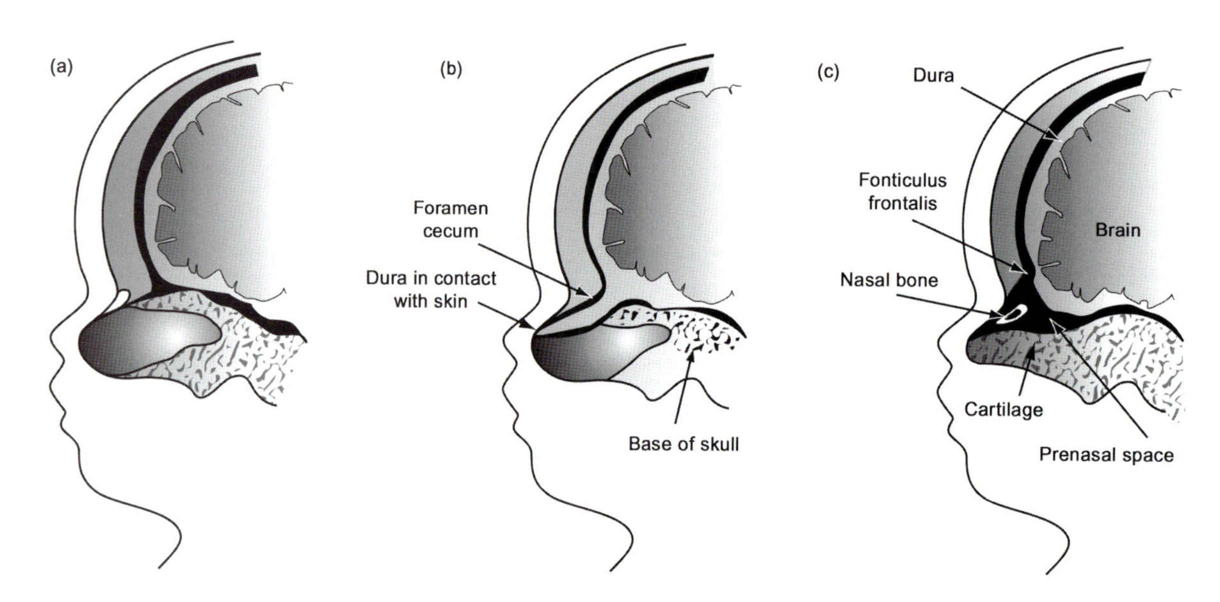

Figure 11.2 *Normal embryological development of the nasofrontal region.* (a) Diagram showing the temporary fonticulus nasofrontalis and prenasal space. (b) Closure of the fonticulus frontalis, formation of the foramen cecum, and a projection of dural diverticulum contacting the tip of the nose. (c) Retraction of the dural diverticulum into the cranium and obliteration of the prenasal space.

other. The nasal prominences subsequently fuse with the frontal prominence to form the frontonasal process. The median nasal prominence and the globular processes then fuse with each other and with the maxillary prominence to form structures around the anterior and inferior aspect of the nose. Surface thickening of the nasal swellings forms the nasal placodes. The placodes invaginate, producing the nasal pits that become the anterior choanae (nostrils) and the primitive posterior choanae. Epithelial plugs initially fill the primitive posterior choanae and are resorbed to form the permanent posterior choanae during the third trimester. The medial nasal and frontal processes give rise to the nasal septum, frontal bones, nasal bones, ethmoid sinus complexes, and upper incisors. The lateral nasal and maxillary processes fuse to form the philtrum and columella (i.e. the septal cartilage at the tip of the nose).

CHOANAL ATRESIA

The posterior choanae connect the posterior nasal cavity with the nasopharynx. Atresia or narrowing of the posterior choanae is a common congenital abnormality, with an incidence of 1 in 5000–8000

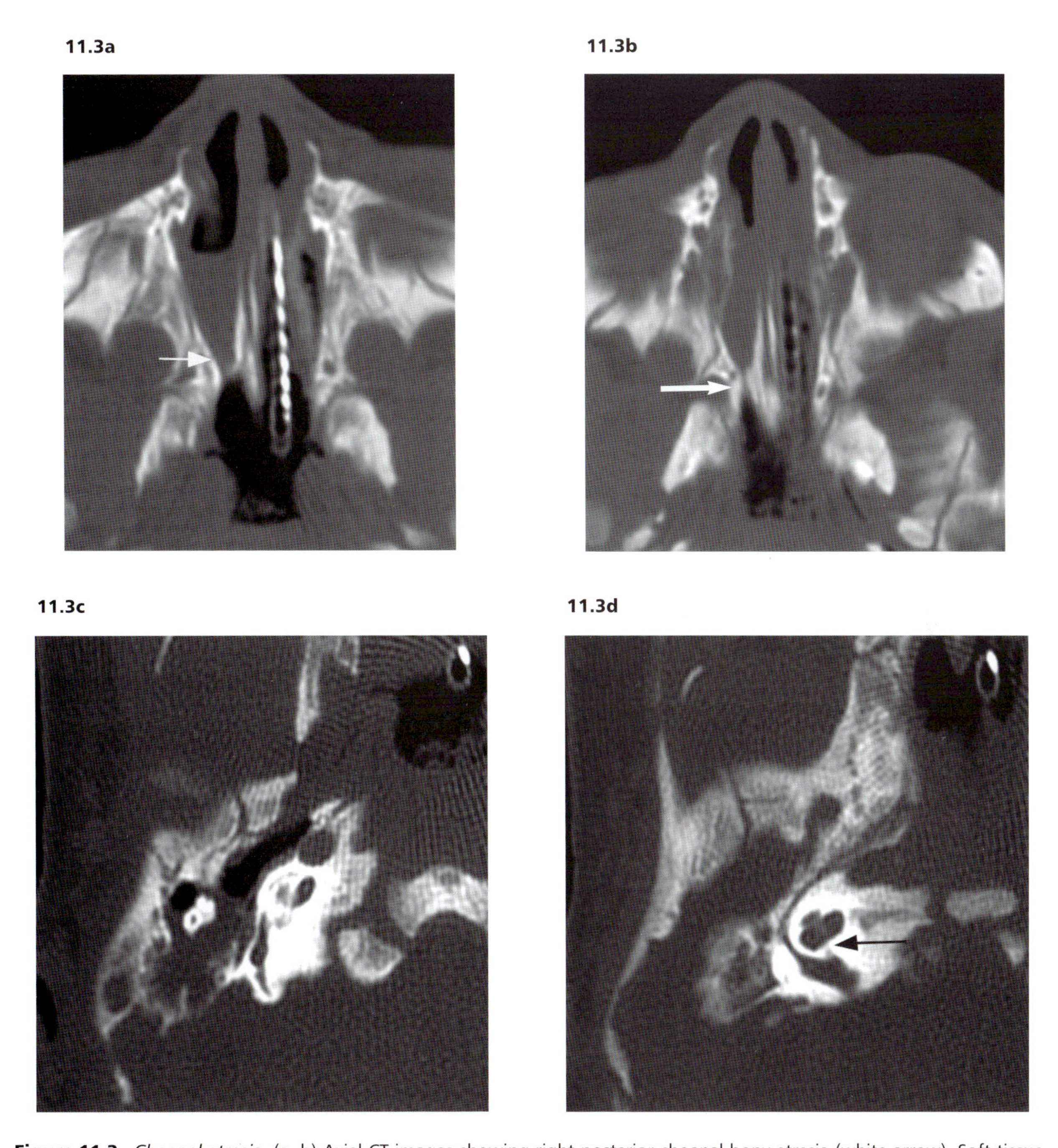

Figure 11.3 *Choanal atresia*. (a, b) Axial CT images showing right posterior choanal bony atresia (white arrow). Soft tissue anterior to the stenosis is membranous component or secretions. (c, d) Axial images through the petrous temporal bone showing absence of the right lateral semicircular canal, and a small cochlear bony canal (black arrow).

newborns. It can be unilateral or bilateral (Figure 11.3).

Bilateral choanal atresia is often associated with other syndromes. Between 50% and 75% of patients have associated congenital malformations, which may include the CHARGE association (colobomas, heart disease, atresia of choanae, retarded growth, genital abnormalities, and ear anomalies) (Figure 11.4), Crouzon's syndrome, Apert's syndrome, Treacher Collins syndrome, facial dysmorphism, fetal alcohol syndrome, and gastrointestinal anomalies. Stenosis is more common than true atresia, and bony atresia is more common than membranous atresia. Atresia results from failure of absorption of the oronasal membrane, which restricts local growth. An alternative theory to

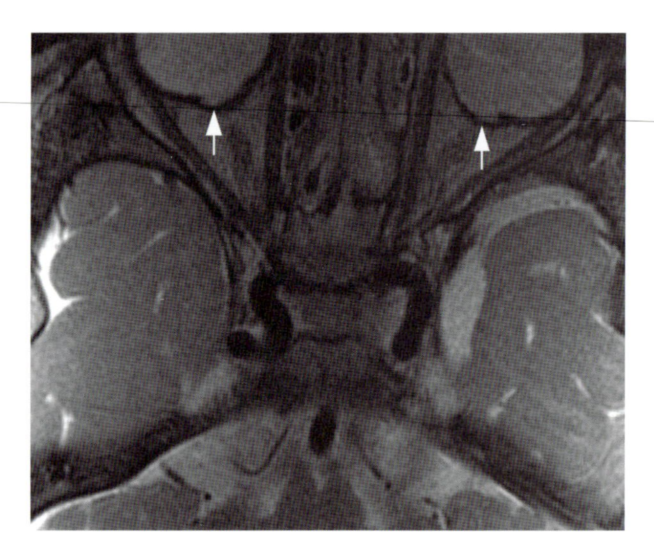

Figure 11.4 *CHARGE syndrome*. Axial T2-weighted MRI in the same child as in Figure 11.3 showing bilateral colobomas (arrows).

explain the pathogenesis of choanal atresia is the abnormal migration of neural crest cells to form the skull base/nasal cavities.

The characteristic finding on CT images is of a thick, club-shaped vomer. The vomer is abnormal if its width is more than 0.34 cm in children under the age of 8 years and more than 0.55 cm in those over 8 years. The posteromedial part of the maxilla and perpendicular plate of the palatine bone are often medially deviated and may be fused with the lateral margins of the vomer. This leads to funneling of the posterior nasal cavity. The width of the posterior nasal cavity is abnormal if it is less than 0.67 cm at birth and less than 0.86 cm by 6 years. The medial pterygoid plates may be expanded and fused with the vomer. In long-standing bony atresias, there can be deviation of the bony hard palate and the nasal septum to the side of the atresia.

ANTERIOR PYRIFORM APERTURE STENOSIS

Congenital anterior nasal (pyriform aperture) stenosis is narrowing of the anterior nasal cavities. It is characterized by hypertrophy of the naso-maxillary processes (Figure 11.5a), with a solitary central incisor occuring in 60% of these cases. When measured, the pyriform aperture typically measures less than 8 mm across and each of the anterior nares measures less than 2 mm. The solitary central incisor tooth is detected on CT (Figure 11.5b, c) before its eruption and can be either of normal size or large (when it is called a mega-incisor). It is important to study the brain for intracranial abnormality, especially for holoprosencephaly and pituitary gland abnormalities, as these can be associated with this condition. Clinically, patients present early in life with nasal obstruction and failure to pass a nasogastric tube. The condition is commonly mistaken for posterior choanal atresia. CT imaging is helpful for diagnosing the abnormality and MRI is useful to look for associated intracranial abnormalities.

FACIAL CLEFTS

Facial clefting disorders are numerous and may be isolated or syndromic. They are either genetic or related to teratogens or problems in the early stage of pregnancy. Several different classification systems for facial clefting are currently in use. The Tessier system documents the topographical location of clefts, with these being numbered from 1 to 14. Clefts 1–7 are below the orbit and 8–14 are above. Other classifications include the DeMeyer and Sedano systems.

The majority of facial clefts are simple clefts involving the upper lip and/or palate. Lip clefting is often associated with palatal clefting, although either may occur in isolation. Lip clefting typically extends from the philtrum to the nostril (Figure 11.6). Palatal clefts are usually located between the incisors and canine teeth, and result from failure of fusion of one side of the primary palatal process with the secondary process of the maxillary prominence. Failure of fusion of the secondary palatal shelves causes a more severe palatal cleft. Other clefts are less common, but are still predicted by the fusion patterns of the facial prominences. Failure of fusion of the mandibular processes leads to a midline mandibular cleft. Persistence of the groove between the maxillary and lateral nasal prominences causes an oblique facial cleft extending from the nasal ala to the medial canthus. When a facial cleft does not respect the embryological pattern, the possibility of amniotic band syndrome must be considered.

11.5a

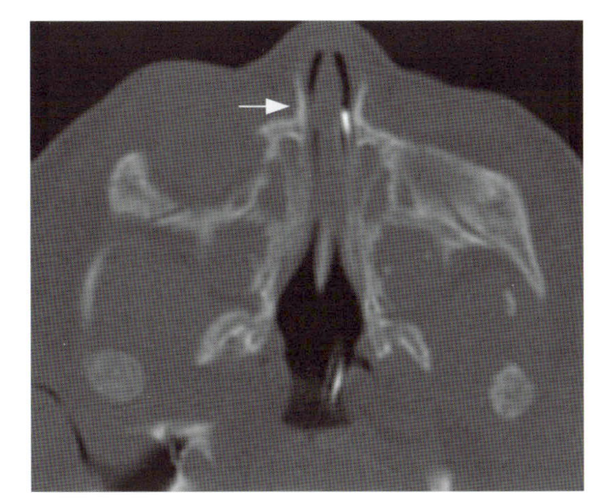

11.5b

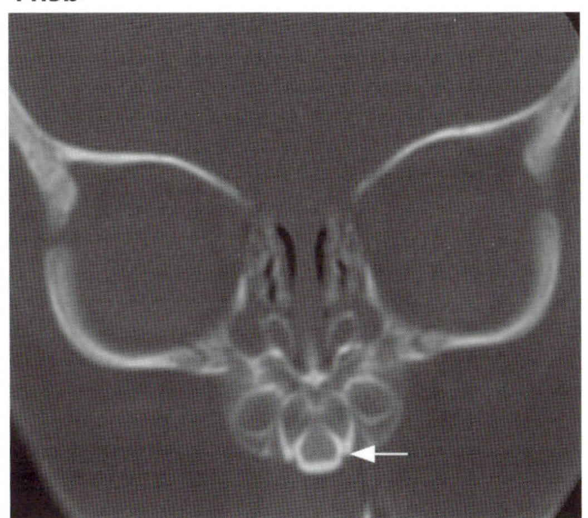

11.5c

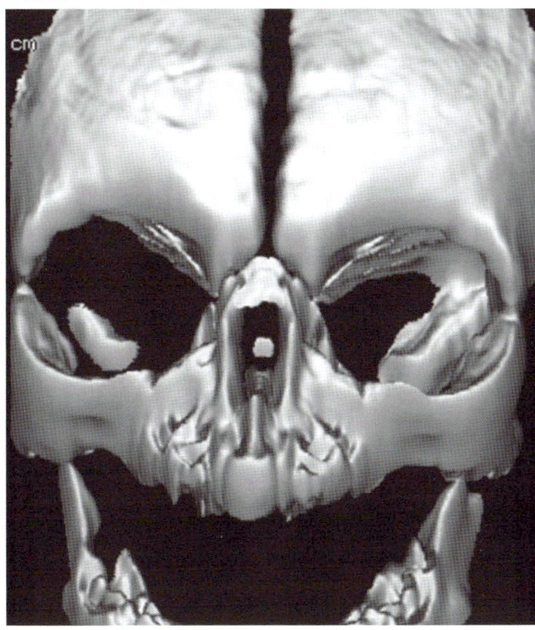

Figure 11.5 *Anterior pyriform stenosis.* (a) Axial CT showing a prominent nasomaxillary process (arrow). (b) Coronal CT showing the central incisor (arrow). (c) 3D CT demonstrating narrowing of anterior aperture (and also showing the central incisor well).

11.6a

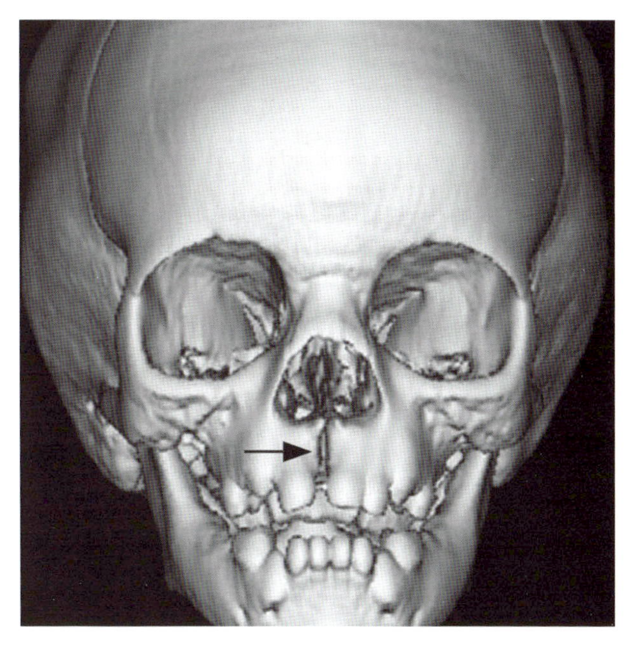

11.6b

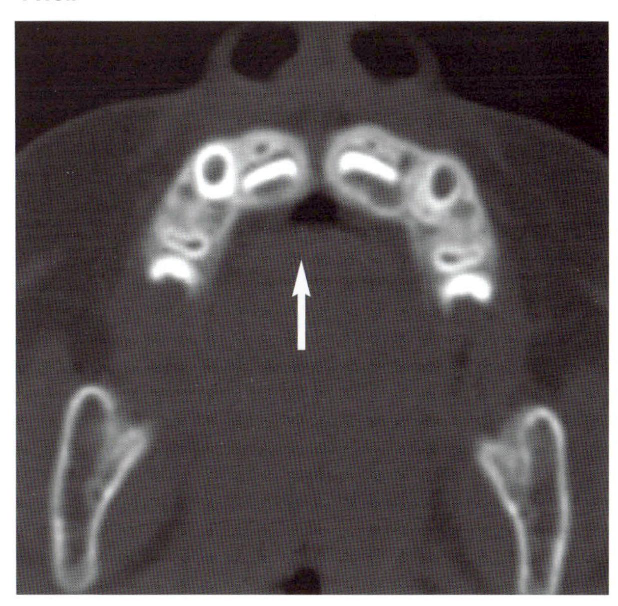

Figure 11.6 *Midline cleft palate.* (a) 3D CT scan of the facial skeleton and (b) axial CT scan showing a midline facial cleft in the maxillary bone (arrow).

Brain anomalies are relatively uncommon in facial clefting syndrome and are usually limited to cases where hypo- or hypertelorism is present. In cases with hypotelorism, the findings can range from alobar holoprosencephaly with near-complete splitting of the telencephalon at one end of the spectrum to a mild form of holoprosencephaly or septo-optic dysplasia. Hypertelorism patients will show a dysgenetic corpus callosum, callosal lipomas, and pituitary anomalies.

CONGENITAL NASOLACRIMAL DUCT OBSTRUCTION

This is not uncommon where there is failure of the nasolacrimal duct to open, with the obstruction usually being at the lower end of the duct. The nasolacrimal apparatus begins to form at 30 days' gestation. It develops along the naso-optic groove. At around the 40th day, surface ectoderm is buried in the underlying mesenchyma, forming an epithelial cord. This cord is canalized from the 3rd to 7th months of intrauterine life. The lacrimal sac forms at the cephalic end of this cord in the medial canthus. Tears drain through the superior and inferior canaliculi into the common canaliculus and then the lacrimal sac and enter the nasolacrimal duct via the valve of Rosenmuller. The nasolacrimal duct forms along the caudal portion of the naso-optic groove and opens below the inferior turbinate bone via Hasner's membrane. Spontaneous rupture of Hasner's membrane to form a mucosal fold known as Hasner's valve usually occurs during the 1st year of life. It is believed that initial crying or attempts to breathe, as well as movement or tear production, are required for membrane perforation.

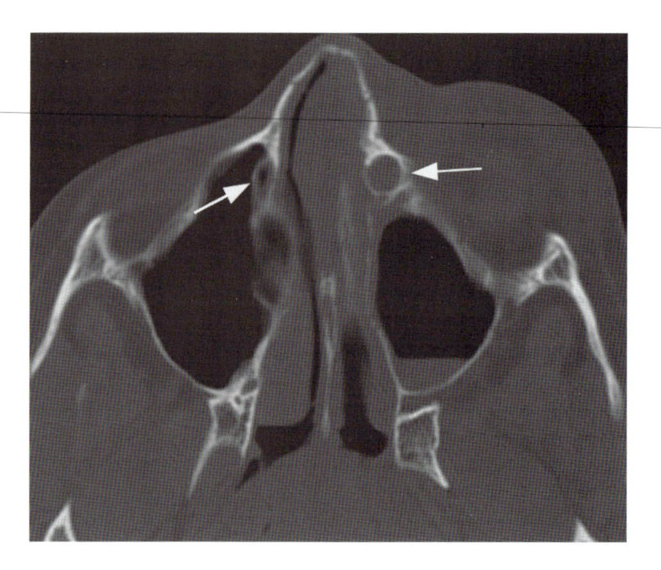

Figure 11.7 *Nasolacrimal duct stenosis*. Enlarged left nasolacrimal duct (right arrow) due to stenosis at Hasner's valve. Note the normal size of the right nasolacrimal duct (left arrow).

NASOLACRIMAL DUCT STENOSIS

Nasolacrimal duct stenosis is common in neonates and is caused by partial persistence of Hasner's membrane. Imaging findings may be normal or may consist of accumulation of secretions within an enlarged nasolacrimal duct (Figure 11.7). With conservative management, ductal stenosis will resolve spontaneously in 90% of children during the 1st year of life. Prophylactic antibiotics may be used during this period to prevent dacryocystitis and periorbital cellulitis.

DACRYOCYSTOCELES

Dacryocystoceles are rare masses manifesting at the medial canthus or in the nasal cavity. They may be unilateral or bilateral. Dacryocystoceles are the second most common cause of neonatal nasal obstruction after choanal atresia. They are caused by obstruction of both the proximal and distal ends of the nasolacrimal duct. An imperforate Hasner's membrane causes the distal blockage, but the cause of proximal obstruction is not clearly understood. Dacryocystoceles can cause nasal obstruction, become infected, or spontaneously rupture into the nose. CT is diagnostic and differentiates dacryocystoceles from other intranasal masses. Imaging features include enlargement of the bony nasolacrimal dilatation and a homogeneous, well-defined, thin-walled mass with fluid attenuation involving the medial canthus or nasal cavity (Figures 11.8 and 11.9). Depending on the size of the dacryocystocele, there may be a superior displacement of the inferior turbinate bone and a contralateral shift of the nasal septum. Cyst wall enhancement is prominent only when there is secondary infection. Adjacent soft tissue enhancement and swelling are also common in dacryocystitis. Unlike nasolacrimal duct stenosis, prompt treatment is usually recommended for dacryocystoceles, due to the possibility of them becoming infected and leading to damage to the nasolacrimal system. The treatment of dacryocystoceles includes manual pressure, probing with irrigation, endoscopic resection, and (in severe cases) marsupialization.

11.8a

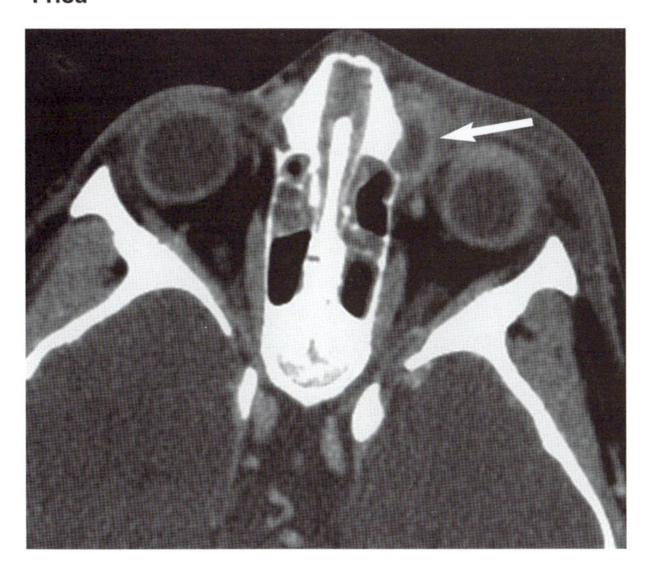

11.8b

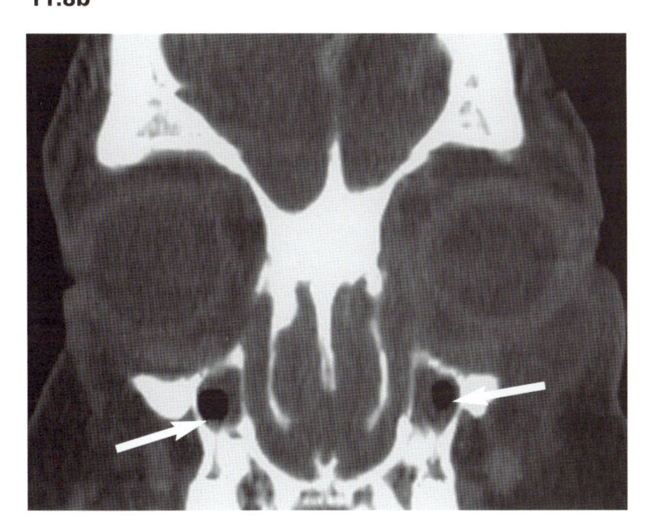

Figure 11.8 *Dacryocystocele*. (a) Axial CT scan with contrast showing an infected left dacryocystocele with left periorbital cellulitis (arrow). (b) Coronal CT scan showing bilateral enlargement of the nasolacrimal ducts (affecting the left side more) (arrows).

CONGENITAL MIDLINE NASAL MASSES

Mesenchymal structures are formed from several elements that eventually fuse and begin to ossify to form the skull base and the nose. Before they fuse, there are recognized spaces between these elements, which are important in the development of congenital midline nasal masses. These include the fonticulus frontalis, the prenasal space, and the foramen cecum. The nasofrontal fontanelle, or fonticulus frontalis, temporarily separates the embryonic nasal and frontal bones. Simultaneously, the transient prenasal space separates the nasal bones and the cartilaginous nasal capsule. A diverticulum of dura mater extends from the anterior cranial fossa through the foramen cecum into the transient prenasal space. It briefly contacts the skin at the tip of the nose before retracting back into the cranium. The tract of this dural diverticulum quickly involutes. The nasal and frontal bones fuse, obliterating the fonticulus frontalis and forming the nasofrontal suture. The prenasal space becomes smaller with growth of the adjacent bone structures, eventually being reduced to a small canal anterior to the crista galli known as the foramen cecum. Finally, the foramen cecum is filled with fibrous tissue and fuses with the prenasal space.

Congenital midline nasal masses are rare anomalies occuring once in 20 000–40 000 live births. The present widely accepted theory suggests that nasal gliomas, dermal sinuses, and encephaloceles result from incomplete regression of the dura that transiently traverses the prenasal space. Dermoid and epidermoid cysts occur when skin elements are pulled into the prenasal space along with the regressing dural diverticulum.

Dermoid and epidermoid cysts

These can occur anywhere along the course of the diverticulum from the columella to the anterior cranial fossa. An intracranial connection is seen in up to 57% of affected patients. Dermoid cysts contain ectoderm with skin appendages, are slightly more common than epidermoid cysts, and are usually midline, with a tendency to occur at the glabella. Epidermoid cysts contain ectodermal elements without skin appendages, are usually paramidline, and tend to occur near the columella. A sinus tract opening, dimple, or tuft of hair is present on the skin surface in up to 84% of dermoid or epidermoid cysts and dermal sinus tracts. Dermoid and epidermoid cysts are firm, non-pulsatile lesions that do not transilluminate and do not change in size with crying or with compression of the jugular veins (negative Furstenberg test). The imaging characteristics of dermoid and epidermoid cysts may overlap, although dermoid cysts are more

11.9a

11.9b

11.9c

11.9d

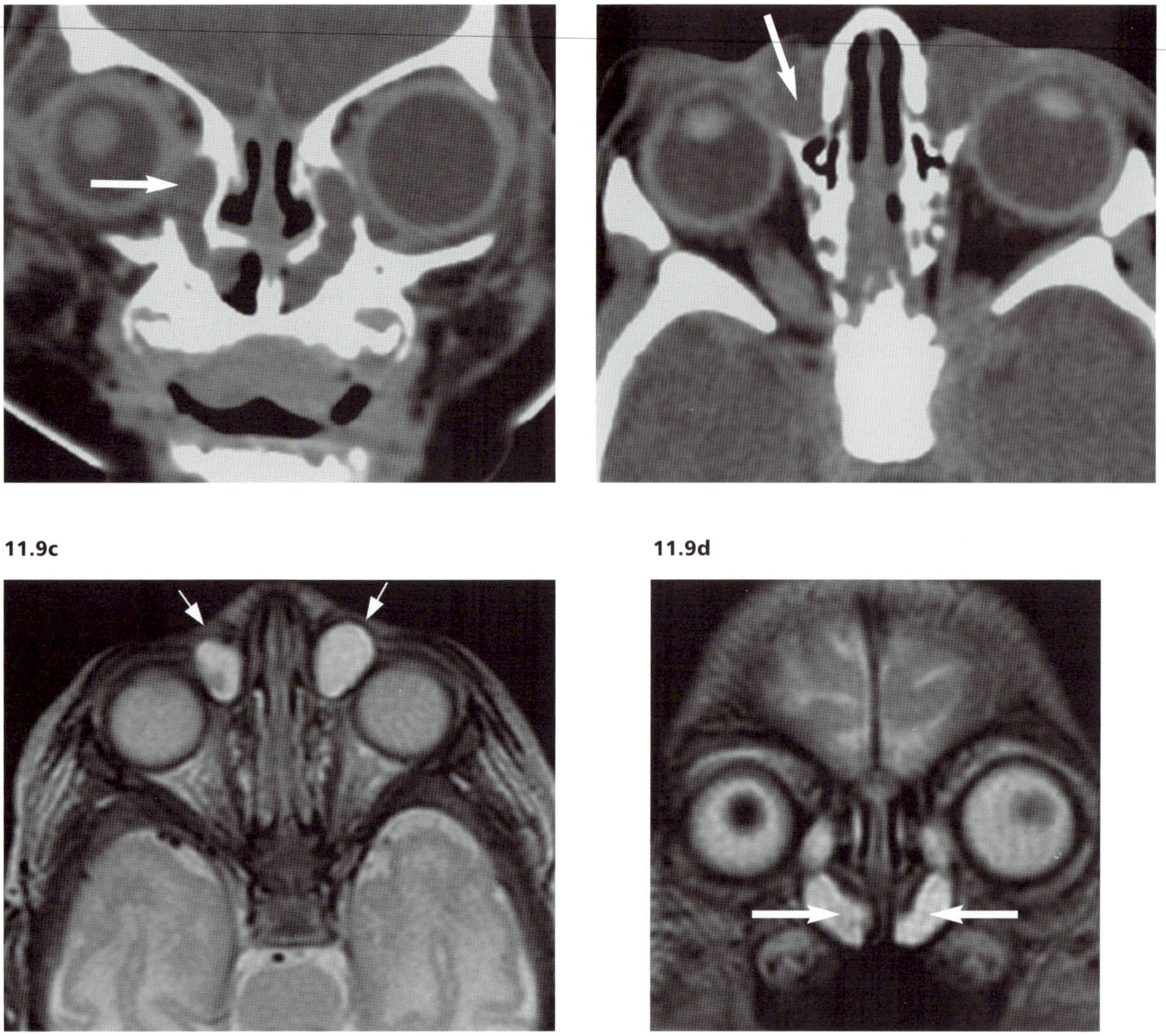

Figure 11.9 *Dacryocystocele.* (a) Coronal and (b) axial CT scans showing cystic lesions along the medial–inferior aspect of the orbits suggestive of dacryocystoceles (arrow). (c) Axial and (d) coronal T2-weighted MRI scans demonstrating these in better detail (arrows).

likely to be midline and fatty, whereas epidermoid cysts usually have fluid attenuation on CT and are isointense relative to fluid on T1- and T2-weighted MRI (Figures 11.10–11.13). Although extracranial epidermoid cysts rarely present a diagnostic dilemma, intracranial lesions may mimic arachnoid cysts (Figure 11.12). Intracranial epidermoid cysts are solid masses that can be identified on MRI with diffusion-weighted images. On diffusion-weighted images, epidermoid cysts have restricted diffusion (Figure 11.13c). Imaging helps to determine whether there is intracranial extension and is therefore important in planning the surgical approach. The treatment of dermoid and epidermoid cysts includes complete resection of the mass and, if present, the sinus tract. Incomplete resection may lead to complications of meningitis or recurrence in up to 15% of cases. When there is intracranial involvement, intracranial–extracranial resection is required to remove the mass and its sinus tract. Resection of the mass may be delayed until 2–5 years of age if possible.

11.10a

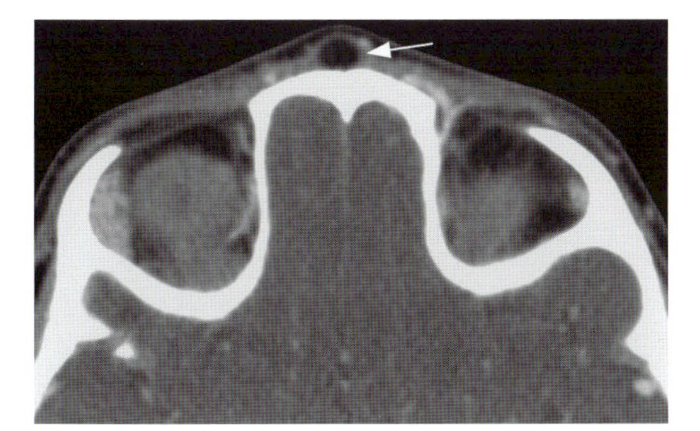

11.10b

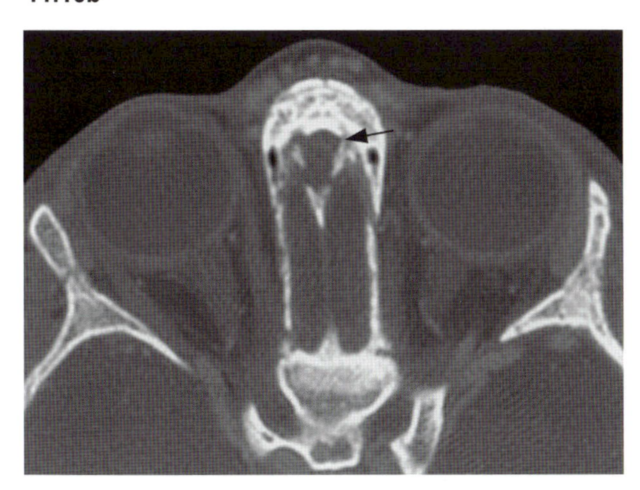

11.10c

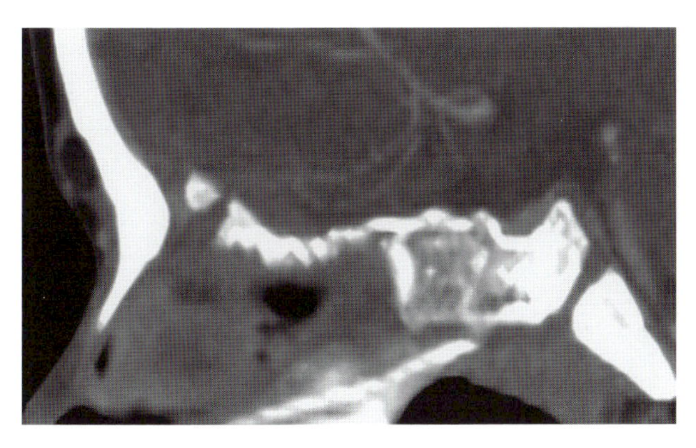

Figure 11.10 *Dermoid cyst.* (a–c) A small dermoid at the base of the nose (white arrow in (a)). Although the foramen cecum appeared enlarged (black arrow in (b)), no obvious intracranial connection (c).

11.11a

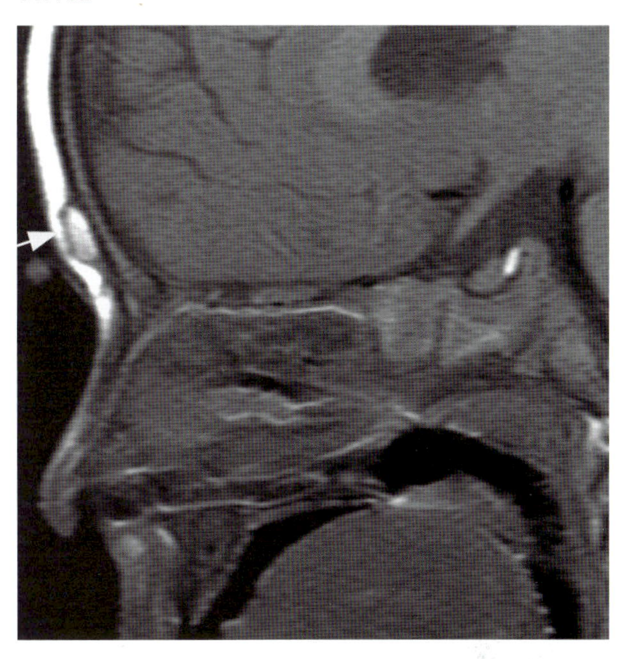

11.11b

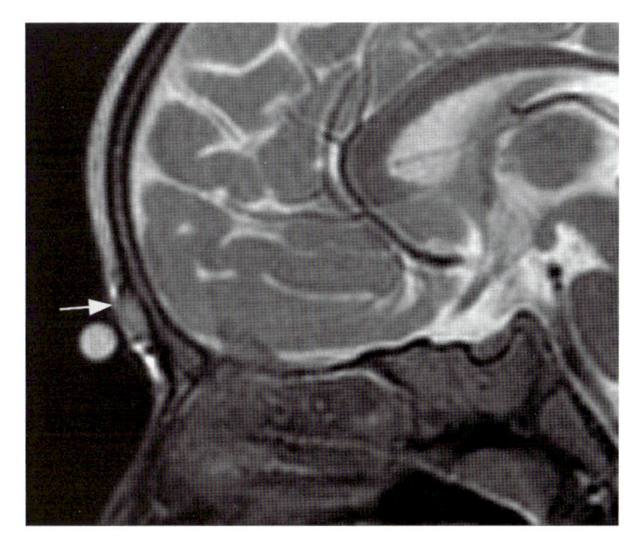

Figure 11.11 *Dermoid cyst.* Sagittal T1-weighted MRI image of the same child as in Figure 11.10 (a). T2-weighted MRI scan (b) shows a lack of intracranial extension in this small dermoid (arrows). The presence of a mildly enlarged foramen cecum may be just a normal variation.

11.12a

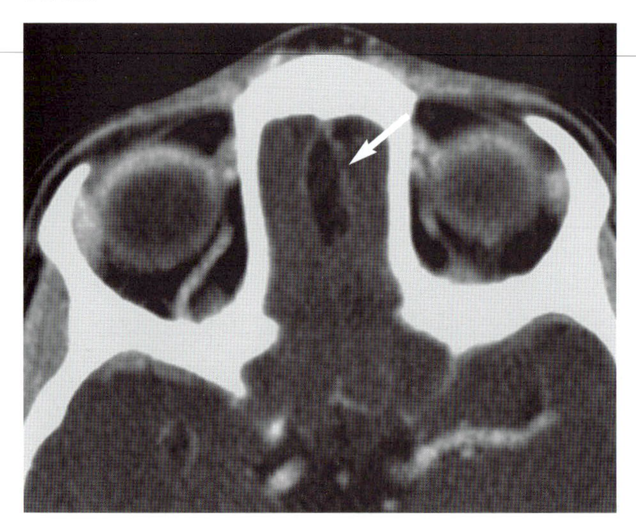

11.12b

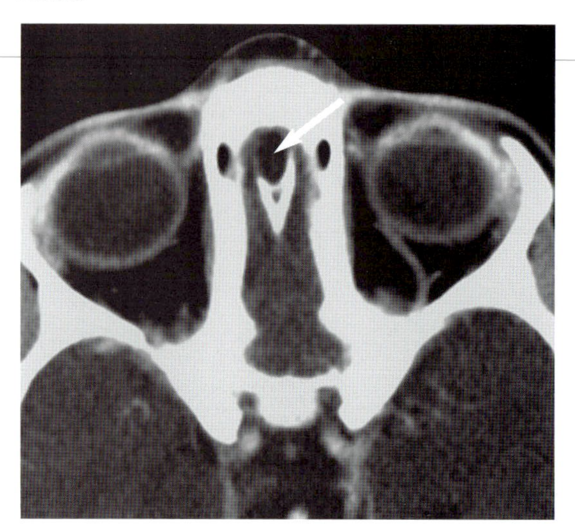

11.12c

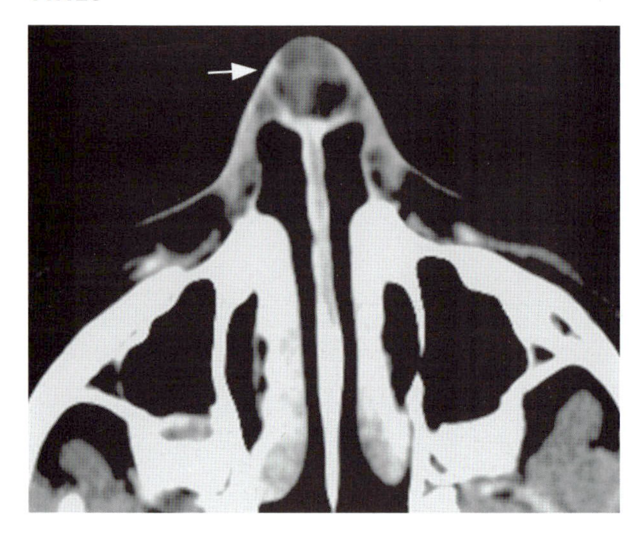

11.12d

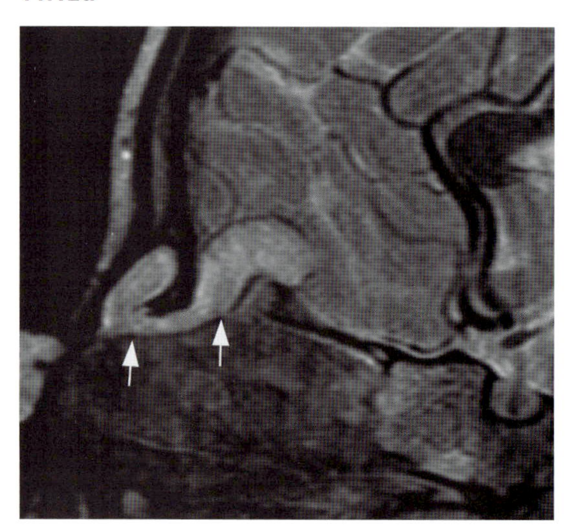

Figure 11.12 *Nasal dermoid cyst.* Nasal dermoid (a, b) note the enlarged foramen cecum in these axial scans (arrow). (c) Axial CT demonstrating nasal dermoid (arrow). (d) Sagittal MRI showing intracranial extension (T2-weighted) (arrows).

Encephaloceles

These occur in one of every 4000 live births and have no sex predilection. They may present as an obvious mass, nasal stuffiness, rhinorrhea, a broad nasal root, or hypertelorism. Depending on the size of the intracranial connection, encephaloceles may be pulsatile or change in size during crying, the Valsalva maneuver, or jugular compression (positive Furstenberg test). Encephaloceles can be classified according to location as occipital (75% of cases), sincipital (15%), or basal (10%). Sincipital encephaloceles involve the midface and occur about the dorsum of the nose, the orbits, and the forehead. The nomenclature used for encephaloceles can also be based on the origin of their roof and floor; thus, for example, the roof and floor of frontonasal encephaloceles are the frontal and nasal bones, respectively. Sincipital encephaloceles can typically be either frontonasal (40–60% of cases) or naso-ethmoid (30%), with the remaining 10% being a combination of the two. Frontonasal encephaloceles result from herniation of dura mater through both

11.13a

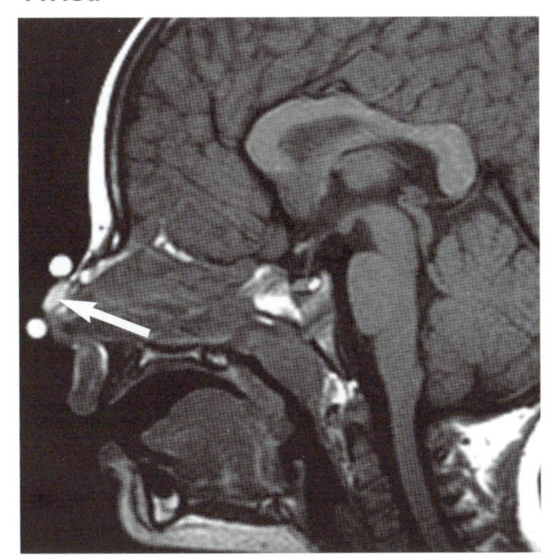

11.13b

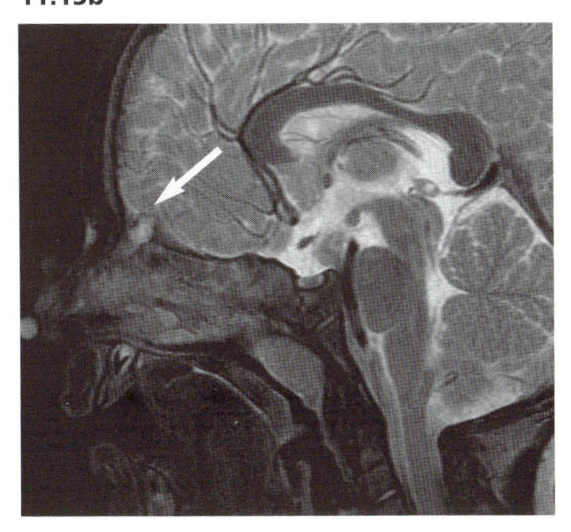

11.13c

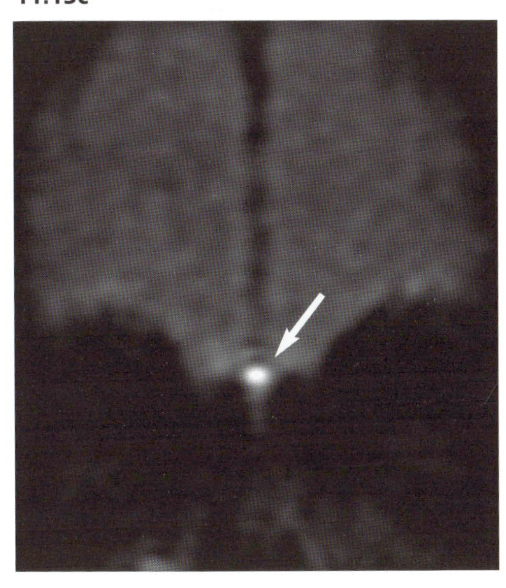

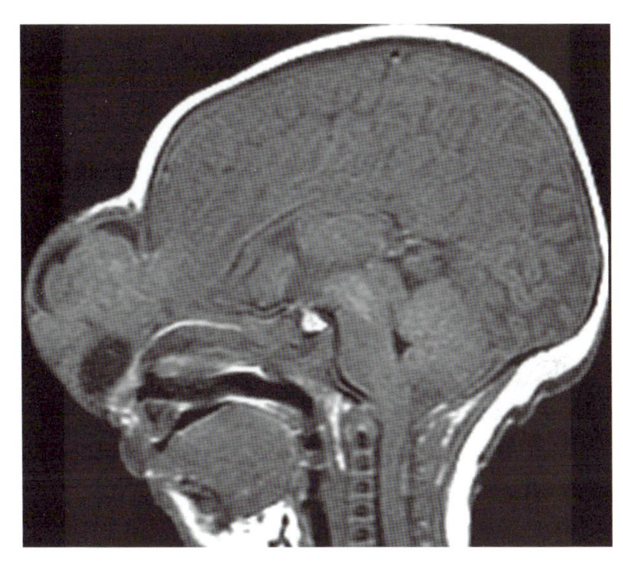

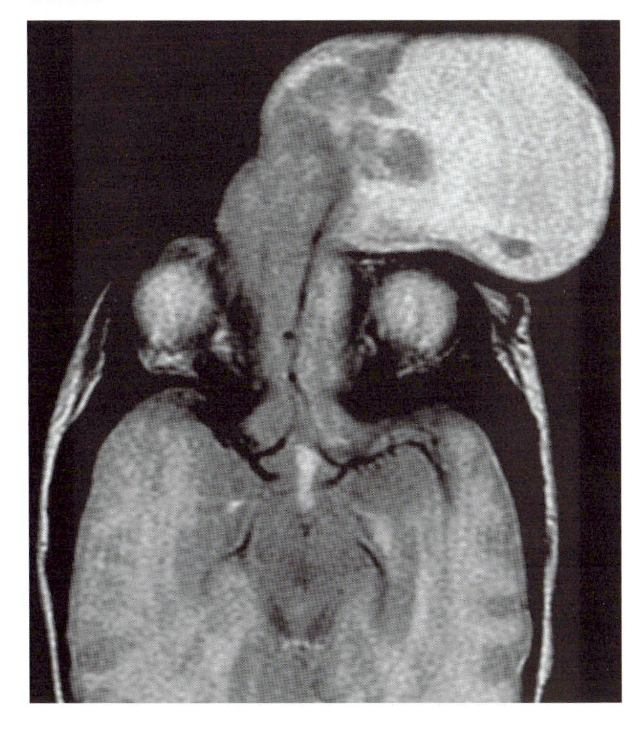

the foramen cecum and the fonticulus frontalis into the glabellar region (Figure 11.14). Nasoethmoid encephaloceles occur when there is persistent herniation of the dural diverticulum through the foramen cecum into the prenasal space and nasal cavity. Encephaloceles have a high prevalence of

11.13a

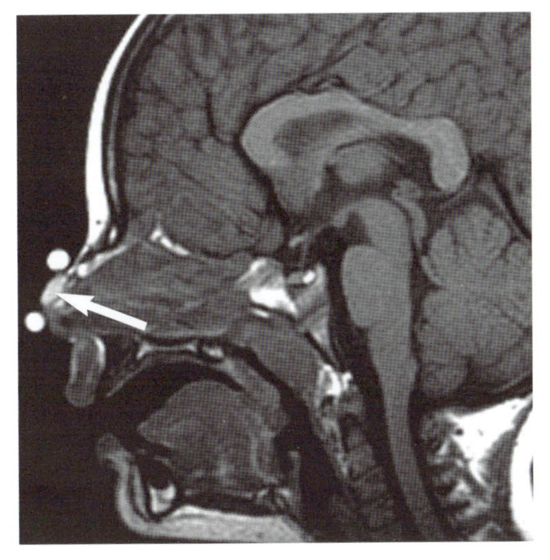

11.13b

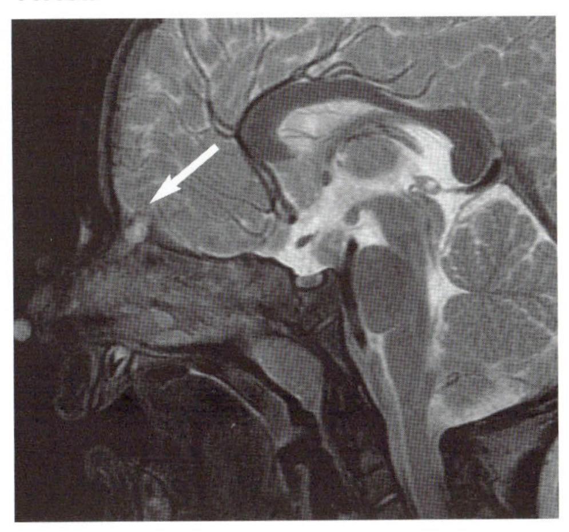

11.13c

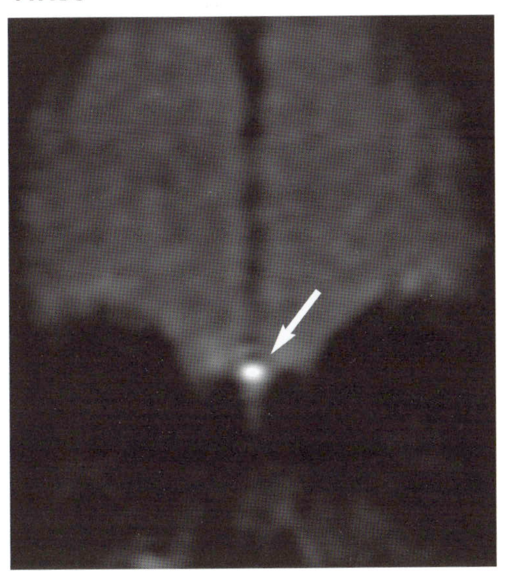

Figure 11.13 *Epidermoid cyst*. Sagittal T1-weighted (a) and T2-weighted (b) MRI scans showing the dermoid tract with an epidermoid cyst intracranially (arrow). (c) Diffusion-weighted image showing restricted diffusion from the epidermoid cyst (arrow).

11.14a

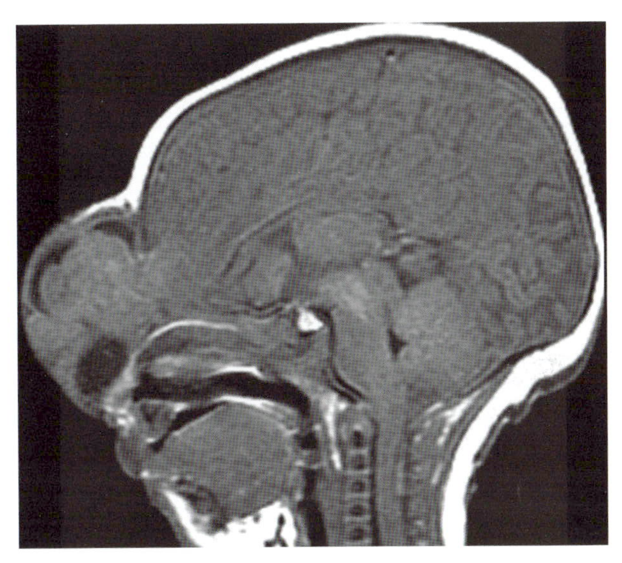

11.14b

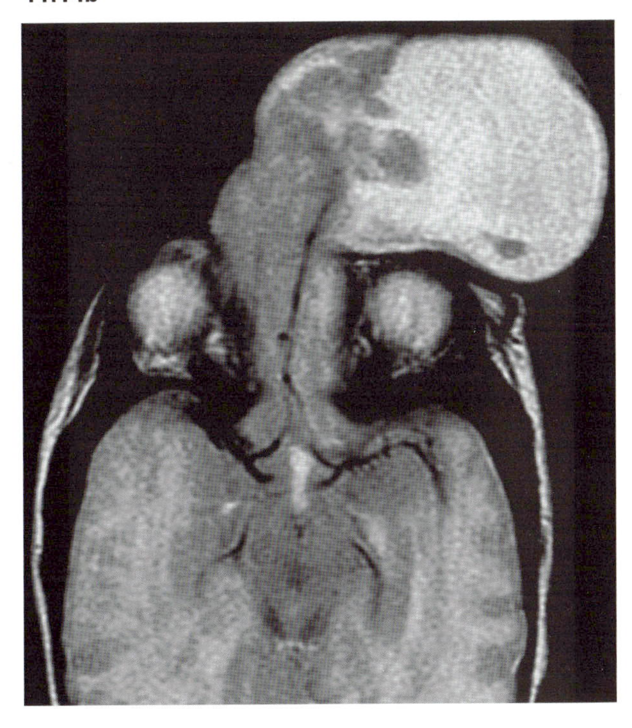

Figure 11.14 *Frontonasal encephalocele*. (a) Sagittal MRI T1-weighted demonstrating large frontonasal encephalocele with brain tissue and cerebrospinal fluid herniating into it. (b) Axial MRI T2-weighted showing the same with gross hypertelorism. Note the anterior displacement of the anterior cerebral arteries towards the frontal bone defect.

associated intracranial anomalies, including intracranial cysts, callosal agenesis, interhemispheric lipomas, facial clefts, and schizencephaly. Subsequent pregnancies have a 6% risk of a congenital central nervous system abnormality. Frontonasal encephaloceles are soft, cystic, and bluish when covered by skin; when not covered, they are usually red and moist. Intranasal encephaloceles are pedunculated and extend downward from the superomedial nasal cavity. Lateral advancement of a nasal catheter may help differentiate encephaloceles from more medially located dacryocystoceles (nasolacrimal mucoceles).

Biopsy is contraindicated in encephaloceles due to the potential for cerebrospinal fluid (CSF) leaks, seizures, or meningitis.

Imaging features of nasal encephaloceles include a soft tissue mass that is connected to the subarachnoid space via an enlarged foramen cecum and extends to the glabella or into the nasal cavity. MRI is the modality of choice for the initial evaluation of encephaloceles because it can help determine the size, extent, and nature of the encephalocele contents as well as the presence of associated intracranial anomalies (Figure 11.15a). If an encephalocele contains only meninges with CSF, it is termed a meningocele; when it also contains brain tissue, it is called a meningoencephalocele. Brain tissue within encephaloceles is usually isointense relative to gray matter with most MRI sequences, but may be hyperintense with T2-weighted sequences due to gliosis. CT is useful in demonstrating bone changes that suggest intracranial extension, such as a bifid or absent crista galli, cribriform plate, or frontal bone. 3D CT scans are useful to show the extent of the bony defect and are very useful for surgical planning (Figure 11.15b, c).

Encephaloceles are treated with complete surgical resection as soon as possible to prevent CSF leakage and meningitis, and to improve facial appearance. Surgery involves repairing the dura mater. Resection of the brain tissue in an encephalocele does not lead to an increased risk of neurological deficits due to the abnormal function of the herniated brain tissue.

Nasal gliomas

Nasal gliomas are usually isolated anomalies. These are benign masses of glial tissue, occurring near the root of the nose and usually without any intracranial connection. However, in 15% of cases, nasal gliomas remain connected with intracranial structures by a stalk of glial or fibrous tissue, usually through a defect in the cribriform plate. They can be thought of as encephaloceles that have lost their intracranial connection. The usual age of presentation of nasal gliomas is in infancy or early childhood. Nasal gliomas can be extranasal (60% lying external to the nasal bones and nasal cavities – usually just lateral to the nasal root), intranasal (30% lying within the nasal cavities – usually in the lateral nasal wall, mouth, or rarely the pterygopalatine fossa), or mixed (10% with both intra- and extranasal components communicating via a defect in the nasal bones or around their edges). Nasal gliomas can cause remodeling and deformities of the adjacent bones, and commonly cause hypertelorism. No microscopic invasion, mitotic figures, or metastases have been reported to date. They usually contain large aggregates of astrocytes (fibrous or gemistocytic) and fibrous connective tissue enveloping the blood vessels.

Nasal gliomas are usually isodense on CT scans. They can deform the bones of the nasal fossa and may have extensions through the glabella, nasal bones, cribriform plate, or foramen cecum. Calcifications are rarely reported in them. Cystic changes may occasionally occur within nasal gliomas. MRI is more reliable for differentiating nasal gliomas from encephaloceles. On MRI, nasal gliomas are usually hyperintense on T2-weighted images. They may appear hypo-, iso-, or hyperintense to the gray matter on T1-weighted images.

Radiological evaluation of congenital midline nasal masses

When a dermoid cyst, glioma, or encephalocele is suspected, a biopsy should not be attempted before an intracranial connection has been ruled out, because of the risk of causing meningitis or CSF leak. CT and MRI can both provide complementary information. CT shows bony abnormalities better,

11.15a

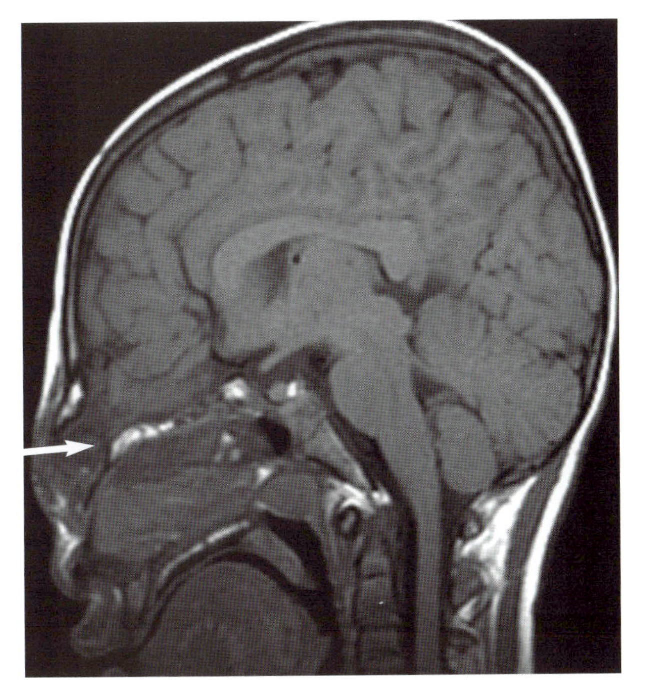

11.15b

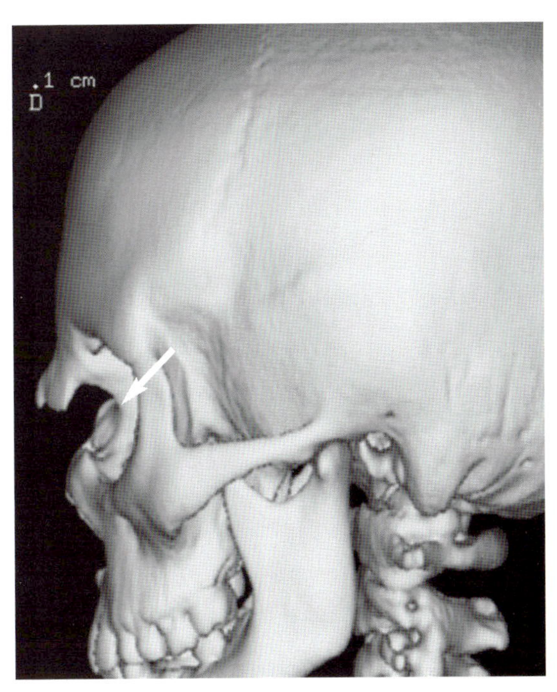

11.15c

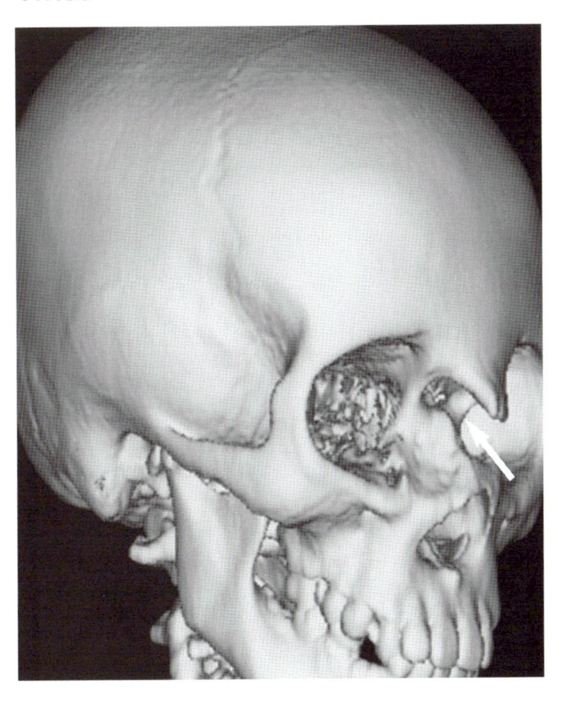

Figure 11.15 *Frontonasal encephalocele*. (a) Sagittal T1-weighted MRI scan showing a frontonasal encephalocele (arrow). (b, c) 3D CT scans showing the extent of the bony defect for surgical planning (arrow).

while MRI is valuable for identifying intracranial connections and any other associated intracranial abnormalities. Due to the added cost of two tests, and the added risk of anesthesia, MRI is often recommended as the initial study, with CT (with 3D reconstructions) being reserved for encephaloceles in the context of surgical planning.

The presence of an enlarged foramen cecum or bifid crista galli on CT images is suggestive of intracranial involvement. It is generally thought that the absence of these findings is more reliable in ruling out intracranial involvement. The presence of these findings is suggestive but not conclusive of intracranial involvement, as false positives have been reported (see Figures 11.10 and 11.11). Thin sagittal MRI scans are very effective at looking for an intracranial connection. The presence of any fat signal intensity in the mass suggests a dermoid cyst. For non-fatty masses, the addition of a diffusion-weighted sequence is useful to confirm an epidermoid cyst, which will typically show diffusion restriction. If any evidence of inflammation is present, gadolinium-enhanced fat-saturated images are useful to show the presence of a dermal sinus tract.

CRANIOSYNOSTOSIS

Craniosynostosis or sutural stenosis is a group of disorders characterized by premature closure of one or more of the cranial sutures from any cause. Primary craniosynostosis occurs in the absence of underlying brain abnormality. Secondary craniosynostosis occurs as an indirect consequence of reduced intracranial volume, often after shunting of hydrocephalus or a cerebral insult. Metabolic causes include vitamin D-related rickets, familial hypophosphatasia, hyperthyroidism, and idiopathic hypercalcemia. Primary craniosynostosis may occur as an isolated phenomenon (non-syndromic craniosynostosis, 85%) or as one part of a syndrome (syndromic craniosynostosis, 15%). Non-syndromic craniosynostosis usually occurs in isolation, whereas syndromic cases show involvement of more than one suture. CT of the craniofacial skeleton with 3D reconstructed images is the modality of choice to image these patients. MRI is not usually required, unless an intracranial abnormality is expected, especially in cases with craniosyndromic synostosis. The general rule about craniosynostosis is that there is no growth perpendicular to the fused suture and the skull grows parallel to the fused suture.

Non-syndromic craniosynostosis

Sagittal craniosynostosis

Sagittal craniosynostosis is produced by premature fusion of the sagittal suture. It gives rise to a dolicocephalic or scaphocephalic appearance of the head (an increase in anteroposterior dimension with no growth in the right–left direction). A well-defined ridge of bone is often seen at the site of the fused suture (Figure 11.16).

11.16a

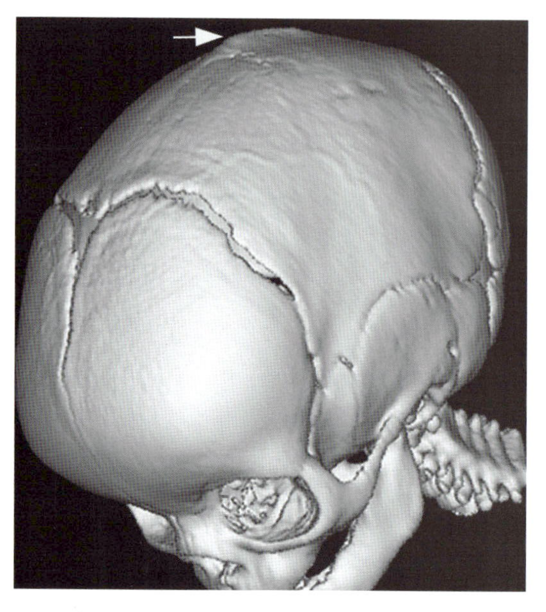

11.16b

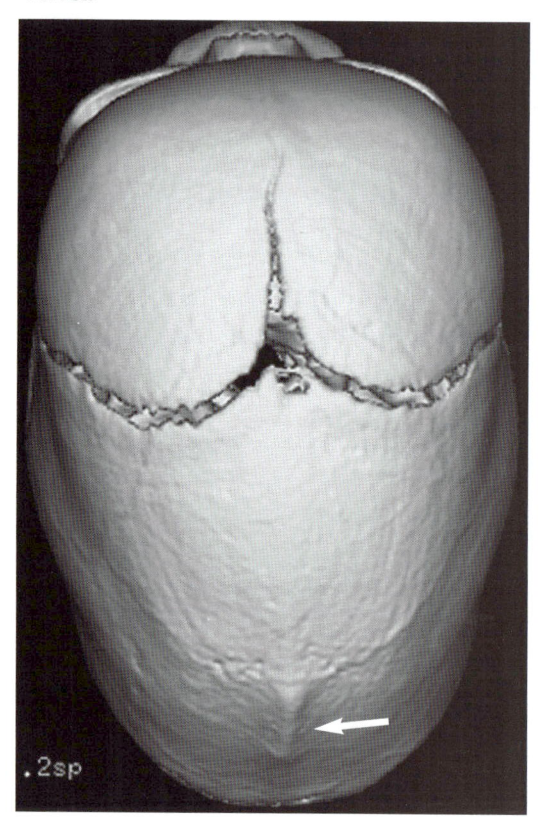

Figure 11.16 *Sagittal craniosynostosis*. (a, b) 3D reconstructed CT scans of sagittal craniosynostosis showing a fused sagittal suture with a scaphocephalic skull vault. Note the ridge of bone along the expected position of the sagittal suture (arrow).

Coronal craniosynostosis

Coronal craniosynostosis is caused by premature fusion of the coronal suture. It can be unilateral or bilateral. Bilateral coronal craniosynostosis causes brachycephaly (increased right–left dimensions and decreased anteroposterior dimensions). There is compensatory bulging at the temporal regions and upward and posterior sloping of the supraorbital ridge (Figure 11.17). This gives rise to the 'harlequin's orbit' appearance. Unilateral coronal craniosynostosis gives rise to asymmetric skull, also known as plagiocephaly.

Metopic craniosynostosis

The metopic suture usually closes by the 2nd year of life. Metopic craniosynostosis occurs due to premature closure of the metopic suture. It gives rise to trigonocephaly (an axe- or pear-shaped skull

11.17a

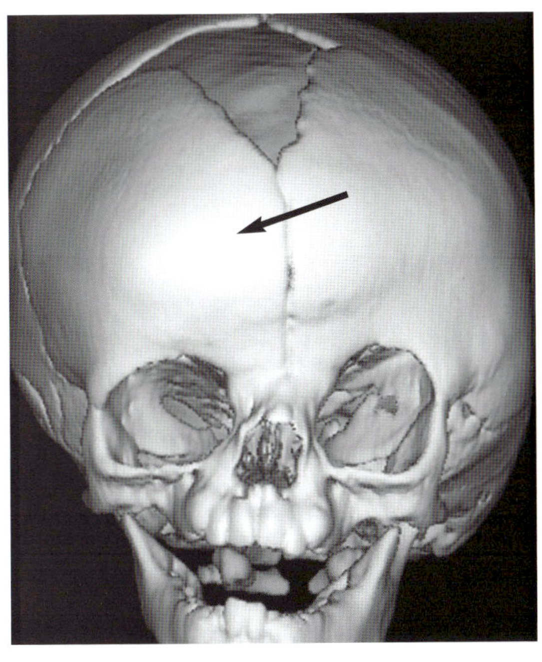

11.17b

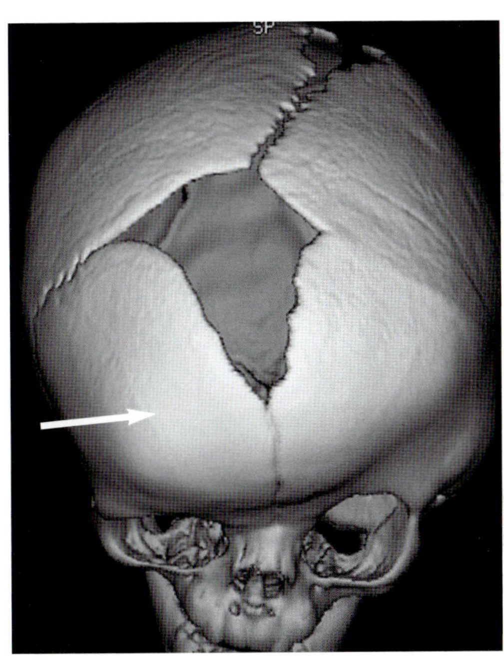

11.17c

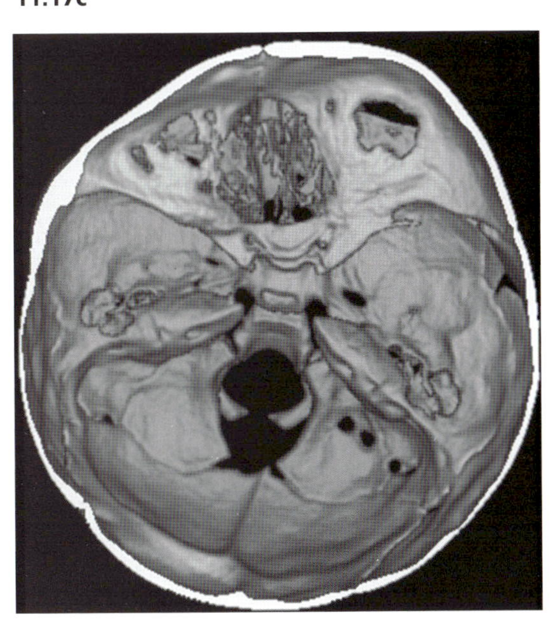

Figure 11.17 *Coronal craniosynostosis*. (a–c) 3D CT scans in unilateral coronal craniosynostosis showing increased frontal bulging on the affected side (arrow), with bulging in the temporal region. The superior orbital ridge is pulled upwards and the lateral wall of the left orbit slants backwards.

on axial views). There is a decrease in the bifrontal diameter and the skull overall looks triangular in appearance anteriorly (Figure 11.18). It is often associated with hypotelorism.

Lambdoid craniosynostosis

Lambdoid craniosynostosis is very rare in comparison with the other craniosynostoses. Lambdoid craniosynostosis shows posterior deviation of the ipsilateral pinna and the petrous temporal bone. This helps to differentiate this entity from the far more common positional plagiocephaly produced due to the child lying on the occiput for a prolonged period of time.

Syndromic craniosynostosis

Apert's syndrome

Apert's syndrome is also known as acrocephalosyndactyly type I and is one of the common causes of syndromic craniosynostosis. It has an incidence of 15.5 cases per million and comprises 4.5% of all cases of craniosynostosis. The major diagnostic criteria include sutural stenosis and syndactyly. There is

11.18a

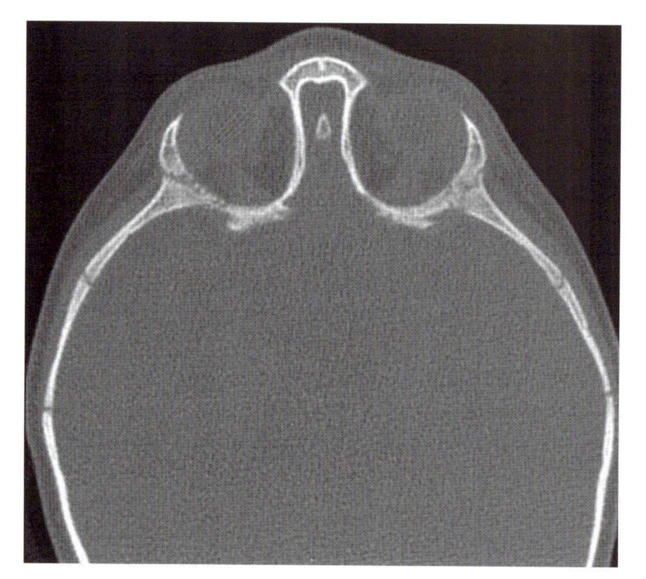

11.18b

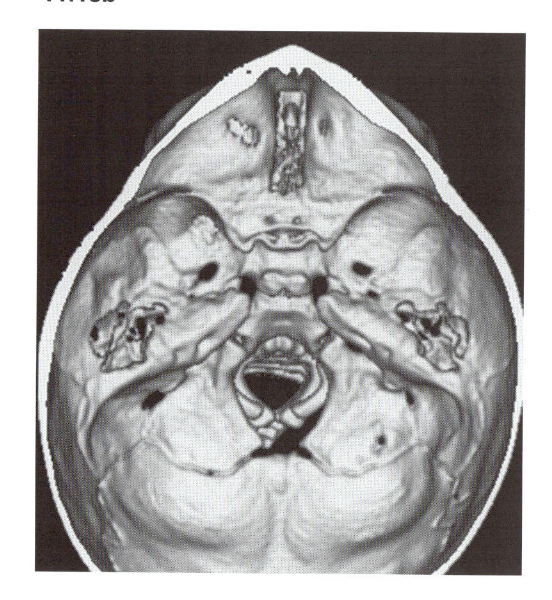

11.18c

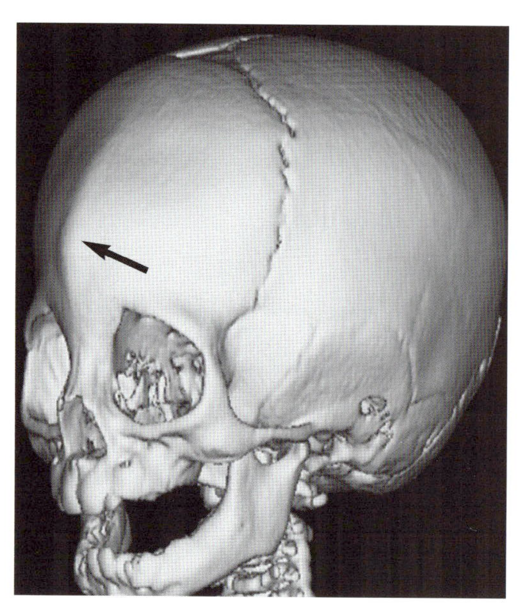

Figure 11.18 *Metopic craniosynostosis*. (a–c) Axial and 3D CT scans of the facial skeleton showing fusion of the metopic suture with a triangular anterior skull vault and hypotelorism. A prominent ridge of bone is located at the normally expected location of the metopic suture (arrow).

bicoronal craniosynostosis, giving the skull a brachycephalic appearance with a shortened anteroposterior diameter and a flat occiput. Sometimes, craniosynostosis can be severe, leading to a cloverleaf deformity of the skull vault (Figure 11.19a). In addition, these patients often show anomalies of the corpus callosum and limbic structures. Dental anomalies with crowding and malocclusion of the teeth are also seen. Normal intelligence is seen in about 70% of patients. Hand findings include syndactyly of the second, third, and fourth fingers, forming a mid-digital mass (Figure 11.19b). The first and fifth fingers may join this hand mass. Syndactyly can also be seen in the feet. Other findings include cervical vertebral segmentation–fusion anomalies, radio-ulnar synostosis, pyloric stenosis, ventricular septal defects, and polycystic kidney disease.

11.19a

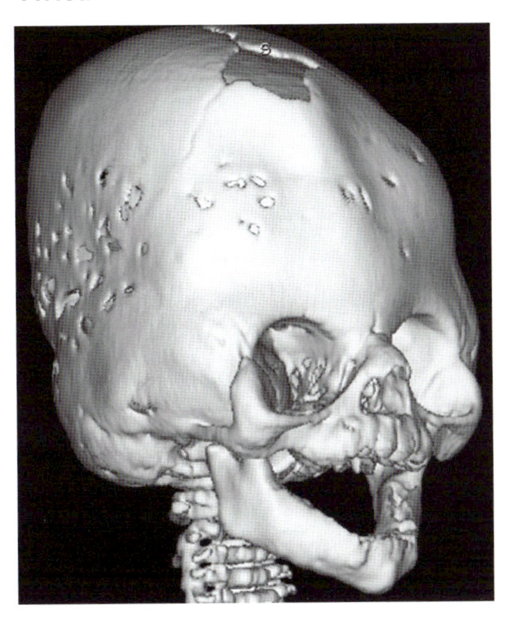

11.19b

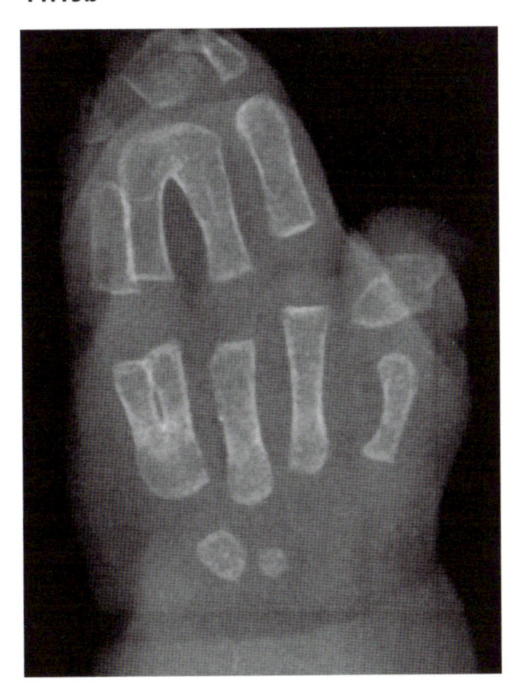

Figure 11.19 *Apert's syndrome.* (a) Bicoronal craniosynostosis with multiple punched-out lesions in the skull vault reflecting raised intracranial pressure. (b) Radiograph of the hand revealing syndactyly.

Crouzon's syndrome

Crouzon's syndrome, or craniofacial dysostosis, is characterized by premature craniosynostosis, with midfacial anomalies, exophthalmos, hypertelorism, and mandibular prognathism (Figure 11.20). The sutures involved are the bicoronal, sagittal, or lambdoid sutures. Unlike Apert's syndrome, there is no finding of syndactyly. However, 30–55% of patients have hearing loss with atretic external auditory canal and cleft palate with bifid uvula. The shallow orbits cause proptosis, leading to exposure keratitis of the cornea. Anomalies of the palate (palatal swellings), nose (often parrot-like), and C2–C3 vertebrae are some of the other associated findings.

Goldenhar's syndrome

Goldenhar's syndrome, or oculoauriculovertebral (OAV) dysplasia, is characterized by anomalies of the facial skeleton, orbits, ears, spine, and central nervous system. The incidence varies from 1 in 3500 to 1 in 25 000 births. In these patients, the mandibular ramus and condyle are hypoplastic, the malar eminence and the temporal bone are small, and the mastoid is underpneumatized (Figure 11.21). Microtia with occasional preauricular tags, anomalies of the middle ear with aberrant facial nerve canal, and ossicular anomalies of the cervical spine are seen. The parotid gland is often agenetic or displaced, and cleft lip/palate is seen in 10% of cases. Mental retardation is variable, the reported incidence being 5–15%.

11.20a

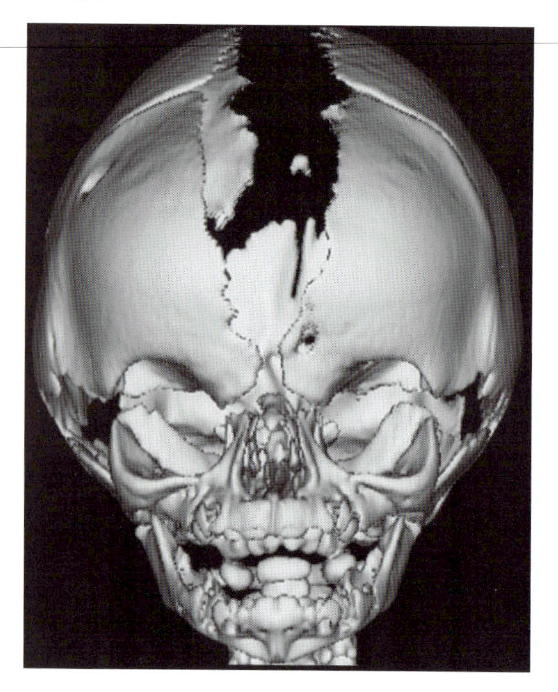

11.20b

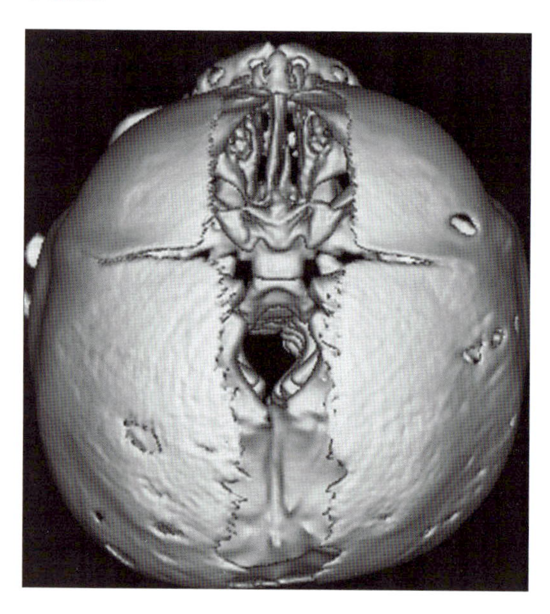

Figure 11.20 *Crouzon's syndrome*. (a, b) 3D CT scans showing an abnormally wide sagittal suture and bicoronal craniosynostosis.

11.21a

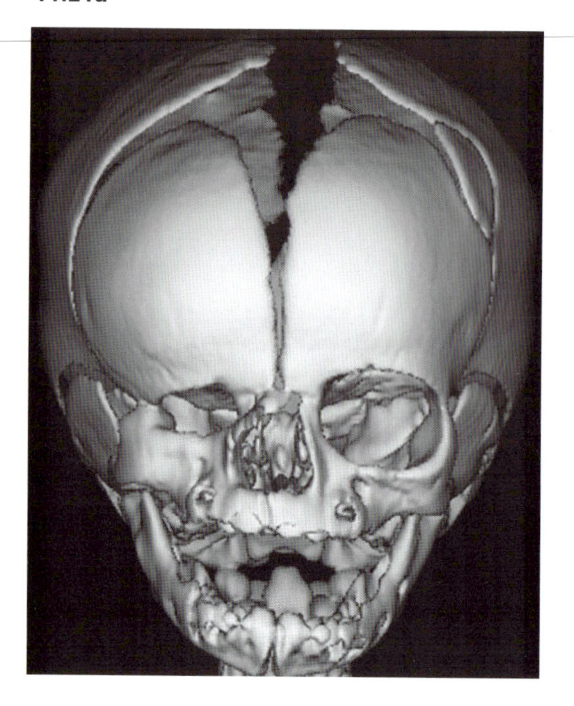

11.21b

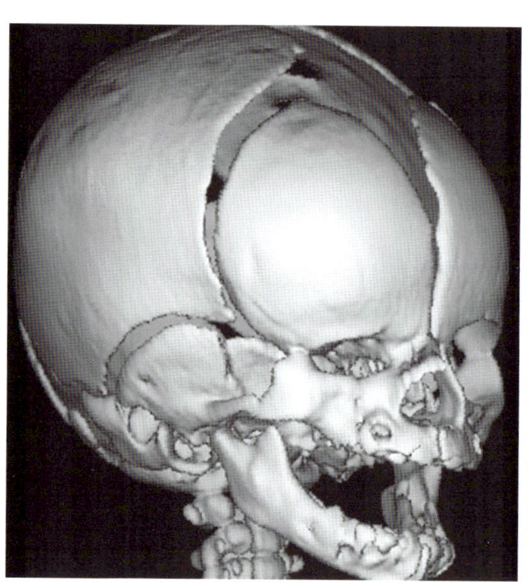

Figure 11.21 *Goldenhar's syndrome*. 3D CT scans showing hypoplasia of the right zygomatic bone, with increased mandibular angle and small right orbit.

Treacher Collins syndrome

First described in 1900, Treacher Collins syndrome, or mandibulofacial dysostosis, is characterized by microtia, malformed ears and midface, downward slanting of the palpebral fissures, coloboma of the outer third or lower eyelids, and micrognathia. The supraorbital ridges are flat. The auricles are malformed and the external auditory canals are stenosed or absent. The major features in Treacher Collins syndrome include:

- Midfacial hypoplasia with hypoplastic malar bones, small zygomatic buttresses, and absent zygomatic arches

11.22a

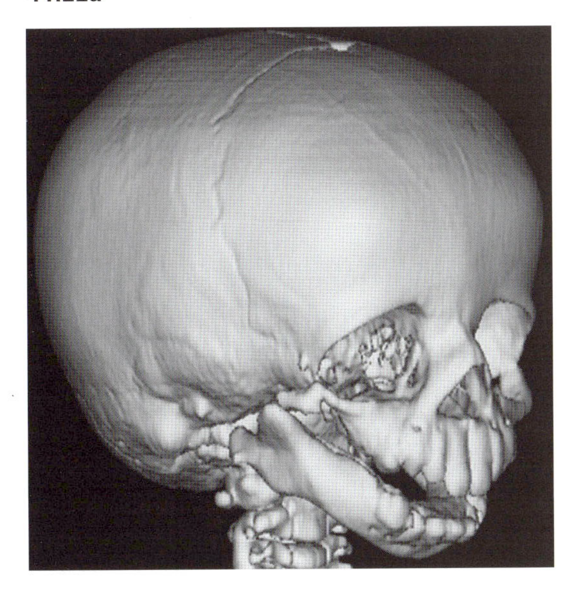

11.22b

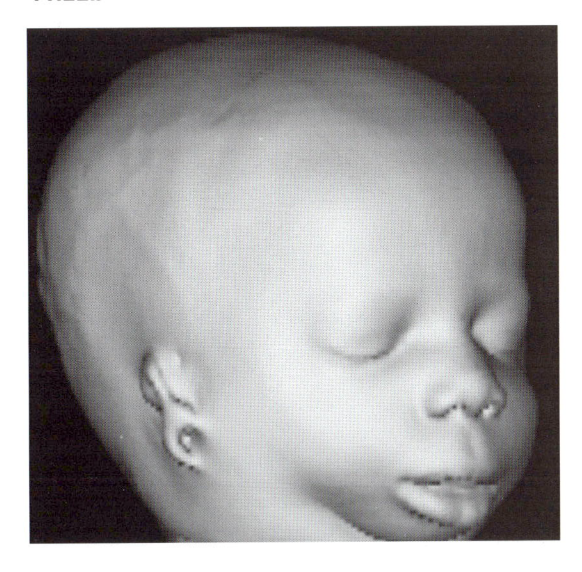

Figure 11.22 *Treacher Collins syndrome*. 3D CT scans in bone (a) and soft tissue (b) showing absence of the zygoma on the right side, with a hypoplastic mandible. On the soft tissue image (b), there is microtia and micrognathia.

- The inferior orbital fissures are hypoplastic with inferolateral slanting
- Micrognathia with a small, dysplastic mandible
- There is no vertical ramus, with the condylar plane being parallel to the horizontal ramus
- Microtia with small pinna that are inferior and forward from their usual positions
- Conductive hearing loss
- Cleft palate

Brain abnormalities in syndromic craniosynostosis

Brain abnormalities are not uncommon in craniosynostosis and should be sought before any definitive surgery. Findings usually include hydrocephalus, due to distortion of the brain, and compression, particularly around the foramen magnum. Small ischemic lesions and cranial neuropathies due to foraminal narrowing are also mentioned. Congenital anomalies such as corpus callosal dysgenesis and hippocampal and optic nerve hypoplasia can also occur, particularly with Apert's syndrome.

CONCLUSION

A wide variety of midface abnormalities occur. Familiarity with midface embryogenesis and developmental anatomy is the key to understanding these anomalies. Midface anomalies in children, although not common, are fairly characteristic in their imaging appearance and features. Modern CT and MR have proved to be extremely valuable in the management of these abnormalities.

12

Imaging of facial and paranasal sinus trauma

The paranasal sinuses develop within and are protected by the facial bones, which also surround and serve to protect both orbits and the nasal and oral cavities. The facial skeleton, which supports the maxillary dental arch and serves as an attachment for the facial musculature, develops into a honeycombed structure of varying thickness in the form of either a fine lattice or a strong buttress, depending on the degree of strength required along the lines of stress exerted by the facial musculature and forces of mastication.

STRUCTURE OF THE FACIAL SKELETON

The facial skeleton tends to be assessed in terms of the supporting buttresses forming its structure in the sagittal, coronal, and axial planes.

Sagittal buttresses

There are two main sagittal buttresses on either side of the face. A medial nasomaxillary buttress extends from the anterior maxillary alveolus up the lateral wall of the pyriform aperture and into the medial wall of the orbit, and is formed by the inferior maxilla, the frontal process of the maxilla, the lacrimal bone, and the nasal process of the frontal bone. A lateral zygomaticomaxillary buttress is formed by the lateral wall of the maxilla, the body of the zygoma, and the orbital process of the frontal bone in the lateral orbital wall. It is augmented by the anterior coronal buttress at the lateral orbital rim–frontal process of the zygoma and the zygomatic process of the frontal bone more anteriorly. Other augmenting sagittal buttresses of less importance include the more posterior pterygomaxillary buttress, extending from the maxillary tuberosity (posterior maxillary alveolus) cranially along the pterygoid plates to the skull base, and the midline (median) buttress formed by the nasal septum, extending from the palate to the crista galli and the skull base. The greatest occlusal masticatory forces are absorbed by the zygomaticomaxillary buttress, as evidenced by its thick cortical bone compared with the fragile medial maxillary wall. The curvature seen within the evolved craniocaudad buttresses (with the exception of the weak median nasal septal buttress) may suggest a need for structural reinforcement, which is supplied by horizontal axial buttresses or struts.

Axial struts

Three levels of axial struts interconnect and reinforce the vertically orientated buttresses: at the level of the maxillary alveolus and hard palate, the orbital floor and zygomatic arches, and the floor of the anterior cranial fossa. In addition, the central skull base, angled at 45° to the maxillary occlusal plane, also acts as an axial buttress.

Coronal buttresses

There are two planes of coronal buttresses: an anterior plane formed by the vertical portion (glabellar region) of the frontal bone, the orbital rims, the anterior maxilla, and the alveolus; and a posterior plane formed by the posterior wall of the maxilla and the pterygoid processes of the sphenoid bone, extending inferiorly from the skull base.

This overall structure of the midface resists the vertical forces of mastication, providing excellent stability. These buttresses are less well structured with regard to resisting stresses due to external forces (e.g. traumatic impact), especially those that are not aligned along the strong directions of the facial skeleton. Disruption of a single buttress weakens the entire lattice and may cause it to collapse. Such potential collapse may be prevented by the strength of the facial buttresses and the support of the skull base. In general, the more superficial aspect of the facial skeleton has thicker buttresses to protect the more fragile central and deeper parts of the face.

FACIAL FRACTURE CLASSIFICATION

An understanding of the major lines of weakness in the facial skeleton allows the prediction of fracture patterns. Traditionally, midfacial fractures are classified according to the specific pattern by which the fracture lines extend through the facial strut system (Tables 12.1 and 12.2). Low-velocity impact forces, as seen in falls, sporting events, and punches, are more consistent with the fracture patterns initially described by Le Fort. The increased forces of high-velocity trauma (due to traffic accidents, assault with a blunt weapon, or gunshot wounds) allow for more significant transfer of stress (injury) to distant sites within the craniofacial skeleton. Multiple sites of impact at the time of facial injury may also result in discrete separate areas of injury. Although such high-velocity impact forces result in the same fracture lines as are found with lower impact forces, the involvement tends to be more extensive, more comminuted, more asymmetric, and in more varied fracture combinations than described in the typical Le Fort classification.

CLINICAL INJURY PATTERNS ASSOCIATED WITH MIDFACIAL FRACTURES

Facial fractures, of which midface injuries were most frequent, occurred in 16% of our patients who experienced multiple blunt trauma and were referred to a regional trauma center (Kassel and Gruss, 1991). Although most of the patients (71%) seen in one trauma referral center presented with midface fractures, only a minority of these patients (16.7%) had their fractures limited to the midface, with approximately 55% also having fractures involving the upper and lower face (Lee, 1987). Fractures of the anterior cranial fossa floor were noted in 14.7% of centrolateral midface fractures, 7.1% of central midface fractures, and 1.1% of lateral midface fractures (Schwenzer and Kruger, 1986).

A 59% incidence of intracranial injury was found among midface injuries related to motor vehicle accidents (high-velocity), compared with only 10% if the midface fractures resulted from falls or assaults (Brandt *et al.*, 1991). The incidence of concurrent intracranial injury was higher if orbitoethmoid, frontal sinus, superior midface, or Le Fort III fractures were present. A small number (1–2%) of patients with facial fractures will have an associated cervical spine fracture. These are almost

Table 12.1 Classification of midfacial fractures

A. Limited (single) strut
   1. Nasal arch
   2. Zygomatic arch
   3. Localized sinus wall (frontal, maxillary)
   4. Orbital floor
   5. Medial orbital wall

B. Complex structure (two anatomically adjacent regions)
   1. Zygomaticomaxillary complex
   2. Nasomaxillary complex
   3. Nasoethmoid–nasofrontoethmoid complex
   4. Sphenotemporal buttress

C. Transfacial fractures (bilateral, require pterygoid plate fracture)
   1. Le Fort I (transverse, Guérin)
   2. Le Fort II (pyramidal)
   3. Le Fort III (craniofacial dysjunction)
   4. Complex Le Fort (asymmetric, combined with zygomaticomaxillary)

D. Multiple strut fractures

E. Midface smash

F. Associated or extended fractures: skull base, mandible

always related to high-velocity motor vehicle accidents and are occasionally seen from falls down stairs. Coexistent mandibular fractures were present in several of those midfacial fracture patients with associated cervical spine fractures.

Improved motoring safety standards over the past decade, including seatbelt legislation and front and side airbag deployment, have helped decrease the number and severity of facial injuries. However, such high-velocity injuries remain disappointingly frequent.

Table 12.2 Complications of midfacial fractures

1. Orbit
   - (a) Visual pathway
     - Traumatic optic neuropathy
     - Optic nerve avulsion
     - Ocular rupture, hyphema, enophthalmitis
     - Lens dislocation
   - (b) Extraocular muscles
     - Entrapment/impaled
     - Contusion, laceration
     - Avulsion
     - Displaced (tugged)
   - (c) Lacrimal system injury
     - Nasolacrimal duct fracture
     - Lacrimal sac, canaliculi injury
     - Medial canthal ligament avulsion
2. Paranasal sinuses
   - Obstructed drainage: mucocele/pyocele
   - Intracranial empyema
   - Meningitis
3. Masticator space/dental/temperomandibular joint
   - Malocclusion
   - Trismus
4. Brain
   - Hematoma
   - Contusion
   - Infarct: post-embolic, post-dissection
   - Vessel occlusion
   - Dural venous thrombus
5. Neurovascular complications
   - (a) Vascular
     - Vessel occlusion, dissection, pseudoaneurysm, carotid cavernous fistula
     - Epistaxis
   - (b) Cranial neuropathy (superior orbital fissure syndrome)
6. Facial bones
   - Infection: osteomyelitis
   - Mal-union, non-union

CLINICAL DIAGNOSIS AND THE USE OF IMAGING (Figure 12.1)

Diagnosis of facial fractures may be made from clinical signs of facial deformity, abnormal mobility, crepitus, malocclusion, facial elongation or flattening, or hypertelorism. Diplopia, visual disturbance, cerebrospinal fluid (CSF) leak, or cranial neuropathy may further suggest the pattern of injury. Overlying edema, hemorrhage, or soft tissue injury may conceal the underlying facial injury. The deeper midface is not accessible to physical examination.

IMAGING TECHNIQUES AND OBJECTIVES

Computed tomography (CT) remains the modality of choice, offering excellent evaluation of the facial skeleton and adjacent facial soft tissues and overcoming most limitations of physical examination. Multidetector-row CT allows isotropic imaging with a concomitant dramatic increase of image data, with more comprehensive interpretation of the extent of fracture and the amount of dislocation or fragmentation. Minimally invasive CT angiography may be performed, where indicated, allowing greater opportunity for a fast emergent assessment. The newer CT techniques can be performed with greater accuracy, less time, less patient discomfort, and lower cost. The speed of helical technology permits thorough studies of patients who may not have tolerated such a study previously. These techniques enable 'one-visit' multiple sequential CT studies in the multitrauma patient. Higher quality results from decreased respiratory misregistration, better enhancement of vascular structures, and greater flexibility in image reconstruction, including multiplanar and three-dimensional (3D) reformations. A small amount of detail is lost as part of the 3D smoothing algorithm, but such images may preferentially visualize fractured segments and their relationship to each other better than are visualized on a series of 2D images.

Orthogonal two-plane CT studies are felt to offer superior detailed information than single-plane CT studies and subsequent reformations; however, with recent CT advances, such reformatting degradation may be eliminated. In either case, visualization of the actual 'source' images, and not just the reformations, remains invaluable. It should be noted, however, that magnetic resonance imaging (MRI) is better in assessing intracranial injury or complications.

Radiological exploration must assess the information necessary to allow appropriate clinical treatment and should answer a number of key questions:

- Does the maxillofacial fracture involve areas that may alter the physiological function of the sinuses (obstruction), orbits (vision, tearing, or diplopia), mouth (occlusion or airway compromise), nasal cavity, or nasopharynx (airway compromise or hemorrhage)?
- Will the fracture result in any cosmetically detectable abnormality?
- Is a foreign body or penetrating injury present?
- Is there any risk of imminent airway compromise or danger of fragments being aspirated?
- Is there any evidence of hyphema or endophthalmitis?
- Is a compound fracture present?
- Is any sizeable fragment of bone missing?
- Is there a potential fracture fragment that may compromise the orbital apex or optic canal?
- Are there any abnormalities in position, number, extent, depression, elevation, impaction, distraction, or rotation that will hinder reduction of the fracture or proper fixation of the fractured bones to one another and to the skull that represents a restriction on surgical restoration of facial form and occlusion?
- Is there any hematoma or soft tissue swelling present that may explain facial deformity or epistaxis clinically suggesting a fracture?

TREATMENT OF FACIAL FRACTURES

Current surgical treatment of facial fractures includes early primary fracture treatment with open reduction and rigid internal fixation, using microplates, miniplates, and lag screws, following wide subperiosteal exposure based on reconstructive craniofacial surgical procedures. Missing bone structures are replaced primarily by autogenous bone grafts or exogenous materials. Such early primary treatment reduces late esthetic and functional sequelae. Multiple small thin comminuted bone fragments – more commonly encountered in fractures of the anterior maxillary wall, orbital floor, orbital roof, and frontal sinuses – are difficult to manage, making accurate reduction with interfragmentary wires difficult. Larger bone fragments may be reconstructed, with the smaller fragments being discarded. Tissue adhesive (n-butyl 2-cyanoacrylate) may be used to maintain these small thin fragmented segments with some success. Gaps in non-buttress midface bony surfaces represent acceptable postsurgical findings.

Infections of a fracture line represent a serious complication of facial fractures. Any fracture should be considered a compound fracture and potentially infected if it traverses the alveolus or the walls of the nasal cavity or the paranasal sinuses, or if it communicates with a soft tissue wound. Antibiotic treatment reduces the chance of infection in maxillary or midfacial fractures to approximately 2%, and the risk of osteomyelitis to 0.5%. The risk of osteomyelitis increases approximately threefold to 1.3% if there is a treatment delay of 2–3 weeks. Post-traumatic sinusitis occurs in 7.25–9% of patients with midfacial fractures, and can be prevented or treated by proper maintenance of sinus drainage.

MIDFACIAL FRACTURES (Table 12.3)

Midfacial fractures are subclassified as central and lateral. They may be further described as localized or transfacial; unilateral or bilateral; and simple (segmental), complex, or compound.

CENTRAL MIDFACIAL FRACTURES

The maxillae, separated by the intervening nasal cavity, form the major volume of the central midface. The maxilla extends superiorly to form a component of the root of the nose superior to the level of the orbital floor. Inferiorly, the maxilla extends to form the maxillary alveolus and the major component of the hard palate. The nasal bones, lacrimal bones, inferior turbinate, vomer, ethmoid bones, and palatal bones also contribute to the central midface. Central midface fractures include all forms of fracture that occur between the root of the nose and the alveolar processes of the maxillae, but do not involve the zygomae.

Table 12.3 Midfacial fractures

1. Central
   - Isolated:
     - Dental alveolus
     - Palate
     - Maxillary
     - Nasal bones
   - Le Fort I transverse (Guérin's)
   - Le Fort II (pyramidal), Wassmund II
   - Wassmund I (nasal bones spared)
   - Nasoethmoid–orbital:
     - Nasoethmoid
     - Naso-orbital
     - Nasoethmoid–orbital
     - Nasofrontal
2. Lateral
   - Zygomaticomaxillary
   - Tripod (trimalar)
   - Zygomatic arch
   - Zygomaticomandibular
   - Orbital wall fracture:
     - Medial wall
     - Orbital floor (blowout/blow-in)
3. Centrolateral
   - Le Fort III
   - Various combinations of central and lateral components

Segmental

Alveolar fractures (Figures 12.2 and 12.4)

Alveolar fractures are the most common type of isolated maxillary fracture. They most frequently result from a blow to the mandible driving the mandibular dentition into the maxillary dental arch. The smaller-diameter mandibular arch forces the maxillary dentition upward and outward, fracturing the dentition or the maxillary alveolus. The strong supporting periodontal and periosteal tissues, tightly adherent to the alveolus, significantly limit displacement of alveolar fractures such that imaging findings are often subtle. In children, occult injury to the developing tooth buds may need to be assessed over time. In our experience, the probability of an associated mandibular fracture (dentition, alveolus, body, or condyle) is high, at approximately 70%. The probability of an associated mandibular fracture is greater if there is no indication of a direct blow to the central midface, suggesting that the maxillary alveolar fracture is caused by the dental arches being slammed together. Fractures of the maxillary tuberosity require more force and usually involve a dentoalveolar segment, bearing the molar teeth, being displaced superolaterally. These fractures may be associated with sagittal fractures of the palate or maxilla.

Palate (Figure 12.3)

Fractures that involve the palate frequently divide it longitudinally adjacent to the midline, at the weakest portion of the palatine process of the maxilla. The midline palate is reinforced by the vomer, while the lateral hard palate is supported by the maxillary alveolus. Midline palatal sagittal fractures imply more violent trauma. Comminuted palatal fractures tend to be associated with other central or centrolateral facial fractures. The presence of palatal fractures permits rotation of dentoalveolar segments, significantly increasing the instability of the fracture, and requires more specific internal fixation.

Synostosis of the palatal suture begins between 15 and 19 years of age. Trauma in younger individuals may separate the suture rather than dividing the palate parasagittally. Incisor tooth avulsion is common in palatal injuries and suggests the possibility of a sagittal fracture of the maxilla.

Fractures of the palate may lead to significant hematoma formation and subsequent airway compromise. A very tightly bound mucoperiosteum limits hematoma formation of the anterior hard palate. However, over the posterior hard palate at the horizontal plate of the palatine bone, the periosteum and mucous membranes are more loosely bound, with potential for significant hemorrhage of the posterior hard palate, soft palate, and pharyngeal walls by a fracture located more posteriorly within the palate. The posterior position of the greater palatine arteries and draining palatine veins, which communicate with the pterygoid and pharyngeal venous plexuses, supplies such hematoma formation.

Segmental fractures of the maxilla

These fractures usually involve the anterior or lateral walls of the maxilla, and result from a low-velocity force, often with a smaller-diameter striking surface. They may extend toward the nasal cavity or into the maxillary alveolus.

Comminuted or transfacial fractures (Figures 12.5, 12.8 and 12.9)

Le Fort I fracture (transverse) (Guérin's) (Figures 12.10 and 12.11)

The Le Fort I fracture results from a blow to the lower midface just superior to the maxillary dental arch. The horizontal (transverse) fracture involves the nasal cavity and maxillary antra bilaterally just superior to the hard palate, with the fracture being characterized by detachment of the caudal portion of the maxillae (including the palate, alveolus, and dentition) from the more superior intact maxillary component. The fracture line traverses all walls of the antra and nasal cavity, as well as the pterygoid processes. The 'floating' palate segment may be intact or comminuted. The lower face fracture lines tend to be less comminuted and more horizontal than for Le Fort II fractures. There may be minimal comminution or displacement of the fracture fragment, making detection difficult on axial CT alone. Clues are the tendency for the fractured component to be displaced posteriorly, creating a malocclusion with an anterior open bite. Occasionally, the Le Fort I transverse fracture may be seen more superiorly in the mid- or even upper maxillary sinus, with typical involvement of the walls of the antra and nasal cavity. This latter finding may be related to a striking force located slightly more superiorly. An altered Le Fort I pattern may also be noticed in denture wearers with full dentures of the maxillary arch protecting the maxillary alveolus from fracture, but a vertical fracture component may be noted passing superiorly from the main transverse fracture, and in those patients whose maxillary appliance has a discontinuity, an alveolar fracture may also be noted at that site.

Le Fort II fracture (pyramidal) (Figures 12.6, 12.7 and 12.12)

This fracture, named because of its triangular configuration, extends inferiorly and laterally from the pyramidal apex at the root of the nose, to involve the lacrimal bone and medial orbital wall (ethmoid) obliquely. The fracture then extends anteriorly along the orbital floor, involving the medial portion of the orbital process of the maxilla near the infraorbital canal, before extending inferiorly down the zygomaticomaxillary suture and the anterior wall of the maxilla. Posteriorly, the fracture extends across the posterolateral (infratemporal) wall of the maxillary sinus to involve the more inferior aspect of the pterygoid plates. The fracture may extend posteriorly along the orbital floor to the inferior orbital fissure and then inferiorly along the posterior maxilla to involve the pterygoid plates. The level of pterygoid plate involvement does not differentiate a Le Fort II from a Le Fort I fracture. The Le Fort II fracture remains inferior and medial to the zygomaticomaxillary suture, with the lateral orbital wall, body, and arch of the zygoma remaining intact. The Le Fort II fracture is a subzygomatic midface fracture in which the central portion of the midface is separated from the skull base superiorly and from the lateral aspect of the midface laterally. The involvement of the naso-ethmoid complex, medial orbital wall, and medial aspect of the orbital floor seen in the Le Fort II fracture are not seen with the Le Fort I fracture, which remains inferior to the level of the orbital floor and ethmoid sinuses. The fracture of the medial wall of the maxillary sinus and of the nasal septum, noted in the Le Fort I fracture, may also be seen in the Le Fort II fracture, especially if a central midface Le Fort II fracture is comminuted secondary to a high-velocity force. The pyramidally shaped Le Fort II central face fragment is displaced posteriorly, relative to the uninvolved lateral midface and skull, with a resultant 'dishface' deformity and malocclusion. Anesthesia or paresthesia of the infraorbital nerve is a frequent occurrence (approaching 80%), due to the intimate relationship of the orbital floor and rim fracture component to the infraorbital nerve. The deep central midface (Wassmund I) fracture spares the nasal bones and extends from the lateral edges of the pyriform aperture posteriorly across the lacrimal bones and the medial orbital walls.

Le Fort III fractures (Wassmund IV) (craniofacial dysjunction) (Figures 12.12 and 12.13)

The Le Fort III fracture is characterized by separation of the entire centrolateral facial skeleton from the skull base as a craniofacial dysjunction. As with the Le Fort II fracture, the medial component has a fracture line that involves the root of the nose, the lacrimal bone, and the medial orbital wall, but then crosses the orbital floor posterolaterally to reach the inferior orbital fissure, at which point the fracture line diverges. One portion of the fracture line continues laterally and superiorly across the lateral orbital wall to terminate near the zygomatic–frontal suture and the lateral orbital rim. The second fracture line extends from the posterior orbital floor posteriorly and inferiorly along the posterior maxilla to the more inferior aspect of the pterygoid plate. The zygomatic arches are also fractured, completing the craniofacial separation. A Le Fort III fracture without inclusion of the nasal bones is called a Wassmund III fracture, with the fracture line extending from each side of the pyriform aperture up to the lacrimal bones, then continuing as seen with the Le Fort III fracture. The Le Fort II fracture tends to involve the orbital floor more medially, in contrast to the more lateral floor involvement seen with the Le Fort III fracture. Both fracture types are associated with infraorbital nerve involvement, which is slightly greater with Le Fort II (89%) than with Le Fort III (70%). A true Le Fort III fracture involves the roof of the maxillary sinus (orbital floor) without disruption of the anterior or lateral maxillary sinus walls as noted with the Le Fort II fracture, and without the medial disruption of the Le Fort I fracture. Le Fort III patients also tend to have a 'dishface' deformity, malocclusion, nasolacrimal drainage disruption, and CSF rhinorrhea. Instability or displacement of the lateral midface may clinically differentiate this fracture from a Le Fort II fracture.

Upper central midfacial fractures: naso-orbital, nasoethmoid, nasoethmoid–orbital fractures (NEO)

The nasoethmoid–orbital region represents the junction between the nasal, orbital, and cranial cavities. The interorbital space posterior to the nasal bones, between the medial wall of the orbit, and beneath the floor of the anterior cranial fossa (ACF) contains the two ethmoid labyrinths, the upper nasal cavity, the nasal septum, and portions of the superior and middle turbinate bones. The roof is formed by the cribriform plate, the fovea ethmoidale, and the orbital plate of the frontal bone from medial to lateral. The junction of the ethmoid roof and cribriform plate is the weakest portion of the ACF floor. The tight adherence of a thinner dura here results in dural lacerations and CSF leaks associated with fractures at this site, with the dura and the skull base functioning as a single unit. Olfactory nerve injury may also be suspected with disruption of the cribriform region. Intracranial pneumocele or infection have an increased incidence related to fractures at this site.

Fractures may be confined to the NEO complex, but more frequently are associated with other facial fractures. The majority of these fractures result from high-velocity motor vehicle trauma, with a tendency to orbital and intracranial complications, and with CNS injury being seen in approximately 50% of cases. The medial wall of the orbit with the lacrimal bone anteriorly and the lamina papyracea more posteriorly is fragile and invariably comminutes from a traumatic force centered over the bridge of the nose, displacing the nasal pyramid posteriorly. Telecanthus, seen in 10–12% of these injuries, is nearly always produced by splitting of the nasomaxillary buttress, which is displaced laterally. The medial canthal ligament tends to be displaced with the buttress, and is rarely torn or avulsed. Injuries to the nasolacrimal apparatus are also common. The thinner medial orbital floor facilitates concomitant orbital floor fractures.

The fine lattice of the ethmoid sinuses allows the nasoethmoid complex to collapse, accordion style, on itself, with the nasal bones being driven posteriorly into the ethmoid sinus. This protective design better maintains the traumatic forces more centrally, with a relatively decreased frequency of bone fragments involving the globes or optic nerves. The crista galli and the nasal septum have a mild buttressing effect and help limit the extent of comminution along the floor of the ACF.

Fractures of the NEO complex may extend posteriorly along the cribriform plate or medial orbital wall to involve the sphenoid sinus, orbital apex, and optic foramen. Subtle alterations in the configuration of the NEO complex, especially a minimal lateral shift of this complex, have significant implications because of its intimate relationship to the optic nerve, the orbital apex, and the parasellar tissues, including anterior cavernous sinus structures. Serious injury to these structures may occur secondary to transmitted forces along the medial orbital wall, with minimal, if any, displacement of bony parts. Extreme caution during reduction of these facial fragments is required to avoid any displacement of an optic canal fragment, resulting in blindness.

Nasoethmoid–orbital trauma tends to fracture the orbital rim at the junction of the medial and supraorbital margins. Inferiorly, the fracture extends to areas of relative weakness at the infraorbital or nasolacrimal canals.

NEO fractures show marked complexity and potential for deformity and dysfunction. An associated orbital rim or floor fracture is seen in approximately 95%, with associated Le Fort II or III or complex maxillary fractures in 75% of cases. Forty percent of these patients have rhinorrhea, and 25% have associated frontal sinus fractures. Severe ocular injury is seen in 30%. The nasolacrimal duct is injured in 66% of comminuted anterior ethmoid fractures. The nasal bone, vomer, perpendicular plate of the ethmoids, and ethmoid labyrinth are thin and predisposed to comminution, significantly restricting the nasal airway. The nasal process of the frontal bone and the frontal process of the maxilla are stronger and offer some stability. Orbital hematomas are relatively frequent. The anterior and posterior ethmoid foramina (at the upper lamina papyracea at the junction of the fronto-ethmoid suture) represent a site of relative fixation, with resultant tears of the transmitted vessels or nerves.

The curved slope of the posterior wall of the frontal sinus onto the floor of the anterior cranial fossa may be assessed poorly by axial images, underestimating fractures or displacement. Posterior displacement of the anterior ethmoid–nasofrontal complex suggests disruption of the floor of the anterior cranial fossa and requires further assessment by coronal and sagittal reconstructions. Fractures of the anterior ethmoid–root of the frontal sinus have a higher incidence of drainage complications than fractures positioned more superiorly.

LATERAL MIDFACIAL FRACTURES

Lateral midfacial fractures include zygomatico-maxillary fractures, tripod–trimalar fractures, zygomatic arch fractures, and zygomaticomandibular fractures, as well as blowout fractures of the orbital floor.

Zygomaticomaxillary and tripod–trimalar fractures

(Figures 12.30–12.39)

The zygoma, as a protective prominence at the superolateral aspect of the midface, is the second most frequently fractured facial bone (after the nasal bone), representing approximately 50% of midfacial fractures, and approximately 70% of midfacial fractures involving the zygomatic complex alone or in conjunction with other mid-facial fractures. These fractures are traditionally referred to as trimalar or tripod fractures related to fractures through the three bony projections of the zygoma, namely the lateral orbital wall, the zygomaticomaxillary interface, and the zygomatic arch. The fracture line through the lateral orbital wall involves both the zygomaticofrontal and zygomaticosphenoidal sutures. The zygomatic arch component most commonly fractures at the weaker temporal component of the arch, approximately 1.5 cm posterior to the zygomaticotemporal suture. Fractures associated with the zygoma frequently involve the abutting bones, with no fracture through the zygoma itself.

The tripod fracture line extends from the lateral orbital wall to the inferior orbital fissure, then along the lateral aspect of the orbital floor near the infraorbital canal, to extend inferiorly at the anterior maxilla near the zygomaticomaxillary suture. The infraorbital nerve is impaired in approximately 95% of tripod fractures. Ocular disorders are seen in one-third of tripod fractures – twice the occurrence of ocular disorders in blowout fractures.

Delayed malpositioning with rotation or tilting of zygomatic fractures may occur in a non-fixed malar fracture due to muscular forces, especially from the masseter muscle. Such delayed onset of displacements may occur post-traumatically for up to 10 days, requiring close clinical follow-up for assessment of these patients. Medially rotated zygomatic body fractures or more complex zygomaticomaxillary fractures have increased instability and greater risk of intraorbital nerve injury. Fractures of the zygomaticomaxillary buttress allow the zygomatic body to tilt downward and inward, causing late depression of the zygomatic prominence.

The zygomaticomaxillary fracture tends to be more complex than the tripod fracture, with the former having more extensive maxillary, orbital, or pterygoid components. The anterior maxillary segment extends more medially near the infraorbital foramen, with the fracture line extending inferiorly toward the premolar region and then extending across the palate to the maxillary tuberosity and the lower pterygoid plates.

The more lateral orbital floor fracture involves less intimate positioning relative to the inferior rectus or inferior oblique muscles unless the orbital component is extensive – which explains the relative infrequency of diplopia or muscle entrapment. Fractures through the zygomatic recess of the maxillary sinus, involving the infraorbital rim, should not be confused with a Le Fort II fracture.

Blowout orbital wall fractures (Figures 12.21–12.29)

Orbital blowout fractures result from blows to the orbit by objects too large to enter the orbit, with the force absorbed by the orbital rim being transmitted to the thinner inferior (orbital floor) or medial orbital wall, which disrupts at its thinnest aspect. The posterior displacement of the globe increases the orbital pressure, directing the fracture fragments outward (blowout). Although the medial wall is thinner than the orbital floor, buttressing by the underlying ethmoid septa offers increased strength to this wall. Conversely, the thin orbital process of the maxilla is further weakened by the infraorbital canal, which is often dehiscent. The floor most commonly fractures at the medial mid-third, in contrast to the tripod fracture, which tends to occur lateral to the infraorbital canal.

Approximately 50% of orbital floor fractures have an associated medial wall fracture. The presence of orbital emphysema suggests a medial wall fracture, with such emphysema rarely originating from the maxillary sinus. Rapid sealing of the orbital floor fracture site by edema, hemorrhage, herniated fat, or muscle components may account for the decreased incidence of orbital emphysema. Medial wall fractures tend not to cause muscle dysfunction or entrapment. An increased incidence of medial orbital wall fractures has been noted in some studies, with medial wall fractures being more common than orbital floor fractures. The most common associated fracture of this pure medial wall fracture is a nasal fracture, seen in approximately 50%, with only one-third of medial wall fractures having an associated orbital floor fracture.

Delayed diagnosis of enophthalmos, which occurs in 14% of orbital floor fractures, leads to fibrosis and chronic changes of lipogranulation of herniated tissues, causing further volume loss, adhesions, and reduced mobility of the globe and extraocular muscles.

FRONTAL SINUS FRACTURES

(Figures 12.14–12.16, 12.18 and 12.19)

Fractures of the frontal sinus may be limited to the anterior table, posterior table, or both, with fractures of the anterior wall being much more common. Fractures of the frontal sinus occur either from direct force or as extensions of a calvarial fracture. Posterior wall fractures may occur as an extension of a skull base fracture. Comminuted depressed fractures of the frontal sinus may be clinically obscured by edema and hemorrhage filling the resultant depression. Complex frontal sinus fractures may be associated with other midfacial fractures, especially nasoethmoid–orbital injuries.

The degree of force associated with fractures of the frontal bone and the frontal sinuses, buttressed within a stronger bony framework, is significantly greater than that noted with fractures of the ethmoid or maxillary sinuses. The required greater traumatic forces and the more intimate relationship to the cranial contents are consistent with the much higher incidence of associated intracranial injury. These fractures are associated with increased involvement of the epidural and subdural spaces, CSF leakage, pneumocephalus, and possible pneumocele formation, as well as intracranial infections. Traumatic forces may be transmitted to the adjacent orbital rim, orbital roof, and skull base. In our experience, fractures involving under-pneumatized frontal sinuses have a greater tendency to extend to the adjacent skull base and orbital apices, suggesting a buffering effect on the traumatic forces with increased pneumatization of these sinuses. Severe comminution of the anterior sinus wall (eggshell deformity) is the most common pattern of frontal sinus injury seen in severe high-velocity blunt trauma. The buffering ability of the aerated frontal sinus as a protective barrier for the brain can be seen in patients who have comminuted anterior sinus wall fractures but minimal posterior sinus wall or cerebral injury. In contrast, forces that strike the forehead more laterally often result in posterior displacement of both anterior and posterior walls at the lateral aspect of the frontal sinus, with fracture extension along the floor of the anterior cranial fossa. Although linear fractures across the forehead may appear to be well visualized on conventional imaging, inferior extension along the orbital roof or skull base may not be appreciated, and may require further CT imaging techniques.

SPHENOID SINUS FRACTURES

(Figure 12.17)

Fractures of the sphenoid sinus are relatively rare owing to the protective function of the more anteriorly located sinuses. Such fractures are usually associated with severe cranial trauma and skull base fractures. Anterior calvarial or forehead trauma from forces obliquely or more laterally directed may involve greater transmission of these forces to the central skull base. Sphenoid sinus fractures are most frequently associated with fractures of the upper third of the face extending posteriorly along the orbital roof to involve the orbital apex and sphenoid sinus, or with fractures of the nasoethmoid complex in which the protective lattice structure favors absorption of the striking force within the central midface, with transmission of the fractures posteriorly along the medial wall of the orbit or cribriform plate to the sphenoid sinus. Fractures of the sphenoid sinus, most frequently involving the lateral walls and roof of the sinus, may be difficult to detect. The majority of such fractures do not show significant, if any, bone displacement. Fractures of the lateral wall of the sphenoid sinus often have a horizontal component and, with minimal displacement, may be difficult to see on axial CT. Fractures, of the sphenoid pterygoid plates, which provide attachments for the pterygoid musculature, may cause muscle dysfunction, especially if comminuted. The intimate relationship between the internal carotid artery and the sphenoid bone suggests possible vascular complications. Dissection, pseudoaneurysm, emboli, or occlusion may result. Carotid–cavernous fistulae may not manifest immediately. CSF leaks related to the sphenoid sinus may be difficult to detect, especially if fractures extend through the lateral recesses of the sinus. Such fractures of the sphenoid sinus may be secondary to zygomaticomaxillary fractures, with extension of forces along the greater sphenoid wing to the lateral sphenoid recess and adjacent skull base, despite minimal displacement of the zygomaticomaxillary component. Fractures involving the sphenoid sinus may be intimately associated with, and cause injury to, the optic canal or superior orbital fissure and its contents. Imaging studies to assess the sphenoid sinus are more frequently performed for assessment or treatment of complications. Such studies tend to be more demanding than for the other paranasal sinuses, with imaging data utilizing thinner axial slices and greater use of reformatted images. CT angiography or definitive catheter angiography may be required. Clinical aspects of masticatory function and cosmesis are generally not factors in sphenoid sinus injuries. Surgical intervention for such fractures is also limited in function.

12.1a

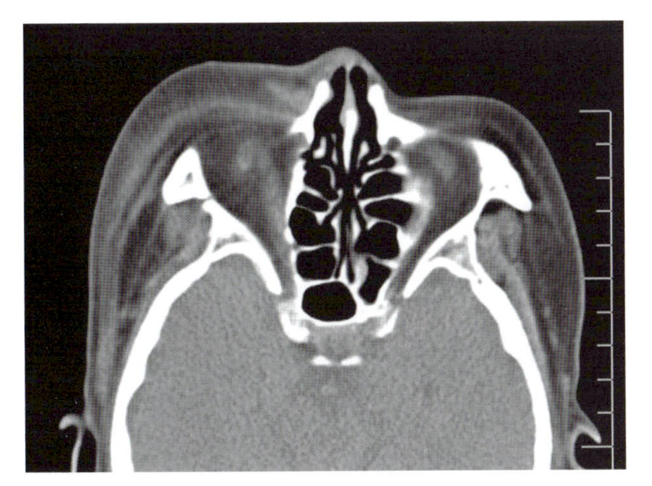

12.1b

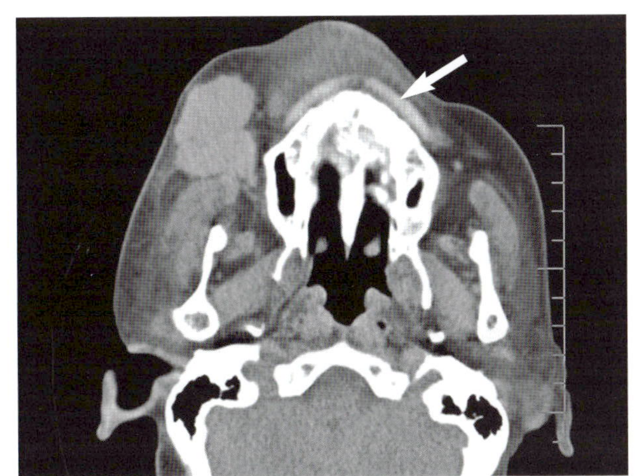

12.1c

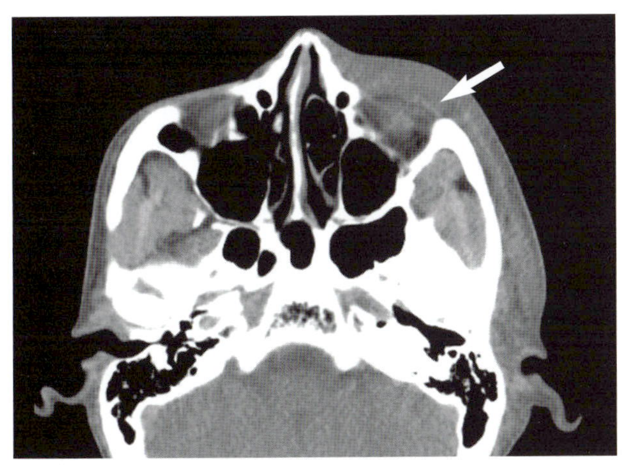

12.1d

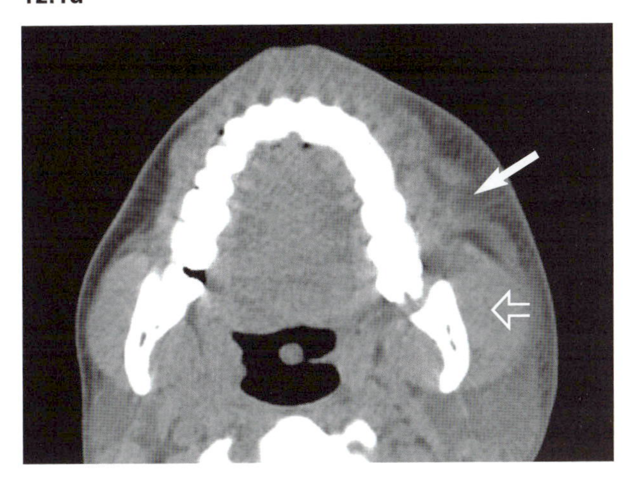

12.1e

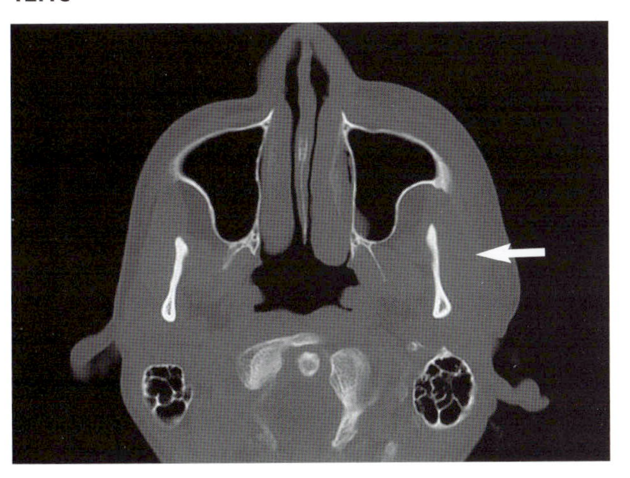

Figure 12.1 *Facial trauma – soft tissue injuries.* (a) Extensive facial soft tissue edema overlies the right midface and orbit, limiting clinical assessment of the underlying facial structures and orbit. (b) A large hematoma in the cheek explains the firm facial finding, clinically felt to be a displaced lateral midface fracture. The linear increased density at the anterior maxilla represents the more superior aspect of the patient's denture (arrow). (c–e) An assaulted patient with suspected left lateral face fracture. Soft tissue swelling overlies the left midface anteriorly and laterally (arrows). Increased interstitial edema is noted within the left lateral facial soft tissues. The left masseter muscle is contused, explaining the patient's trismus and a significantly larger than normal right masseter muscle (open arrow). No abnormality of the underlying midface or mandible is present.

12.2a

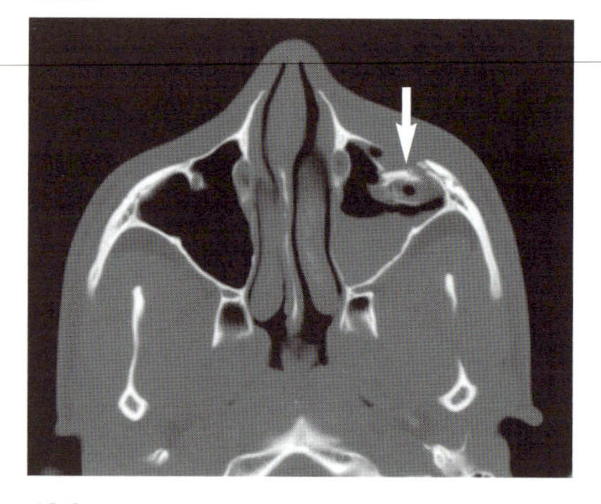

12.2b

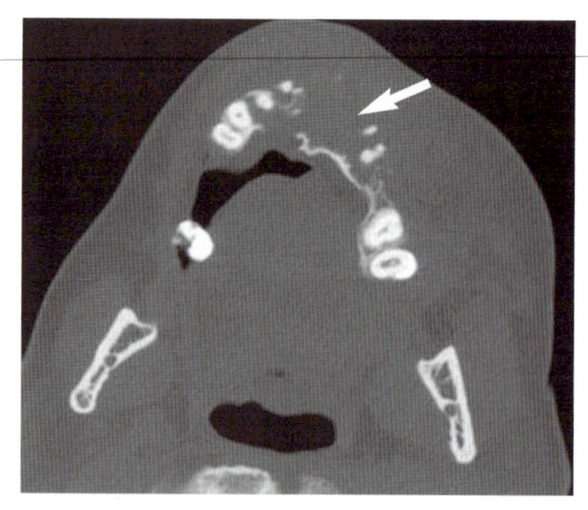

12.2c

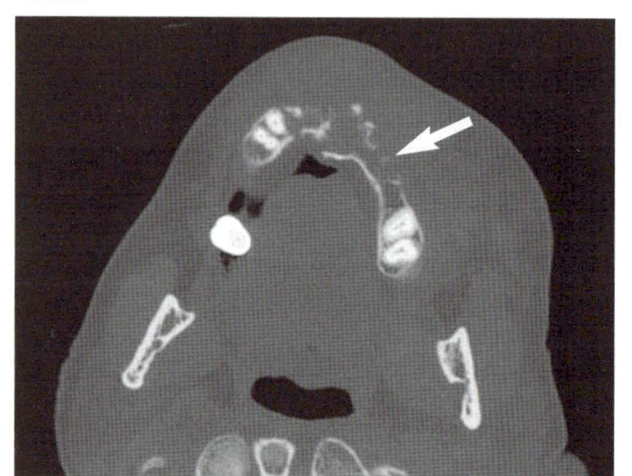

12.2d

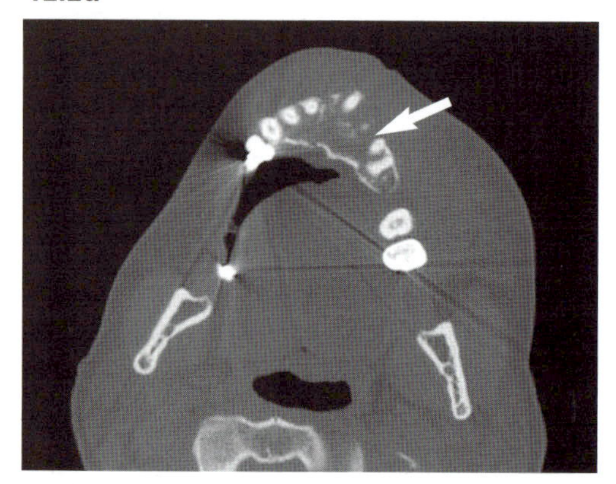

12.2e

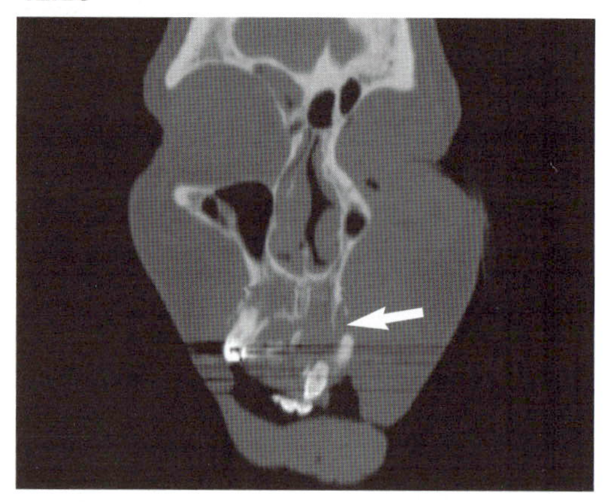

12.2f

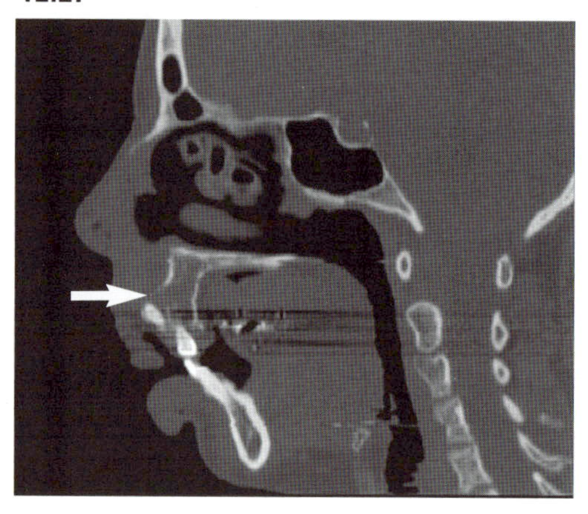

12.2g

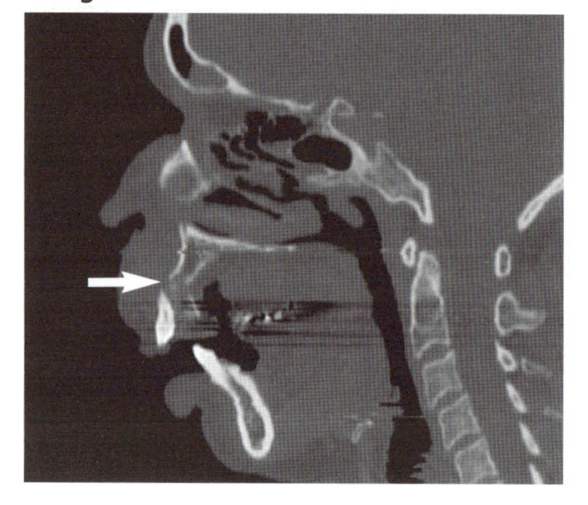

Figure 12.2 *Segmental fractures of the midface.* (a) Isolated depressed fracture of the anterior wall of the left maxilla resulting from a lower velocity focal force of smaller diameter (arrow). No abnormality of the zygoma or nasal structures is present. (b–g) A comminuted fracture of the anterior maxillary dental arch with disruption of the labial and lingual cortex (arrow). (b–d) Axial images showing expanded anterior–posterior dimension of the anterior maxillary arch. (e) Coronal reformation showing displacement of the anterior dentition with a fracture through the anterior maxillary dental arch. (f, g) Sagittal reformations showing a fracture through the alveolus at and superior to the dentition, with displaced and avulsed teeth and bone fragments. No injury to the midface is otherwise seen (arrows).

12.3a

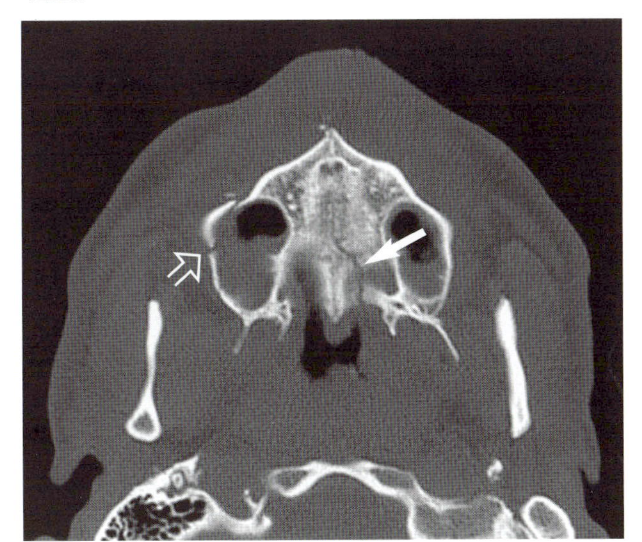

12.3b

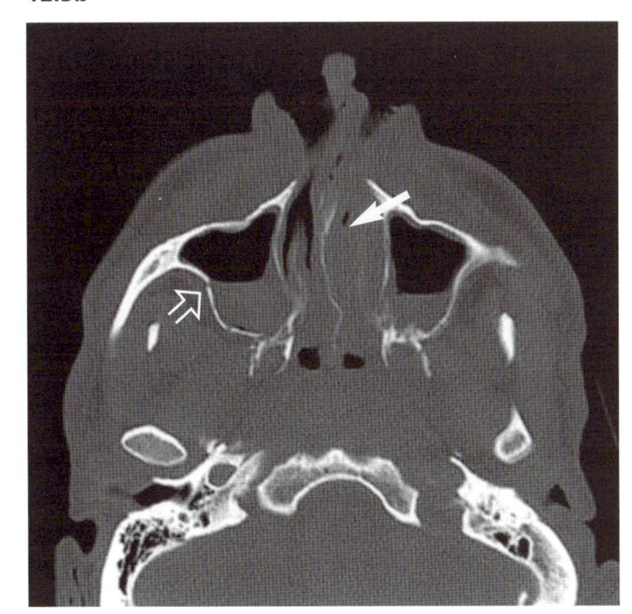

12.3c

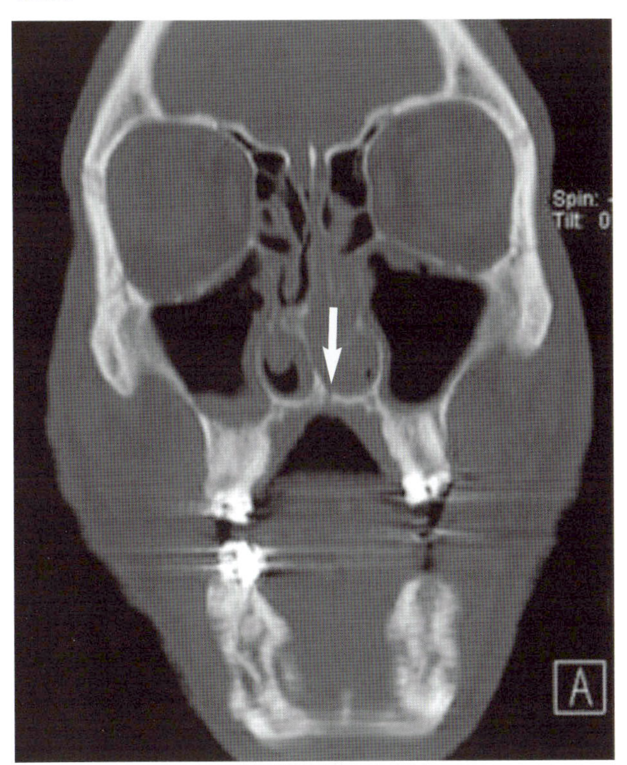

12.3d

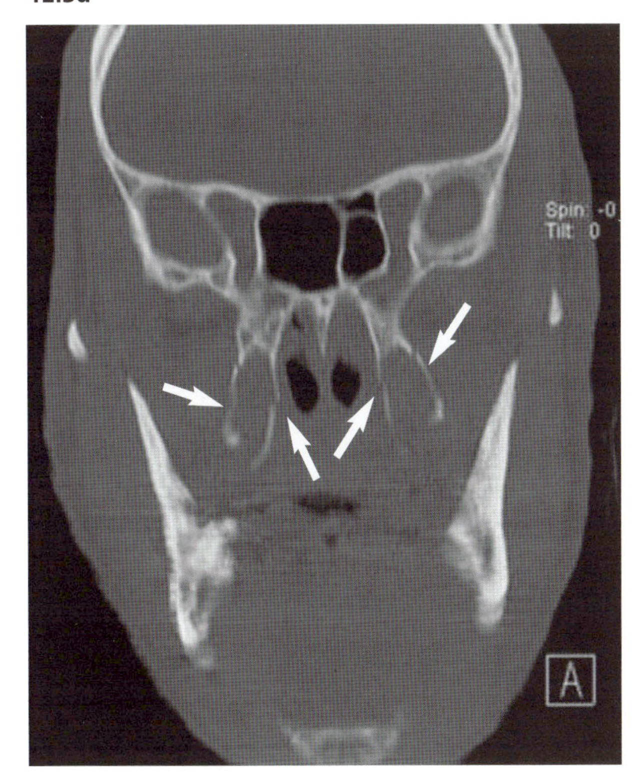

Figure 12.3 *Segmental fracture of the palate and pterygoids.* An undisplaced fracture of the palate just to the left of the midline posteriorly, shown on axial (arrow) (a, b) and coronal (c) images, is associated with an undisplaced fracture of the right lateral wall of the maxilla (open arrow) and bilateral fractures of the pterygoid plates, the latter being seen on the coronal reformation (d) (arrows).

12.4a

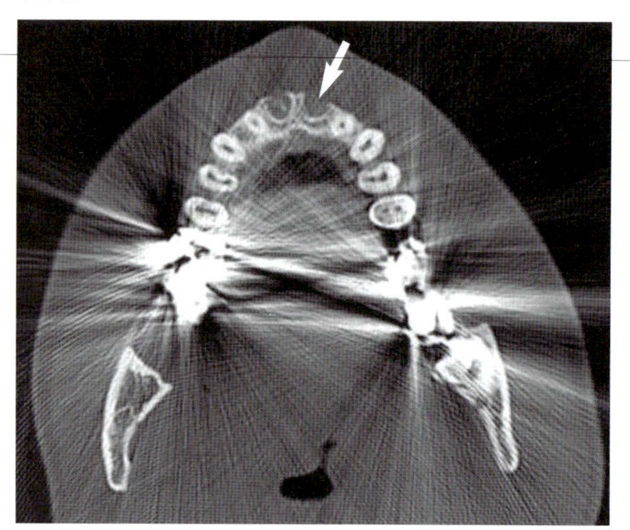

12.4b

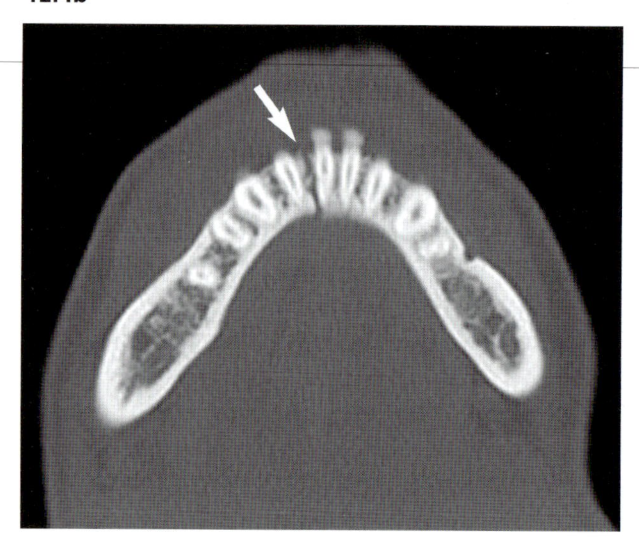

12.4c

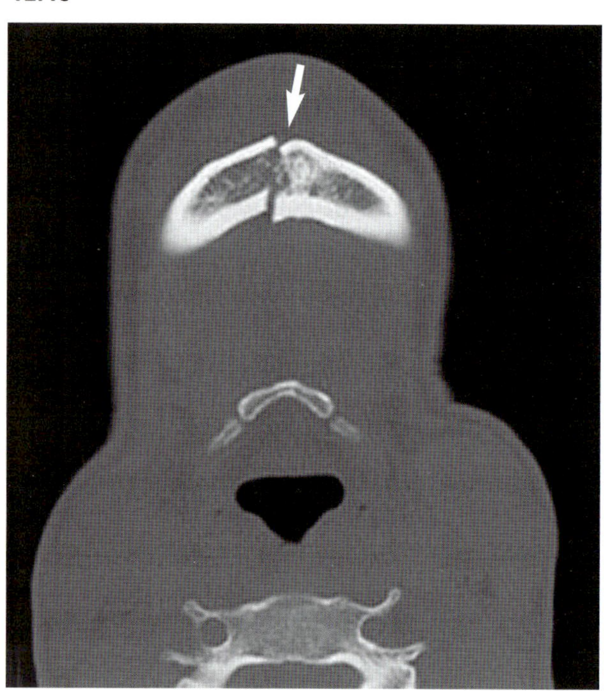

Figure 12.4 *Maxillary injury from mandibular force*. (a–c) Avulsed maxillary central incisors secondary to an occlusal force to the maxillary dentition from a blow to the the mandible. A parasymphyseal fracture of the mandible is present (arrows).

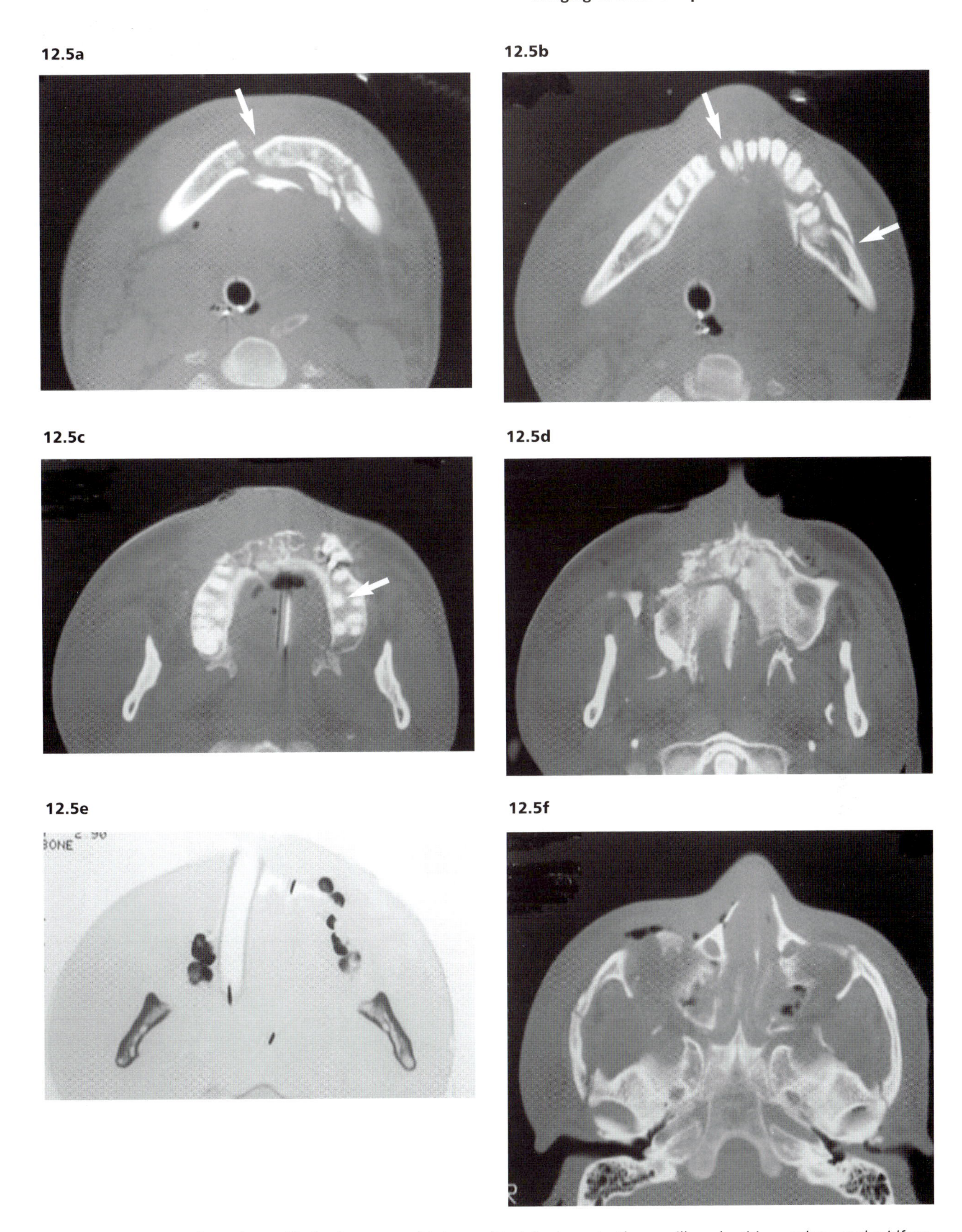

Figure 12.5 *Comminuted mandibular fractures with transmitted fractures to the maxillary dentition, palate, and midface.* (a–f) Axial images from inferior to superior. (a) Comminuted fracture of the anterior inferior mandible (arrow). (b) Comminuted fractures of the mandible, including a fracture through the left mandibular first molar (arrows). Avulsed maxillary anterior dentition, with the left maxillary bicuspid teeth displaced lateral to their dental sockets (c) (arrow). Sheared crowns of the left maxillary dentition. (d) Comminuted palatal fractures. (f) Bilateral maxillary and zygomatic fractures (clinically bilateral Le Fort III fractures).

12.6a

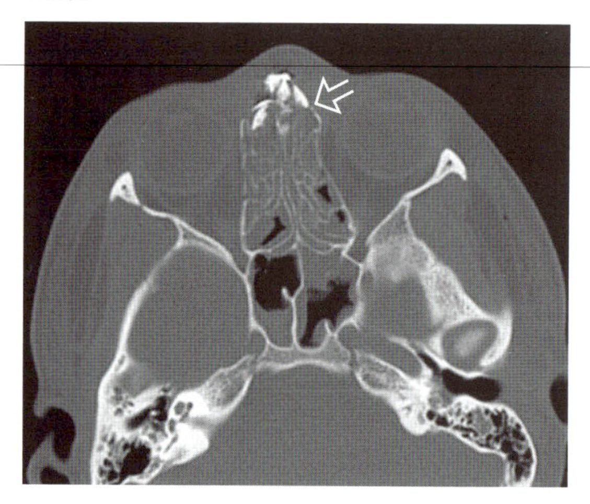

12.6b

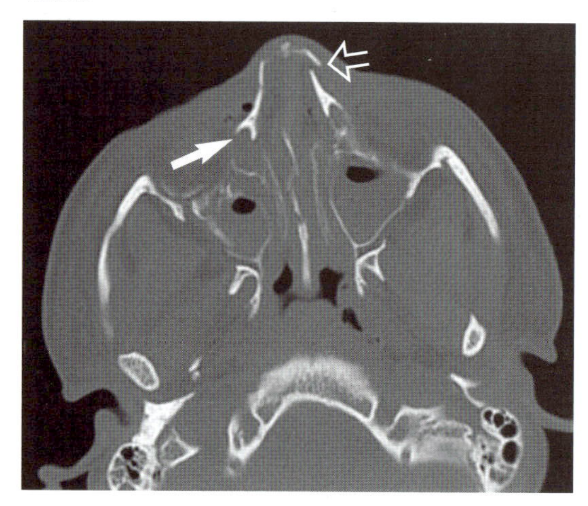

Figure 12.6 *Bilateral Le Fort II (pyramidal) fracture extending into the nasolacrimal canal* (arrow). (a, b) Axial images showing comminution through the anterior nasoethmoid complex bilaterally (open arrows), with no posterior displacement of the bony fragments. Fractures extend into the medial wall of the left nasolacrimal canal and split the anterior aspect of the right nasolacrimal canal from its posterior component. Comminuted fractures of the nasal septum as well as the right lateral maxillary sinus wall are noted. The lateral bony facial structures are normal.

12.7a

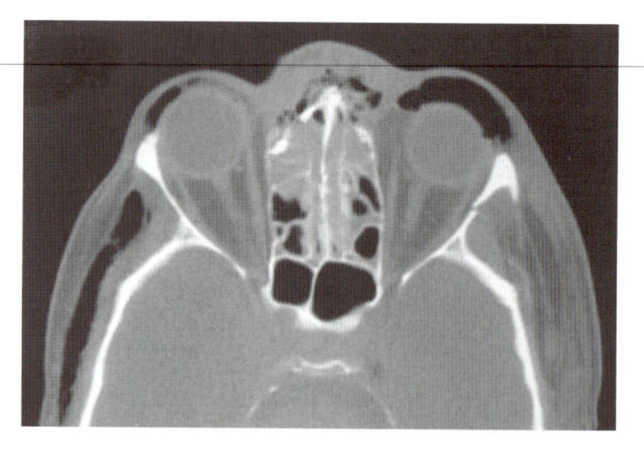

12.7b

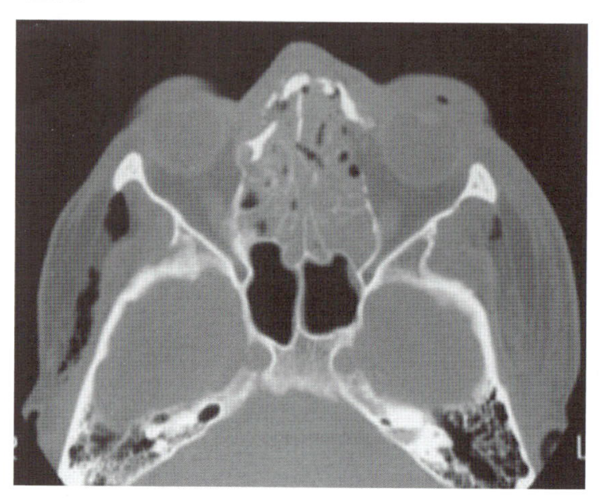

12.7c

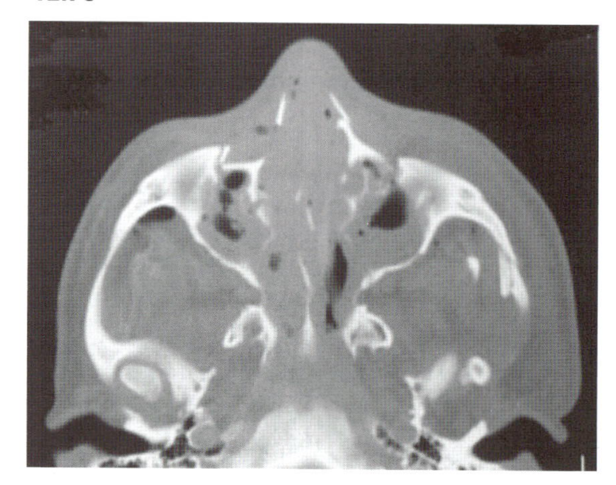

Figure 12.7 *Combined right Le Fort II–left Le Fort III fracture*. (a–c) Axial images (from superior to inferior) showing a comminuted fracture of the anterior nasoethmoid complex with an undisplaced fracture of the left lateral orbital wall. At the inferior orbital level, there is greater comminution of the nasoethmoid complex, including a fracture of the right nasolacrim canal and focal avulsion of bone at the insertion of the left medial canthal tendon. At the level of the midface, fractures extend down the anterior maxilla, with posterior displacement of the central face relative to the lateral facial structures. A comminuted fracture of the mid left zygomatic arch is present.

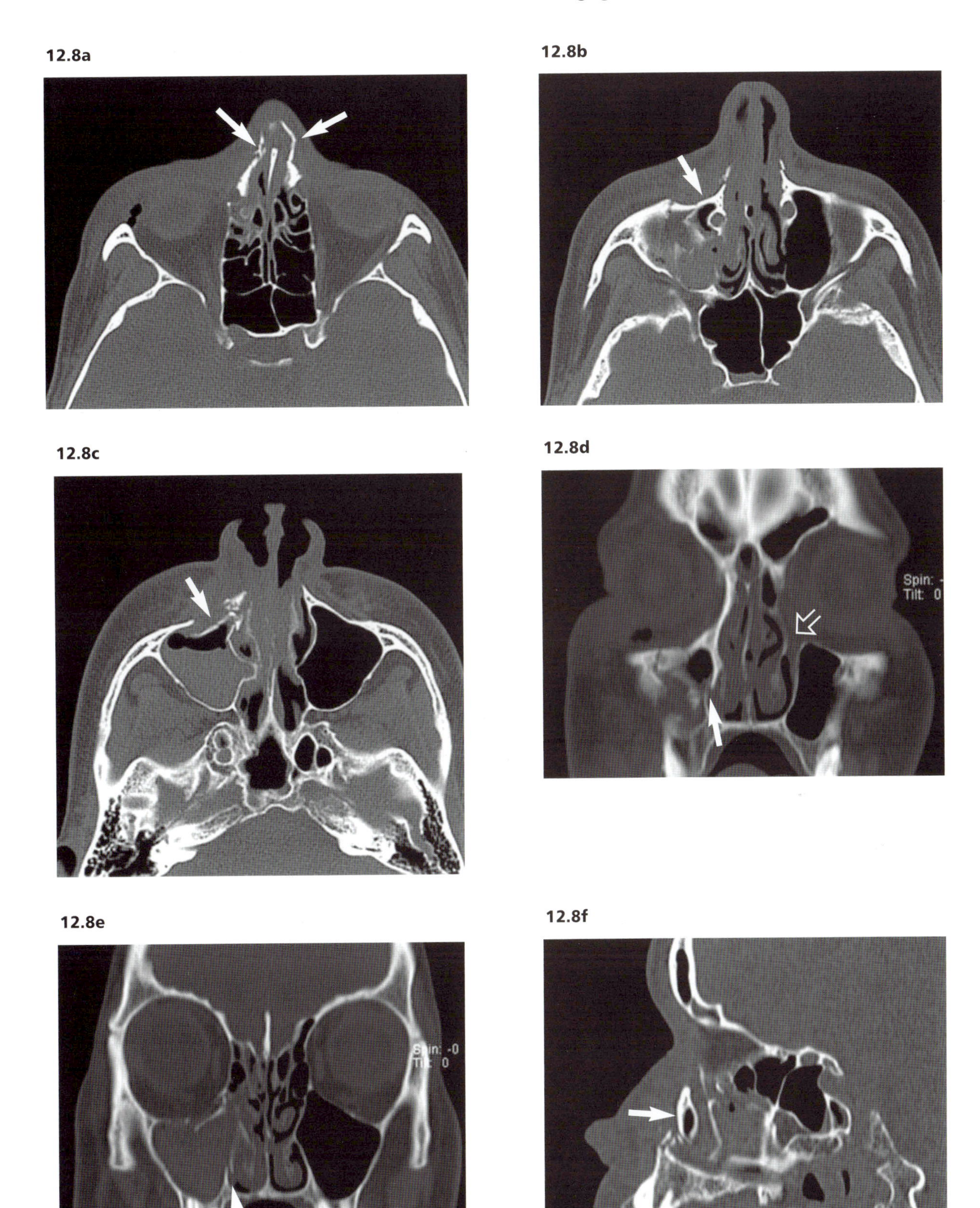

Figure 12.8 *Right nasomaxillary focal fracture fragment displaced posteriorly with the nasolacrimal canal (NLC) remaining patent*. (a–c) Axial images showing bilateral nasal bone fractures (arrows (a)), with a right nasomaxillary–nasolacrimal segment displaced posteriorly, including the right NLC (arrow (b)). Comminution of the bone fragment is noted more inferiorly, including bone fragmentation projecting into the inferior meatus, at the inferior aspect of the NLC (arrow). (d–e) Coronal images showing the right bone fragment displaced posteriorly, compromising the right inferior meatus (arrow) (see the normal left nasolacrimal canal (open arrow) (d)). (f) Sagittal reformation showing a patent NLC despite posterior displacement and fragmentation of the adjacent anterior maxilla (arrow).

12.9a

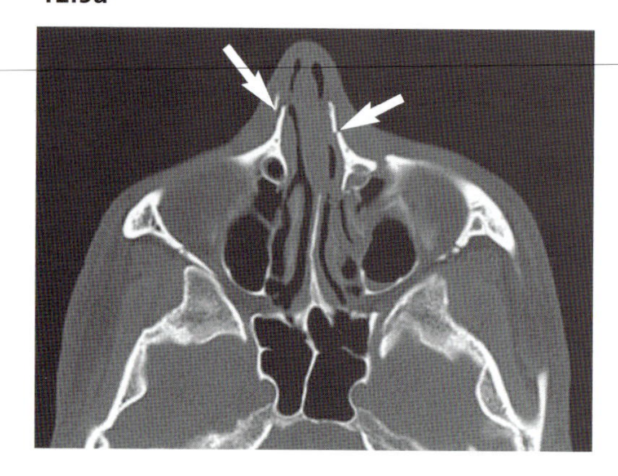

12.9b

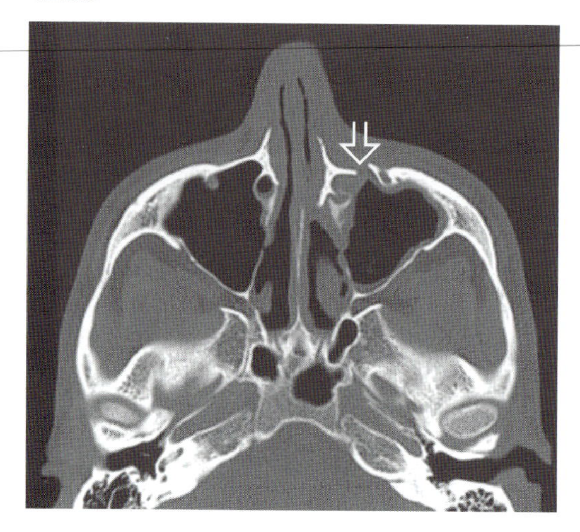

12.9c

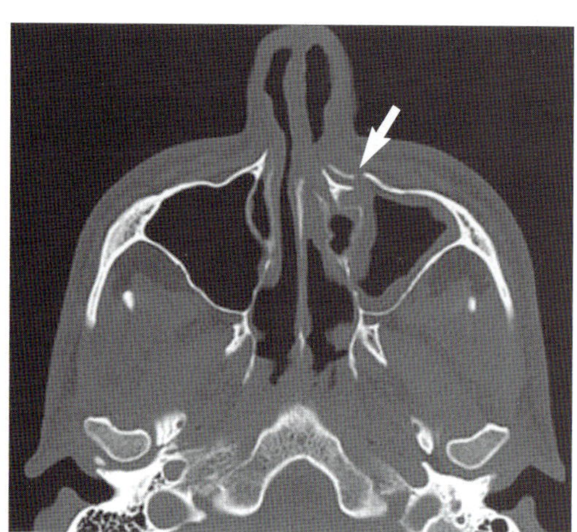

12.9d

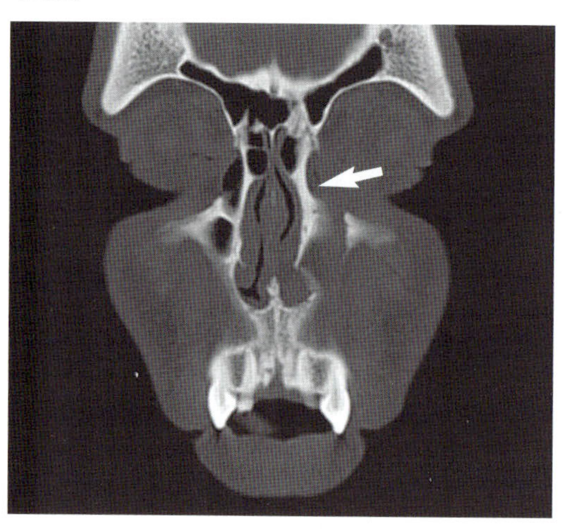

12.9e

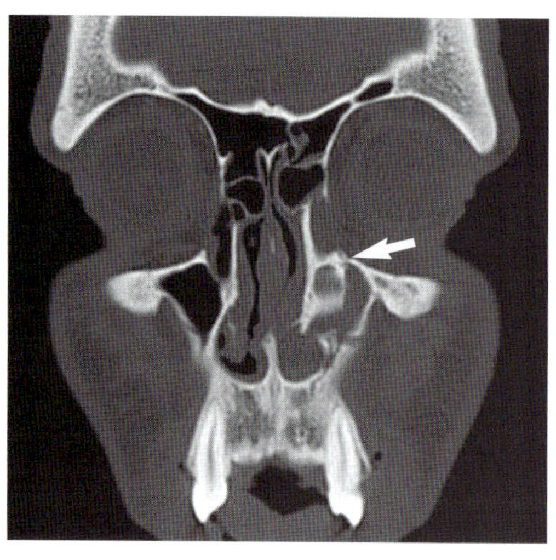

12.9f

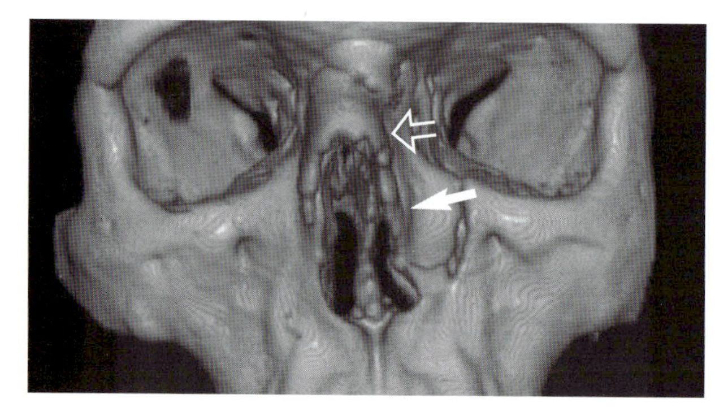

Figure 12.9 *Comminuted left anteromedial maxilla displaced into the nasolacrimal canal (NLC).* (a–c) Axial images showing bilateral nasal fractures, more comminuted on the left (arrows). A separate bone fragment surrounds the comminuted left nasolacrimal canal (open arrow). (d, e) Coronal CT does not show the relationship to the NLC so well, with the canal being obscured by the displaced bone fragment (arrow). (f) Frontal 3D view showing a bone fragment at the left anteromedial superior maxilla (arrow), with displacement of the nasal bones (open arrow).

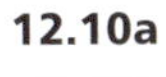

12.10a

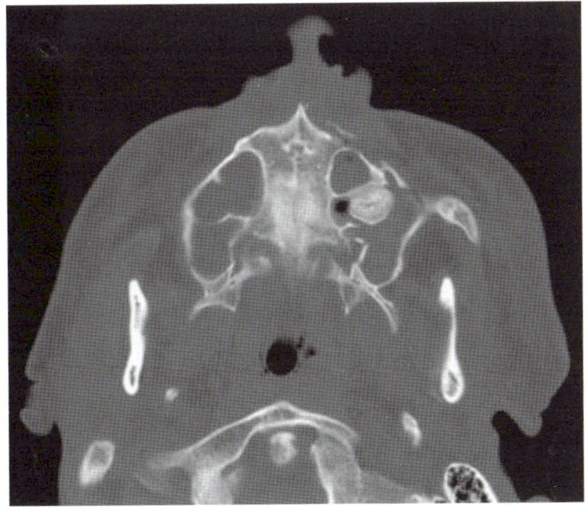

12.10b

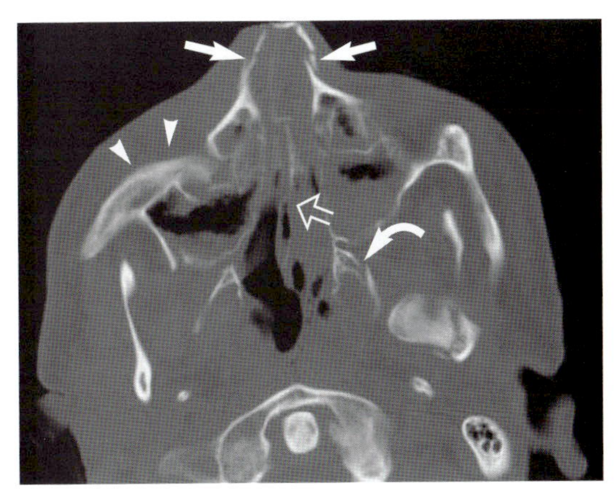

12.10c

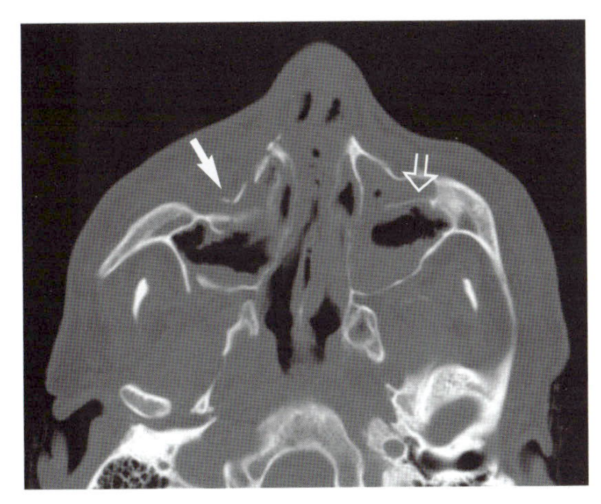

12.10d

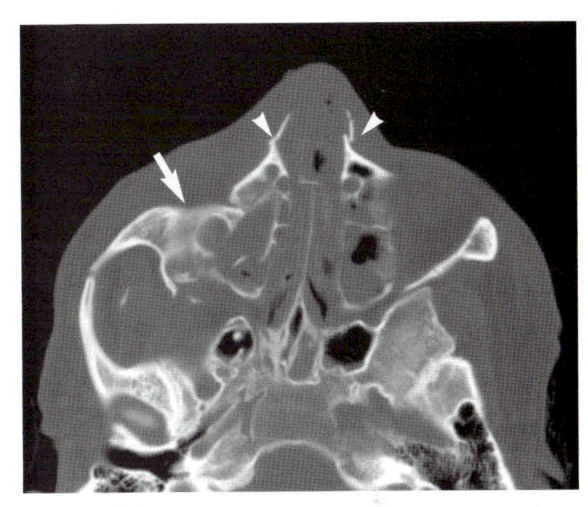

12.10e

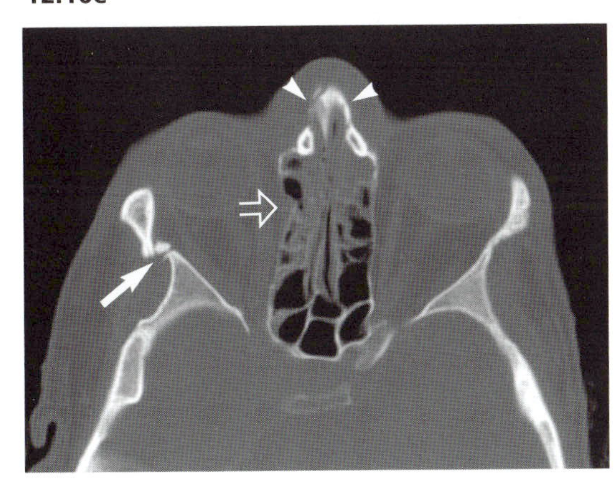

12.10f

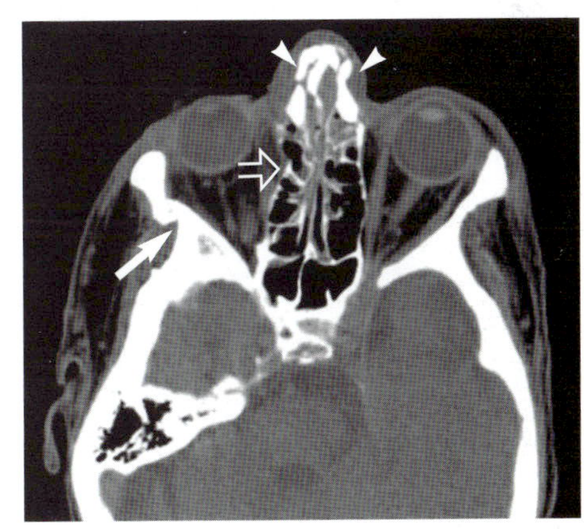

Figure 12.10 *Complex bilateral asymmetric Le Fort fractures.* Axial (a–f) and coronal (g–i) images displaying multiple bilateral facial fractures. Note the previous right temporal craniotomy for subdural hematoma. Fracture–dislocation of the left mandibular condylar head (temporomandibular joint, TMJ) appears subacute, with periostial bone reaction present. Incidental osteoma is present at the inferior left maxillary sinus. (a–f) Axial images from inferior to superior. (a) A fracture of the inferior anterior wall of the left maxillary sinus. (b) Bilateral nasal bone fractures (arrows) and a comminuted nasal septal fracture (open arrow), a posteriorly displaced right zygoma with associated fracture of the anterior and lateral walls of the right maxillary sinus (arrowheads), a fracture of the left pterygoid process (curved arrow), and a bone fragment within the left maxillary sinus. (c) Comminuted fractures of the anterior right maxillary sinus (arrow). The bone fragment within the left maxillary sinus is seen better here (open arrow)). (d) Bilateral nasal bone (arrowheads), and nasal septal fractures and a posteriorly displaced right zygomaticomaxillary fracture (arrow). (e, f) Fractures of the right lateral orbital wall (arrow), right medial orbital wall (open arrow), and the bilateral nasoethmoid complex (arrowheads).

12.10g

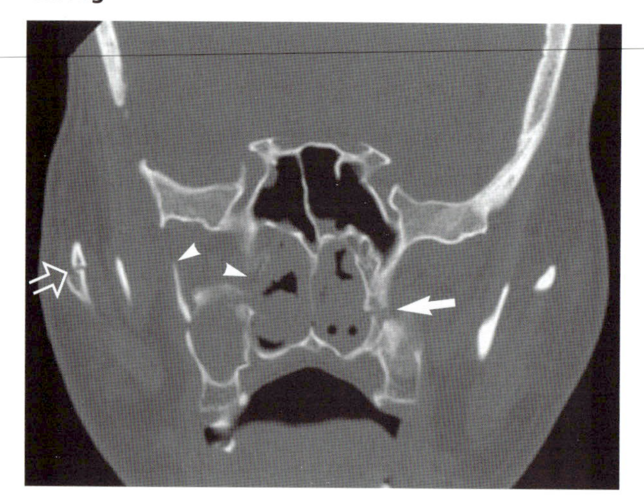

12.10h

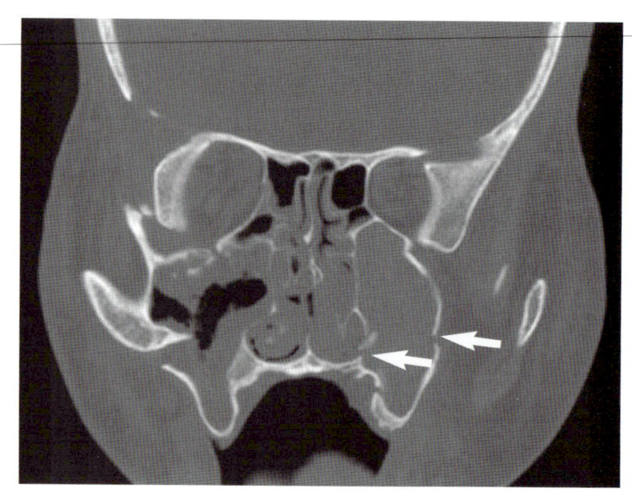

12.10i

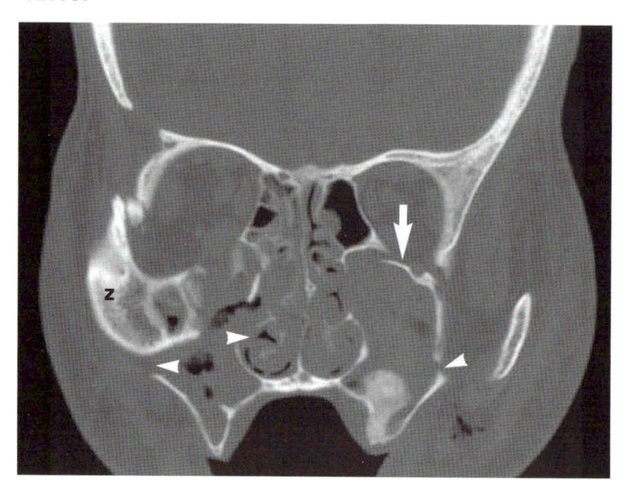

Figure 12.10 *continued* (g–i) Coronal images from posterior to anterior. (g) Fractures of the right zygomatic arch (open arrow), the medial and lateral walls (arrowheads), and the posterior right maxillary sinus, and a horizontal fracture of the left pterygoid process (arrow). (h) Fractures of the medial and lateral walls of the inferior left maxillary sinus (arrows). (i) Superior displacement of the right zygomatic body (z), a fracture of the left orbital floor (arrow), and fractures of the medial and lateral maxillary sinus walls bilaterally (arrowheads) – this combination of fractures represents right Le Fort I, II, and III fractures and a left Le Fort I and II combination.

12.11a

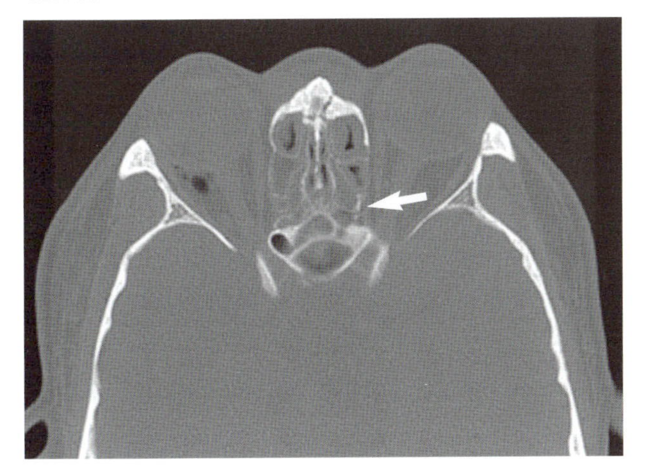

12.11b

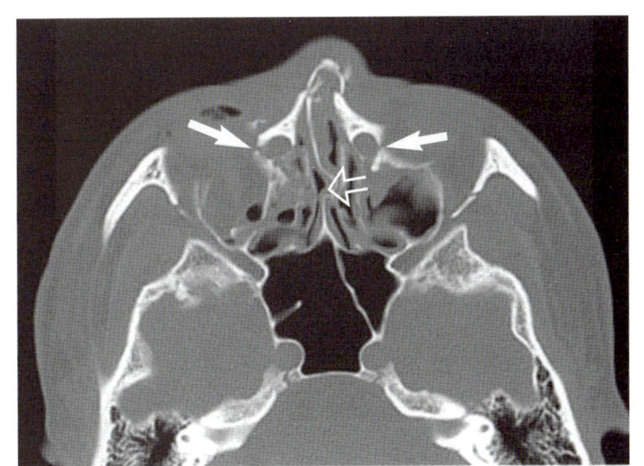

12.11c

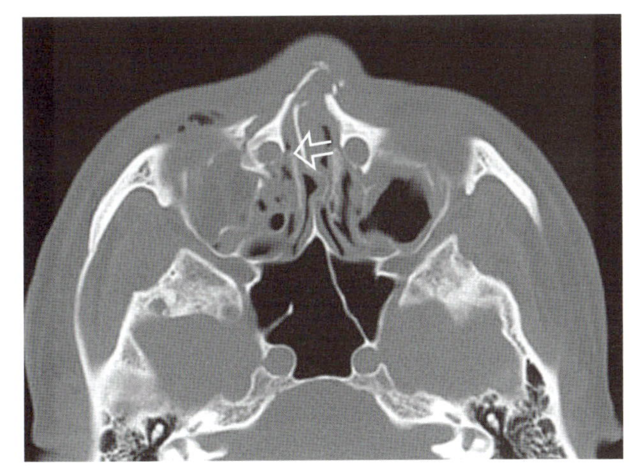

12.11d

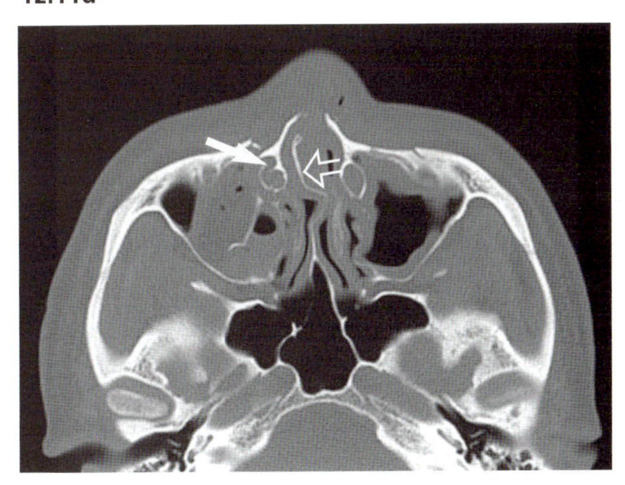

12.11e

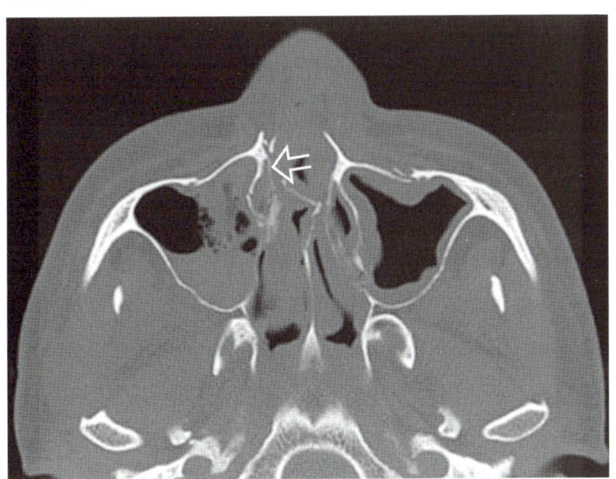

Figure 12.11 *Complex nasoethmoid maxillary fractures.* (a–e) Axial images. The axial images from superior to inferior (a–e) show a fracture of the nasoethmoid complex, with subtle buckling of the lamina papyracea bilaterally (on the most superior image (arrow) (a)). The nasal septum is buckled and deviated (open arrows). The nasoethmoid complex is displaced posteriorly relative to the lateral face structures. Fractures extend through the nasolacrimal canals bilaterally (arrows) (d). The right nasal bones, nasolacrimal canal (NLC), and nasal process of the maxilla are fractured as a unit and rotated to the left. The left NLC and nasal process of the maxilla are fractured as a separate unit and rotated to the right.

12.11f

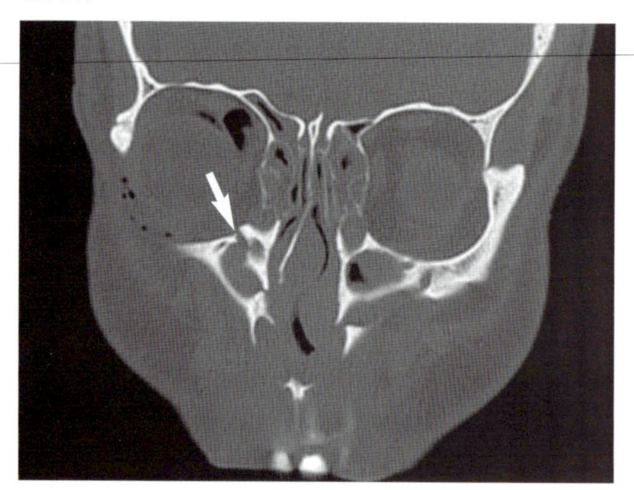

12.11g

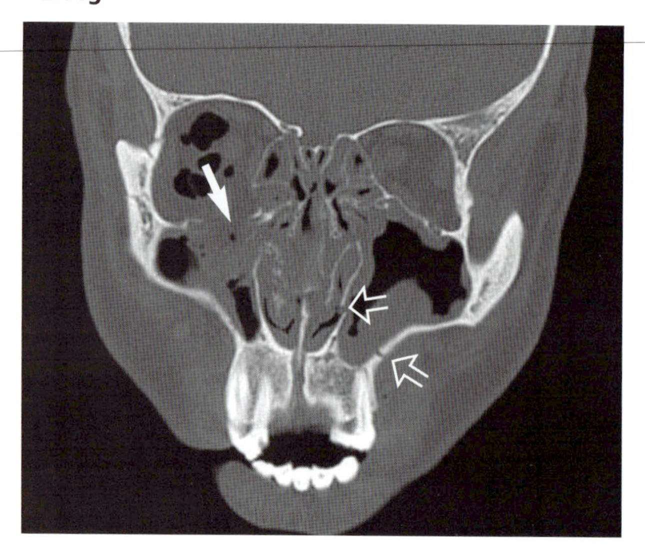

12.11h

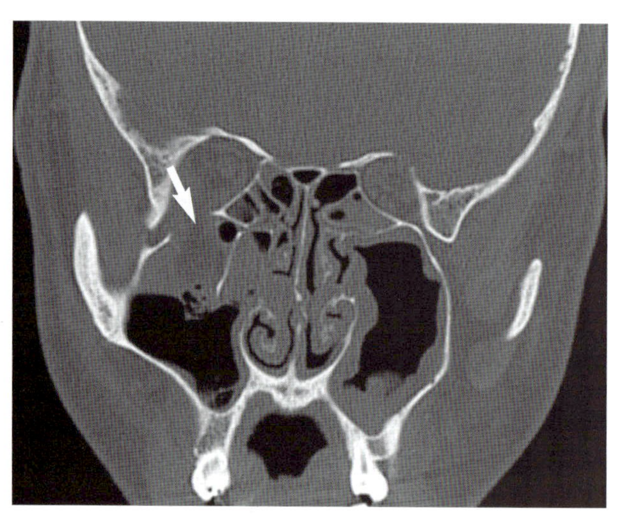

Figure 12.11 *continued* (f–h) Coronal images. The left infraorbital rim and the anterior wall of the maxilla are displaced posteriorly. There is a large right orbital floor fracture (arrows). The right lateral face remains intact, with no evidence of Le Fort II or Le Fort III components. On the left, there is a fracture of the medial and lateral wall of the maxilla consistent with a Le Fort II fracture (open arrows).

12.12a

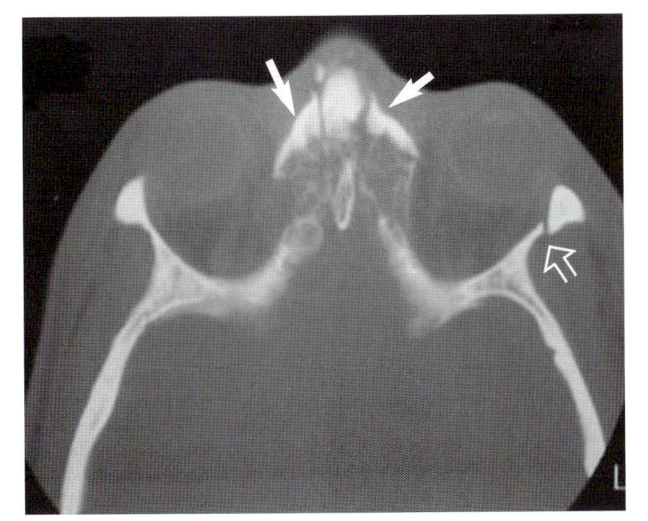

12.12b

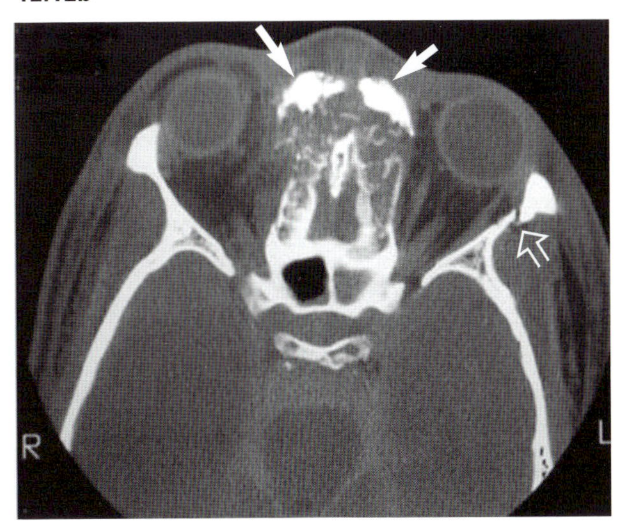

12.12c

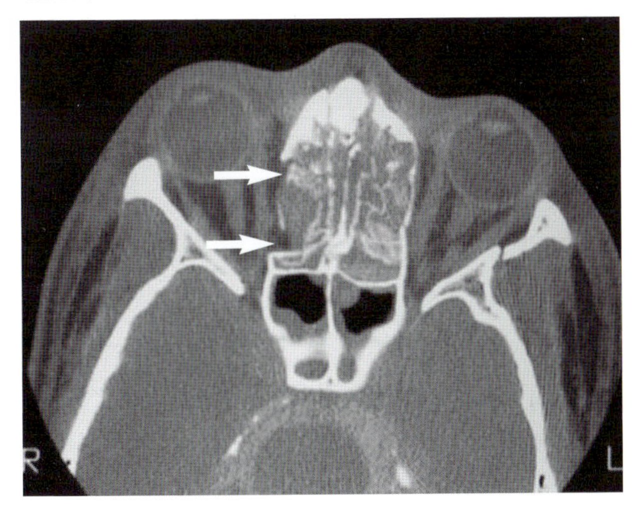

12.12d

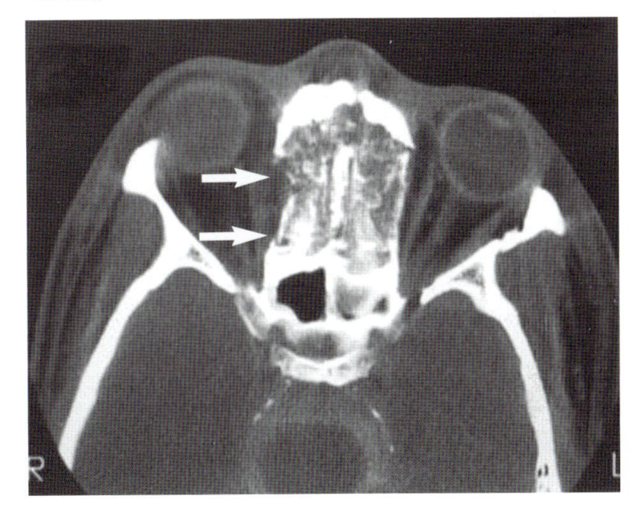

12.12e

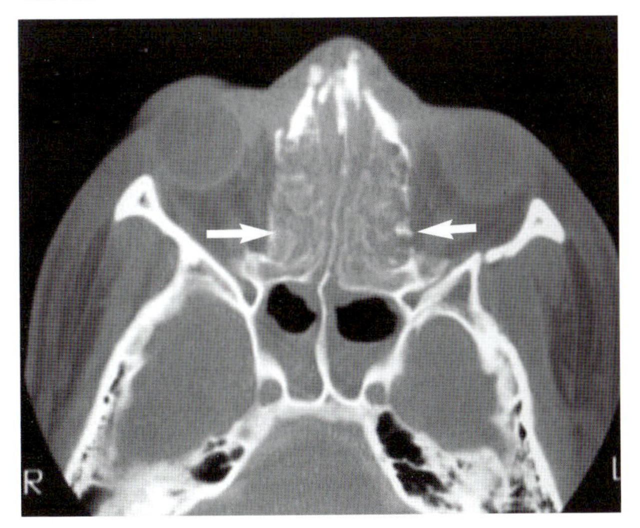

Figure 12.12 *Complex midface fractures: comminuted nasoethmoid, right Le Fort II, left Le Fort III fractures, with splaying of nasoethmoid and nasomaxillary complexes.* (a–g) Axial images from superior to inferior. (a, b) Comminuted fractures with splaying of the anterior nasoethmoid fragments, including the nasolacrimal canals (arrows). The crista galli remains in its normal position. A fracture of the left lateral orbital wall with lateral displacement of the lateral orbital rim is present (open arrows). The right globe is displaced laterally by the bone fragments. (c–e) At the level of the sphenoid sinus and skull base, comminuted nasoethmoid fragments (arrows) represent an unstable bone complex. Extensive subarachnoid hemorrhage is present.

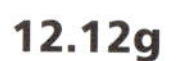

12.12f

12.12g

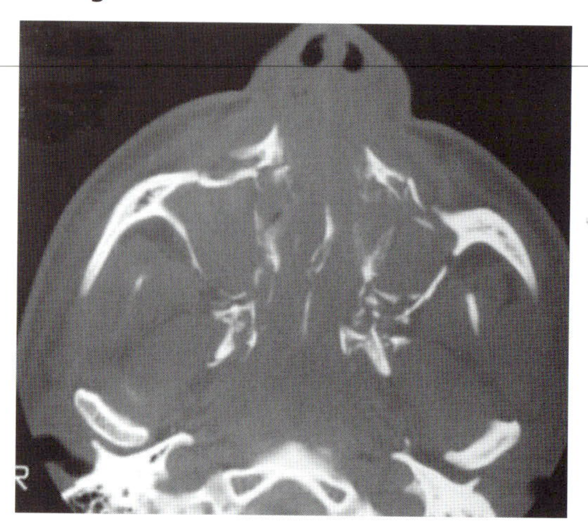

Figure 12.12 *continued* (f, g) At the inferior midface, complex nasoethmoid fractures extend toward the inferior orbital apex. Comminuted fractures of the posterior orbital floor are present bilaterally. There are subtle fractures of the left zygomatic arch. The fracture patterns represent complex nasoethmoid fractures with a right Le Fort II and a left Le Fort III fracture.

12.13a

12.13b

12.13c

12.13d

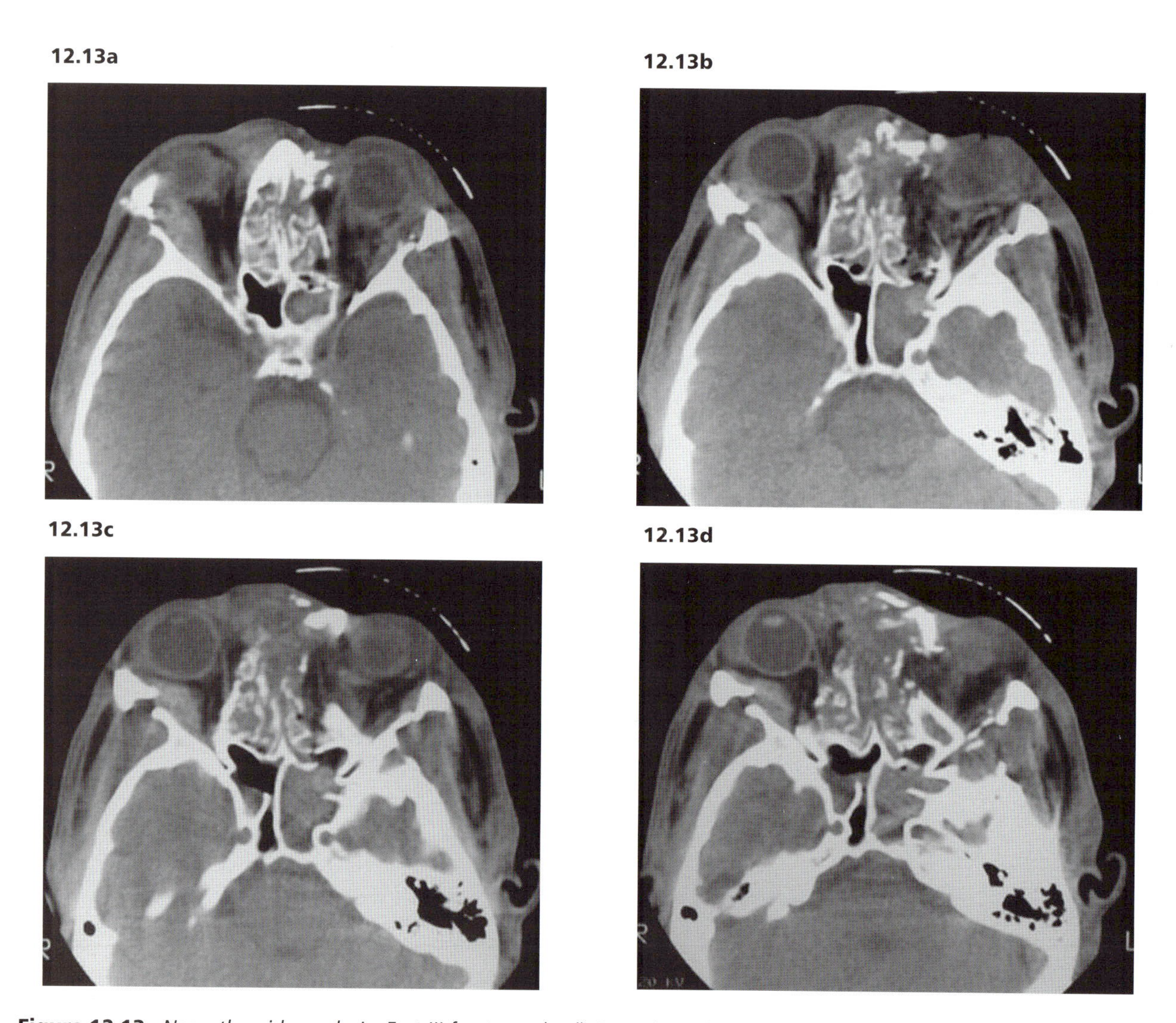

Figure 12.13 *Nasoethmoid smash, Le Fort III fractures.* (a–d) Comminuted nasoethmoid fractures with associated fractures of the lateral face (Le Fort III fractures). Traumatic hypertelorism is noted at the mid to inferior orbital levels. A subperiosteal hematoma is noted with the right lateral orbital wall fracture.

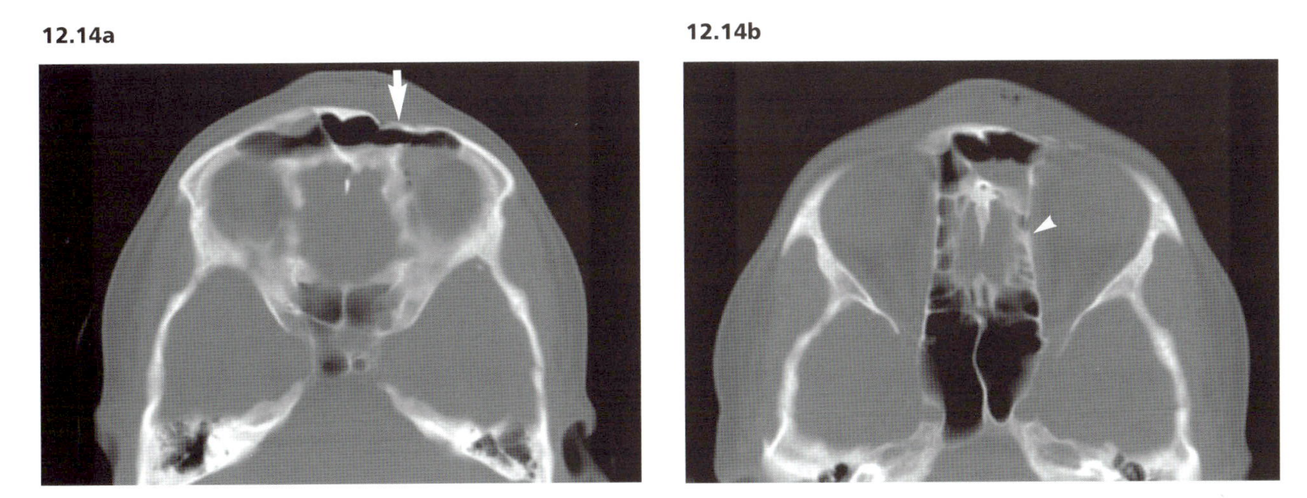

Figure 12.14 *Frontal sinus: frontoethmoid fracture*. (a, b) Despite a minimally displaced fracture of the anterior table of the left frontal sinus (arrow), there is transmission of the fracture force with resultant minimal displacement and subtle fractures of the lateral wall of the left ethmoid sinus (arrowhead). The posterior table of the frontal sinuses is intact.

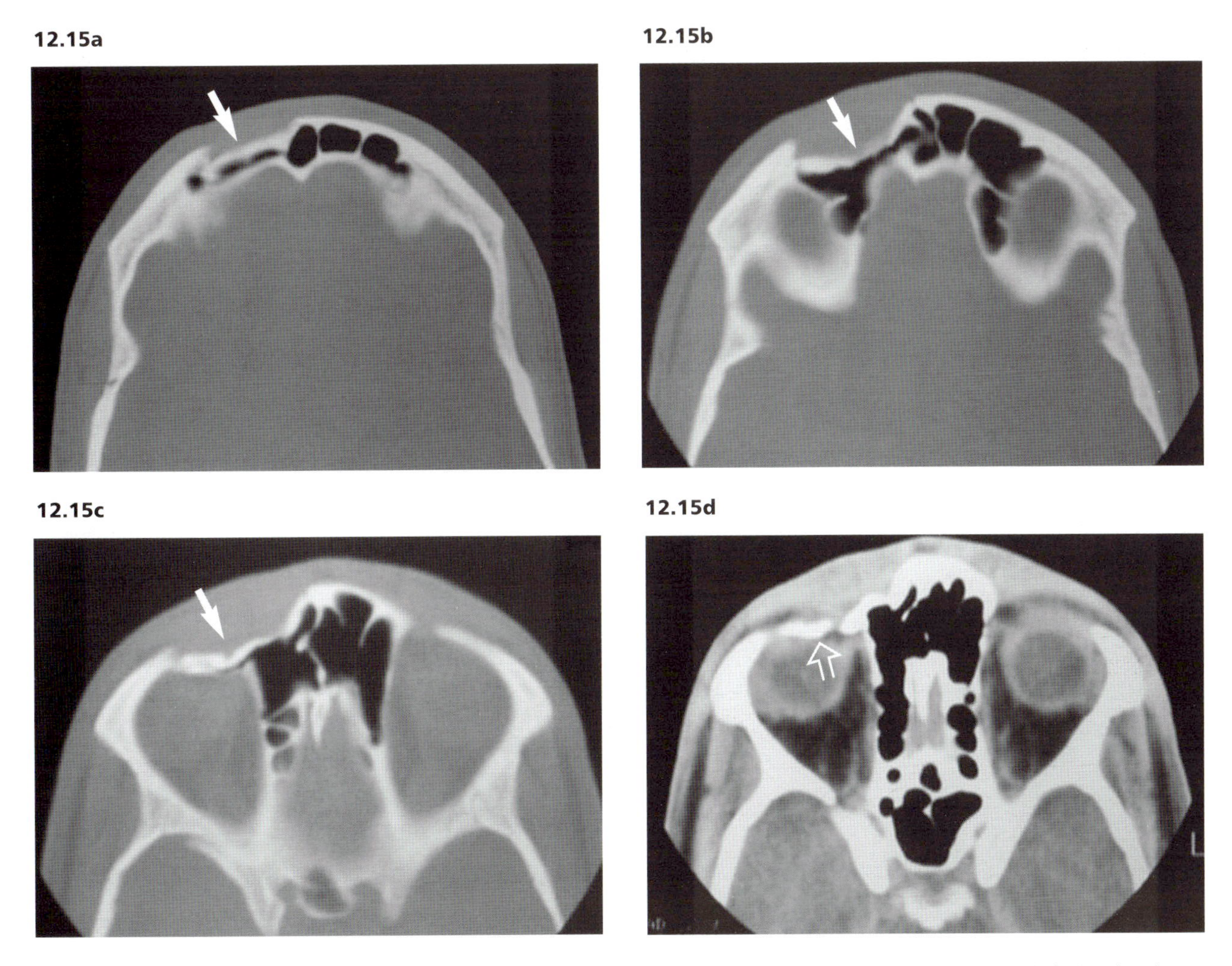

Figure 12.15 *Well-aerated frontal sinus with anterior wall fracture*. (a–d) Axial images from superior to inferior showing a depressed fracture of the anterior wall of the right frontal sinus (arrows), with no transmission of the fracturing force to the posterior wall of the frontal sinus or to the adjacent skull base. On the most inferior image (d), the fracture fragment includes the superior orbital rim, which minimally encroaches on the superior anterior orbit (open arrow).

12.16a

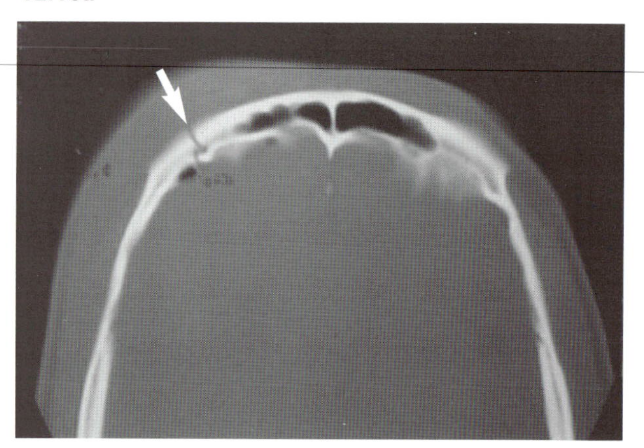

12.16b

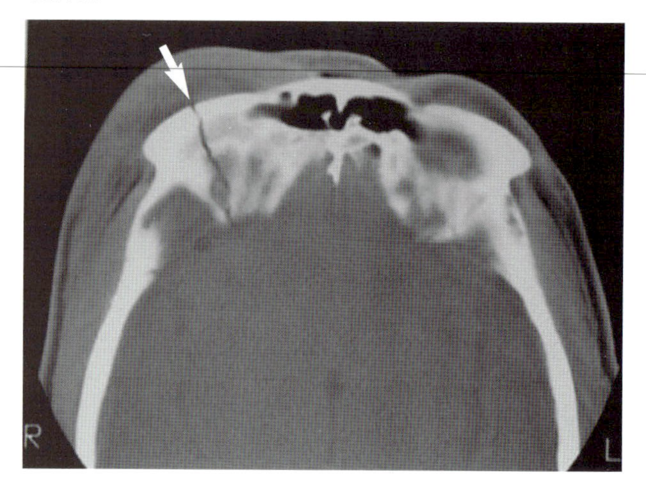

12.16c

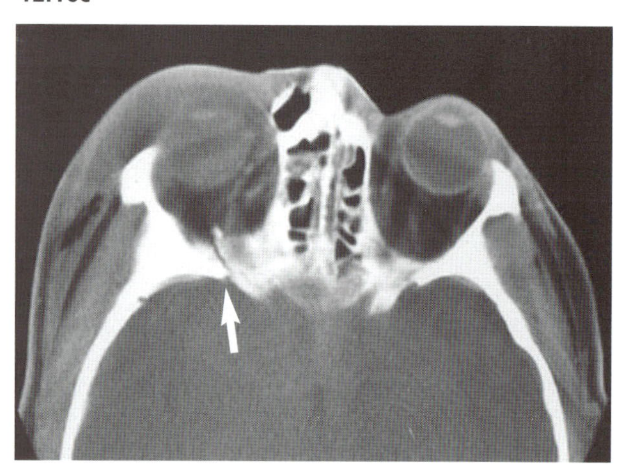

Figure 12.16 *Lateral forehead or hypoplastic frontal sinus fracture*. (a–c) An undisplaced fracture through the lateral aspect of the frontal bone, lateral to the frontal sinus, extending posteriorly along the right orbital roof and lesser wing of the sphenoid wing (arrows). Such fractures tend to extend deeper into the central skull base, because there is a relative lack of a buffering as associated with an aerated frontal sinus.

12.17a

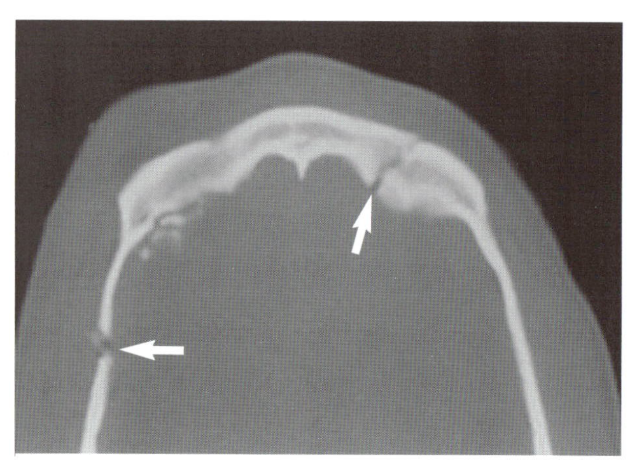

12.17b

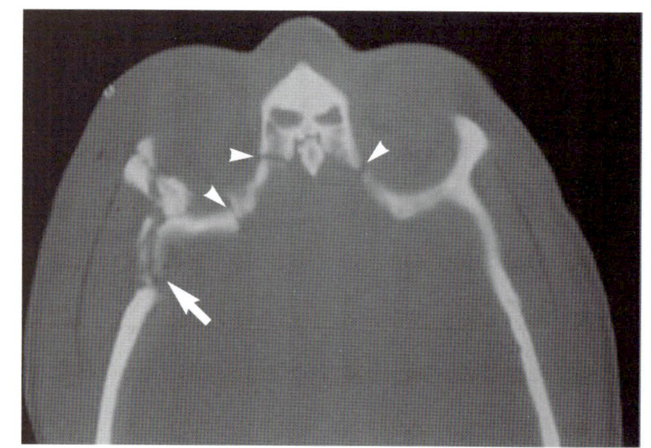

Figure 12.17 *Trauma to the upper face with fractures to the central and lateral skull base and the orbit. There is sparing of the midface (a–f)*. (a) At the level of the inferior forehead (note the frontal sinus hypoplasia), a fracture is present at the left anterior and right posterior lateral aspects of the forehead (arrows). (b) At the level of the superior orbit, there is a comminuted right lateral orbital wall fracture extending to include the floor of the temporal fossa (arrow), as well as bilateral medial orbital wall fractures and a right ethmoid roof fracture (arrowheads).

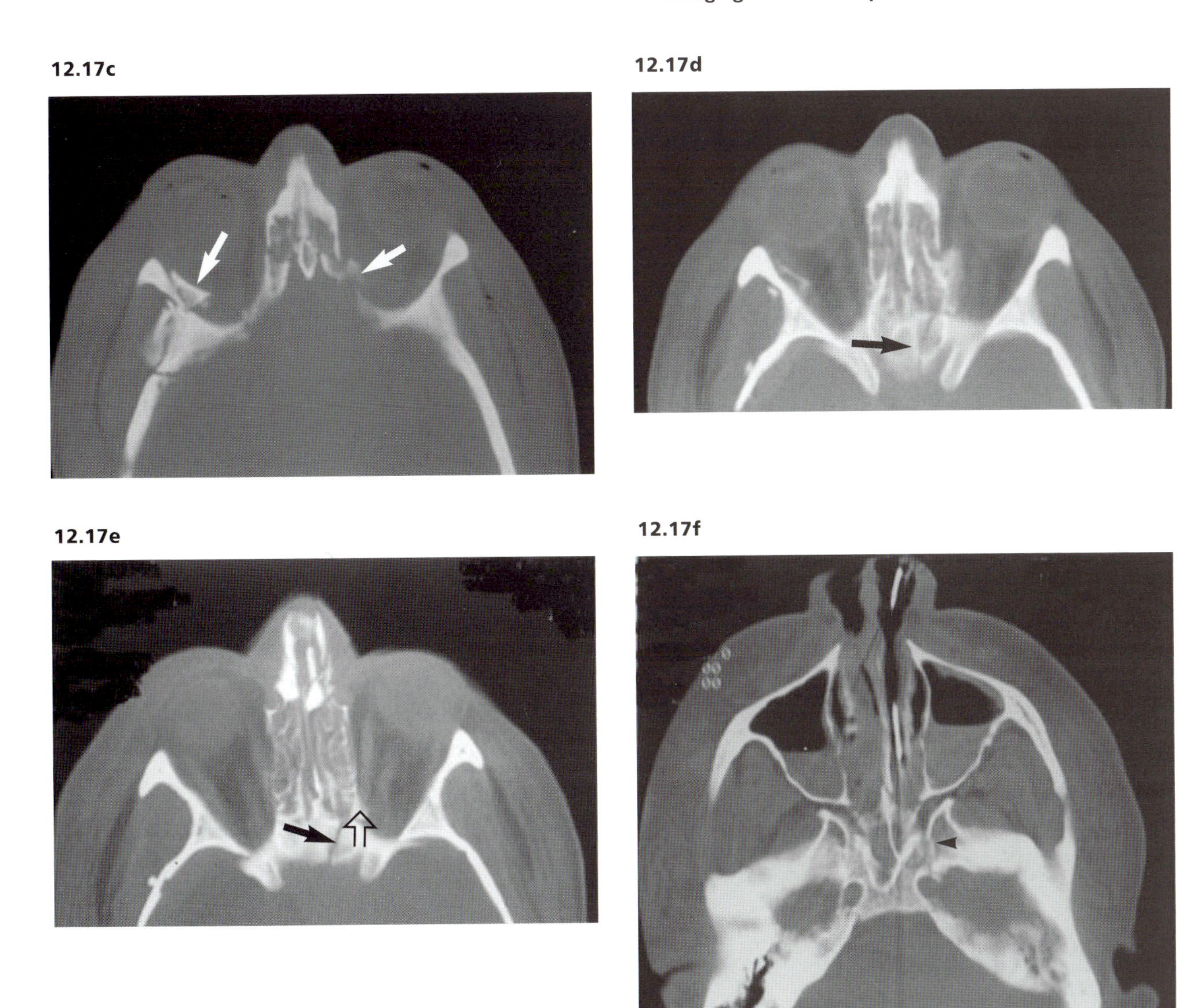

Figure 12.17 *continued* (c) Displaced bone fragments extend into the right lateral and left posteromedial orbits (arrows). (d, e) A fracture extends from the posterior left ethmoid into the left sphenoidal roof, and the planum sphenoidale. The posterior aspect of the medial orbit fragment abuts the optic nerve (open arrow). Left nasal fractures remain more superiorly. (f) A linear fracture extends into the anterior margin of the left carotid canal (arrowhead). No midface fractures are seen other than the more superior nasoethmoidal and left lateral orbital wall fractures.

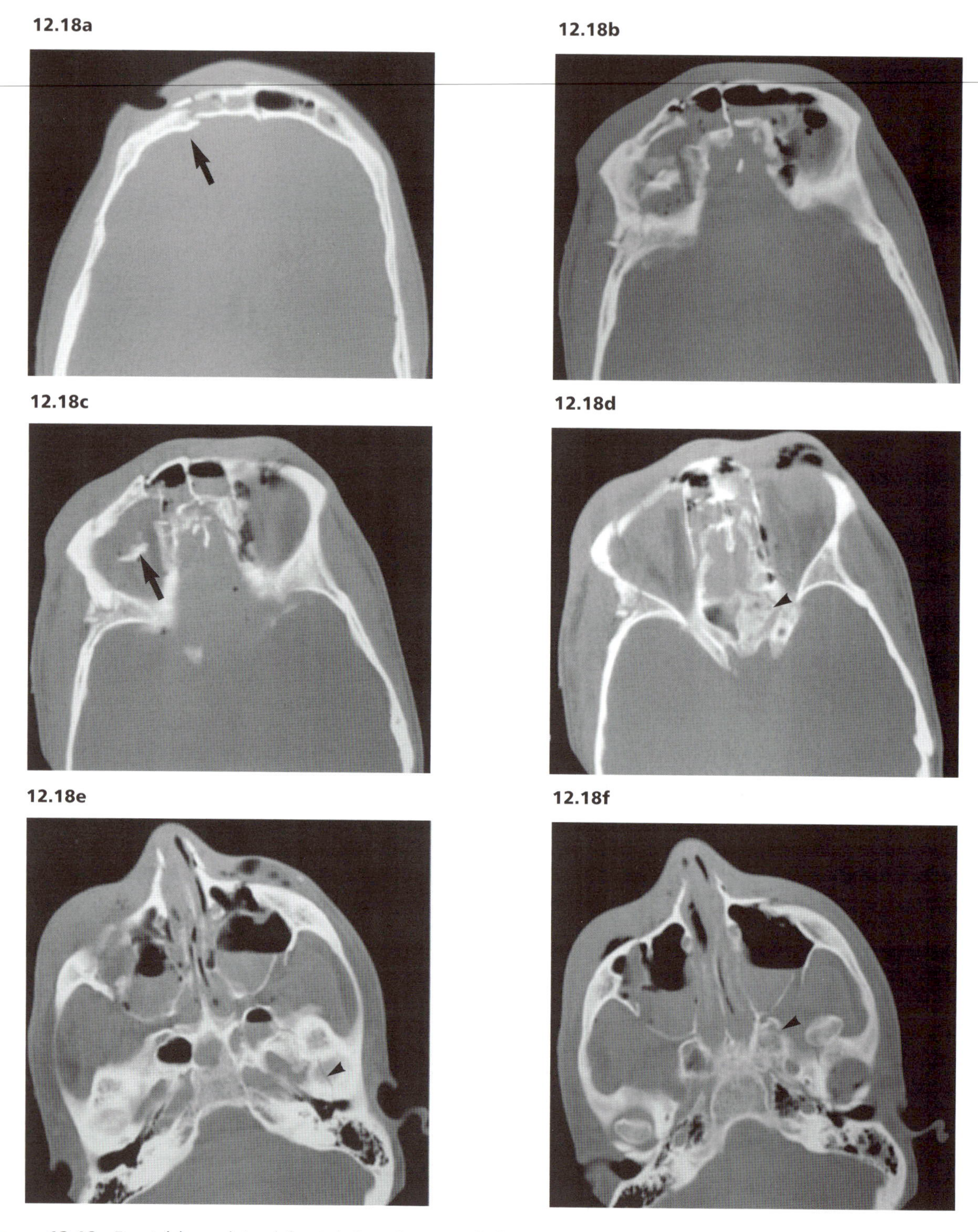

Figure 12.18 *Frontal bone–lateral frontal sinus fractures (tobogganing injury) extending to the anterior skull base, the orbital roof, the orbital apices, the floor of the left middle cranial fossa, and the left temporomandibular joint (TMJ).* (a–f) Axial images from superior to inferior. (a) Comminuted fracture of the lateral aspect of the right frontal sinus (arrow), including anterior and posterior sinus walls, with mild posterior displacement of the right lateral forehead. (b) Comminuted fracture of the orbital roof bilaterally, greater on the right, where the fracture extends through the lesser wing of the sphenoid. There are comminuted frontal sinus fractures. (c) At the level of the superior orbit, a bone fragment is displaced into the orbit from the orbital roof (arrow). There is a superior orbital rim fracture and bilateral fractures into the superior aspect of the medial orbital walls. (d) Medial orbital wall comminuted fractures. A skull base fracture extends through the planum sphenoidale and left optic nerve canal (arrowhead). (e) Anterior midface nasomaxillary fracture – just inferior to the level of the orbit. There is a subtle fracture of the floor of the left middle cranial fossa from the left lateral recess of the sphenoid sinus to the left glenoid fossa (arrowhead). (f) Anterior midface fractures as well as fractures of the left pterygoid plate (arrowhead). There is a left mandibular condylar fracture–dislocation.

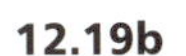

12.19a

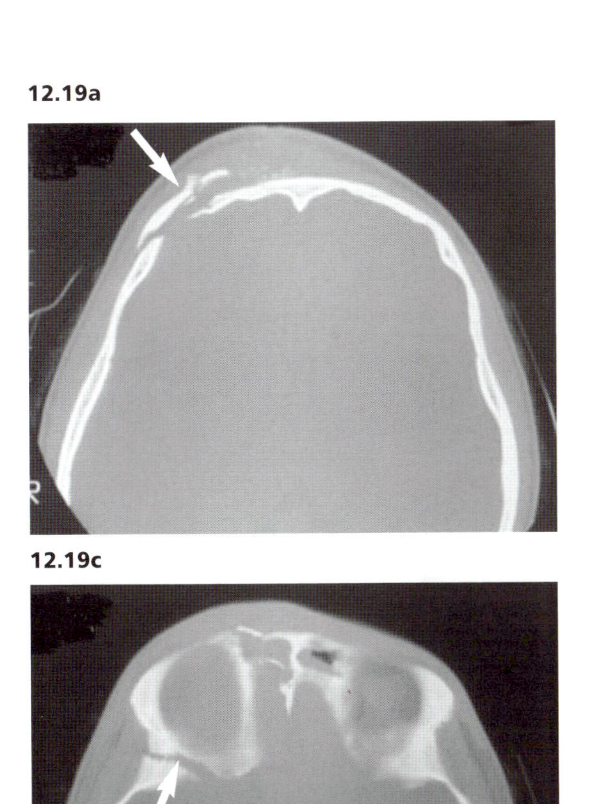

12.19b

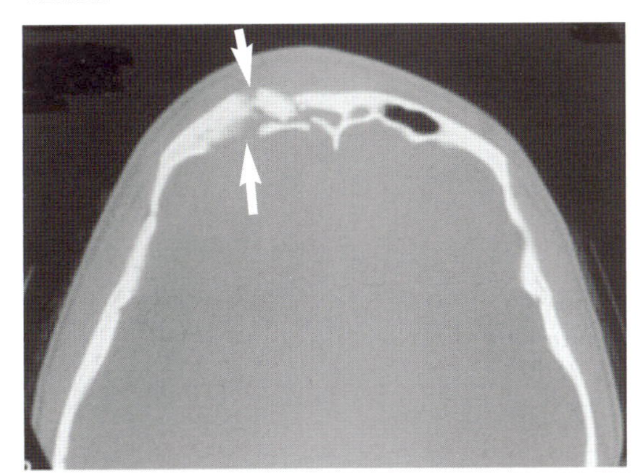

12.19c

12.19d

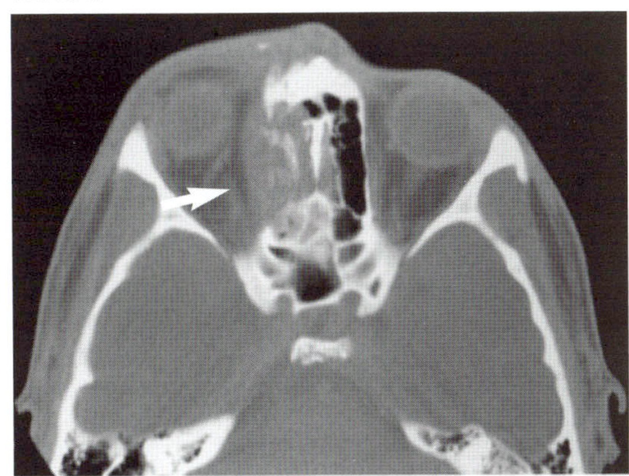

12.19e

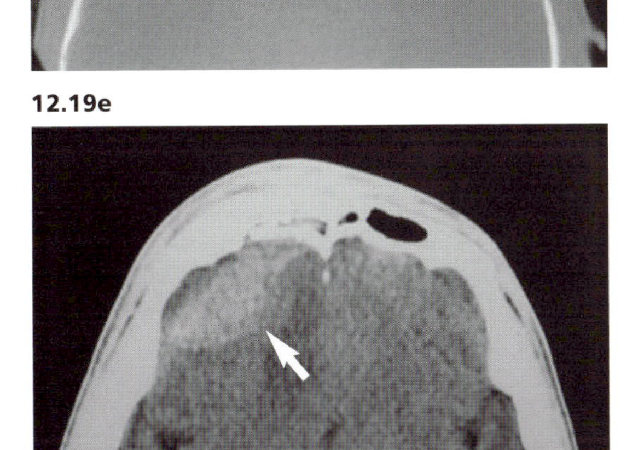

12.19f

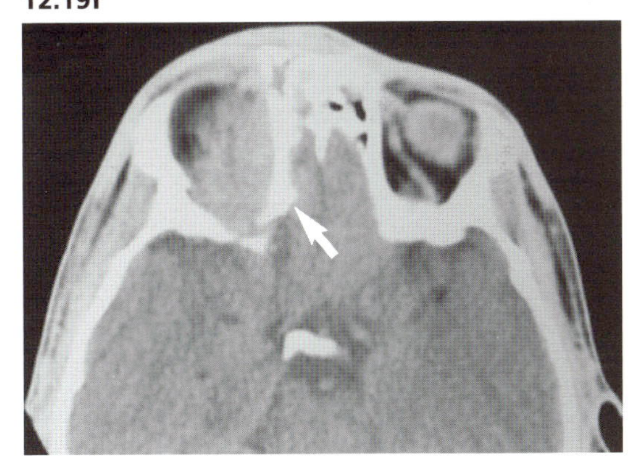

12.19g

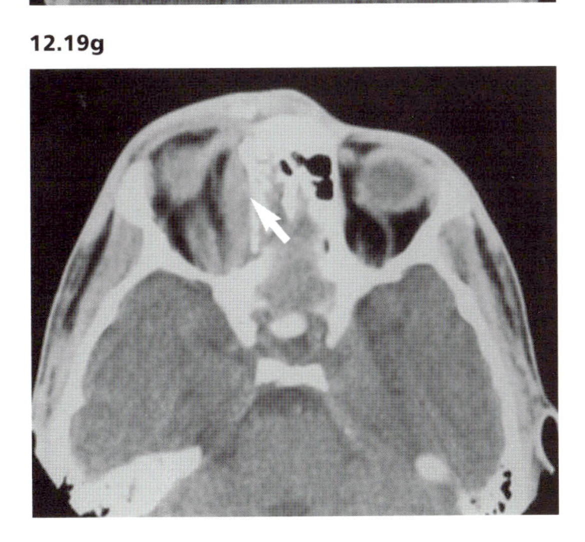

Figure 12.19 *Fracture of the lateral forehead and the lateral aspect of the frontal sinus. This allows greater transmission of the fracture force to the frontoethmoid, orbital roof, orbit, or brain.* (a–g) Axial images. (a) Comminuted fracture of the lateral aspect of the right forehead (arrow). (b) Comminuted fractures of the anterior and posterior walls of the relatively hypoplastic right frontal sinus (arrows). (c) Fracture extending to the posterior aspect of the floor of the anterior cranial fossa (arrow), suggesting that the orbital roof represents a large fracture fragment. (d) Displaced bone at the medial wall of the right orbit, with adjacent periorbital soft tissue consistent with hematoma. (e) Associated contusion, hemorrhage, and edema of the right frontal lobe (arrow). (f, g) Soft tissue prominence at the superior aspect of the right orbit, extending along the medial aspect, representing periorbital hematoma (arrows).

12.19h

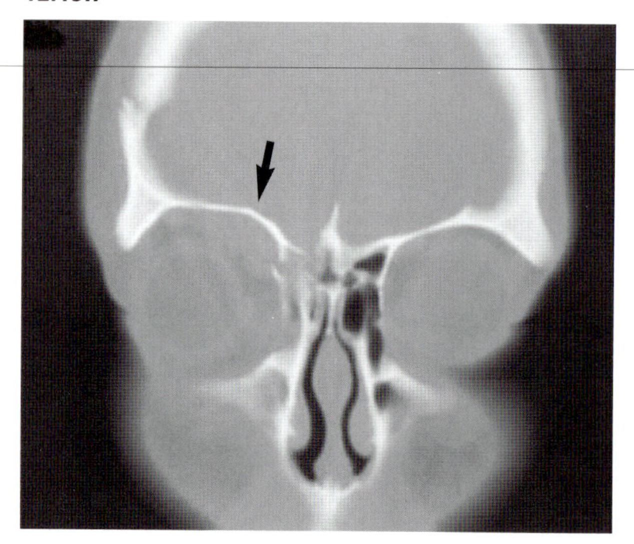

12.19i

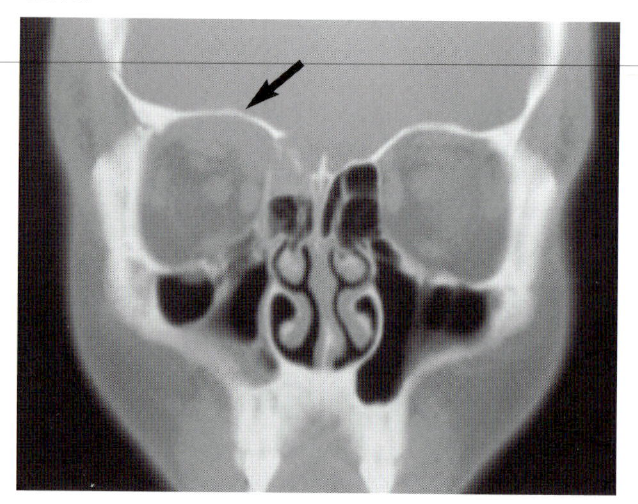

12.19j

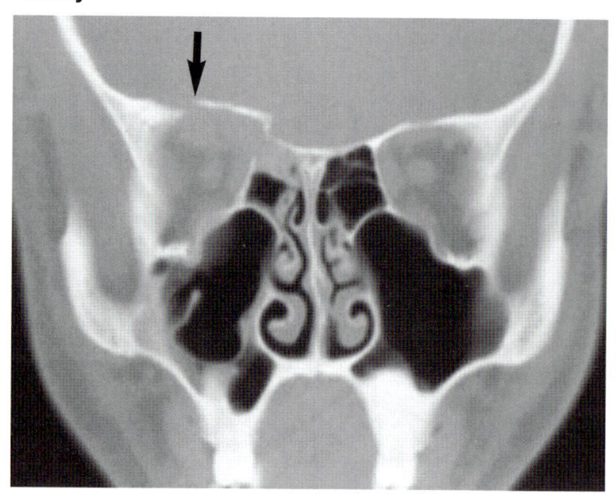

Figure 12.19 *continued* (h–j) Coronal bone images. The roof of the right orbit represents a large bone fragment separated from the ethmoid complex by a medial fracture plane (arrows). The right orbital roof fragment is elevated – more diffusely anteriorly and more focally posteriorly.

12.19k

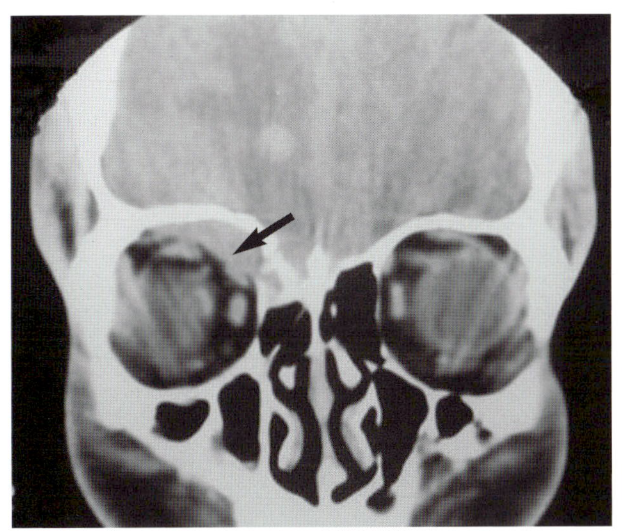

12.19l

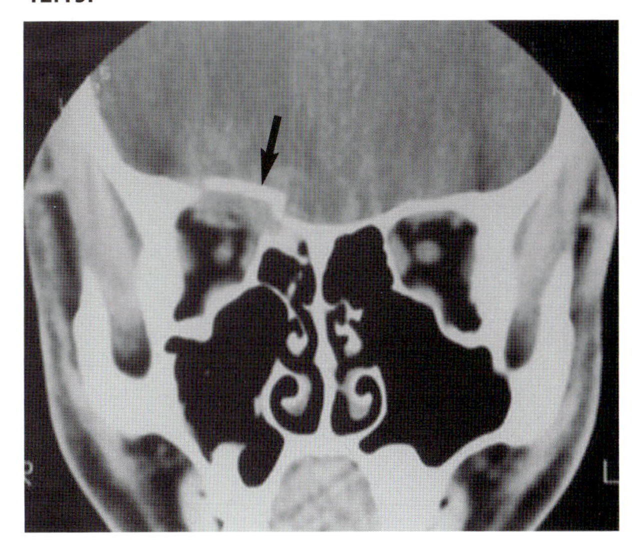

Figure 12.19 *continued* (k, l) Coronal soft tissue images. A periorbital hematoma is seen under the orbital roof, with associated elevation of the roof fracture fragment (arrows). Cerebral injury is also noted.

12.20a

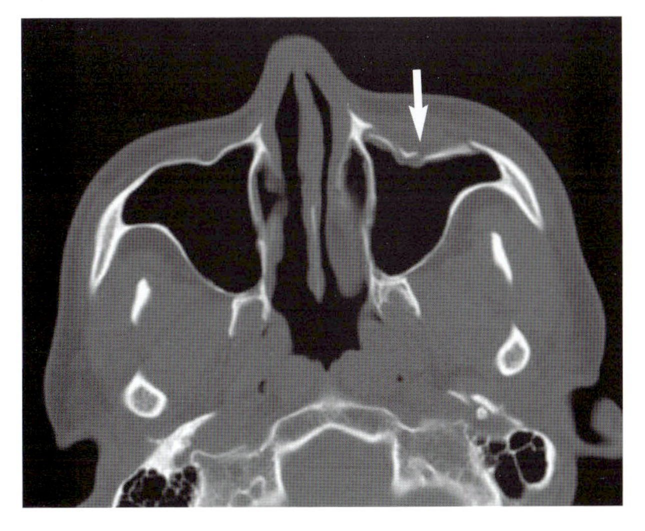

12.20b

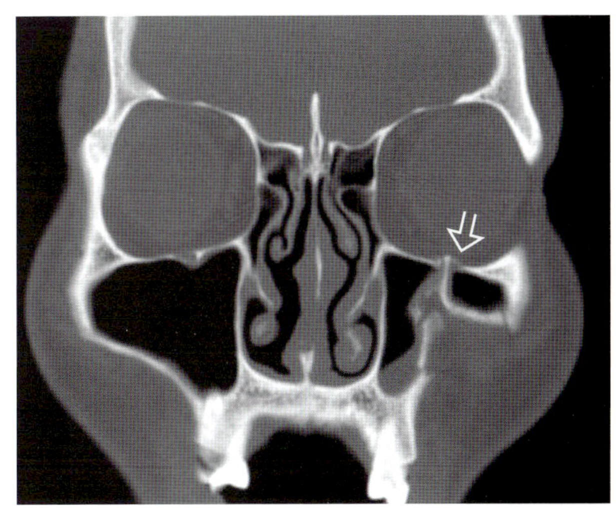

Figure 12.20 *Segmental fracture with infraorbital nerve paresthesia*. A segmental fracture of the left anterolateral maxillary sinus wall is present. The patient presented with infraorbital nerve paresthesia. A fracture fragment impaled the left infraorbital nerve canal. (a) Axial image showing a comminuted fracture of the anterior wall of the left maxillary sinus (arrow). (b) Coronal image showing a fragment extending into the left infraorbital canal (open arrow). No fractures of the orbital floor were present. No other facial fractures were noted.

12.21a

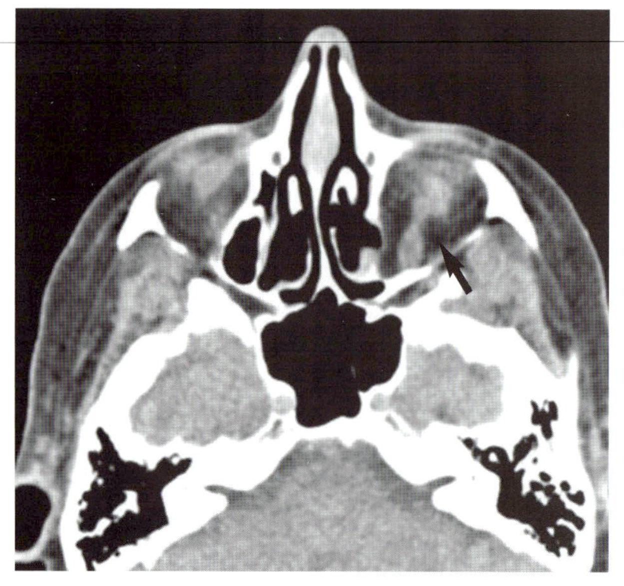

12.21b

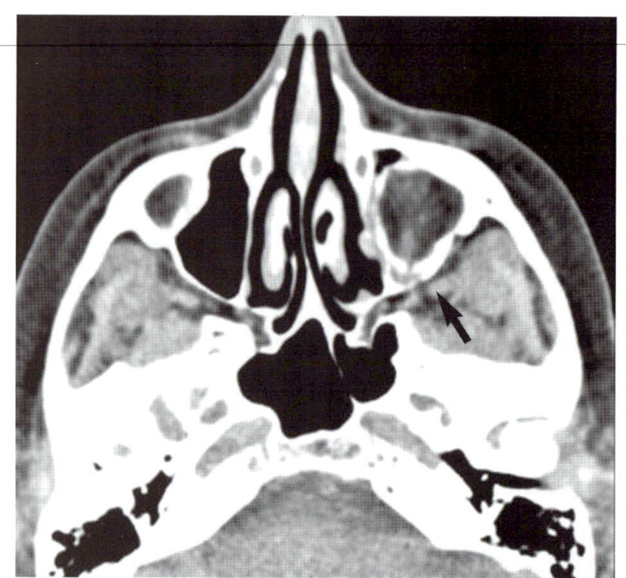

12.21c

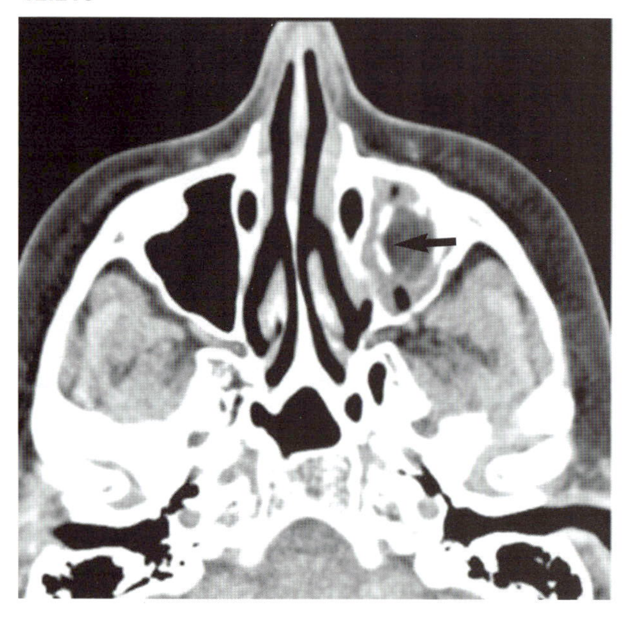

12.21d

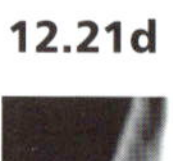

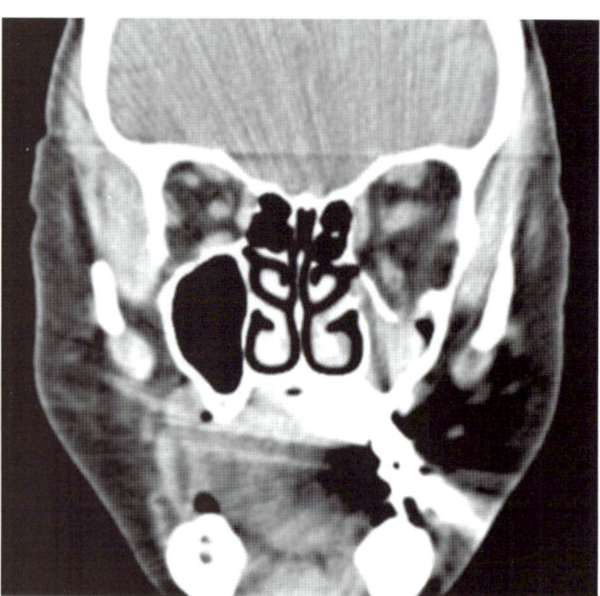

12.21e

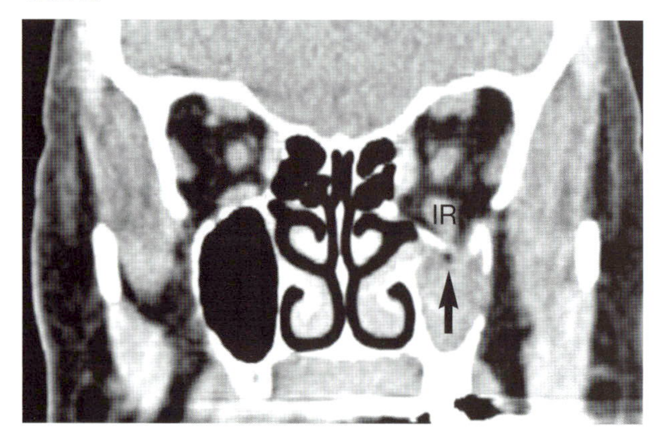

Figure 12.21 *Direct axial, coronal and images reformations of orbital floor blowout fracture*. (a–c) Axial images. (a) Inferior displacement of the left orbital floor is subtle, with the posterior superior aspect of the maxillary sinus obscured by orbital contents, including inferior rectus muscle when compared with the right (arrow). (b) More inferior image showing bony margins of the orbital floor fracture extending into the maxillary sinus (arrow). (c) Bone fragments within the maxillary sinus (arrow). (d–g) Coronal images. (d) Direct coronal image detail through the retrobulbar orbit is partially obscured by a metallic artifact from dental restoration. (e) Coronal reformatted image showing an orbital floor blowout fracture (arrow). Note the altered configuration of the left inferior rectus muscle (IR), with its inferior aspect tugged by soft tissue attachment to the displaced fracture. The dental artifact, now seen in the horizontal direction, is below the fracture site on the reformatted image.

12.21f

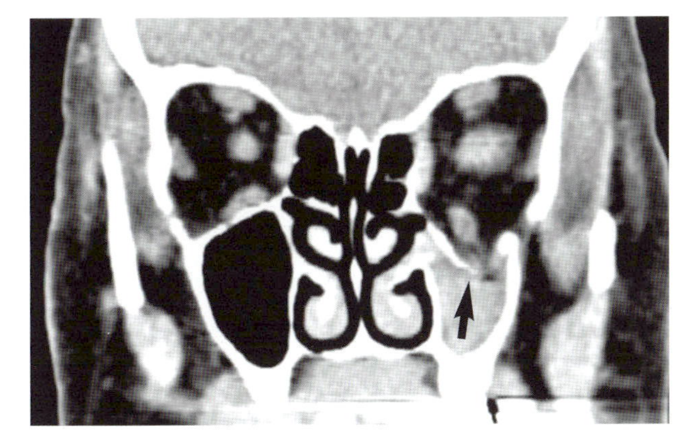

12.21g

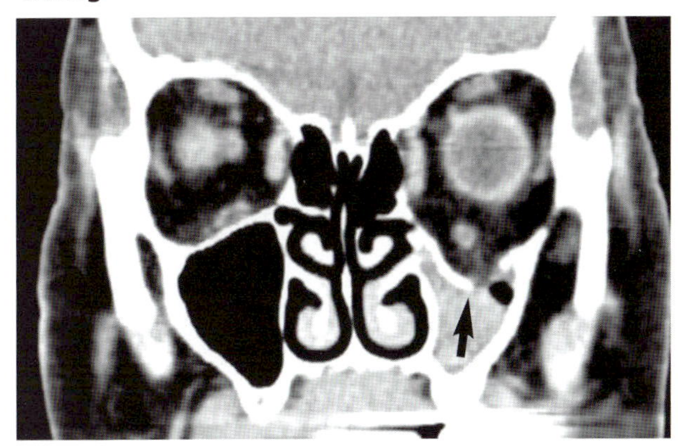

Figure 12.21 *continued* (f, g) More anterior images showing the inferior rectus muscle with soft tissue connection to the displaced orbital floor (arrows).

12.22a

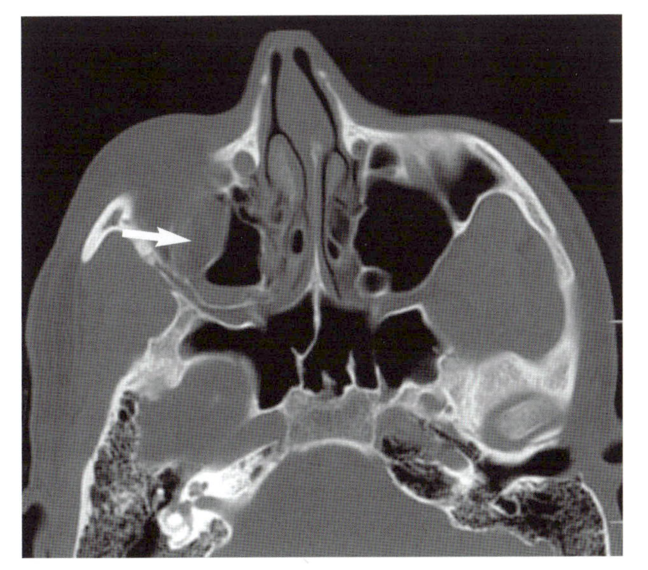

12.22b

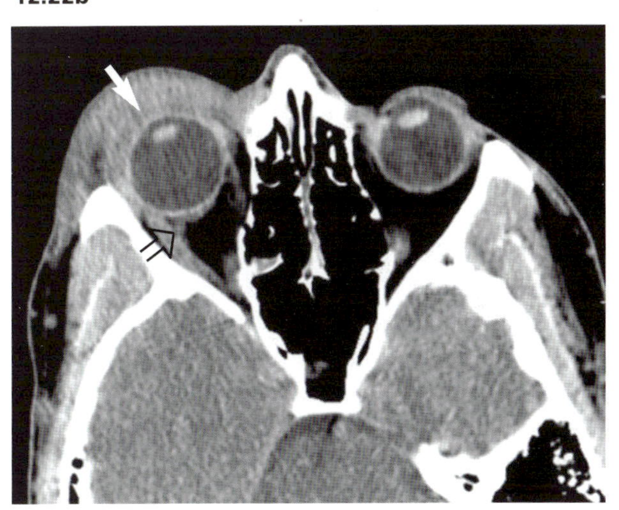

12.22c

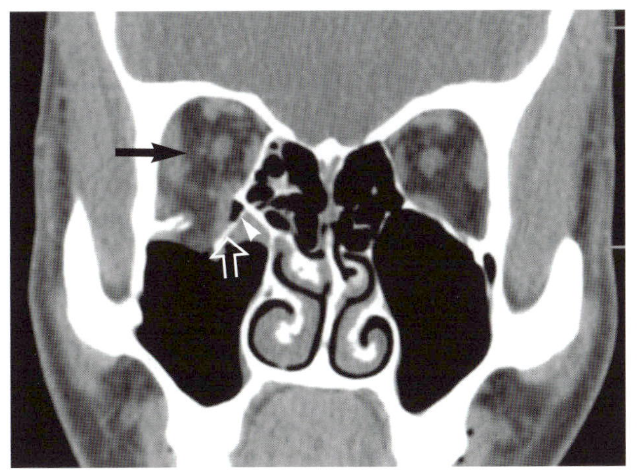

Figure 12.22 *Orbital floor blowout fracture, entrapped inferior rectus muscle, and contused lateral rectus muscle.* (a) Axial bone image showing inferior displacement of the right orbital floor, encroaching on the maxillary sinus (arrow). (b) More superior axial soft tissue image showing preseptal soft tissue swelling (arrow), and an enlarged contused right lateral rectus muscle (open arrow). (c) The enlarged lateral rectus muscle is further visualized on coronal image (arrow). The inferior rectus muscle remains entrapped by the medial orbital floor displaced bone fragment, and has a more vertical axis in this midorbital image (open arrow). The infraorbital canal is just lateral to the fracture fragment. A small collection of air is seen within the medial inferior orbit (arrowhead).

12.23a

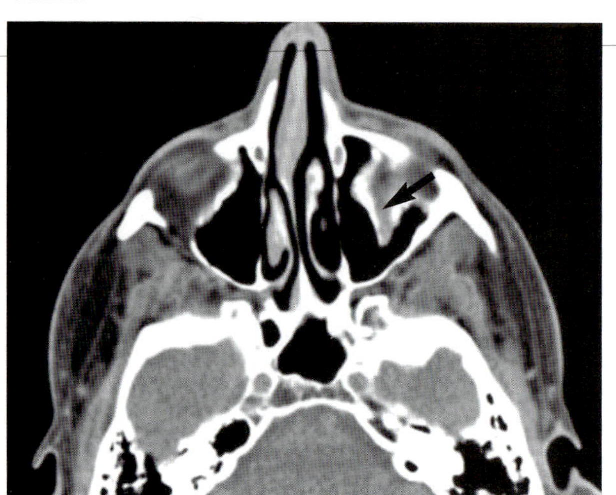

12.23b

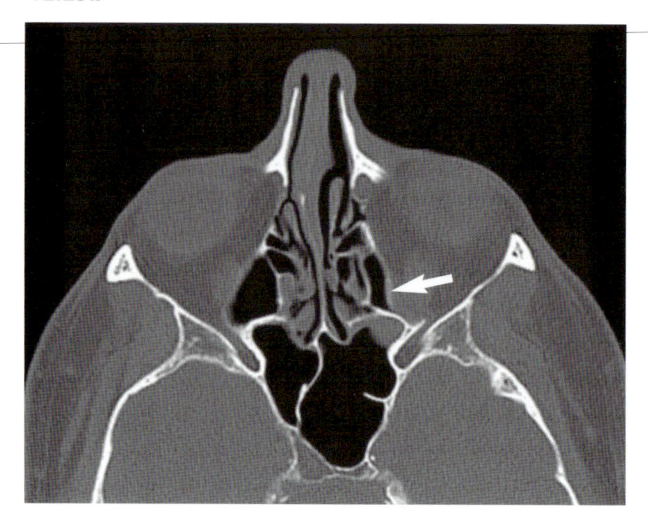

12.23c

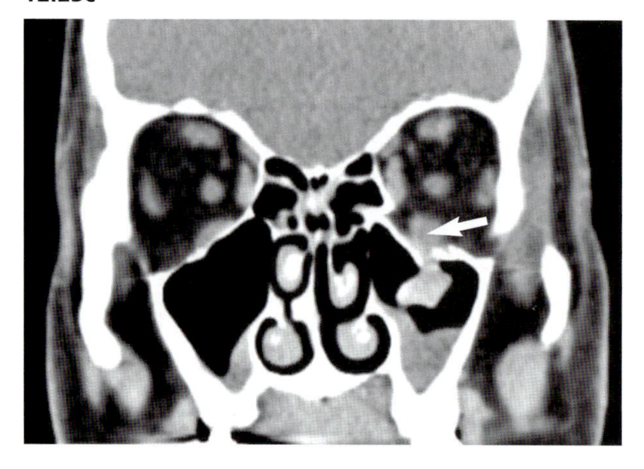

12.23d

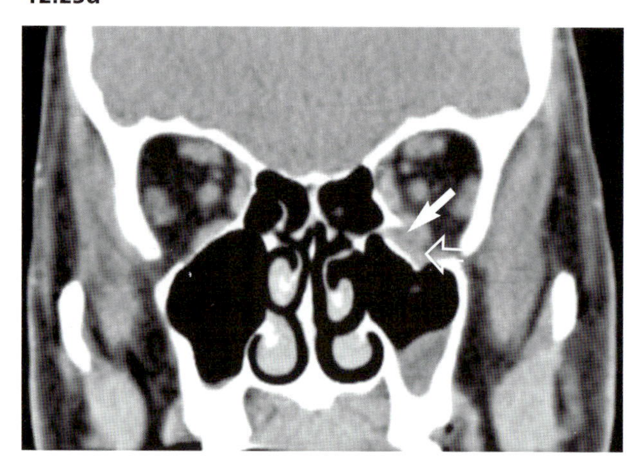

Figure 12.23 *Orbital floor blowout fracture – entrapped inferior rectus muscle*. (a) Axial soft tissue image showing bone fragments at the superior aspect of the left maxillary sinus (arrow). (b) Axial bone image showing an abnormal position of the left orbital floor, posteromedially displaced (arrow). (c, d) Coronal soft tissue images showing an enlarged left inferior rectus muscle (arrow) extending into the traumatic dehiscence of the orbital floor. Submucosal hematoma is present at the superior aspect of the maxillary sinus. Slightly more posteriorly, the left orbital floor fragment is more inferiorly displaced (open arrow). An enlarged left inferior rectus muscle is impaled by the lateral edge of the medial orbital floor remnant.

12.24a

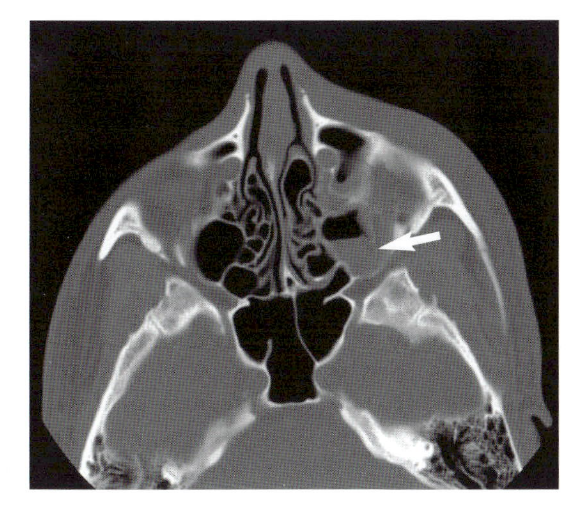

12.24b

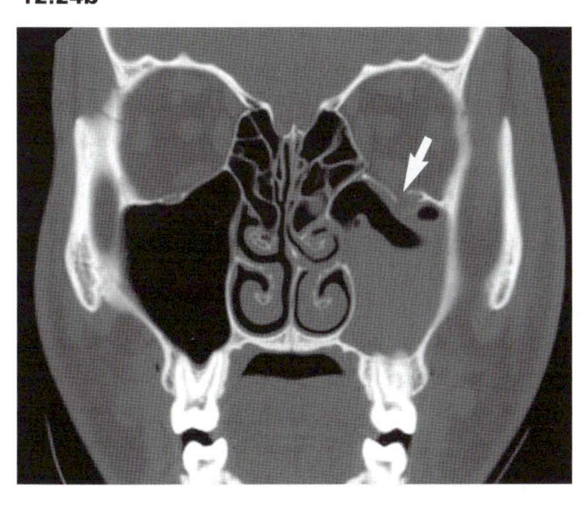

12.24c

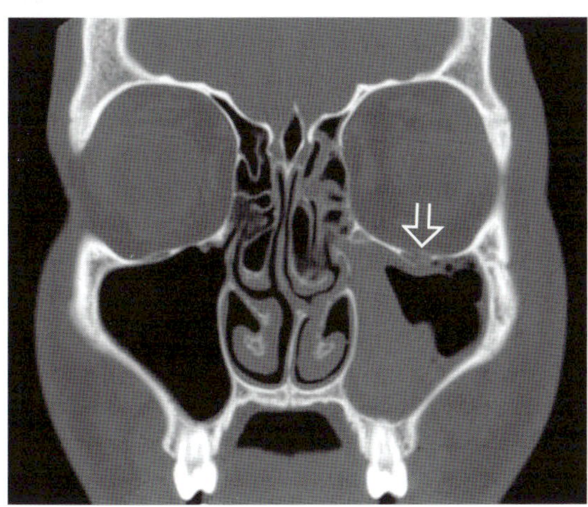

Figure 12.24 *Isolated left orbital floor blowout fracture, extending through the infraorbital canal.* (a) Axial bone image through the orbital floor showing widened left infraorbital canal. Hemorrhage is seen within the left maxillary sinus (arrow). (b, c) Coronal images showing the left orbital floor fracture extending through the medial aspect of the left infraorbital canal more posteriorly (arrow) and the central aspect of the canal more anteriorly, with a resultant enlarged canal (open arrow).

12.25a

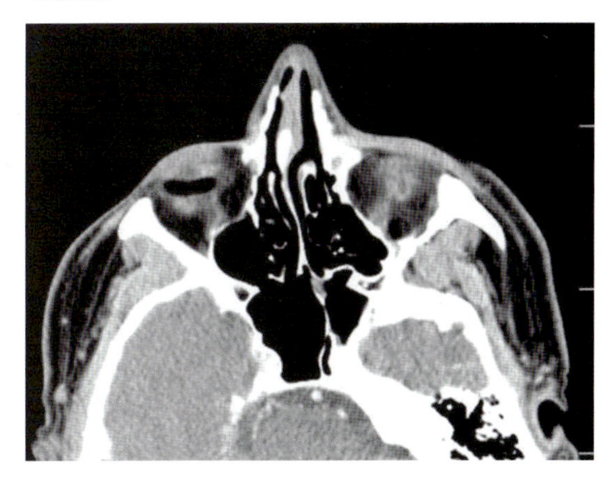

12.25b

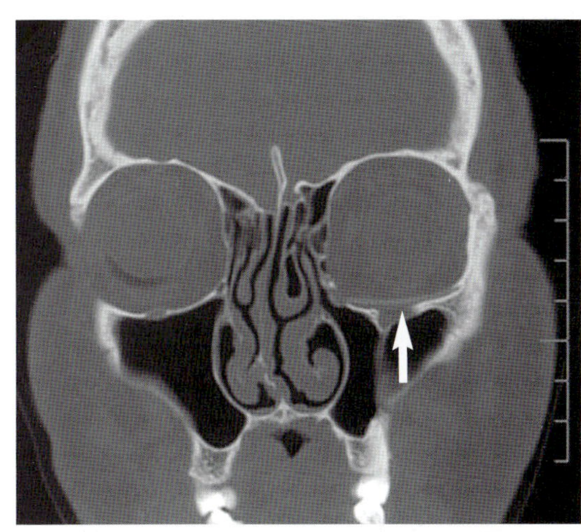

12.25c

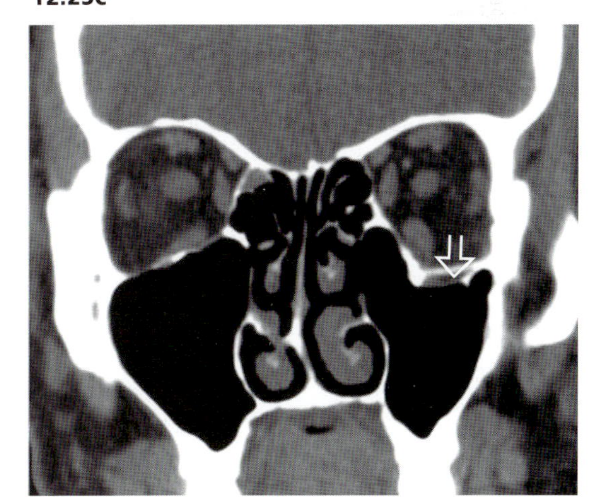

Figure 12.25 *Silastic graft for orbital floor blowout fracture.* Post orbital floor repair CT study showing an incidental right scleral band in place. (a) Axial image showing the posterior left orbital floor to be slightly inferior in position compared with the right. (b, c) Coronal images showing that the graft is in a good position anteriorly (arrow) but that it has slipped inferiorly on the image through the mid-orbit (open arrow). The left inferior rectus muscle is tugged inferiorly by strands of tissue connecting the muscle to the orbital floor or the silastic implant.

12.26a

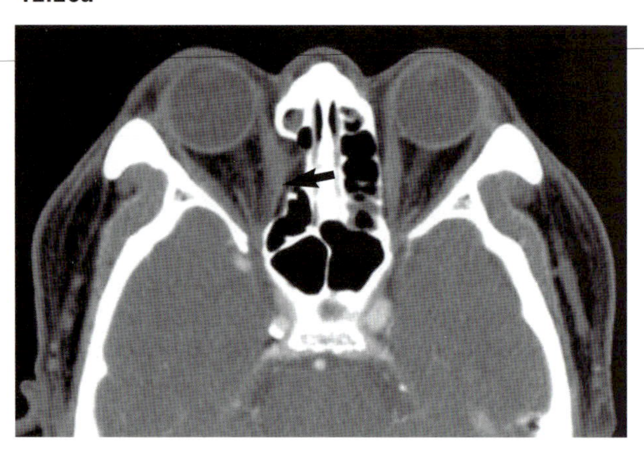

12.26b

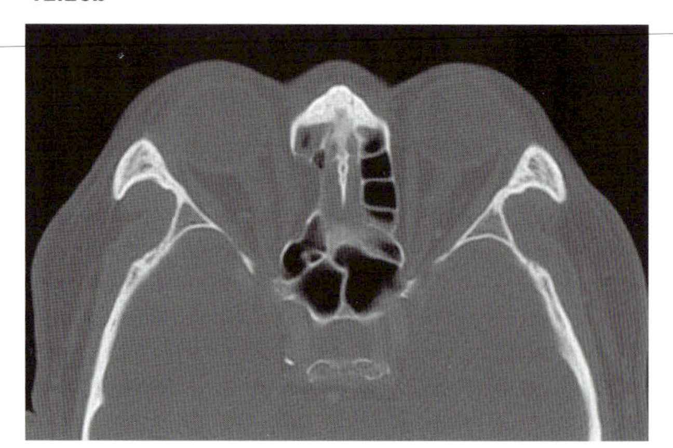

12.26c

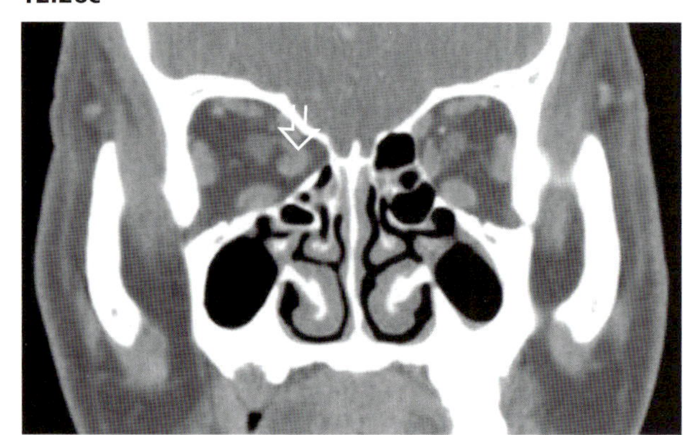

12.26d

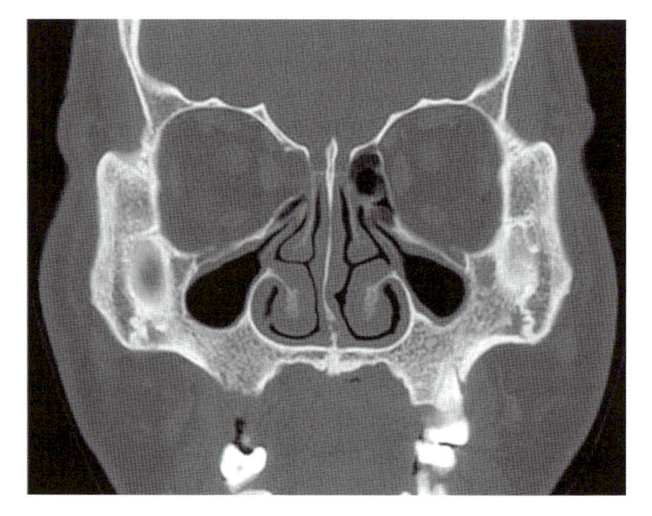

Figure 12.26 *Right medial blowout fracture*. (a, b) Axial soft tissue and bone images showing a defect in the medial wall of the right orbit. The soft tissue image (a) shows the medial rectus muscle to be thickened and pulled into the defect (arrow) – consistent with a previous medial blowout fracture rather than congenital medial wall dehiscence. Minimal mucosal changes in the adjacent ethmoid air cells suggest previous injury. (c, d) Coronal images showing the altered configuration of the medial rectus muscle – oval with a horizontal rather than its usual vertical longer axis, dipping into the blowout segment (open arrow).

12.27a

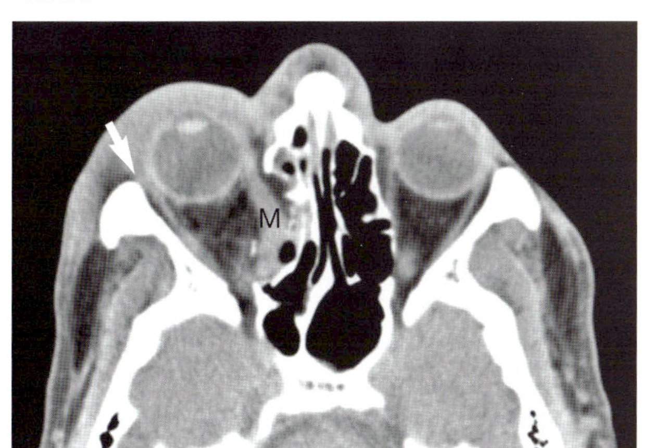

12.27b

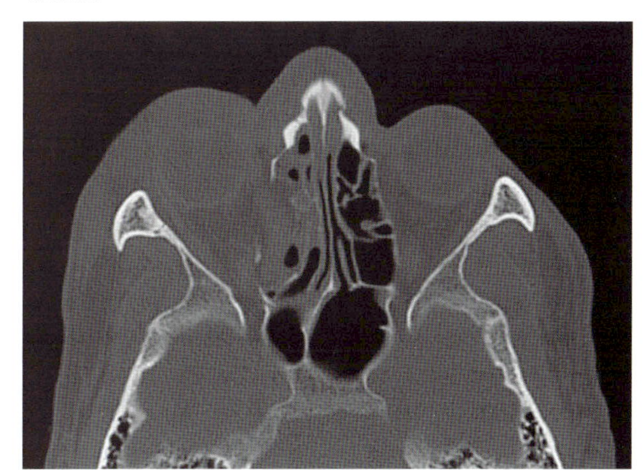

12.27c

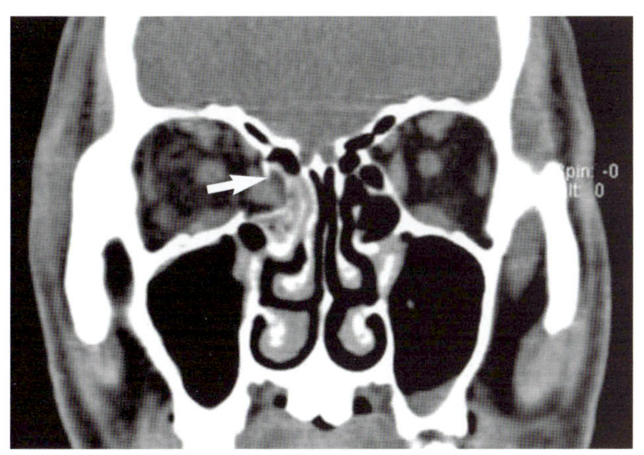

12.27d

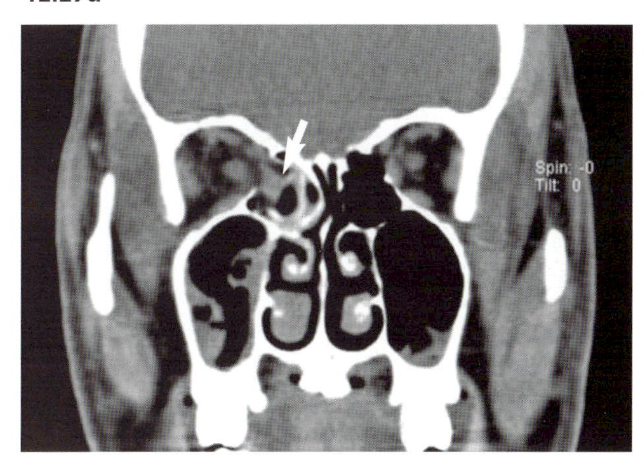

12.27e

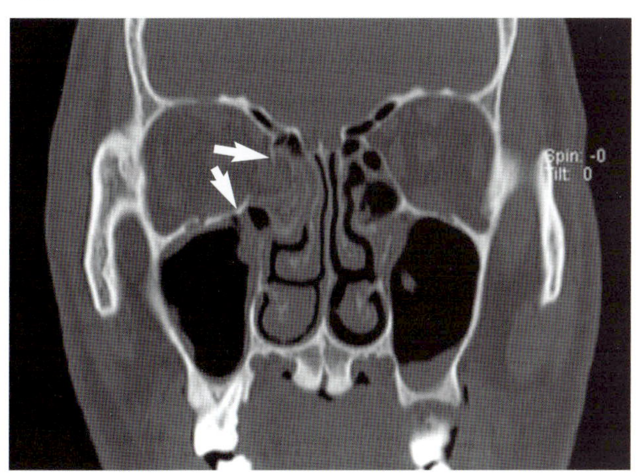

12.27f

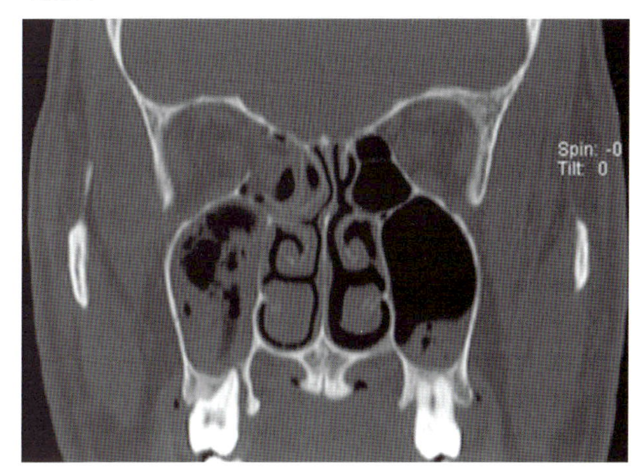

Figure 12.27 *Right medial blowout fracture – displaced medial rectus muscle, with adjacent bone spicules superiorly and inferolaterally*. (a, b) Axial soft tissue and bone images showing a large right medial blowout fracture with an enlarged medial rectus muscle (M) extending into the fracture site. Soft tissue swelling overlying the orbit (arrow) plus mucosal reactive changes in the ethmoid sinus, suggest a recent injury. (c) More anterior coronal soft tissue image showing a bone spicule indenting the superior aspect of the enlarged medial rectus muscle. (d) More posterior coronal image showing tethering of the medial rectus muscle to the displaced medial wall (arrow). (e, f) Coronal bone images showing more clearly the fracture fragments above and inferolateral to the medial rectus muscle (arrows).

12.28a

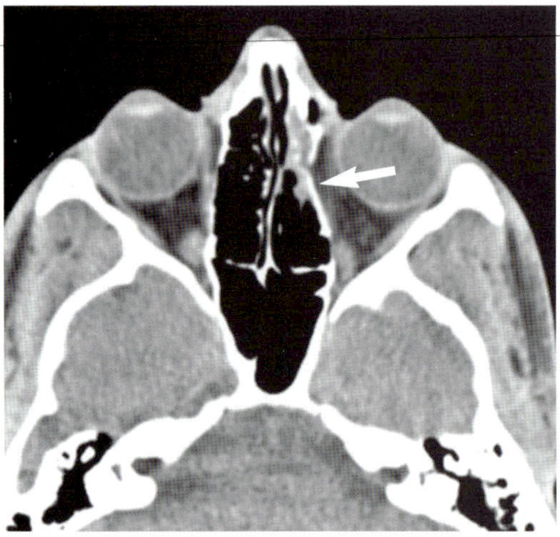

12.28b

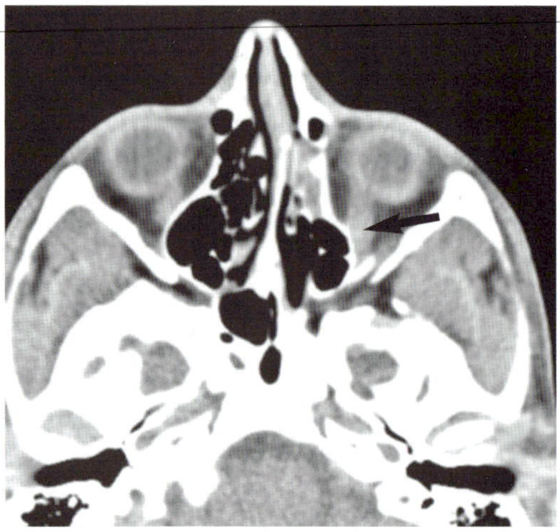

12.28c

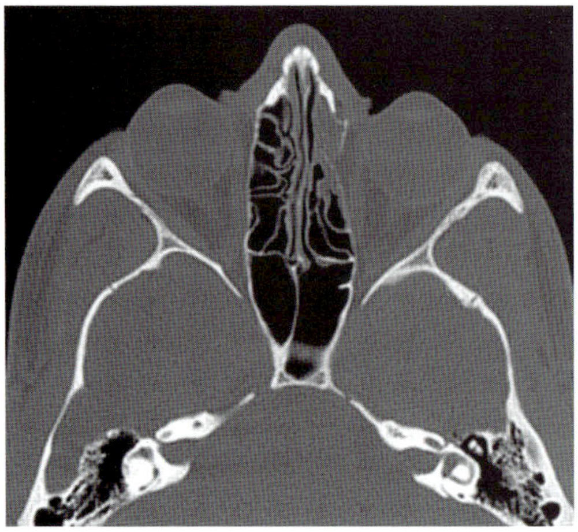

12.28d

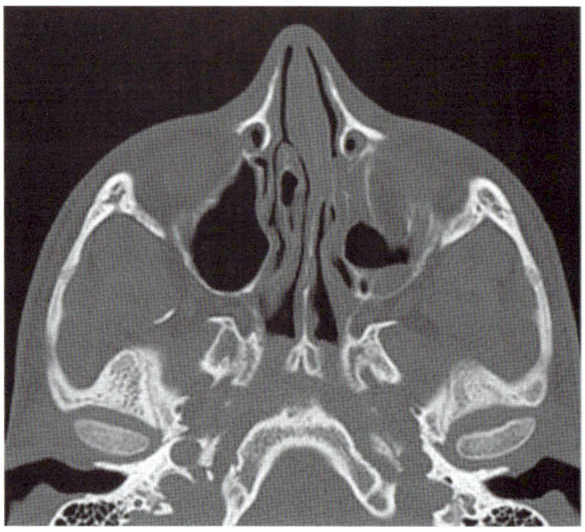

12.28e

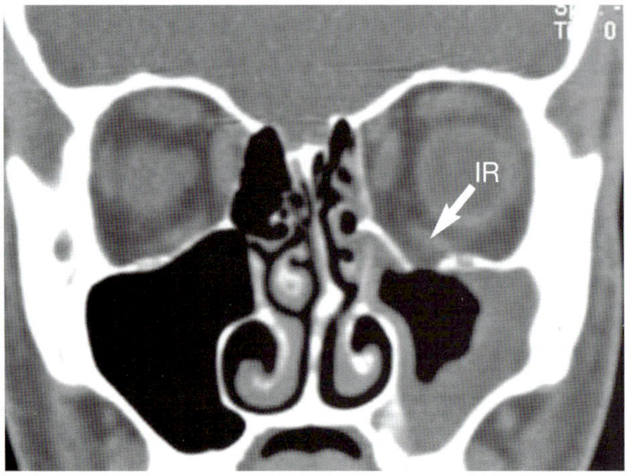

IR

12.28f

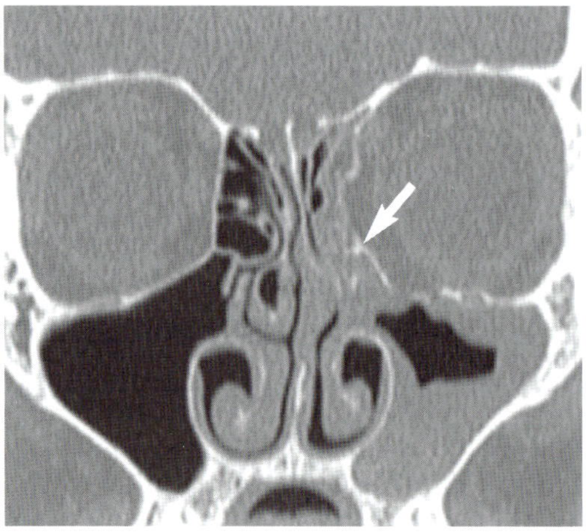

Figure 12.28 *Left combined medial wall–orbital floor blowout fracture*. (a, b) Axial soft tissue images showing mild left enophthalmos and irregularity of the left medial orbital wall (arrow), with opacified anterior left ethmoid air cells. The more inferior image (b) shows prominence of the left inferior rectus muscle and the more posteriorly positioned orbital floor – suggesting an orbital floor blowout fracture (arrow). (c, d) These fractures are further detailed on the axial bone algorithm images. The orbital floor fracture is medial to the infraorbital canal. (e) Coronal soft tissue image showing a small amount of fat tissue displaced into the fracture site (arrow). The muscle is of normal caliber with no evidence of entrapment inferior rectus (IR). (f) Coronal bone image showing irregularity and displacement of the inferior aspect of the medial wall, contiguous with the fragmented medial aspect of the orbital floor (arrow).

12.29a

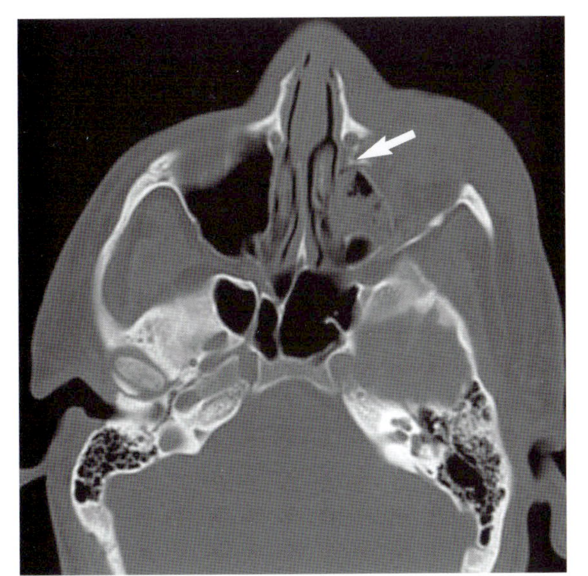

12.29b

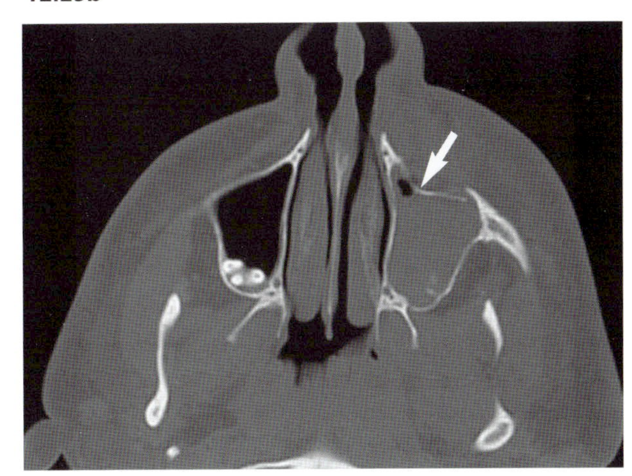

12.29c

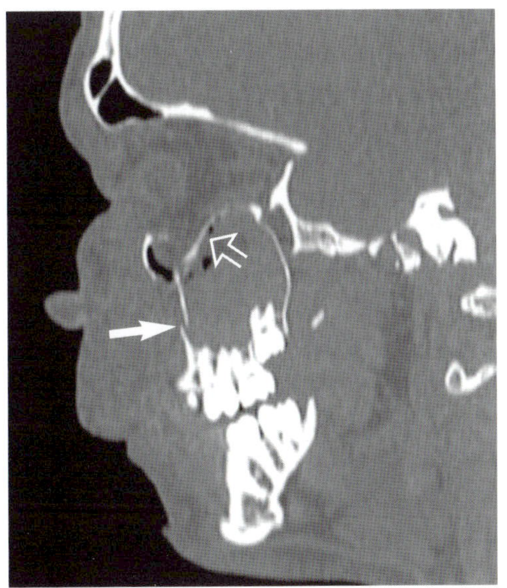

12.29d

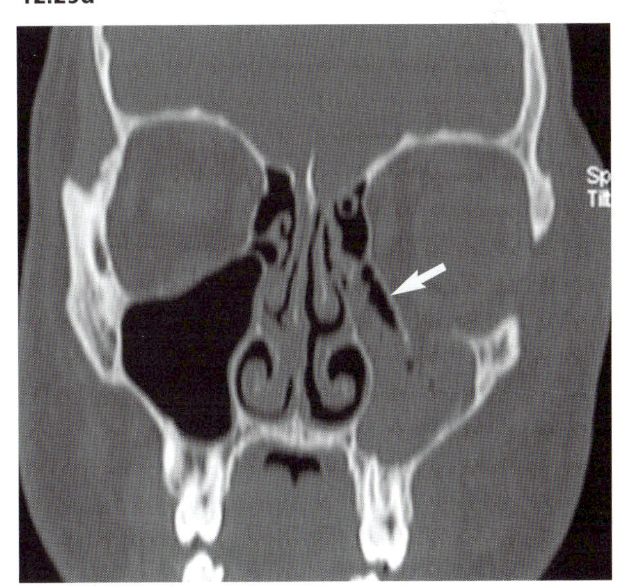

Figure 12.29 *Left comminuted orbital floor blowout fracture*. (a) Axial bone image showing a left orbital floor fracture. A comminuted fragment is noted just posterolateral to the nasolacrimal canal (arrow). (b) Just inferiorly, a depressed fragment of the anterior wall of the maxilla is shown (arrow). (c) Sagittal reconstruction shows posterior displacement of the anterior maxillary wall fragment (arrow), as well as pronounced depression of the anterior orbital floor (open arrow). (d) Coronal bone image showing a large hinge-type blowout component (arrow).

12.30a

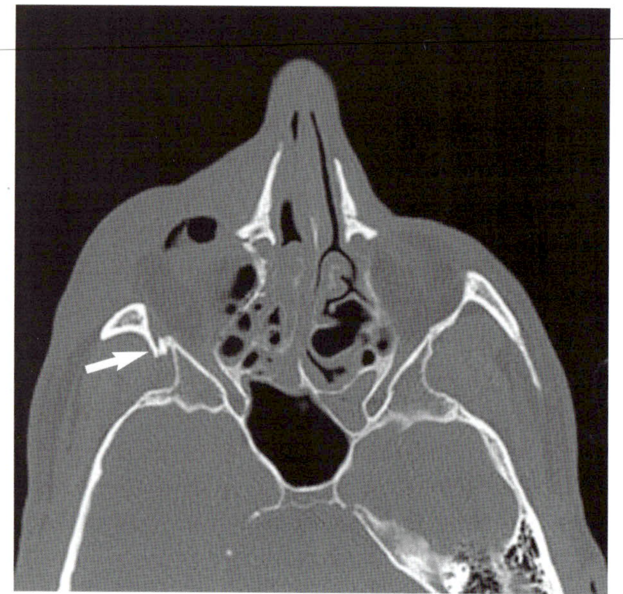

12.30b

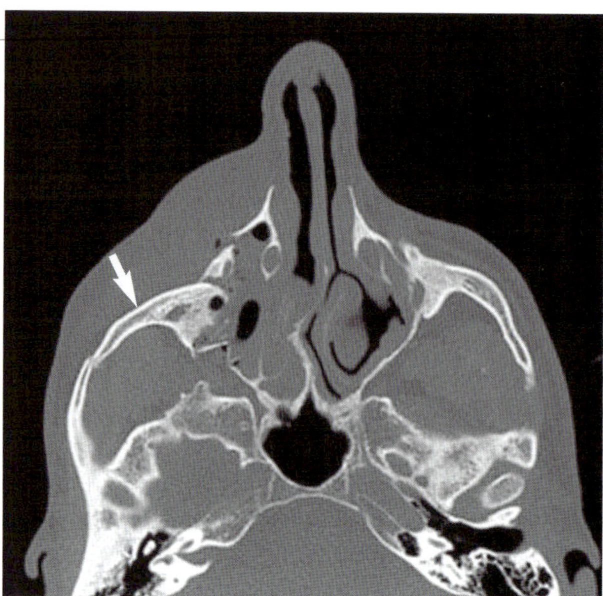

12.30c

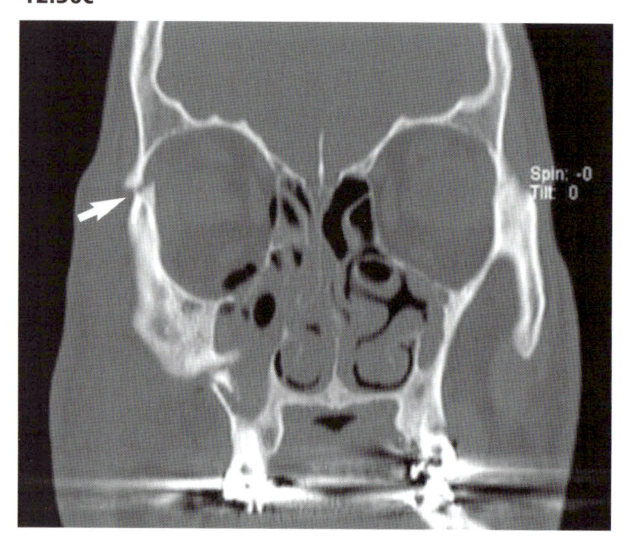

Figure 12.30 *Right zygomaticomaxillary fracture*. (a) Axial image through the orbit showing posterior displacement of the right lateral orbital rim with overlapping and comminution of the lateral orbital wall at the zygomaticosphenoid suture (arrow). (b) Axial image through the face showing the body of the zygoma displaced medially and posteriorly (arrow), with associated fractures of the anterior and lateral walls of the right maxillary sinus. There is exaggerated curvature of the zygomatic arch due to posterior displacement of the zygomatic body, with a fracture at the midzygomatic arch. Note that the body of the zygoma itself remains intact, with the fractures tending to occur at its attachments or extensions. (c) Coronal image showing the fracture of the frontal extension of the zygoma at the zygomaticofrontal suture (arrow). No abnormality of the nasoethmoid complex is noted.

12.31a

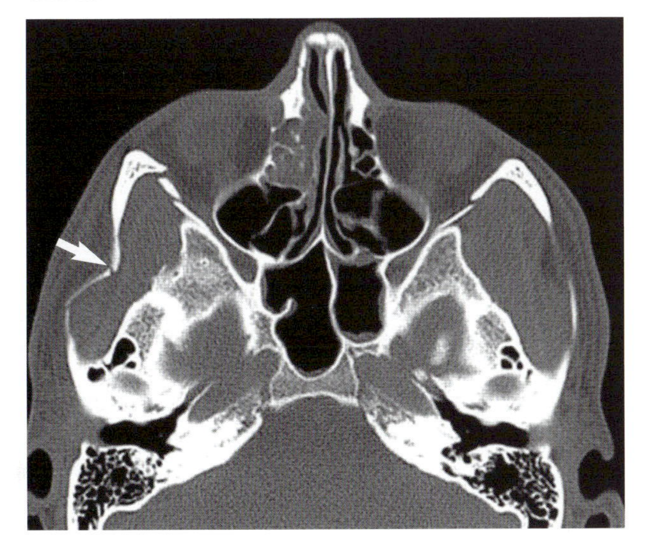

12.31b

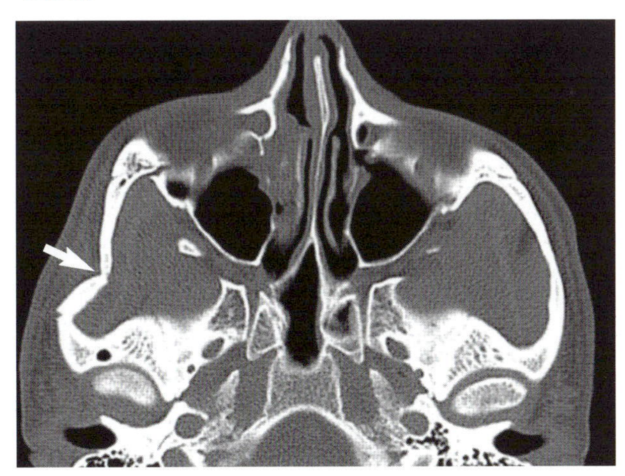

12.31c

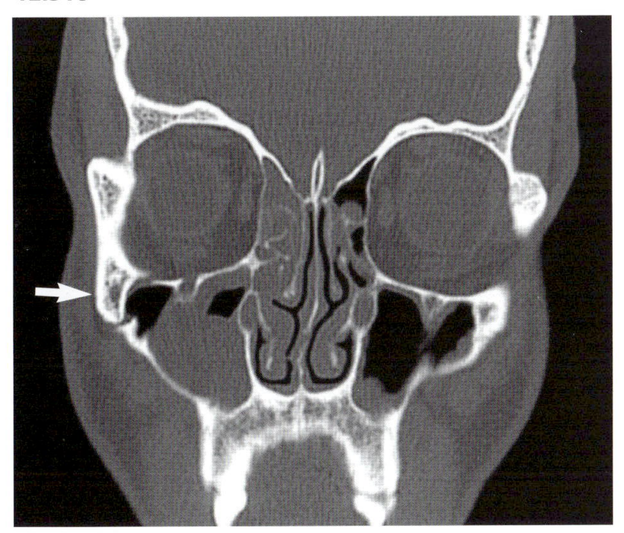

Figure 12.31 *Right tripod fracture with associated depressed zygomatic arch fracture*. Axial (a, b) and coronal (c) images showing a comminuted depressed fracture of the midzygomatic arch with a comminuted fracture of the lateral orbital wall (arrows). No significant displacement of the zygoma is noted. The lateral orbital rim is intact, with the fracture extending just medial to the rim, at the most lateral aspect of the orbital floor, and just inferior to the zygomatic body through the lateral wall of the maxillary sinus and at the adjacent anterior aspect of the lateral orbital wall.

12.32a

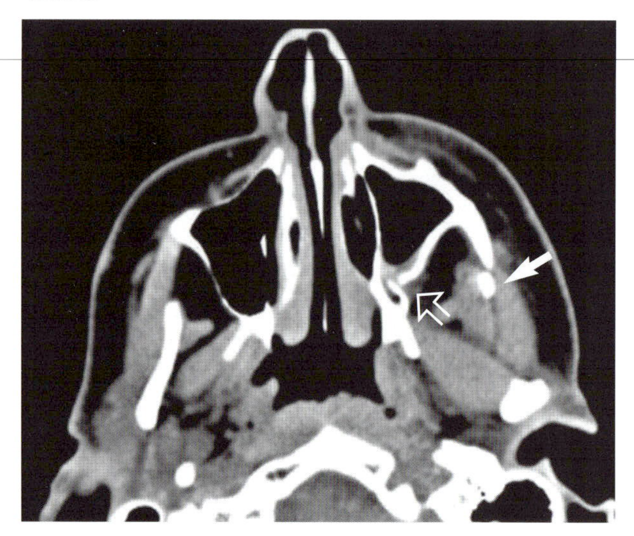

12.32b

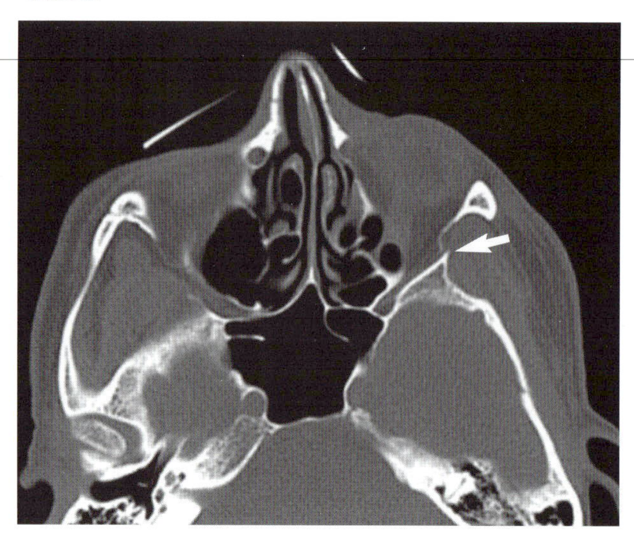

12.32c

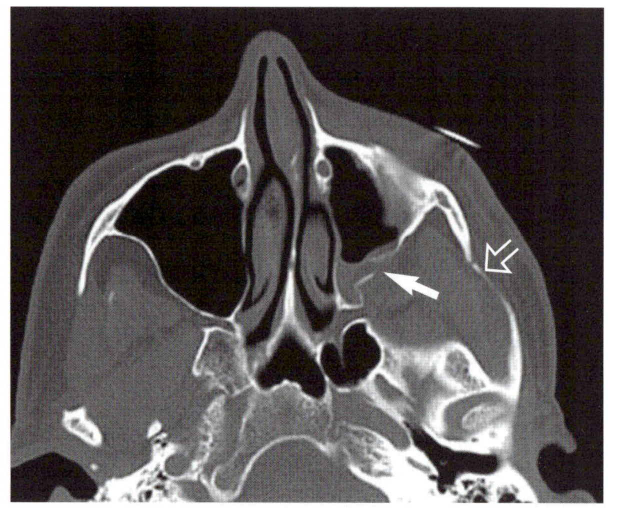

12.32d

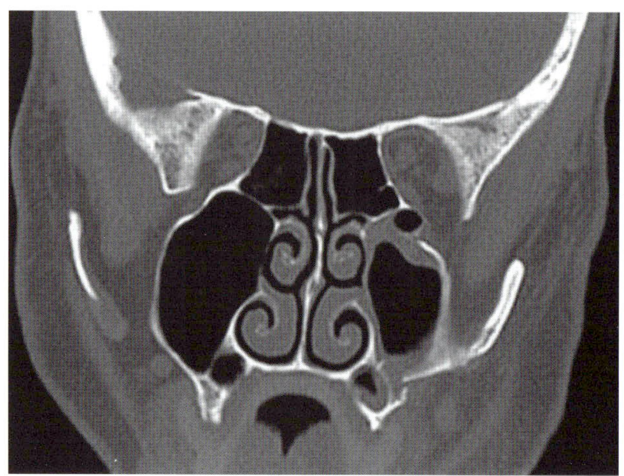

Figure 12.32 *Left zygomatic arch fracture abutting the coronoid process, with mild rotation and minimal displacement of the zygoma*. (a) Axial soft tissue image showing the zygomatic arch abutting the left coronoid process (arrow). A fracture of the posterior lateral aspect of the left maxillary sinus is also present (open arrow). (b, c) Axial bone images showing a fracture of the lateral orbital wall (arrow) and orbital floor, as well as mild depression of the zygomatic arch (open arrow). (d) Coronal image showing slight inferior displacement and mild rotation of the zygomatic component.

12.33a

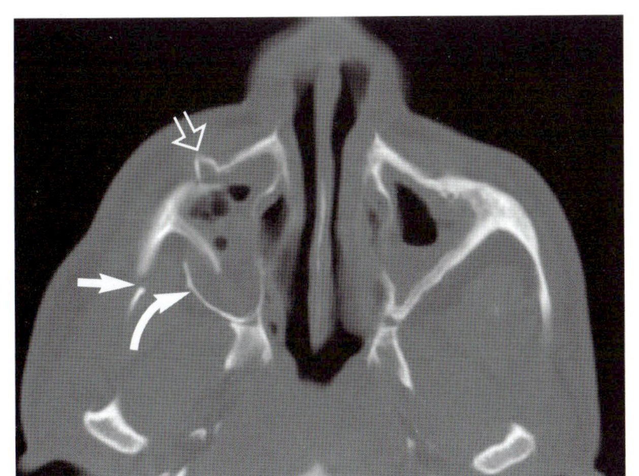

12.33b

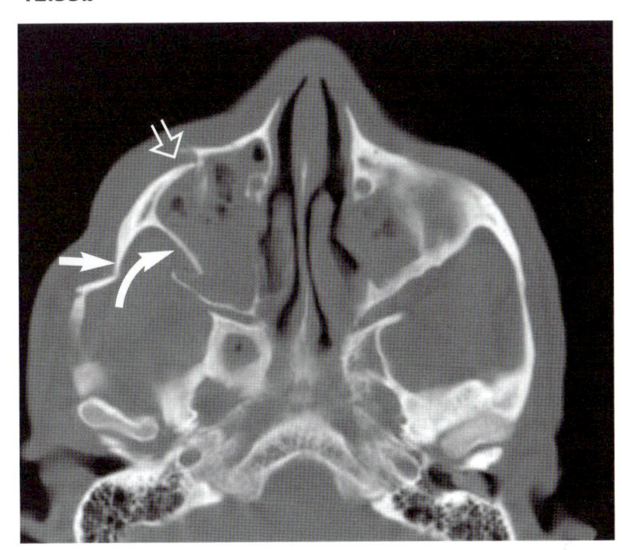

12.33c

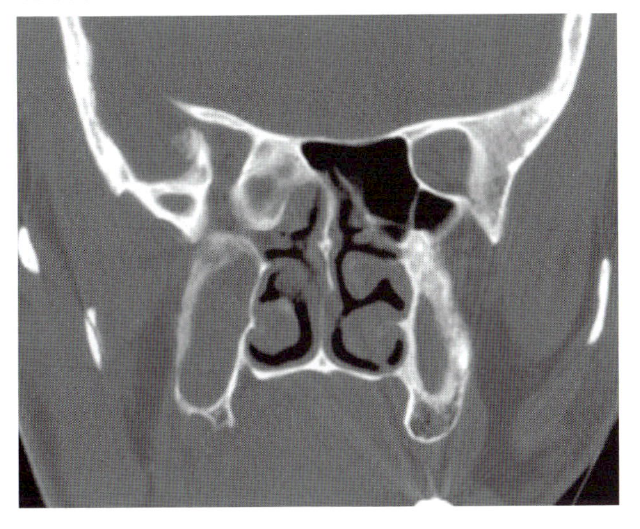

12.33d

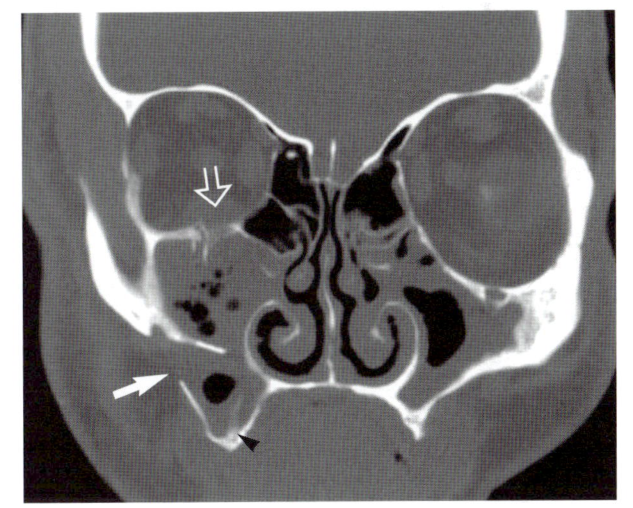

Figure 12.33 *Right tripod fracture with comminution of the infraorbital canal and fracture of the coronoid process.* (a, b) Axial images showing the right medially displaced zygoma (arrow) with a comminuted fracture of the anterior wall of the maxilla at the site of the infraorbital foramen (open arrow). The coronoid process lies adjacent to the displaced zygomatic component of the zygomatic arch. The more superior slice (a) shows the medially displaced zygoma buckling the lateral sinus wall posteriorly (curved arrow) and penetrating the infraorbital foramen anteriorly. (c) More posterior coronal image showing an undisplaced fracture of the coronoid process. (d) More anteriorly, the disruption of the infraorbital canal and displacement of the lateral sinus wall can be seen (arrows). The right inferior rectus muscle is enlarged (open arrow). A bone fragment lies in the inferior aspect of the right maxillary sinus (arrowhead).

12.34a

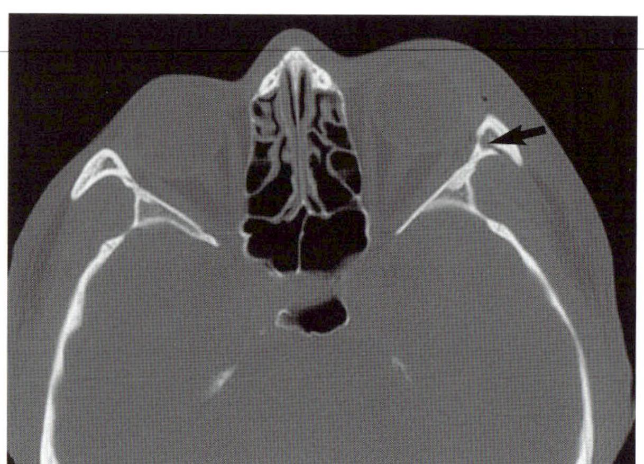

12.34b

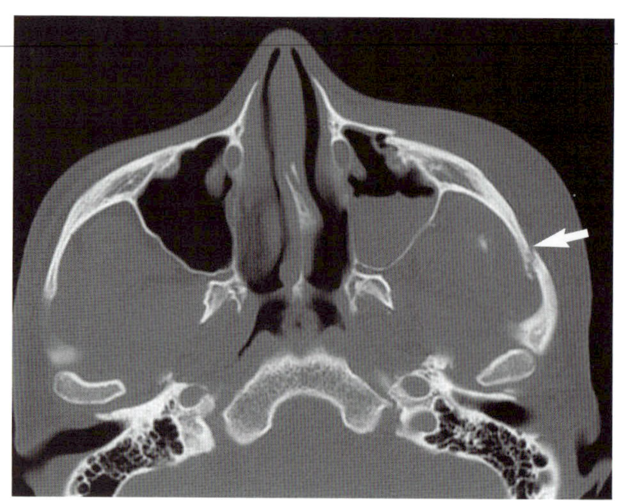

12.34c

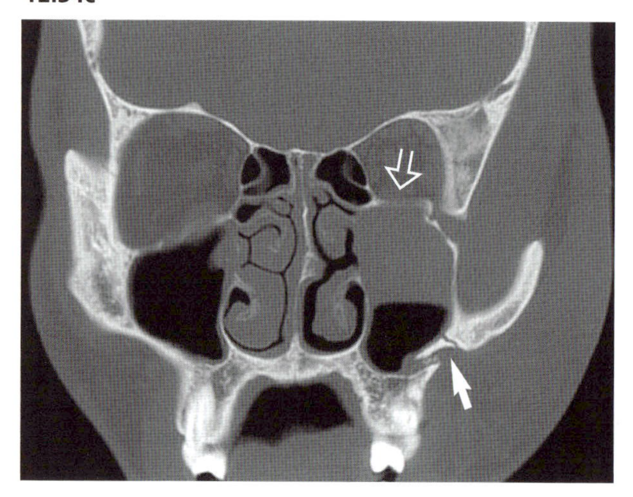

Figure 12.34 *Left tripod fracture with elevation of the orbital floor.* (a) Axial bone image through the orbit showing fractures through the lateral orbital wall anteriorly (arrow), soft tissue swelling overlying the left lateral face, and a suspected left proptosis. (b) Image through the maxillary sinuses showing a fracture of the zygomatic arch and minimal medial displacement of the zygoma (arrow). (c) Coronal image showing slight elevation of the bone fragment (arrow), with mild elevation of the left orbital floor more posteriorly (open arrow).

12.35a

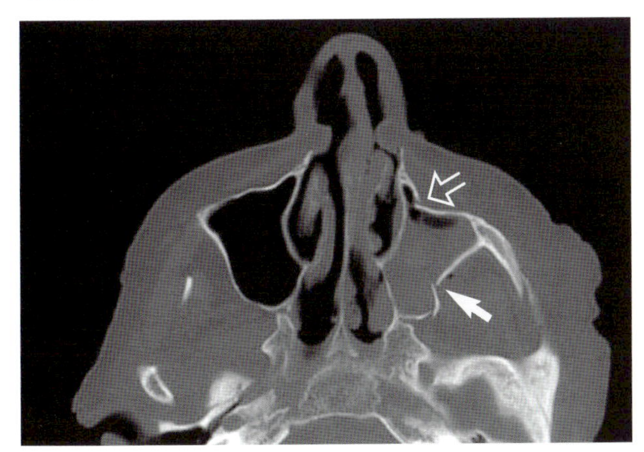

12.35b

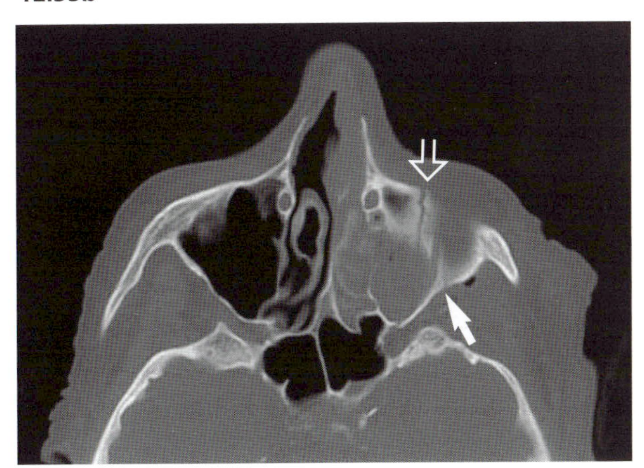

12.35c

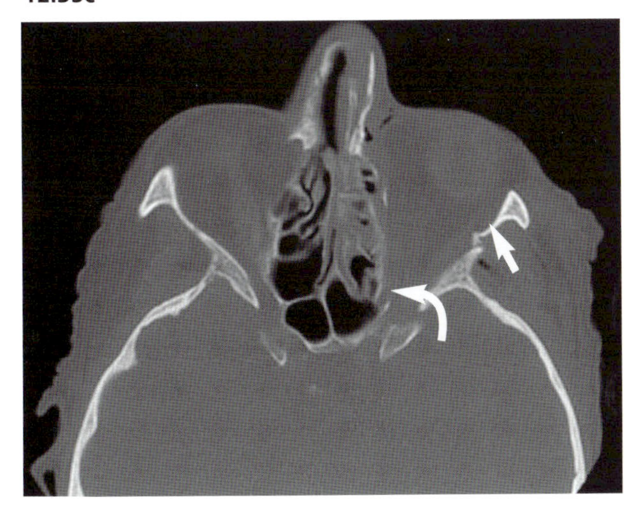

12.35d

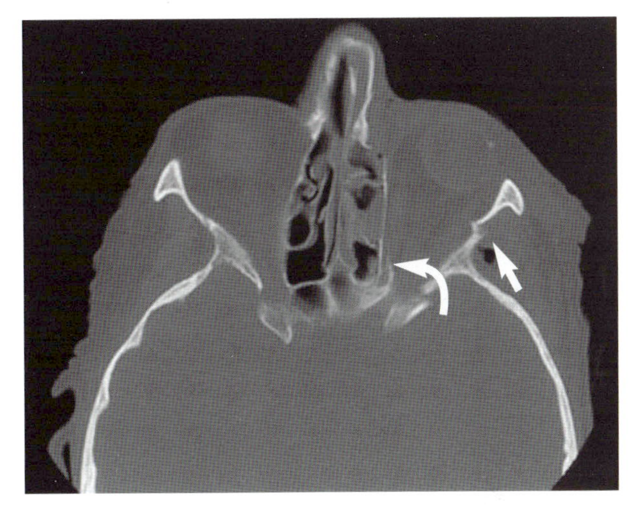

12.35e

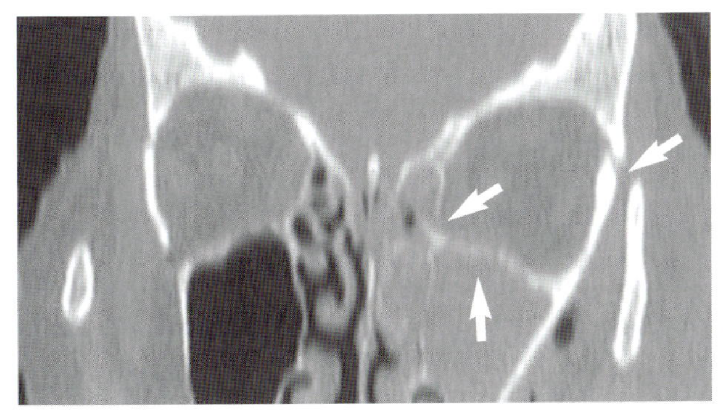

Figure 12.35 *Left zygomaticomaxillary fracture extending to the left medial orbital wall (unilateral Le Fort III).* (a–d) Axial images from inferior to superior. There is a tripod-type fracture with posterior displacement of the body of the zygoma, and associated fractures of the anterior (open arrow) and lateral walls (arrow) of the left maxillary sinus and zygomatic arch are present. Fractures are seen extending along the left orbital floor, medial to the infraorbital canal, with subtle fractures of the anterior wall of the left pterygopalatine fossa. At the level of the inferior orbit, there is mild overlap of the lateral orbital wall fracture. There is a displaced left nasal bone fracture, as well as fractures of the ethmoid septations and the medial orbital wall. The displaced left medial orbital wall fragment is more easily defined at the mid- to upper-orbital level and resembles a unilateral Le Fort III fracture (curved arrow). Caution is necessary in reducing this fracture to ensure that the medial orbital wall component does not impale or compress the optic canal, contained nerve, or vessels. (e) Coronal reformation showing the transmission of force along the left orbital floor into the ethmoid sinus and lamina papyracea (arrows).

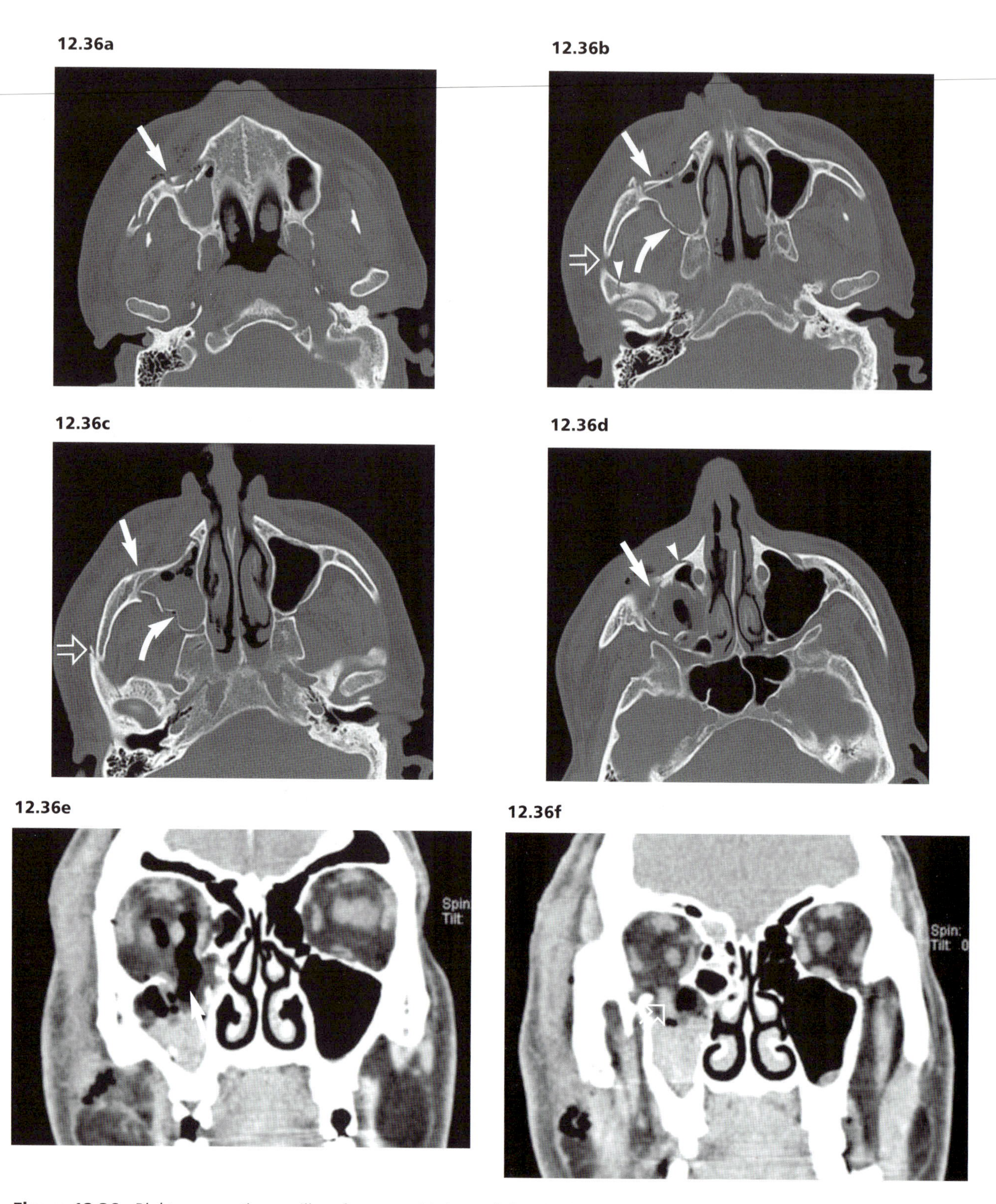

Figure 12.36 *Right zygomaticomaxillary fracture with large defect in the orbital floor*. (a–d) Axial images from inferior to superior showing fractures of the anterolateral wall of the right maxillary sinus (arrow), including the zygomatic recess of the maxillary sinus, and the zygomatic arch; there is an undisplaced fracture through the articular eminence of the right temporomandibular joint (b) (arrowhead). A posterior displacement of the zygoma is present, with overlapping of the zygomatic arch components (open arrow) and buckling of the lateral wall of the maxillary sinus (d) (curved arrow). There is a fracture of the infraorbital rim. Subtle bone fragments are noted within the superior maxillary sinus. (e, f) Coronal images through the mid-orbit just posterior to the globe showing a large defect in the right orbital floor (arrow), with orbital emphysema extending from the maxillary sinus. There is a hematoma within the inferior maxillary sinus. Soft tissue swelling overlies the right face and scalp with a hematoma in the right cheek. The inferior rectus muscle is pulled inferiorly into the superior aspect of the maxillary sinus (open arrow). The right maxillary sinus has a decreased transverse diameter due to the mild medial displacement of the zygoma.

12.36g

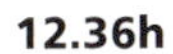

12.36h

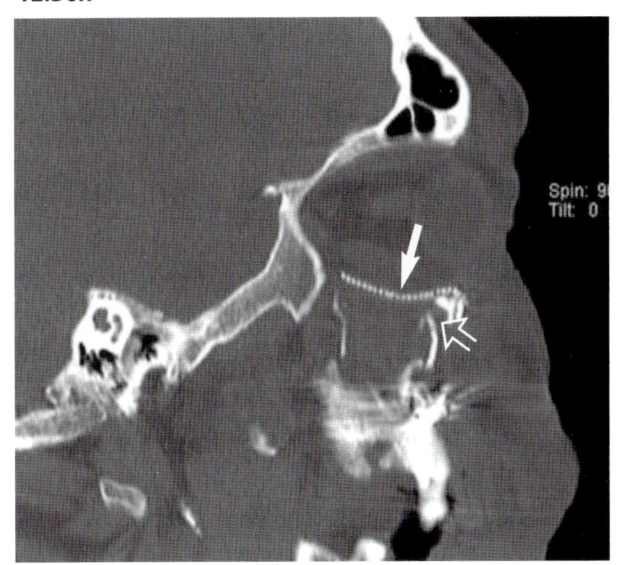

12.36i

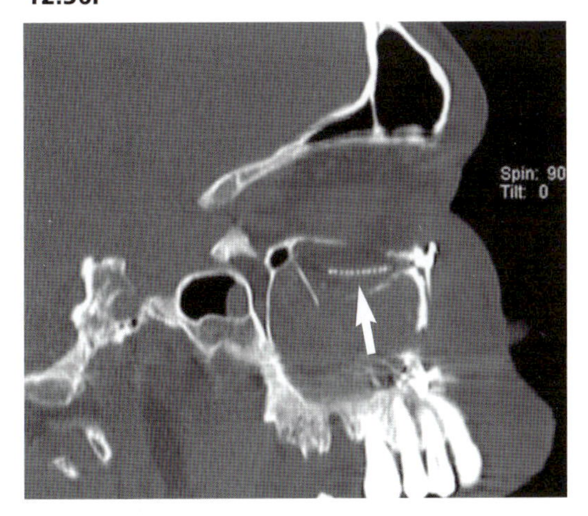

12.36j

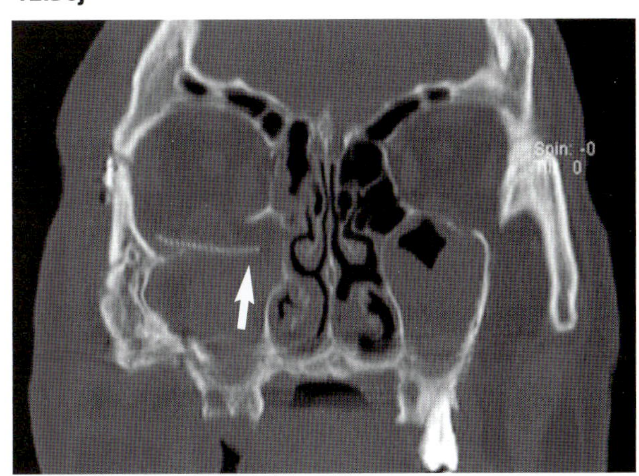

Figure 12.36 *continued* (g–j) Postoperative assessment of the same patient. (g) Axial image showing a wire mesh implant at the right orbital floor (arrow). Note that the axial image cannot assess adequacy of the graft position in this plane. (h) More lateral sagittal reformation showing the graft to be in a good position (arrow). A fragment of bone at the anterior maxilla remains posteriorly displaced. (i) More medial sagittal reformation showing an inferior displacement of the graft below the level of the orbital floor (arrow). (j) Coronal reformation providing a better display of the inferior position of the graft medially (arrow).

12.37a

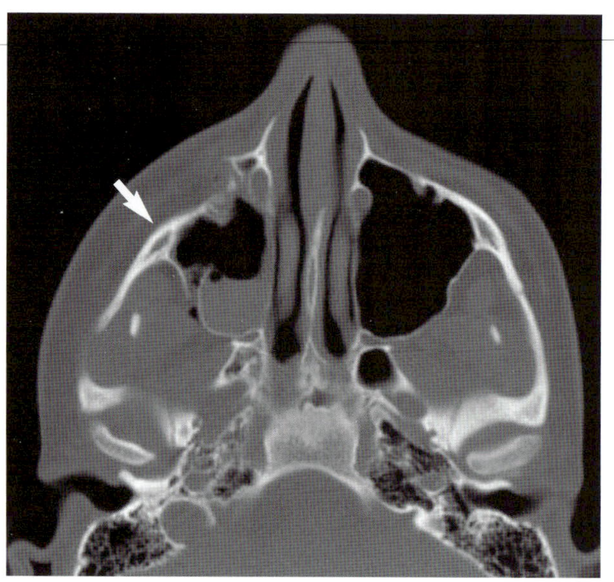

12.37b

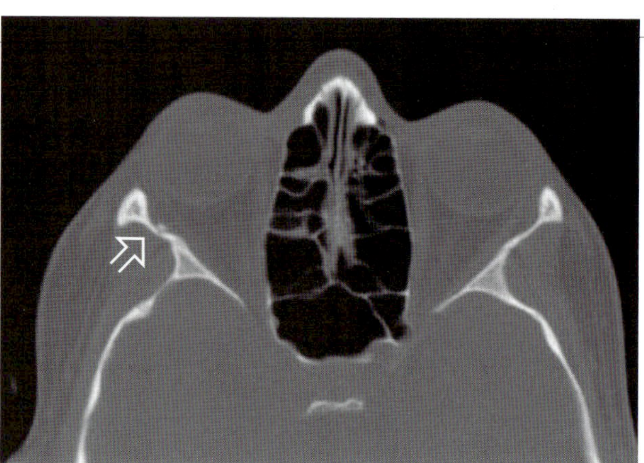

12.37c

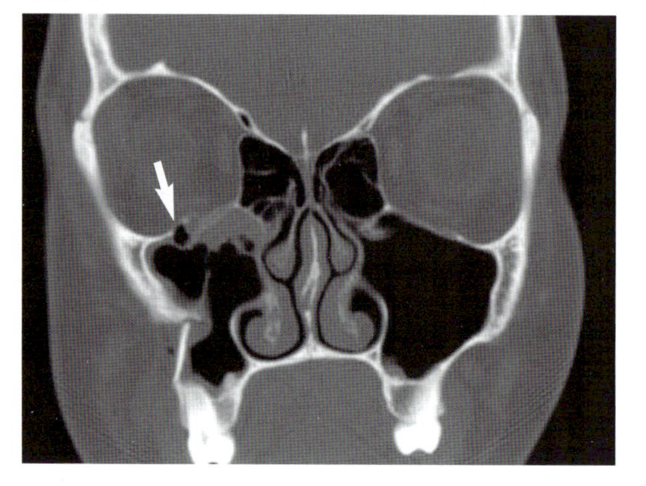

12.37d

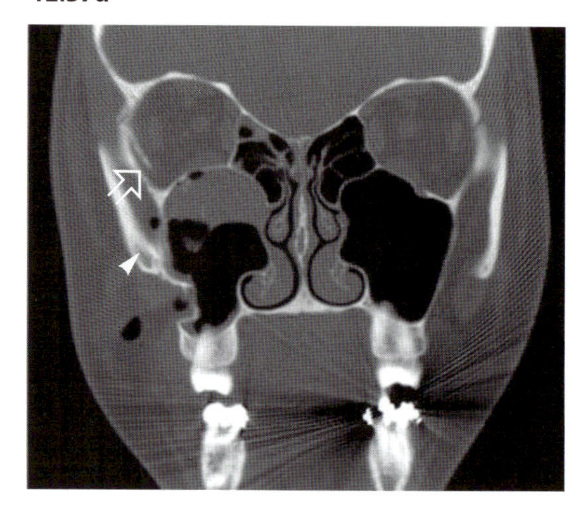

Figure 12.37 *Right tripod fracture – body of zygoma displaced posteriorly*. (a, b) Axial images showing the body of the zygoma displaced medially and posteriorly (arrow), encroaching on the lateral anterior aspect of the right maxillary sinus. A tiny bone fragment is present at the lateral wall of the orbit (open arrow). (c, d) Coronal images showing encroachment on the lateral aspect of the maxillary sinus. A subtle orbital floor fracture is present (arrow). More posteriorly, overlap of bone fragments at the lateral orbital wall is noted (open arrow), as well as elevation of the orbital floor by the posteromedial displacement of the zygoma, as seen by its presence in this plane (arrowhead).

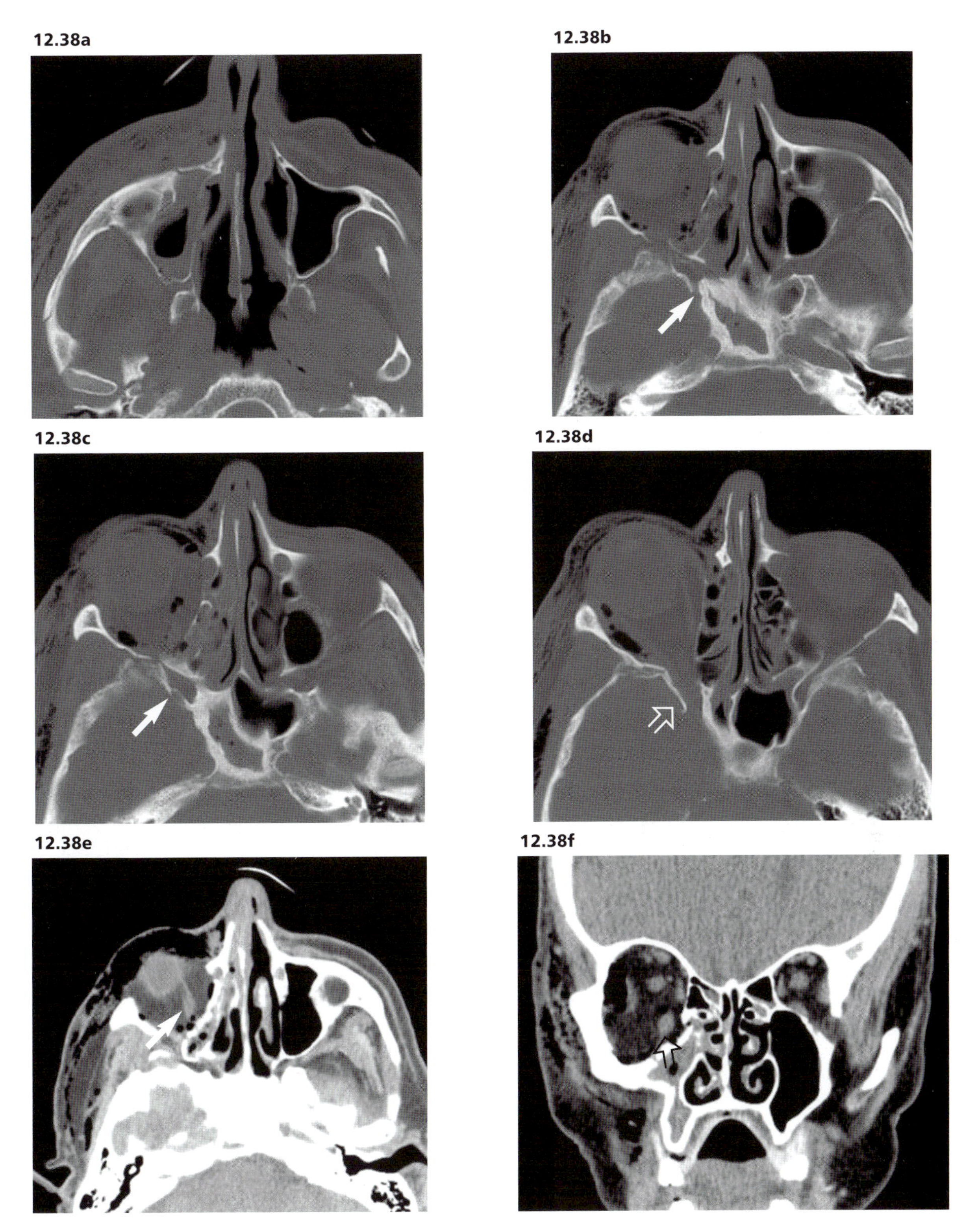

Figure 12.38 *Right zygomaticomaxillary fracture with forces transmitted to the greater wing of the sphenoid.* (a–d) Axial bone images from inferior to superior showing fractures of the right zygoma, with slight exaggeration of the curvature of the zygomatic arch. Subtle fractures of the anterior and posterolateral walls of the maxillary sinus are present. On the image (a) through the inferior orbit, orbital floor fractures are noted with the inferior rectus muscle maintaining a close relationship to the displaced orbital floor. The immediately superior image (b) shows a fracture of the right greater wing of the sphenoid extending into the anterior aspect of the middle cranial fossa (arrow). The orbital floor fracture encroaches on the superior posterior aspect of the left maxillary sinus. Deformity of the greater wing of the sphenoid lateral to the superior orbital fissure is noted (open arrow). (e) Axial soft tissue image showing a suspected entrapped inferior rectus muscle (arrow). The lateral wall of the orbit is shortened, suggesting posterior displacement. (f) Coronal soft tissue image showing an altered appearance of the right inferior rectus muscle, tethered to the orbital floor (open arrow). The orbital floor in this plane is displaced infero-medially.

12.38g

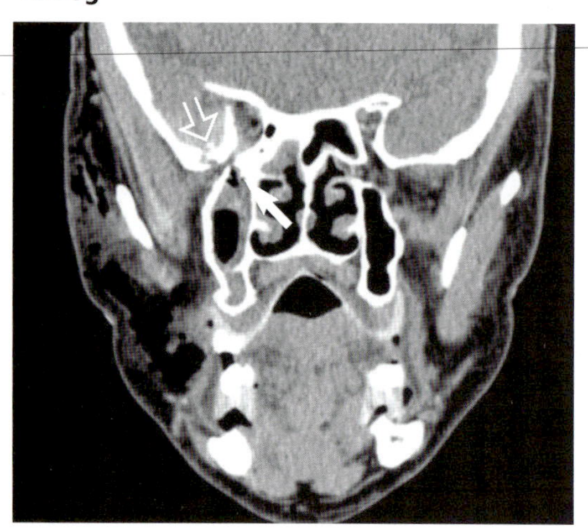

12.38h

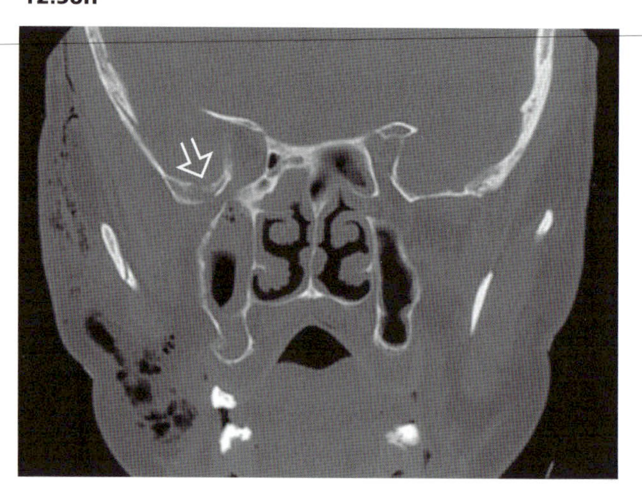

12.38i

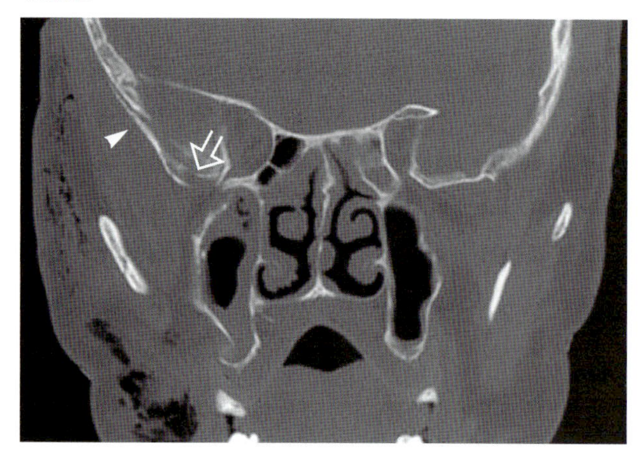

12.38j

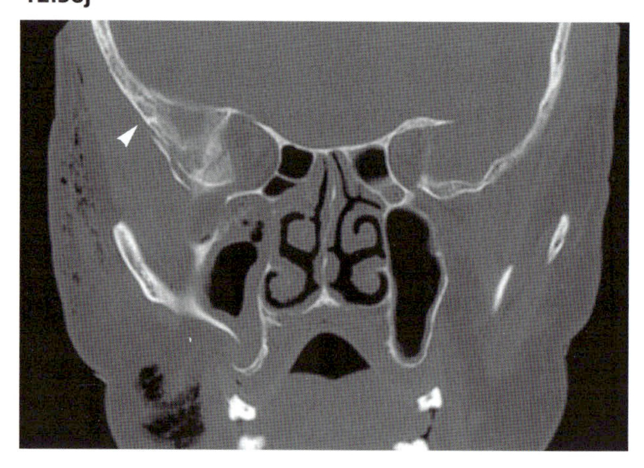

12.38k

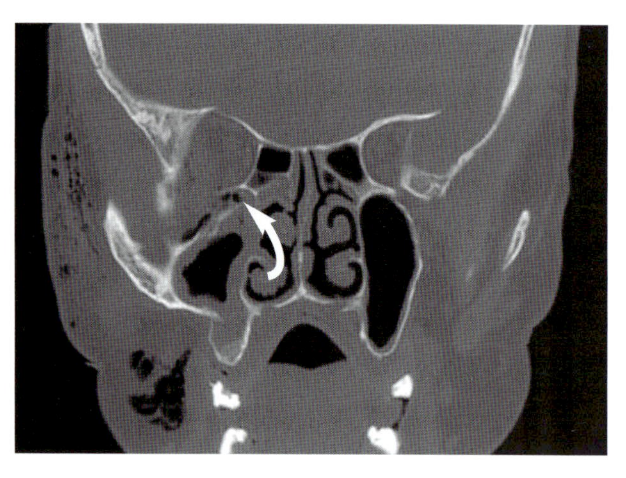

12.38l

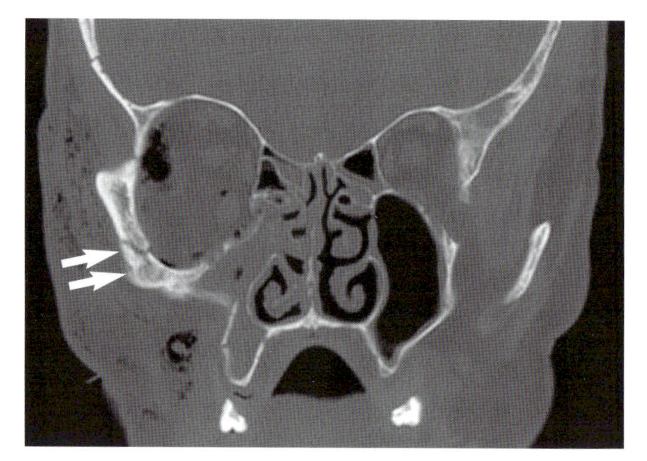

Figure 12.38 *continued* (g) More posterior coronal soft tissue image showing a fracture at the posterior superior aspect of the maxillary sinus, extending into the inferior orbital fissure (arrow) and through the greater wing of the sphenoid at the floor of the middle cranial fossa (open arrow). (h–l) Coronal bone algorithm images, from posterior to anterior, showing fractures through the greater wing of the sphenoid, a fracture (open arrow) of the zygomatic arch, and subtle fractures at the lateral aspect of the middle cranial fossa vault (arrowheads), noted just superior to the level of the orbits. The right orbital floor is displaced inferiorly (curved arrow). There is a fracture of the inferior aspect of the frontal process of the zygoma, at the lateral orbital rim (double arrow).

12.39a

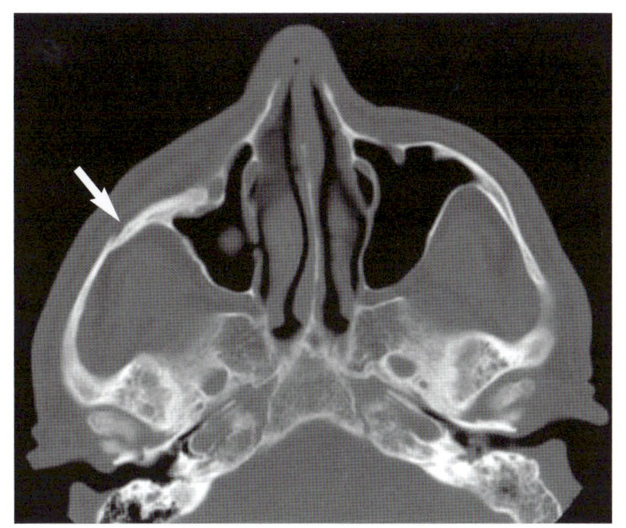

12.39b

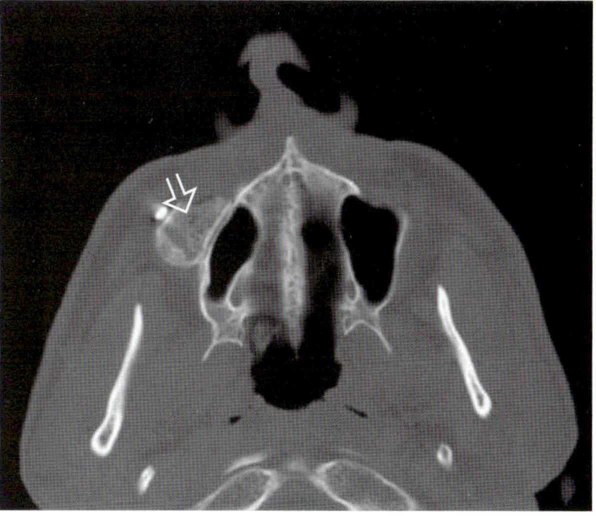

Figure 12.39 *Right unreduced tripod fracture with an onlay bone graft.* (a) Axial image showing exaggerated curvature of the zygomatic arch (arrow) in an unreduced right tripod fracture with the body of the zygoma displaced posteriorly and medially. (b) More inferior axial image showing an onlay bone graft placed to improve the cosmetic appearance of the lower mid-face (open arrow).

Bibliography

Alden TD, Lin KY, Jane JA. Mechanisms of premature closure of cranial sutures. Childs Nerv Syst 1999; 15: 670–675

al-Qurainy IA, Stassen LF, Dutton GN, et al. Diplopia following midfacial fractures. Br J Oral Maxillofac Surg 1991; 29: 302–307

al-Qurainy IA, Stassen LF, Dutton GN, et al. The characteristics of midfacial fractures and the association with ocular injury: a prospective study. Br J Oral Maxillofac Surg 1991; 29: 291–301

Astor FC, Donegan O, Glugman JL. Unusual anatomic presentations of inverting papilloma. Head Neck Surg 1985; 7: 243–245

Babbel R, Harnsberger HR, Nelson B, et al. Optimization of techniques in screening CT of the sinuses. AJNR Am J Neuroradiol 1991; 12: 849–854

Balter S. An introduction to the physics of magnetic resonance imaging. Radiographics 1987; 7: 371–383

Bassoiouny A, Newlands WJ, Ali H, et al. Maxillary sinus hypoplasia and superior orbital fissure asymmetry. Laryngoscope 1982; 92: 441–448

Bassoiouny A, Newlands WJ, Ali H, et al. Maxillary sinus hypoplasia and superior orbital fissure asymmetry. Laryngoscope 1982; 92: 441–448

Beahm E, Teresi L, Lufkin R, Hanafee W. MR of the paranasal sinuses. Surg Radiol Anat 1990; 12: 203–208

Behrman RE, Kuelman R, Jenson H. Craniosynostosis. In: Kliegman R, ed. Nelson Textbook of Pediatrics, 16th edn. Philadelphia: WB Saunders, 2000: 1831–1832

Berlinger NT. Sinusitis in immunodeficient and immunosuppressed patients. Laryngoscope 1985; 95: 29

Bingham B, Shankar L, Hawke M. Pitfalls in computed tomography of the paranasal sinuses. J Otolaryngology 1991; 20: 414–418

Black CM, Dungan D, Fram E, et al. Potential pitfalls in the work-up and diagnosis of choanal atresia. AJNR Am J Neuroradiol 1998; 19: 326–329

Blaser S, Armstrong D. Congenital Malformations of the Face. In: King SJ, Boothroyd AE, eds. Pediatric ENT Radiology. New York: Springer Verlag, 2002: 99–118

Bolger WE, Butzin CA, Parsons DS. Paranasal sinus bony anatomic variations and mucosal abnormalities: CT analysis for endoscopic sinus surgery. Laryngoscope 1991; 101: 56–64

Bolger WE, Woodruff WW, Morehead J. Maxillary sinus hypoplasia: classification and description of associated uncinate process hypoplasia. Otolaryngol Head Neck Surg 1990; 103: 759–765

Borges A, Fink J, Villablanca P, et al. Midline destructive lesions of the sinonasal tract: simplified terminology based on histopathologic criteria. AJNR Am J Neuroradiol 2000; 21: 331–336

Bradley WG Jr. Fundamentals of magnetic resonance image interpretation. In: Bradley WG, Adey WR, Hasso AN, eds. Magnetic Resonance Imaging of the Brain, Head, and Neck: A Text Atlas. Rockville, MD: Aspen, 1984: 1–16

Brandt KE, Burruss GL, Hickerson WL, et al. The management of mid-face fractures with intracranial injury. J Trauma 1991; 31: 15–19

Bridger MWM, van Nostrand AWP. The nose and paranasal sinuses – applied surgical anatomy. J Otolaryngol 1978; 7(Suppl 6)

Brockbank MJ, Brookes GB. The sphenoiditis spectrum. Clin Otolaryngol 1991; 16: 15–20

Buchwald C, Nielsen LH, Ahlgren P, et al. Radiologic aspects of inverted papilloma. Eur J Radiol 1990; 10: 134–139

Burm JS, Chung CH, Oh SJ. Pure orbital blowout fracture: new concepts and importance of medial orbital blowout fracture. Plast Reconstr Surg 1999; 103: 1839–1849

Carter BL, Bankoff MS, Fisk JD. Computed tomographic detection of sinusitis responsible for intracranial and extracranial infections. Radiology 1983; 147: 739–742

Castillo M. Congenital abnormalities of the nose: CT and MR findings. AJR Am J Roentgenol 1994; 162: 1211–1217

Catalano PJ, Lawson W, Som P, Biller HF. Radiographic evaluation and diagnosis of the failed frontal osteoplastic flap with fat obliteration. Otolaryngol Head Neck Surgery 1990; 104: 225–234

Centeno RS, Bentson JR, Mancuso AA. CT scanning in rhinocerebral mucormycosis and aspergillosis. Radiology 1981; 140: 383–389

Chan LL, Singh S, Jones D, et al. Ginsberg imaging of mucormycosis skull base osteomyelitis. AJNR Am J Neuroradiol 2000; 21: 828–831

Coker NJ, Brooks BS, El Gammal T. Computed tomography of orbital medial wall fractures. Head Neck Surg 1983; 5: 383–389

Conner BL, Roach ES, Laster W, Georgitis JW. Magnetic resonance imaging of the paranasal sinuses: frequency and type of abnormalities. Ann Allergy 1989; 62: 457–460

Cooke LD, Hadley DM. MRI of the paranasal sinuses: incidental abnormalities and their relationship to symptoms. J Laryngol Otol 1991; 105: 278–281

Cooke LD, Hadley DM. MRI of the paranasal sinuses: incidental abnormalities and their relationship to symptoms. J Laryngol Otol 1991; 105: 278–281

Crain MR, Dolan KD, Maves MD. Maxillary sinus mucocoele. Ann Otol Rhinol Laryngol 1990; 99: 321–322

Curtin HD, Williams R, Johnson J. CT of perineural tumor extention: pterygopalatine fossa. AJR Am J Roentgenol 1985; 144: 163–169

Curtin HD, Williams R. Computed tomographic anatomy of the pterygopalatine fossa. Radiographics 1985; 5: 429–435

Danemann F, Pereira P, Laniado M, et al. Inverted papilloma of the nasal cavity and the paranasal sinuses: using CT for primary diagnosis and follow-up. AJR Am J Roentgenol 1999; 172: 543–548

Daniels DL, Pech P, Kay MC, et al. Orbital apex: correlative anatomic and CT study. AJR Am J Roentgenol 1985; 145: 1141–44

Daniels DL, Rauschning W, Lovas J, et al. Pterygopalatine fossa: computed tomographic studies. Radiology 1983; 149: 511–516

DeLone DR, Goldstein RA, Petermann G, et al. Disseminated aspergillosis involving the brain: distribution and imaging characteristics. AJNR Am J Neuroradiol 1999; 20: 1597–1604

Deutsch JH, Hudgins PA, Siegel JL, et al. The paranasal sinuses of patients with acute graft-versus-host disease. AJNR Am J Neuroradiol 1995; 16: 1287–1291

Dillon WP, Som PM, Fullerton GD. Hypointense MR signal in chronically inspissated sinonasal secretions. Radiology 1990; 174: 73–78

Dolan K, Smoker WRK. Paranasal sinus radiology, Part 4B: Maxillary sinus. Head Neck Surg 1983; 5: 428–446

Dolan KD, Smoker WRK. Paranasal sinus radiology, Part 4A: Maxillary sinuses. Head Neck Surg 1983; 5: 345–362

Fascenelli Maj FW. Maxillary sinus abnormalities. Arch Otolaryngol 1969; 90: 98–101

Felsberg GJ, Tien RD, McLendon RE. Frontoethmoidal giant cell reparative granuloma. AJNR Am J Neuroradiol 1995; 16: 1551–1554

Fullerton GD. Magnetic resonance imaging signal concepts. Radiographics 1987; 7: 579–596

Furin MJ, Zinreich SJ, Kennedy DW. The atelectatic maxillary sinus. Am J Rhinology 1991; 5: 79–83

Gentry LR, Manor WF, Turski PA, Strother CM. High resolution CT analysis of facial struts in trauma. 1. Normal anatomy. AJR Am J Roentgenol 1983; 140: 523–532

Gentry LR, Manor WF, Turski PA, Strother CM. High resolution CT analysis of facial struts in trauma. II. Osseous and soft tissue complications. AJR Am J Roentgenol 1983; 140: 533–541

Gentry LR. Facial trauma and associated brain damage. Radiol Clin North Am 1989; 27: 435–446

Gonsalves CG, Briant TDR. Radiologic findings in nasopharyngeal angiofibromas. J Canadian Assos Radiol 1978; 29: 209–213

Gordon AR, Loevner LA, Sonners AI, et al. Post-transplantation lymphoproliferative disorder of the paranasal sinuses mimicking invasive fungal sinusitis: case report. AJNR Am J Neuroradiol 2002; 23: 855–857

Gorlin RJ, Cohen MM Jr, Levin LS. Syndromes of the Head and Neck. New York: Oxford University Press, 1990

Goss CM, ed. Gray's Anatomy. Philadelphia: Lea & Febiger, 1973

Gotwald TF, Sprinzl GM, Fischer H, Rettenbacher T. Retained packing gauze in the ethmoidal sinuses after endonasal sinus surgery: CT and surgical appearances. AJR Am J Roentgenol 2001; 177: 1487–1489

Grossman RJ, Gomori JM, Goldberg HL, et al. MR imaging of hemorrhagic conditions of the head and neck, Radiographics 1988; 8: 441–454

Gruss JS, Kassel EE, Bubak P. Clinical, surgical, and treatment perspectives in the management of craniomaxillofacial trauma. Neuroimag Clin North Am 1991; 1: 341–355

Gruss JS. Naso-ethmoid-orbital fractures: classification and the role of primary bone grafting. Plast Reconstr Surg 1985; 75: 303–315

Han MH, Chang KH, Lee CH, et al. Cystic expansile masses of the maxilla: differential diagnosis with CT and MR. AJNR Am J Neuroradiol 1995; 16: 333–338

Harris J, Robert E, Kallen B. Epidemiology of choanal atresia with special reference to the CHARGE association. Pediatrics 1997; 99: 363–367

Hasso AN. CT of tumours and tumour like conditions of the paranasal sinuses. Radiol Clin North Am 1984; 22: 119–130

Havas TE, Motbey Å, Gullane PJ. Prevalence of incidental abnormalities on Computed tomographic scans of the paranasal sinuses. Arch Otolaryngol Head Neck Surg 1988; 114: 856–859

Hsu L, Fried MP, Jolesz FA. MR-guided endoscopic sinus surgery. AJNR Am J Neuroradiol 1998; 19: 1235–1240

Hudgins PA, Browning DG, Gallups J, et al. Endoscopic paranasal sinus surgery: radiographic evaluation of severe complications. AJNR Am J Neuroradiol 1992; 13: 1161–1167

Hudgins PA, Mukundan S. Screening sinus CT: a good idea gone bad? AJNR Am J Neuroradiol 1997; 18: 1850–1854

Hunink MGM, de Slegte RGM, Gerritsen GJ, et al. CT and MR assessment of tumors of the nose and paranasal sinuses, the nasopharynx and the parapharyngeal space using ROC methodology. Neuroradiology 1990; 32: 220

Hurst RW, Judkins A, Bolger W, et al. Mycotic aneurysm and cerebral infarction resulting from fungal sinusitis: imaging and pathologic correlation. AJNR Am J Neuroradiol 2001; 22: 858–863

Jackson IT. Classification and treatment of orbitalo-zygomatic and orbitalo-ethmoid fractures. Clin Plast Surg 1989; 16: 77–91

Jacobs M, Som PM. The ethmoidal 'polypoidal mucocoele'. J Comput Assist Tomogr 1982; 6: 721–724

Jorgensen RA. Endoscopic and computed tomographic findings in ostiomeatal sinus disease. Arch Otolaryngol Head Neck Surg 1991; 117: 279–287

Kassel EE, Gruss JS. Imaging of midfacial fractures. Neuroimaging Clin North Am 1991; 1: 259–283

Katsantonis GP, Friedman WH, Sivore MC. The role of computed tomography in revision sinus surgery. Laryngoscope 1990; 100: 811–816

Kennedy DW, Josephson JS, Zinreich SJ, et al. Endoscopic sinus surgery for mucocoeles: a viable alternative. Laryngoscope 1989; 99: 885–895

Kennedy DW, Zinreich SJ, Shaalan H, et al. Endoscopic middle meatal antrostomy: theory, technique and patency. Laryngoscope 1987; 94 (Suppl 43): 1

Khalek AA, Razek A, Elasfour AA. MR appearance of rhinoscleroma. AJNR Am J Neuroradiol 1999; 20: 575–578

Khanobthamchai K, Shankar L, Hawke M, Bingham B. The ethmo-maxillary sinus and hypoplasia of the maxillary sinus. J Otolaryngol 1991; 20: 425–427

Khanobthamchai K, Shankar L, Hawke M, Bingham B. The secondary middle turbinate. J Otolaryngol 1991; 20: 412–413

Kim HJ, Kim JH, Kim JH, Hwang EG. Bone erosion caused by sinonasal cavernous hemangioma: CT findings in two patients. AJNR Am J Neuroradiol 1995; 16: 1176–1178

Koichi Y, Watanabe M, Nakamura T. Age-related expansion and reduction in aeration of the sphenoid sinus: volume assessment by helical CT scanning. AJNR Am J Neuroradiol 2000; 21: 179–182

Kopp W, Stammberger H, Fotter R. Special radiologic imaging of paranasal sinuses. Eur J Radiol 1988; 8: 153

Kopp W, Stammberger H, Fotter R. Special radiologic imaging of paranasal sinuses. Eur J Radiol 1988; 8: 153

Kramer GS, Gatenby RA. Malignant plasmacytoma appearing as invasive paranasal sinus disease after cardiac transplantation. AJNR Am J Neuroradiol 1996; 17: 1582–1584

Lai PH, Yang CF, Pan HB, et al. Recurrent inverted papilloma: diagnosis with pharmacokinetic dynamic gadolinium-enhanced MR imaging. AJNR Am J Neuroradiol 1999; 20: 1445–1451

Lang J. Clinical anatomy of the nose, nasal cavity and paranasal sinuses. New York: Thieme, 1989

Lanzieri CF, Shah M, Krauss D, Lavertu P. Use of gadolinium-enhanced MR imaging for differentiating mucoceles from neoplasms in the paranasal sinuses. Radiology 1991; 178: 425–428

Lauffer RB. Magnetic Resonance contrast media: principles and progress. Magn Reson Q 1990; 6: 65–84

Lee JH, Lee MS, Lee BH, et al. Rhabdomyosarcoma of the head and neck in adults: MR and CT findings. AJNR Am J Neuroradiol 1996; 17: 1923–1928

Lee KF. High resolution computed tomography in facial trauma associated with closed head injury. In: Toombs BD, Sandler CM. eds. Computed Tomography in Trauma. Philadelphia: WB Saunders, 1987: 187–209

LeFort R. Etude experimental sur les fractures de la machoire superieure, Parts I, II, III. Rev Chir (Paris) 1901; 23: 208–227

Lewin JS, Curtin HD, Eelkema E, Obuchowski N. Benign expansile lesions of the sphenoid sinus: differentiation from normal asymmetry of the lateral recesses. AJNR Am J Neuroradiol 1999; 20: 461–466

Lidov M, Behin F, Som PM. Calcified sphenoid mucocoele. Arch Otolaryngol Head Neck Surg 1990; 116: 718–720

Littlejohn MC, Stiernberg CM, Hokanson JA, et al. The relationship between the nasal cycle and mucociliary clearance. Laryngoscope 1992; 102: 117–120

Lloyd GAS, Lund VJ, Phelps PD, et al. Magnetic resonance imaging in the evaluation of nose and paranasal sinus disease. Br J Radiol 1987; 60: 957–968

Lloyd GAS. CT of the paranasal sinuses: study of a control series in relation to endoscopic sinus surgery. J Laryngol Otol 1990; 104: 477–481

Loevner LA, Yousem DM, Lanza DC, et al. MR evaluation of frontal sinus osteoplastic flaps with autogenous fat grafts. AJNR Am J Neuroradiol 199; 16: 1721–1726

Lowe LH, Booth TN, Joglar JM, Rollins NK. Midface anomalies in children. Radiographics 2000; 20: 907–922

Lund VJ, Lloyd GAS. Radiological changes associated with inverted papilloma of the nose and paranasal sinuses. Br J of Radiol 1984; 57: 455–461

Mackay IS, Bull TR. Scott Brown's Otolaryngology, Vol 4: Rhinology, 5th edn. London: Butterworths, 1987

Mafee MF. Endoscopic sinus surgery. role of the radiogist. AJNR Am J Neuroradiol 1991; 12: 855–860

Mafee MF. Endoscopic sinus surgery. role of the radiogist. AJNR Am J Neuroradiol 1991; 12: 855–860

Maniglia AJ. Fatal and major complications secondary to nasal and sinus surgery. Laryngoscope 1989; 99: 276–283

Manson PN, Glassman D, Vanderkolk C, et al. Rigid stabilization of sagittal fractures of the maxilla and palate. Plast Reconstr Surg 1990; 85: 711–717

Manson PN, Markowitz B, Mirvis S, et al. Toward CT-based facial fracture treatment. Plast Reconstr Surg 1990; 85: 202–12; discussion 1990: 213–214

Maran AGD, Lund VJ. Clinical Rhinology. New York: Thieme, 1990

Martello JY, Vasconez HC. Supraorbital roof fractures; a formidable entity with which to contend. Ann Plast Surg 1997; 38: 223–227

Masala W, Perugini S, Salvolini U, Teatini GP. Multiplanar reconstruction in the study of ethmoid anatomy. Neuroradiology 1989; 31: 151–155

Masala W, Perugini S, Salvolini U, Teatini GP. Multiplanar reconstruction in the study of ethmoid anatomy. Neuroradiology 1989; 31 :151–155

McLean FM, Ginsberg LE, Stanton CA. Perineural spread of rhinocerebral mucormycosis. AJNR Am J Neuroradiol 1996; 17: 114–116

Melhem ER, Oliverio PJ, Benson ML, et al. Optimal CT evaluation for functional endoscopic sinus surgery. AJNR Am J Neuroradiol 1996; 17: 181–188

Merkes J, Sarnat H. Child Neurology, 6th edn. Philadelphia: Lippincott Williams & Wilkins, 2000: 351–354

Miaux Y, Ribaud P, Williams M, et al. MR of cerebral aspergillosis in patients who have had bone marrow transplantation. AJNR Am J Neuroradiol 1995; 16: 555–562

Mitchell MR, Tarr RW, Conturo CL, et al. Spin echo technique selection: basic principles for choosing MRI pulse sequence timing intervals. Radiographics 1986; 6: 245–260

Mitchell MR, Tarr RW, Conturo CL, et al. Spin echo technique selection: basic principles for choosing MRI pulse sequence timing intervals. Radiographics 1986; 6: 245–260

Modic MT, Weinstein WA, Berlin J, Duschesneau PM. Maxillary sinus hypoplasia visualised with computed tomography. Radiology 1980; 135: 383–385

Moloney JA, Badham NJ, McRae A. The acute orbit: preseptal (periorbital) cellulitis subperiosteal abscess and orbital cellulitis due to sinusitis. J Laryngol Otol 1987; 12(Suppl): 1

Moser FG, Panush D, Rubin JS, et al. Incidental paranasal sinus abnormalities on MRI of the brain. Clin Radiol 1991; 43: 252–254

Nass RL, Holliday RA, Reede DL. Diagnosis of surgical sinusitis using nasal endoscopy and computed tomography. Laryngoscope 1989; 99: 1158–1160

Nolasco FP, Mathog RH. Medial orbital wall fractures: classification and clinical profile. Otolaryngol Head Neck Surg 1995; 112: 549–556

Noyek AM, Zizmor J. Radiology of the maxillary sinus after Caldwell-Luc surgery. Otolaryngol Clin North Am 1976; 9: 135–151

Ojiri H, Ujita M, Tada S, Fukuda K. Potentially distinctive features of sinonasal inverted papilloma on MR imaging. AJR Am J Roentgenol 2000; 175: 465–468

Olson EM, Wright DL, Hoffman HT, et al. Frontal sinus fractures: evaluation of CT scans in 132 patients. AJNR Am J Neuroradiol 1992; 13: 897–902

Ooi GC, Chim CS, Liang R, et al. Nasal T-cell/natural killer cell lymphoma: CT and MR imaging features of a new clinicopathologic entity. AJR Am J Roentgenol 2000; 174: 1141–1145

Pace Balzan A, Shankar L, Hawke M. Computed tomographic findings in atrophic rhinitis. J Otolaryngol 1991; 20: 428–432

Patel RS, Yousem DM, Maldjian JA, Zager EL. Incidence and clinical significance of frontal sinus or orbital entry during pterional (frontotemporal) craniotomy. AJNR Am J Neuroradiol 2000; 21: 1327–1330

Phillips CD, Platts-Mills TA. Chronic sinusitis: relationship between CT findings and clinical history of asthma, allergy, eosinophilia, and infection. AJR Am J Roentgenol 1995; 164: 185–187

Provenzale JM, Allen NB. Wegener granulomatosis: CT and MR findings. AJNR Am J Neuroradiol 1996; 17: 785–792

Rak KM, Newell JD, Yakes WJ, et al. Paranasal sinuses on MR images of the brain: significance of mucosal thickening. AJNR Am J Neuroradiol 1990; 11: 1211

Raymond HW, Zwiebel WJ, Harnesberger HR. Essentials of screening sinus. Comput Tomogr 1991; 12: 526

Robinson JD, Crawford SC, Teresi LM, et al. Extracranial lesions of the head and neck: Preliminary experience with Gd-DTPA-enhanced MR imaging. Radiology 1989; 172: 165–170

Rohen JW, Yokochi C. Color Atlas of Anatomy. Schattauer Verlag, 1983

Rontal M, Rontal E. Studying whole-mounted sections of the paranasal sinuses to understand the complications of endoscopic sinus surgery. Laryngoscope 1991; 101: 361–366

Rumboldt Z, Castillo M. Indolent intracranial mucormycosis: case report. AJNR Am J Neuroradiol 2002; 23: 932–934

Russell EJ, Czervionke L, Huckman M, et al. CT of the inferomedial orbit and the lacrimal drainage apparatus: normal and pathologic anatomy. AJR Am J Roentgenol 1985; 145: 1147–1154

Saini S, Modic MT, Hamm B, Hahn PF. Advances in contrast-enhanced MR imaging. AJR Am J Roentgenol 1991; 156: 235–254

Schatz CJ, Becker TS. Normal and CT anatomy of the paranasal sinuses. Radiol Clin North Am 1984; 22: 107–118

Schuknecht B, Simmen D, Yuksel C, Valavanis A. Tributary venosinus occlusion and septic cavernous sinus thrombosis: CT and MR findings. AJNR Am J Neuroradiol 1998; 19: 617–626

Schwenzer N, Kruger E. Midface fracture. In: Kruger E, Schilli W, Worthington P, eds. Oral and Maxillary Facial Traumatology. Vol 2. Chicago: Quintessence, 1986: 107–136

Scuderi AJ, Harnsberger HR, Boyer RS. Pneumatization of the paranasal sinuses: normal features of importance to the accurate interpretation of CT scans and MR images. AJR Am J Roentgenol 1993; 160: 1101–1104

Shankar L, Hawke M. Principles and objectives of functional endoscopic sinus surgery and CT of the paranasal sinuses. ENT J 1991; 4: 1

Shankar L, Hawke M. Principles and objectives of functional endoscopic sinus surgery and CT of the paranasal sinuses. ENT J 1991; 4: 1

Shetty PG, Shroff MM, Fatterpekar GM, et al. A retrospective analysis of spontaneous sphenoid sinus fistula: MR and CT findings. AJNR Am J Neuroradiol 2000; 21: 337–342

Shetty PG, Shroff MM, Sahani DV, Kirtane MV. Evaluation of high-resolution CT and MR cisternography in the diagnosis of cerebrospinal fluid fistula. AJNR Am J Neuroradiol 1998; 19: 633–639

Shockley WW, Stucker FJ Jr, Gage-White L, Antony SO. Frontal sinus fractures: some problems and some solutions. Laryngoscope 1988; 98: 18–22

Silver AJ, Beredes S, Bello JA, et al. The opacified maxillary sinus: CT findings in chronic sinusitis and malignant tumors. Radiology1987; 163: 205–210

Silverman CS, Mancuso AA. Periantral soft-tissue infiltration and its relevance to the early detection of invasive fungal sinusitis: CT and MR findings. AJNR Am J Neuroradiol 1998; 19: 321–325

Silverman FN, Caffey J, Kuhn JP. Essentials of Caffey's Pediatric X-Ray Diagnosis. St Louis, MO: Mosby-Year Book, 1990: 11–19

Slovis TL, Renfro B, Watts FB, et al. Choanal atresia: precise CT evaluation. Radiology 1985; 155: 345–348

Som PM, Bergeron RT. Head and Neck Imaging, 2nd edn. St Louis MO: Mosby-Year Book Inc, 1991

Som PM, Brandwein MS. Facial fractures and postoperative findings. In: Som PM, Curtin HD, eds. Head and Neck Imaging, 4th edn. St. Louis, MO: Mosby, 2003: 374–438

Som PM, Dillon WP, Curtin HD, et al. Hypointense paranasal sinus foci: differential diagnosis with MR imaging and relation to CT findings. Radiology 1990; 176: 777

Som PM, Dillon WP, Fullerton GD, et al. Chronically obstructed sinonasal secretions: observations on T1 and T2 shortening. Radiology 1989; 172: 515–520

Som PM, Dillon WP, Sze G, et al. Benign and malignant sinonasal lesions with intracranial extention: differentiation with MR imaging. Radiology 1989; 172: 763–766

Som PM, Lawson W, Biller HF, Lanzieri CF. Ethmoid sinus disease: CT evaluation in 400 cases. Part 1: Nonsurgical patients. Radiology 1986; 159: 591–597

Som PM, Lawson W, Biller HF, Lanzieri CF. Ethmoid sinus disease: CT evaluation in 400 cases. Part 2: Postoperative findings. Radiology 1986; 159: 599–604

Som PM, Lawson W, Lidov MW. Simulated aggressive skull base erosion in response to benign sinonasal disease. Radiology 1991; 180: 755–759

Som PM, Sacher M, Lawson W, Biller HF. CT appearance distinguishing benign nasal polyps from malignancies. J Comput Assist Tomogr 1987; 11: 129–133

Som PM, Shapiro MD, Biller HF, et al. Sinonasal tumors and inflammatory tissues: differentiation with MR imaging. Radiology 1988; 167: 803–808

Som PM, Silvers AR, Catalano PJ, et al. Adenosquamous carcinoma of the facial bones, skull base, and calvaria: CT and MR manifestations. AJNR Am J Neuroradiol 1997; 18: 173–175

Som PM. CT of the paranasal sinuses. Neuroradiology 1985; 27: 189–201

Stammberger H. Functional Endoscopic Sinus Surgery: The Messerklinger Technique. Philadelphia: BC Decker, 1991

Stammberger HR, Kennedy DW. Paranasal sinus: anatomic terminology and nomenclature. The Anatomic Terminology Group. Ann Otol Rhinol Laryngol 1995; 104 (Suppl 167): 7–16

Stankiewicz JA. Complications of endoscopic nasal surgery: occurrence and treatment. Am J Rhinol 1987; 1: 45–49

Stranc MF. The pattern of lacrimal injuries in naso-ethmoid fractures. Br J Plast Surg 1970; 23: 339–346

Suojanen JN, Regan F. Spiral CT scanning of the paranasal sinuses. AJNR Am J Neuroradiol 1995; 16: 787–789

Tassel PV, Lee Y, Jing B, De Pena CA. Mucoceles of the paranasal sinuses: MR imaging with CT correlation. AJR Am J Roentgenol 1989; 153: 407–412

Terrier F, Weber W, Ruenfenacht D, et al. Anatomy of the ethmoid: CT, endoscopic and macroscopic. AJR Am J Roentgenol 1985; 144: 493–500

Tewfik TL, Der Kaloustian VM. Congenital Anomalies of the Ear, Nose, and Throat. New York: Oxford University Press, 1997

Toriumi DM, Berktold RE. Multiple frontoethmoid mucocoeles. Ann Otol Rhinol Laryngol 1989; 98: 831–833

Towbin R, Han BK, Kaufman RA, Burke M. Postseptal cellulitis: CT in diagnosis and management. Radiology 1986; 158: 735

Unger JM, Shaffer K, Duncavage JA. Computed tomography in nasal and paranasal sinus disease. Laryngoscope 1984; 94: 1319–1324

Valvassori GE, Buckingham RA, Carter BL, et al. Head and Neck Imaging. New York: Thieme, 1988

Van Tassell P, Lee YY, Jing BS, De Pena CA. Mucocoeles of the paranasal sinuses: MR with CT correlation. AJR Am J Roentgenol 1989; 153: 407–412

Vogl T, Dresel S, Bilaniuk LT, et al. Tumors of the nasopharynx and adjacent areas: MR imaging with Gd-DTPA. AJNR Am J Neuroradiol 1990; 11: 187–194

Wallace R, Salazar JE, Cowles S. The relationship between frontal sinus drainage and ostiomeatal complex disease. A CT study in 217 patients. AJNR Am J Neuroradiol 1990; 11: 183–186

Weber AL, Mikulis DK. Inflammatory disorders of the paraorbital sinuses and their complications. Radiol Clin North Am 1987; 3: 615–630

Weber AL. Inflammatory diseases ofthe paranasal sinuses and mucoceles. Otolaryngol Clin North Am 1988; 21: 421–438

Weber AL. Tumors of the paranasal sinuses. Otolaryngol Clin North Am 1988; 21: 439–454

Weissman JL, Snyderman CH, Hirsch BE. Hydroxyapatite cement to repair skull base defects: radiologic appearance. AJNR Am J Neuroradiol 1996; 17: 1569–1574

Wigand ME. Endoscopic Surgery of the Paranasal Sinuses and the Anterior Skull Base. New York: Thieme, 1990

Yonetsu K, Bianchi JG, Troulis MJ, Curtin HD. Unusual CT appearance in an odontogenic keratocyst of the mandible: case report. AJNR Am J Neuroradiol 2001; 22: 1887–1889

Yoon JH, Na DG, Byun HS, et al. Calcification in chronic maxillary sinusitis: II comparison of CT findings with histopathologic results. AJNR Am J Neuroradiol 1999; 20: 571–574

Youngs R, Evans K, Watson M. The Paranasal Sinuses. A Handbook of Applied Surgical Anatomy. Taylor & Francis, 2006

Yousem DM, Galetta SL, Gusnard DA, Goldberg HI. MR findings in rhinocerebral mucormycosis. J Comput Assist Tomogr 1989; 13: 878–882

Zimmerman RA, Bilaniuk LT, Hackney DB, et al. Paranasal sinus hemorrhage: evaluation with MR imaging. Radiology 1987; 162: 499–503

Zinreich SJ, Kennedy DW, Kumar AJ, et al. MR imaging of the normal nasal cycle: comparison with sinus pathology. J Comput Assist Tomogr 1988; 12: 1014–1019

Zinreich SJ, Kennedy DW, Malat J, et al. Fungal sinusitis: diagnosis with CT and MR imaging. Radiology 1988; 169: 439–444

Zinreich SJ, Kennedy DW, Rosenbaum AE, et al. Paranasal sinuses: CT imaging requirements for endoscopic surgery. Radiology 1987; 163: 769–775

Zinreich SJ, Mattox DE, Kennedy DW. Concha bullosa: CT evaluation. J Comput Assist Tomogr 1988; 12: 778–784

Zinreich SJ. Paranasal sinus imaging. Otolaryngol Head Neck Surg 1990; 103: 863

Zinreich SZ. Paranasal sinus imaging. Radiology 1990; 103; 5: 863–869

Index